FRONTIERS IN ARTERIAL CHEMORECEPTION

ADVANCES IN EXPERIMENTAL MEDICINE AND BIOLOGY

Recent Volumes in this Series

Volume 401
DIETARY PHYTOCHEMICALS IN CANCER PREVENTION AND TREATMENT
Edited under the auspices of the American Institute for Cancer Research

Volume 402
AIDS, DRUGS OF ABUSE, AND THE NEUROIMMUNE AXIS
Edited by Herman Friedman, Toby K. Eisenstein, John Madden, and Burt M. Sharp

Volume 403
TAURINE 2: Basic and Clinical Aspects
Edited by Ryan J. Huxtable, Junichi Azuma, Kinya Kuriyama, Masao Nakagawa, and Akemichi Baba

Volume 404
SAPONINS USED IN TRADITIONAL AND MODERN MEDICINE
Edited by George R. Waller and Kazuo Yamasaki

Volume 405
SAPONINS USED IN FOOD AND AGRICULTURE
Edited by George R. Waller and Kazuo Yamasaki

Volume 406
MECHANISMS OF LYMPHOCYTE ACTIVATION AND IMMUNE REGULATION VI: Cell Cycle and Programmed Cell Death in the Immune System
Edited by Sudhir Gupta and J. John Cohen

Volume 407
EICOSANOIDS AND OTHER BIOACTIVE LIPIDS IN CANCER, INFLAMMATION, AND RADIATION INJURY 3
Edited by Kenneth V. Honn, Lawrence J. Marnett, Santosh Nigam, Robert L. Jones, and Patrick Y-K. Wong

Volume 408
TOWARD ANTI-ADHESION THERAPY FOR MICROBIAL DISEASES
Edited by Itzhak Kahane and Itzhak Ofek

Volume 409
NEW HORIZONS IN ALLERGY IMMUNOTHERAPY
Edited by Alec Sehon, Kent T. HayGlass, and Dietrich Kraft

Volume 410
FRONTIERS IN ARTERIAL CHEMORECEPTION
Edited by Patricio Zapata, Carlos Eyzaguirre, and Robert W. Torrance

---

A Continuation Order Plan is available for this series. A continuation order will bring delivery of each new volume immediately upon publication. Volumes are billed only upon actual shipment. For further information please contact the publisher.

FRONTIERS IN ARTERIAL CHEMORECEPTION

Edited by

Patricio Zapata
Catholic University of Chile
Santiago, Chile

Carlos Eyzaguirre
University of Utah School of Medicine
Salt Lake City, Utah

and

Robert W. Torrance
University of Oxford
Oxford, England

PLENUM PRESS • NEW YORK AND LONDON

Library of Congress Cataloging-in-Publication Data

Frontiers in arterial chemoreception / edited by Patricio Zapata,
Carlos Eyzaguirre, and Robert W. Torrance.
p. cm. -- (Advances in experimental medicine and biology ; v.
410)
"Proceedings of the XIIth International Symposium on Arterial
Chemoreceptors, held March 25-29, 1996, in Santiago, Chile"--T.p.
verso.
Includes bibliographical references and index.
ISBN 0-306-45490-4
1. Arteries--Innervation--Congresses. 2. Chemoreceptors-
-Congresses. 3. Carotid body--Congresses. I. Zapata, Patricio.
II. Eyzaguirre, Carlos, 1923- . III. Torrance, R. W.
IV. International Symposium on Arterial Chemoreceptors (12th : 1996:
Santiago, Chile) V. Series.
[DNLM: 1. Chemoreceptors--physiology--congresses. 2. Carotid
Body--physiology--congresses. 3. Oxygen--physiology--congresses.
W1 AD559 v.410 1996 / WL 102.9 F935 1996]
QP106.2.F76 1996
612.1'33--dc21
DNLM/DLC
for Library of Congress 96-49626
CIP

Proceedings of the XIIIth International Symposium on Arterial Chemoreceptors, held March 25 – 29, 1996, in Santiago, Chile

ISBN 0-306-45490-4

A Division of Plenum Publishing Corporation
233 Spring Street, New York, N. Y. 10013

10 9 8 7 6 5 4 3 2 1

Printed in the United States of America

PREFACE

This volume, *Frontiers in Arterial Chemoreception*, originated in the presentations given at the XIIIth International Symposium on Arterial Chemoreceptors, held in the Extension Center of the Catholic University of Chile, Santiago, Chile, from March 25–29, 1996. At the symposium, 74 participants from 15 different countries gave 75 presentations, of which 44 were oral and 31 were posters. Some authors who gave more than one presentation at the symposium have condensed their results into a single chapter for this book. The papers of three authors who did not manage to get to the symposium have also been included in the book.

Dan Cunningham died shortly before the symposium. He was a key scientist in the study of arterial chemoreceptors in the control of ventilation in man, and, as an obituary tribute to him, we print an oration delivered at his funeral service by Brian Lloyd, who collaborated with him over many years.

This symposium on arterial chemoreceptors was the first to be held in the southern hemisphere. The International Society for Arterial Chemoreception (ISAC) decided, at its XIth meeting (Chieti, Italy, 1991), to hold the XIIIth meeting in Chile, and confirmed the decision at its next meeting, the XIIth (Dublin, Ireland, 1993). Since most ISAC members work in the northern hemisphere, this decision represents the intention of the society to extend its borders, or frontiers of interest, in the coming century. Thus, when we were selecting a title for this volume, the term "frontiers" appeared to us not only as a meaningful word for the present state of the art and for future perspectives on the understanding of arterial chemoreception, but also as a geographical and chronological reference mark.

The success of a symposium depends on at least four factors. The first is an interesting subject capable of attracting modern research. The second is the organising of the meeting. The third is the financing of such a meeting. The fourth is the active participation of expert scientists in the proceedings of the meeting.

The actuality of arterial chemoreceptors as a lively subject for research is well demonstrated by the increasing number of papers being published on the subject. It is also confirmed by its power of attracting scientists with a wide range of different expertises to work on it: Apart from its classical interest for anatomists, physiologists, pharmacologists, pathologists, and clinicians, it is now increasingly attracting biophysicists and molecular biologists, as well as scientists interested in multidisciplinary approaches.

The organisation of the symposium was a challenge for the small community of biologists in Chile. Patricio Zapata, who was then President of ISAC, is especially grateful to all the members of the local organising committee: Drs. Julio Alcayaga, Hugo Cárdenas, Jaime Eugenin, Rodrigo Iturriaga, and Beatriz Ramírez. He is particularly indebted to his wife, Mrs. Carolina Larraín, for her unfailing help: She dreamed up ways to manage the organisation, she solved innumerable difficult problems, and she did it so willingly, whatever it was that turned up.

The patronage of the President of the Catholic University of Chile, Prof. Juan Vial, and the backing of the Dean of the Faculty of Biological Sciences, Prof. Renato Albertini, were crucial for holding this meeting, and we thank them. The advice of Prof. Daniel McQueen, who had served as Honorary Treasurer of ISAC since it was founded, was also of immense help.

The problems of financing scientific events in a developing country merit special consideration. We are grateful for the generous financial support provided by the higher authorities of the Catholic University of Chile, the National Commission for Scientific and Technological Research (CONICYT), the Andes Foundation, and the Third World Academy of Sciences (TWAS). Additional support was also provided by the subsidiaries of Merck and Nestlé located in Chile.

The attendance at a symposium is the final measure of its success. The distance of Chile from most scientific centres proved no obstacle to the enthusiastic participation of a relatively small but very distinguished group of researchers. We must mention here that the opening address of the symposium was given by the President of the Catholic University of Chile, Prof. Juan Vial, and it forms the first chapter of this book. Prof. Vial, a pupil of Prof. Fernando De Castro, presented a vivid picture of the beginning of modern research on arterial chemoreceptors. We also must mention that all who attended the symposium and their accompanying guests were received at Palace "*La Moneda*" (the seat of the presidency of the Republic) by the Minister-General Secretary of the Presidency, Mr. Genaro Arriagada, who gave a brief speech on the similarities between the functioning of arterial chemoreceptors for the well-being and adaptation of higher living organisms and his State Secretary for the well-balanced functioning and development of the country.

The external fruits of a symposium are usually presented in the form of a book. Here, again, the editors of this volume were fortunate in being able to count on the experience of Mrs. Carolina Larraín, this time in the technical editing of scientific manuscripts. The agreement of Plenum Press to produce a new volume in its prestigious series *Advances in Experimental Medicine and Biology* — as on three previous occasions — assures a book of high quality. We are particularly grateful to Miss Joanna Lawrence — of the London office of Plenum Press — and to Mr. Robert Wheeler and Mr. Jeffrey Gruenglas — of its New York office — for their expert management of the production of this book.

Patricio Zapata
Carlos Eyzaguirre
Robert W. Torrance

CONTENTS

A TRIBUTE TO FERNANDO DE CASTRO ON THE CENTENNIAL OF HIS BIRTH

Juan D. Vial

Catholic University of Chile
Santiago, Chile

1. OPENING REMARKS

I welcome this opportunity to address the opening session of this symposium of the International Society for Arterial Chemoreception. It is a pleasure to greet you in the name of the Catholic University of Chile, and to wish you all that you may enjoy an interesting meeting and a pleasant stay in this country.

I am grateful and honored by the invitation to speak on Fernando De Castro on this year of the centennial of his birth. It is fitting that he should be now remembered. It was him who about seventy years ago, made a major advance in the knowledge of chemoreceptors by discovering that the glomus caroticum should be counted among them. I myself have a large debt of gratitude toward De Castro who initiated me in research work as a histologist, and I feel thankful to have the occasion of acknowledging this debt and paying tribute to his memory.

2. DE CASTRO'S DISCOVERY OF CAROTID BODY FUNCTION

The story of De Castro's discovery has been told a number of times. A short time after becoming an assistant of Santiago Ramón y Cajal, he began studies on what was called at the time the "intercarotideal gland", an organ which was commonly believed to be comparable to the adrenal medulla. De Castro had become at that time interested in the structure of the sympathetic nervous system and related structures. I suspect that behind this choice lay the desire to find some field of neurohistology which might have been left comparatively unexplored by Cajal. De Castro revered his master, but as will happen with creative disciples he wanted his own place in the sun. And this did not seem easy to achieve. Cajal's contribution had been incredibly extensive and varied, and the weight of his authority was immense. On the other hand, his neuron theory was being seriously challenged in the autonomic nervous system. Complex networks of exceedingly fine fibers are found here, which were rendered visible mainly by silver impregnation techniques well-

Frontiers in Arterial Chemoreception, edited by Zapata *et al.*
Plenum Press, New York, 1996

known to be fraught with artifacts. These fields of uncertain structure and difficult study were of course paradise for a legion of fanciful anatomists inclined to see things to the very limit of the visible, and then far beyond. In this case the distinction was often not made between preganglionic and postganglionic processes, and they were all interpreted as parts of a web of anastomosing cytoplasmic outgrowths. Figure 1 is taken from one of De Castro's early papers (1926) and shows the entanglement of dendrites of two sympathetic neurons with a very fine fiber correctly identified as preganglionic.

De Castro's work soon showed that the intercarotideal gland differed from the adrenal medulla. He found that the granules inside the cells did not stain in the same way as in the adrenal, and he discarded the idea that the glomus was a paraganglion. His histochemistry was quite primitive, and he was probably wrong when he dismissed any kinship between glomus caroticum and adrenal medulla, but in a sense this was a lucky mistake, because it raised the obvious question of what the main role of this small gland might be.

De Castro was struck by the unusual fact that this seemingly glandular tissue was very richly innervated, both in the parenchymal cells proper and in the blood vessels. Figures 2 and 3 taken from De Castro's work (1926) show abundant fine axons and nerve endings together with bundles of myelinated fibers. Serial sections by the thousands made on cranial structures of mice which had been block-stained by notoriously capricious silver impregnation techniques, resulted in images beautifully reproduced in the drawings made by De Castro himself. In Figure 4, the "intercarotideal" (carotid sinus) nerve, a branch of the glossopharyngeal, is shown to provide the major part of the fibers to the glomus. It is apparent that De Castro had availed himself of a trick introduced by Cajal. He chose very young small animals, even foetuses, which afforded a chance of getting a view of a large territory in a single adequately oriented section.

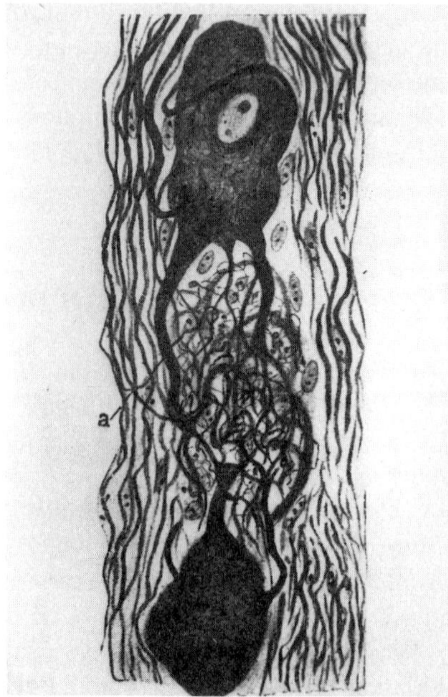

Figure 1. Sympathetic microganglion. *a*, preganglionic fibers. Cajal's reduced silver stain. Reproduced from De Castro (1926).

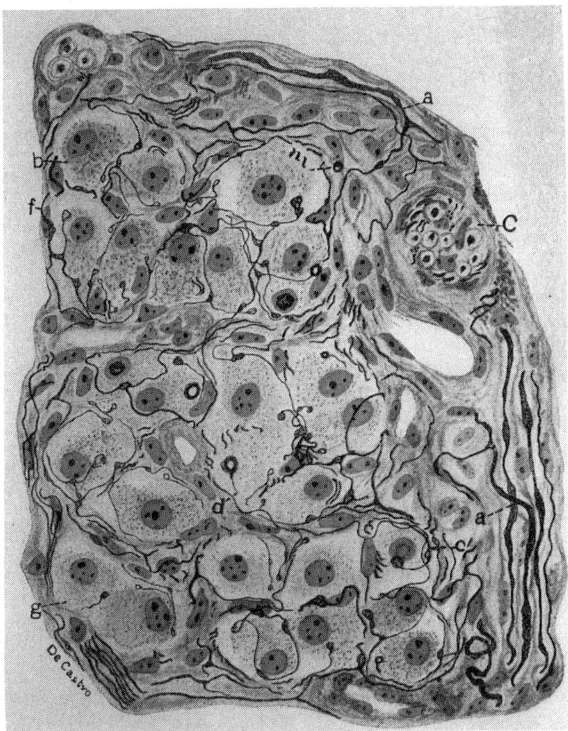

Figure 2. Human "intercarotideal gland". *C*, nervous bundle containing both medullated and non-medullated fibers. *a*, branching of medullated fiber. *d,f*, various aspects of contacts between glandular cells and nervous expansion. Cajal's reduced silver stain. Reproduced from De Castro (1926).

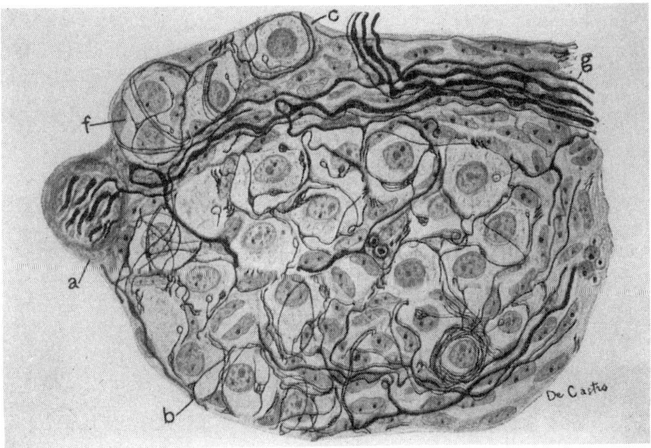

Figure 3. "Intercarotideal gland" of cat, 25 days after excision of the cervical sympathetic chain on both sides. No significant differences can be detected in the aspect of the nervous branches when compared to those of Figure 2. Cajal's reduced silver stain. Reproduced from De Castro (1926).

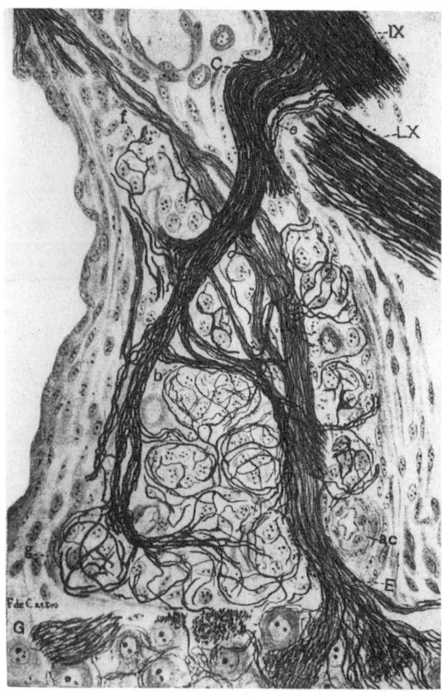

Figure 4. Approximately horizontal section of the head of a 35 day old mouse. *LX*, pharyngeal branch of the vagus. *IX*, glossopharyngeal nerve. *C*, intercarotideal nerve branching into the "gland". *G*, superior cervical ganglion. *E*, branch of the sympathetic chain which traverses the "gland". Cajal's reduced silver stain after fixation in De Castro's "somniphene" fixative. Reproduced from De Castro (1926).

The myelinated bundles constituted a puzzle. De Castro appears to have thought at first that the glossopharyngeal innervation of the gland did not pass through an extracranial synaptic relay, and was consequently an exception in the organization of the autonomic nervous system. On second thoughts, however, he tested the hypothesis that these branching myelinated fibers might be sensory in nature, with the corresponding cell bodies located at the petrosal ganglion. In successive papers, De Castro (1928, 1929, 1940) showed that the nervous endings in the gland were not affected by extirpation of the sympathetic chain, that they were completely wiped out by extra cranial section of the glossopharyngeal, and that they did not suffer after intracranial section of the nerve. Thus the whole of the evidence pointed toward their being sensory fibers, and toward the glomus being a receptor, probably connected to reflex arcs involved in circulatory regulation. De Castro saw also that the endings were entirely different from the pressoreceptors in the arterial wall. Based on anatomical considerations, he attributed to them a role in the detection of qualitative changes in the blood. On the whole, this was a brilliant achievement.

The success of this work rested upon a judicious use of the degeneration undergone by nerves after experimental sectioning. It is easy from our perspective to think that this was mainly an achievement of surgical skill. But one should remember that some very influential anatomical schools raised at the time serious objections against the neuron theory and consequently against the validity of Wallerian degeneration as an experimental tool for exploring the finest nervous plexuses. De Castro's contribution showed that severing of the sympathetic chain, as well as of the glossopharyngeal at various levels enabled him to assign the proper labels to different components of the plexuses.

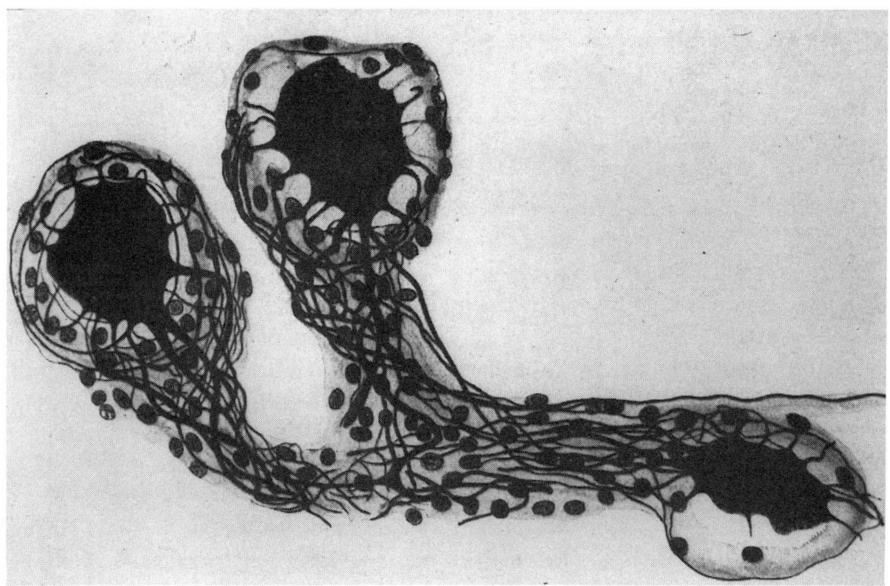

Figure 5. Three nerve cells which build up a tangled ball of processes. Human superior cervical ganglion. Bielschowsky's silver impregnation. Reproduced from Stöhr (1928).

For many years De Castro was part in a heated discussion on the organization of the peripheral territory of the vegetative system. Men no lesser than Max Bielschowsky, professor in Berlin, Germany, and Philip Stöhr Jr, Professor at Bonn, Germany, were extremely skeptical about the neuron theory as proposed by Cajal, and they tended to subscribe the idea that nerve processes built up a network of anastomosing fibers. Some researchers even thought that there was cytoplasmic continuity with effectors, much along the same lines followed by the famous Dutch histologist Jan Boeke for the motor end plate. From this belief in a terminal reticulum of processes, they were dubbed the "reticularists", an expression which amounted almost to a four letter word in the Cajal Institute. These views were put forward even in the most authoritative histological treatise of the late twenties and early thirties, the mammoth "*Handbuch der Mikroskopischen Anatomie*" edited by von Möllendorff, and which came to number if I am not mistaken about twenty volumes. Their arguments rested on superb staining methods for neurons, which were interwoven with general biological theoretical considerations. I show here Figure 5, taken from one of Stöhr's papers (1928), which shows an arrangement comparable to the one in the figure (Fig 1) by De Castro which I presented earlier. You may notice that processes do not end anywhere, neither are any preganglionic fibers to be found. The image is similar to that of De Castro but it represents an entirely different interpretation.

The period of intense activity around 1930, which had ended by the proposal of the idea that the glomus was a chemoreceptor, was followed by a lull. This may be due to the fact that his contribution was widely ignored as coming from Spain. He opened the way to Heymans' discoveries but did not receive due credit, even at the moment when the latter was awarded the Nobel Prize. I never heard De Castro himself refer to that circumstance, but his disciples and friends often did, and were somewhat bitter about it. These were also the years of Cajal's death, and of organizational changes in his Institute.

3. WORKING WITH DE CASTRO

Then in 1936, the black period for Spanish science set in. It was first the civil war. Life in Madrid was rendered very difficult by the advance of the armies of Franco that came to camp on the outskirts of the city within sight of the laboratory. There were also waves of terror by irregular forces of the defenders inside the capital. The Cajal Institute - the new building that Cajal had never really liked - had been placed on top of a small hill, the "*cerro de Atocha*" which commanded a grandiose view of the Castillian highlands, which at that time were not hidden by the tremendous outgrowth of the suburbs which set in the course of later years. On one occasion the defenders of the city believed that messages had been sent to the enemy by means of mirrors, and they came to search the Institute. De Castro's account of the incident was interesting in that it showed the immense respect for the name of Cajal - a sort of scientific saint - that was prevalent among the Spanish people at the time. Upon becoming aware that these men were the collaborators of that glory of Spanish science the aggressive mood of the visitors changed. What might easily have become a punitive raid, ended as a guided tour for the "*milicianos*", led by De Castro, which included a visit to the heart of the sanctuary, Cajal's museum itself. A sort of bond became established between that group of irregular forces and the occupants of the institute, which was of considerable help on the occasion of other emergencies.

The end of the civil war was followed by political persecution. The Cajal group was dispersed and its remains were denied the means for research work to the point that this brilliant center of neuroanatomy became almost extinct. When one recalls that De Castro's political views were extremely moderate, it becomes possible to take full measure of how stupid and blind men can become in the exercise of power. The consequences for Spain were sad indeed. The civil war was followed by the isolation of the country during World War II and during the post war period, all of which caused cruel poverty and cultural stagnation. Only in the early fifties, almost fifteen years after the onset of the civil war, was De Castro made Professor of Histology in Madrid. But even though better years lay ahead, for him most of the damage had already been done.

In January 1950, I went to the Institute to begin my training as a histologist. My previous experience had been practically nihil, and I wished to convey an impression of commendable eagerness at the distinguished place where I was to start. So I ascended the modest Atocha hill at the south of Madrid, at what seemed a reasonable time of day for a first call. At about 10 AM I rang the bell, and had to do it for so long, so long that I was on the point of giving up when a sleepy employee clad in his pajamas opened the door and courteously observed that it was far too early and that if I wanted to talk to the professor in person, I was to come back in the evening. Thus I discovered that De Castro was forced by necessity to pursue his research in the laboratory by working till late in the night, while his living came from surgical practice which he performed by day. For many months to come I was to hear every evening the hurried strides of the tall athletic mountain climber, entering as a whirlwind, his loud voice rallying around him the small group of dedicated staff who made their utmost efforts to help him go along with his research.

De Castro's style of work was highly individualistic. You were expected to work hard, and to achieve something. In the measure in which you did, De Castro would care for you and for your results and provide with valuable suggestions. If you didn't, nobody would take notice of you. I came to know that I wasn't doing bad when he let me have a share of some mysterious fixatives the formulae of which were only known to him. It makes one smile to-day, but this was a common practice in many European histology laboratories of the time, which thus kept their small amounts of classified information which I suspect was not especially valuable. None of their great contributions may be rightly attributed to the power of the secrets they kept so well.

Some weeks after my arrival, he suggested for me some work on the innervation of the gastric glands, and I became immersed in that cordial atmosphere of hard work which was pursued with very straightened means. The passion put by De Castro on his work made a lasting impression on me and was extremely useful for my beginnings. When I came back to Chile, I was given a painfully ill-equipped laboratory in a university that did not number more than five or six full-time staff members, and where according to a good friend who represented a great foundation in this country there was not the slightest chance that scientific research could ever become established. My memory of De Castro and of his style of work was an important inspiration, because I knew then that interesting research could be performed even if conditions might seem appalling. Moreover, my contact with gastric glands turned to be a very useful circumstance when some years later I became interested in the electron microscopy of the hydrochloric acid secreting cells.

A large room in the Madrid laboratory was occupied by cages with cats that had been subjected to some kind of cross anastomosis of cranial nerves. I think that with the dispersion of the Spanish physiologists, De Castro was forced to find some means of exploring the functions of the structures he loved. And he hit upon a most ingenious procedure, which was to manufacture artificial reflex arcs, one of which is shown here (Fig 6), with the nodose ganglion of the vagus sending its peripheral branch through the sinus nerve, and its central branch to the superior cervical ganglion. When either blood pressure or CO_2 content of the blood were altered, the pupil in that cat's eye changed its diameter.

This is only an instance of the variety of these distorted nervous systems that De Castro had built. This particular experiment had considerable theoretical interest in that it showed that the response to a specific stimulus was due to the function of the glomus cells and could not be attributed to the type of the nerve fibers supplying it.

As for me, these cross-anastomoses bring back pleasant associations. The contact with these techniques bore fruit in my own work when some years later, together with Vera and Luco (Vera et al, 1957) we showed that adrenergic endings could be replaced by regenerating cholinergic fibers after suitable cross-anastomoses had been established.

Under the conditions prevailing in Spain and in the Cajal Institute, the gathering together of such a large number of skillfully operated animals amounted to a real treasure. At least that is how De Castro looked upon it. I will not readily forget the night in which one of the cats - an exceptionally prized one, a sort of *Madonna* of the cats - managed to slip away from the cage into darkness. De Castro was frantic, he literally bellowed, and under his leadership the surroundings of the institute became bristling with panicked collaborators, employees and students searching after the animal. The beast was finally discovered passably terrified and cornered near its own room. One of the employees engaged it in a fierce hand to claw battle putting all the time great care not to wound or damage the cat, and after much biting and scratching he managed to get it back unhurt (the cat unhurt of course!) into its empty cage. I did not think that any one could have tackled a cornered cat with his bare hands, but the impassioned voice of De Castro forbade any attempt to retreat.

De Castro loved Madrid; he was "*madrileño*" to the bones. He could not really envisage living at any other place. He loved mountain climbing. He had made a short trip to Chile and had remained with an overpowering feeling of the immensity and the abruptness of the Andean mountain range. The passionate strain in his personality kept him active, hard-working and aggressive, even when for years the isolation in which he worked made him embark upon some dubious hypotheses. As he tried hard to improve the knowledge

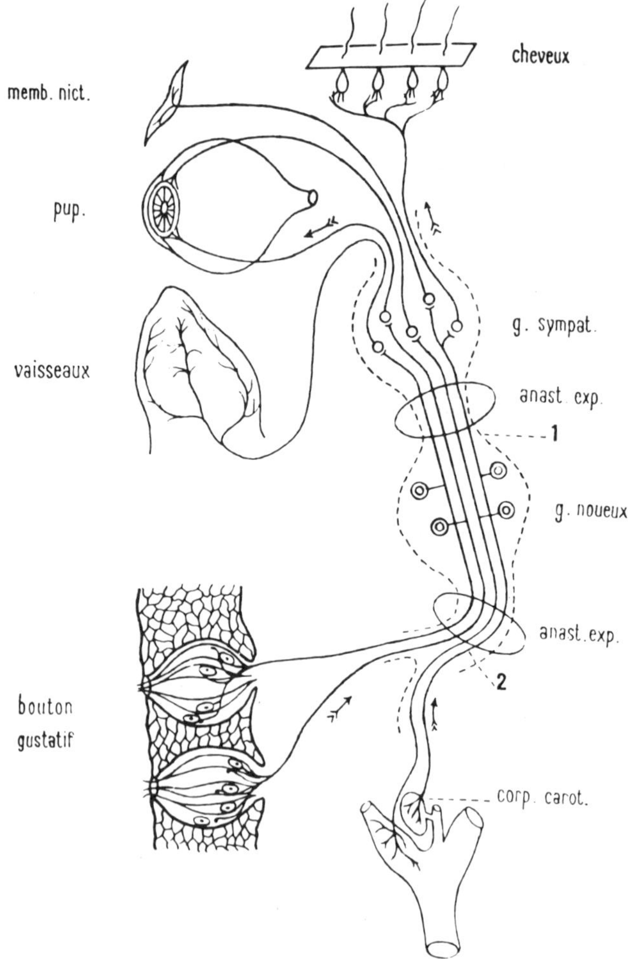

Figure 6. Diagram of artificial reflex arc obtained by double crossed anastomoses: (**1**) between central processes of nodose ganglion neurones (*g. noeux*) and cervical preganglionic sympathetic trunk, to reinnervate the superior cervical ganglion (*g. sympat.*), whose postganglionic fibers innervate the scalp, nictitating membrane, pupil and tongue vessels; (**2**) between peripheral processes of nodose ganglion neurones and peripheral stump of glossopharyngeal nerve, innervating the carotid body and sinus, and gustatory corpuscles, through its carotid (sinus) and lingual branches, respectively. Arrows indicate direction of nerve impulses. Reproduced from De Castro (1951).

about the structure of nervous endings in the glomus, he came to believe that the nerve fiber entered the glomus cell (Fig 7), even though remaining in full trophic dependence from thc neuron. The electron microscope has shown (as De Castro himself lived to study), that this was a mistaken view, possibly due to superposition of planes in the microscopical image. Unfortunately the error fitted well the idea of a bipolar glomus cell, and De Castro fell a victim to the temptation of seeing things which he believed should be there, a temptation alas to which many, many distinguished anatomists have succumbed.

His new idea induced De Castro to think that in many, if not all synapses there was cytoplasm of glial cells interposed. He spent much time and effort in the pursuit of a dem-

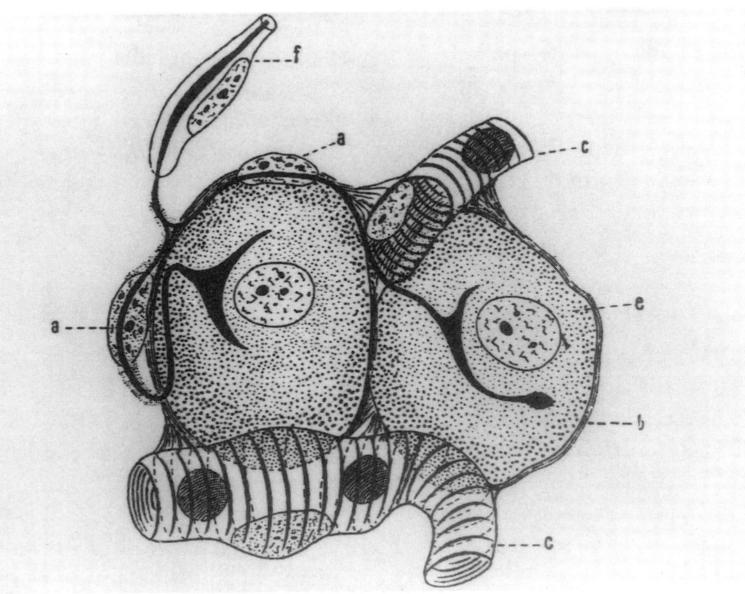

Figure 7. Diagram of synapses between glomus cells ("epithelioid" cells, **ec**) and a sensory nerve fiber (**f**). Capillaries (**c**) and Schwann-type sustentacular cells (**a**) are also depicted. Reproduced from De Castro (1951).

onstration for this hypothesis which did not survive the first electron microscopic images of synaptic boutons. This phase of his research required extremely refined silver impregnation techniques and in the early fifties his laboratory afforded an ideal place to become proficient in these. I remember it well because the technical ability acquired in the Cajal Institute was a good presentation card when I came to other research laboratories to continue with my training. For many years I remained interested in nervous tissue, Wallerian degeneration and relationship of axon and glia in peripheral nerves. I mention this and other work in which I became involved only to show how a comparatively short period with a man like De Castro could go a long way toward shaping your research interests for years to come.

An account of life in the Cajal Institute in the forties and early fifties would be incomplete if nothing was said of the shadow of Santiago Ramón y Cajal which loomed upon the place. Cajal had not only been a formidable genius in nervous system research. He had served as the voice of conscience calling his country and his countrymen to the austere delights of rigorous science. A man of retiring habits, confined to his small laboratory, shunning honors and bored with fame, he had exerted a tremendous influence upon the whole of the cultural life in Spain. His influence on his collaborators had been of course enormous. De Castro's first contact with Cajal had been as an undergraduate student in Histology. He used to tell a story about his exam, when asked a difficult question he developed an elaborate and - he thought- brilliant answer. Cajal looked at him from beneath his thick eyebrows and said: "Very interesting, very interesting ... if only there was some support for it". When one reads the papers written by De Castro in the twenties, one finds the spirit of Ramón y Cajal: sturdy common sense, summary dismissal of nebulous theories, fine, precise technical achievements and a passion for discovery, all of this together with an almost unlimited capacity for work.

Some time after Cajal's death, De Castro was approached by a man, who had risen to wealth coming from the poverty of the Spanish lower middle class and who said he wanted to make a substantial contribution to the Institute. He had no knowledge of scientific matters, and was certainly not of an intellectual turn of mind. His explanation of his feelings for the group of Cajal was simply "*Creo en la virtud del trabajo*" ("I believe in the virtue of work"). In this De Castro also believed and this faith helped him to shape a life full of zest and creative contributions in very difficult times.

4. CONCLUDING REMARKS

I would like to finish with a small anecdote. De Castro was superb at drawing from the microscope. He claimed to be very good at photomicrography. But I think he was a rather poor portraitist. Once when asked for a photograph of himself, and being as he was, extremely careful about his personal appearance, he engaged in a session of experiment with a big bellows camera, and requested his collaborators to sit for trial exposures. Thus it came to pass that the present speaker had a photograph of himself (Fig 8, left) taken sitting at the hallowed place of the professor's microscope, just before De Castro obtained a plate (Fig. 8, right) which is not perhaps very good as photographs go, but which is for me a reminder of the time I spent with a great scientist and a great man.

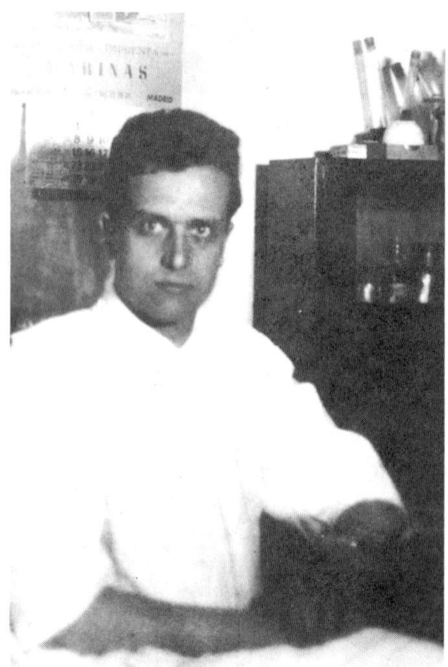

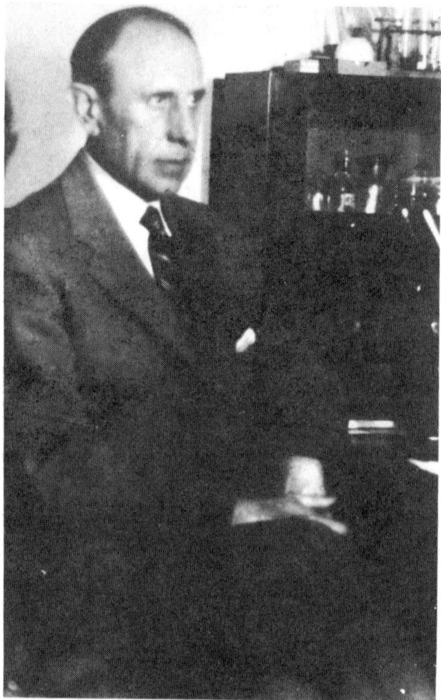

Figure 8. *Left:* Photograph of Juan D. Vial, sitting at De Castro's laboratory chair, taken in 1950. (See text). *Right:* Photograph of Fernando De Castro, in his laboratory at Cajal Institute, taken in 1950. (See text).

5. REFERENCES

De Castro F (1926) Sur la structure et l'innervation de la glande intercarotidienne (*glomus caroticum*) de l'homme et des mammifères, et sur un nouveau système d'innervation autonome du nerf glosso-pharyngien. Trab Lab Invest Biol Univ Madrid 24: 365–432

De Castro F (1928) Sur la structure et l'innervation du sinus carotidien de l'homme et des mammifères. Nouveaux faits sur l'innervation et la fonction du *glomus caroticum*. Trab Lab Invest Biol Univ Madrid 25: 331–380

De Castro F (1929) Über die Struktur und Innervation des Glomus caroticum beim Menschen und bei den Säugetieren. Z Anat Entwickl Gesch 89: 250–265

De Castro F (1940) Nuevas observaciones sobre la inervación de la región carotídea. Los quimio- y preso-receptores. Trab Lab Invest Biol Univ Madrid 32: 297–384

De Castro F (1951) Sur la structure de la synapse dans les chemorecepteurs: leur mécanisme d'excitation et rôle dans la circulation sanguine locale. Acta Physiol Scand 22: 14–43

Stöhr Ph, Jr (1928) Das peripherische Nervensystem. In: Handbuch der mikroskopischen Anatomie des Menshen. Herausgegeben von Wilhelm von Möllendorff. 4 Band. 1 Teil. pp 202–447

Vera CL, Vial JD & Luco JV (1957) Reinnervation of nictitating membrane of cat by cholinergic fibers. J Neurophysiol 20: 365–373

2

PROLEGOMENA

Chemoreception Upstream of Transmitters

R. W. Torrance

St. John's College
Oxford OX1 3JP, United Kingdom

1. INTRODUCTION

This essay will discuss the early stages in the setting up of nerve impulses in arterial chemoreceptors by respiratory gases, an excess of CO_2 and a deficit of O_2. At that stage of the process, the dimensions used in the discussion are usually those of the physiology of respiration, of PO_2, PCO_2 and (H^+), rather than those of the biophysics of excitable membranes, and the equations are those of Henderson and Hasselbalch rather than those of Hodgkin and Huxley. A host of reviews (*e.g.*, Peers & Buckler, 1995; Gonzalez et al, 1995; very recently) discusses recent advances in the study of the later, biophysical, stages of excitation. This essay may serve as a preface to the reviews and to some of the papers in this book.

But before the mechanisms of the responses of chemoreceptors to respiratory gases are considered, the responses themselves will first be outlined, both when the stimuli are steady and when they are changing, and some remarks on the relation between the discharge and the reflexes it produces will be in place. After all, the first test of any hypothesis is whether it seems to account for the behaviour of the chemoreceptors that is already known and then the experiments it suggests are carried out to test it further.

1.1. Sensitivity to Oxygen Lack

It was recognised in the 19th century that the breathing may be increased in acute experiments by lack of oxygen in the air breathed and so there must be some receptor mechanism for O_2 lack, but the range of PO_2 over which O_2 lack has any effect is best determined by studying the long term effects of changes in PO_2 in subjects who are fully acclimatised to various altitudes, for, as the height increases, so does the partial pressure of O_2 in the air breathed fall. Such a study was done by Mabel FitzGerald (1913) when she was a member of JS Haldane's Pikes Peak expedition to Colorado in 1911. She studied men and women who were fully acclimatised to life at altitudes up to 14,000 ft (4,300 m),

Frontiers in Arterial Chemoreception, edited by Zapata *et al.*
Plenum Press, New York, 1996

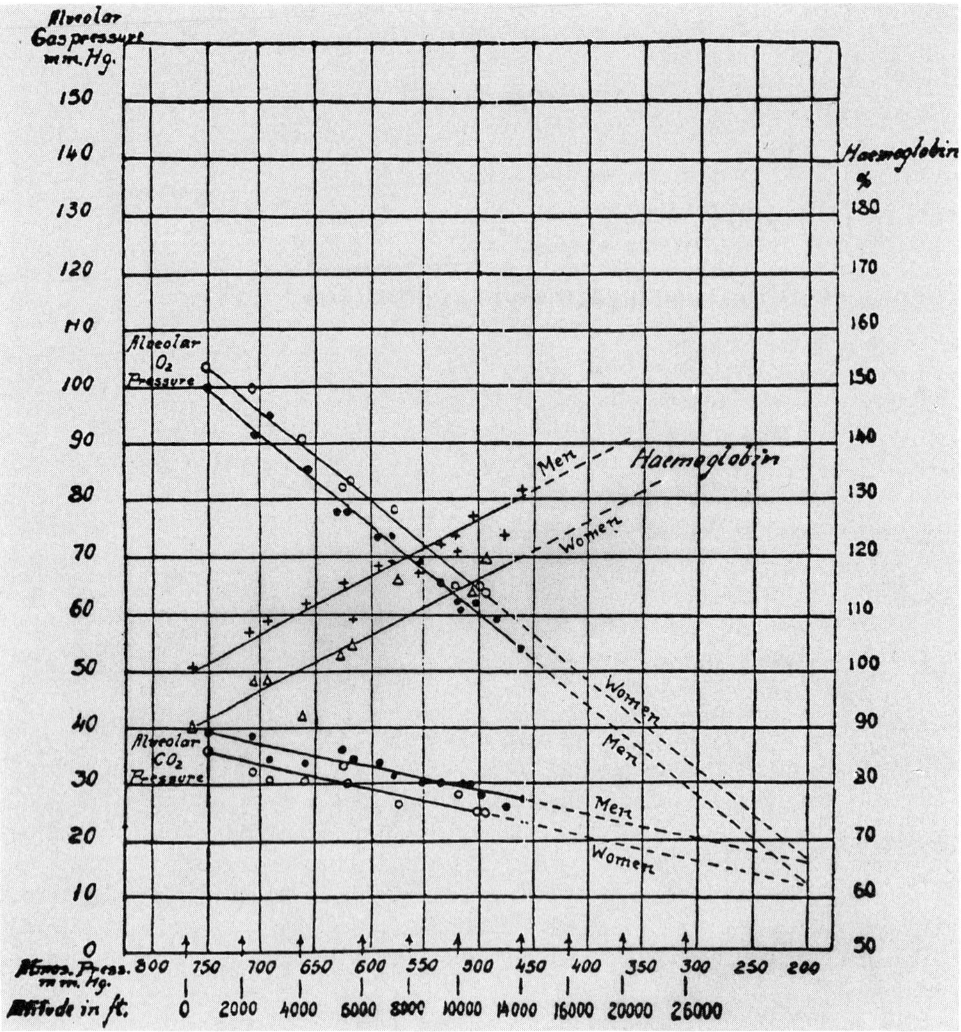

Figure 1. Alveolar pressures of oxygen and CO_2 and percentages of haemoglobin in the blood of persons acclimatised to altitudes from sea level to 14,000 feet, —barometric pressures from 760 to 450 mm Hg. (From JS Haldane (1917) Silliman Lectures: Organism and Environment. Yale University Press).

measuring their alveolar PCO_2, P_ACO_2, and haemoglobin, Hb%, and calculating alveolar PO_2, P_AO_2 (Fig 1). P_ACO_2 fell linearly with barometric pressure and it was this fall of PO_2 that caused the rise in breathing that blew off CO_2 and so lowered P_ACO_2, also linearly, with barometric pressure. Breathing was affected by changes in PO_2 within the range of PO_2 encountered near to sea level. This demonstration that there is a hypoxic drive to breathe even at sea level has now been confirmed in acute experiments in the laboratory with the transient, two breaths, test (Dejours, 1968) and also in steady state experiments such as those of Lloyd et al (1958).

The above experiments show, then, that there is some receptor mechanism that increases breathing in hypoxia and that it responds to changes in P_AO_2 around the region typical of sea level and above, and that the increase in ventilation that it causes is greater when the PO_2 is lower. The receptor does not always evoke the same constant all or nothing reflex response to hypoxia: rather it gives rise to a graded reflex response, and it does that because its own response to PO_2 is graded. It has a threshold at a lesser degree of hypoxia than exists at sea level and its response increases as PO_2 falls.

This range of sensitivity in the steady state seems to be belied by the slight effect on breathing of acutely making the inspired air short of O_2, but that effect is slight because any increase in breathing that an acute fall in PO_2 may initiate causes a blowing off of CO_2 which reduces the CO_2 drive to breathe and so conceals the hypoxic drive. When Mabel FitzGerald studied this at altitude, the blood HCO_3 had been reduced as part of acclimatisation and that had cancelled the effect that lowering PCO_2 has through pH in reducing breathing in the acute experiment.

How intensely the body should respond to the signal about hypoxia is for the heavenly neuromodeller to decide. For if he raises ventilation, he has to trade the advantage of raising P_AO_2 against a fall in HCO_3 buffering when he chooses his connections in the CNS. That is because the immediate effect on breathing of a fall of PCO_2 and so a rise in blood pH is compensated with time by the kidney by reducing blood HCO_3. Apparently the more intense the hypoxia, the more does the body eventually accept the loss of buffering power that a greater fall in HCO_3 produces.

The response should not be regarded as a rugged one from an insensitive receptor. Rather the receptor should be regarded as an appropriate one because it provides a graded message indicating PO_2 over the whole range of PO_2 from sea level upwards. The size of the response that the nervous system chooses to make to the message is a different matter. It is a compromise between single issue fanatics, one lot pressing for the maintenance of PO_2, another for a large buffering power, and no doubt many others pressing their own particular nostrums as well. In the short term, CO_2 seems to win out and to restrain PO_2 greatly but, in the long haul, PO_2 gets its way because the kidney hushes up CO_2 — a political compromise in a pluralistic society.

1.2. The Carotid Body Arrives

At the time of the Pikes Peak expedition in 1911 (Douglas et al, 1913), the carotid body was not known to be a receptor for hypoxia. Rather it was then supposed that the CO_2 receptors in the medulla responded to a local acidity and that the acidity became more intense in hypoxia because some acid, perhaps lactic acid, was made in larger amounts and further excited the CO_2 receptors.

It emerged around 1930, however, that there is a quite distinct receptor for hypoxia, the carotid body. The carotid body had long been known as a small, very vascular, innervated structure at the bifurcation of the common carotid artery. De Castro (De Castro & Rubio, 1968) used classical methods of neurohistology to show that it is a receptor organ. It is made up of many glomeruli, its functional units, which are groups of about six neurosecretory Type I cells, surrounded by another sort of cell, the "glial" Type II cell. Between and around the Type I cells are the endings of glossopharyngeal nerve fibres. De Castro showed that the endings are connected to sensory nerve cells in the glossopharyngeal petrosal ganglion and so suggested that the carotid body is a receptor for something in the blood. The Type I cells taste the blood and then they set up nerve impulses at the nerve endings. De Castro's model of the action of the carotid body is still used today. Shortly afterwards, Heymans found that it is for respiratory gases that the carotid body tastes the blood, first showing this for large changes of PCO_2 and then later for PO_2 (Heymans & Neil, 1958). The carotid body and other similar peripheral receptors soon came to be regarded as the only receptors for O_2 lack whilst the central receptors in the medulla were thought to be much more sensitive than the carotid body is to CO_2 excess.

1.3. The Nerve Impulse

The receptors were first found by recording their reflex effects but their behaviour can be studied much more quantitatively by recording the electrical activity of the nerve fibres than run from the receptors in the carotid sinus nerve to the glossopharyngeal nerve and so on to the medulla. The nerve impulses of a single fibre are studied and that shows that CO_2 and hypoxia both affect all fibres. There is not one set of fibres for hypoxia only and a distinct set for CO_2. And if two fibres are recorded simultaneously in the same cat, their discharges rise and fall in parallel, whether the stimulus changed is O_2 or CO_2. This means that the relative effectiveness of CO_2 and O_2 as stimuli varies little between fibres (Goodman, 1974).

1.4. Impulse Timing

A chemoreceptor fibre does not discharge regularly like, for example, a vagal stretch fibre from the lungs. Even when the stimulus is quite steady, the intervals between the impulses of a train vary randomly and show a near Poisson distribution but with a deficit of the shortest intervals (Fig 2). After an impulse, there is a dead time -a refractory period- which differs from fibre to fibre and is about 20 msec. During the dead time, an impulse only very rarely occurs. Then, over a similar period, the chance, or condition probability, of an impulse occurring increases and then holds steady (Stein, 1968). If the discharge is low, it satisfies quite well the criterion of a Poisson process that the standard deviation of the intervals between impulses, s, is equal to their mean, m, but at mean intervals less than 100 msec,

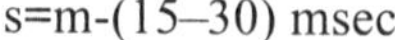

$$s=m-(15\text{–}30)\ \text{msec}$$

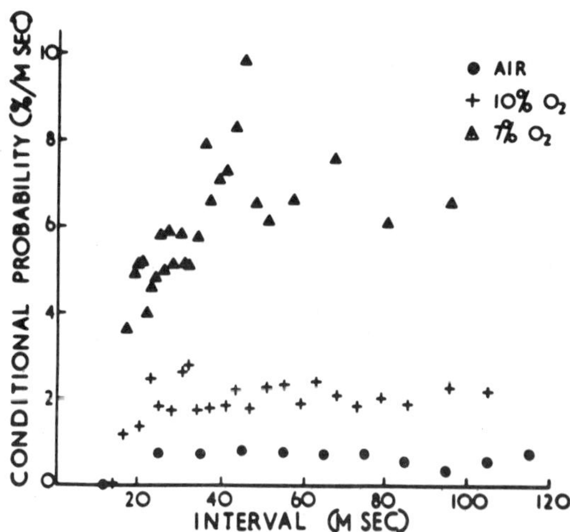

Figure 2. Discharges of a single chemoreceptor fibre at the three steady levels of stimulus indicated. Conditional probability of an impulse occurring plotted at increasing intervals since the previous impulse. (Silk, 1967).

as is to be expected from the apparent absolute and relative refractory periods. As the equation states, a plot of s against m in this range (Fig 3) is quite strikingly linear for any one fibre. Plots for other single fibres are parallel to it but to the right or left.

This near random behaviour has interesting consequences. At the level of reporting the intensity of the stimulus, a single fibre, impulse by impulse, inevitably gives a varying frequency simply because of the randomness of the timing of its impulses. It can only give a good mean intensity if its discharge is averaged over time. If however the discharge of many fibres is averaged, the problem is alleviated. n fibres over 1 sec are as good as one fibre over n sec. But with n fibres, the time resolution of the stimulus is increased. Time resolution is what the CNS often needs and it gets it. It matters, for example, because it has been argued that the time course of discharge within one breath is important in respiratory control (Black & Torrance, 1971). It can only be so if many fibres such as those seen in a single fibre preparation are averaged. There are several hundred fibres in the two carotid sinus nerves. A single fibre, averaged over many respiratory cycles, reveals a respiratory cycle in its discharge (Goodman et al, 1974), and many similar fibres, taken over a single cycle, must do the same. This does depend on the fibres behaving similarly, and that is what was found when two fibres were studied simultaneously.

1.5. Cause of Randomness

At the level of the mechanism of excitation in the carotid body, the fact that the impulses occur randomly, just as do miniature endplate potentials, mepps, in skeletal muscle, immediately suggests that the timing of the impulses, like that of mepps, results from the random release of typical packets of a transmitter from a presynaptic element. But the sensory nerve endings and fibres in the carotid body are very much smaller than skeletal muscle fibres, and their membrane capacity is much less, and so a typical packet of transmitter

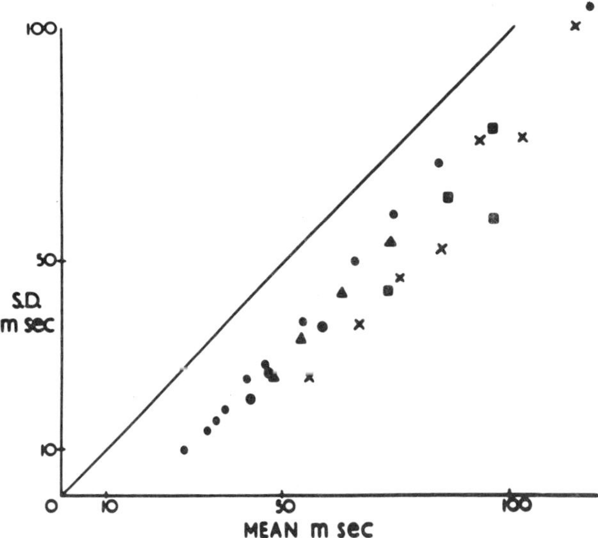

Figure 3. Analysis of variability of intervals between impulses in discharge of single cat carotid chemoreceptor fibres during periods with their stimulus steady. Standard deviation of interval length plotted against mean interval, with each type of symbol indicating discharge of one single fibre at various intensities of stimulus. At lower rates of discharge than those shown, mean and standard deviation not significantly different. (Silk, 1967).

would have a huge effect, way above what is needed to excite (Stein, 1968). The random discharge of chemoreceptor fibres is better attributed to the random opening of single channels in a membrane and the summing of their actions to give impulses randomly. Randomness of discharge does not prove that chemical transmission takes place.

2. STEADY STATE RESPONSES TO RESPIRATORY GASES

Three variables, the stimuli, PO_2 and PCO_2, and the response, f, are being considered, and when all three are presented, f is usually taken as the dependent variable, PCO_2 as the independent one, and PO_2 as a parameter. This gives a fan of straight CO_2 response lines: reducing PO_2 raises the slope of the response line to CO_2. Hypoxia increases the sensitivity of the receptor to CO_2. This type of change is commonly referred to as a multiplicative effect, or a positive interaction, of the stimuli, whereas if the lines had been parallel it would have been called an additive interaction.

To determine the steady state effects of stimuli, the discharge of a single fibre, or of a small group of fibres, dissected from the side of the carotid sinus nerve, is recorded and

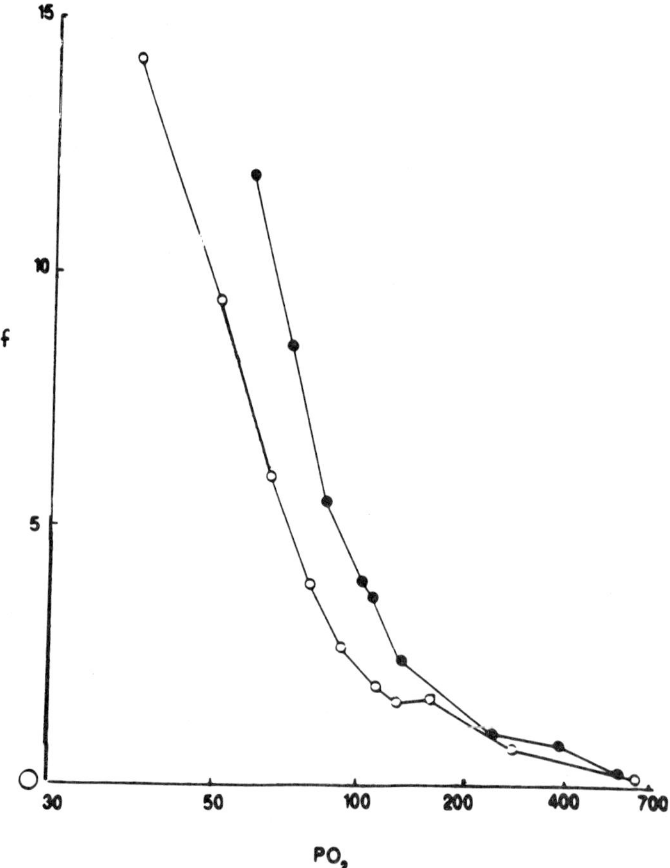

Figure 4. Effect of alveolar PO_2 (Torr) upon steady discharge, f (impulses/sec), of two single carotid chemoreceptor fibres at constant PO_2 (35 Torr). (Hayes, 1974).

the alveolar gas tensions, P_AO_2 and P_ACO_2, are measured. An occasional arterial blood sample is analysed to check that the alveolar measurements are satisfactory.

2.1. Oxygen

The discharge is plotted against P_AO_2 at a fixed P_ACO_2 (Fig 3). As the PO_2 is lowered, so the discharge frequency increases and it does so at an increasing rate as the PO_2 is taken lower. The relation looks like a hyperbola if the discharge is plotted as a frequency (Hayes et al, 1976). If instead the mean interval between impulses is plotted against P_AO_2 (Hayes, 1974), a reasonably straight line results which only breaks at a very low PO_2. Frequency may be plotted against $1/(PO_2\text{-}C)$, if an indicator of the intensity of hypoxia is wanted, and a value for C can be chosen that gives a straight line. The relation of O_2 content of the blood to discharge also is linear — Zotterman showed that in 1939 in the first quantitative study ever of chemoreceptor discharge (von Euler et al, 1939).

Single chemoreceptor fibres do not all have exactly the same response curves but they form a much more homogenous group than the lung stretch fibres of the vagus nerve or the afferents of the phrenic nerve, some of which may only be recruited when the overall activity of the nerve is quite intense. Most chemoreceptor fibres are active in modest hypoxia and seldom is a new fibre recruited as the PO_2 falls below 60–70 Torr. The activity of a single fibre does then give a fair indication of the activity of the whole nerve. Recruitment does occur but it is not very important.

2.2. Tissue PO_2 in the Carotid Body

Why does discharge, or ventilation for that matter, relate to $1/(PO_2 - C)$ rather than $1/PO_2$? Any basic process of chemoreception in the tissue of the carotid body would be expected to be set off by the local tissue PO_2, P_tO_2, rather than by the PO_2 of the arterial blood, P_aO_2, or of the alveoli, P_AO_2. P_tO_2 is lower than P_aO_2 for two reasons:

1. The capillary blood PO_2 is lower than P_aO_2 because O_2 is removed from the blood as it traverses the capillaries; and
2. the mean P_tO_2 is less than capillary PO_2 because there is a diffusion drop of PO_2 from the blood to the tissue where O_2 is consumed.

The overall drop of PO_2 from P_AO_2 in the alveoli to P_tO_2 in the carotid body has been calculated and it also has been measured directly with O_2 microelectrodes. It is interesting that the calculations and Whalen's measurements (Whalen & Nair, 1977) give a drop of PO_2 from blood to tissue of the same order, 30 Torr, as the value of C in the reciprocal expression for hypoxia in the discharge, and also in the ventilation, equations. But an agreement of more than this order can hardly be expected; for example, the first difference of PO_2, the $(a\text{-}\bar{v})$ difference one, must be greater at a high PO_2 because of the sigmoid shape of the O_2 dissociation curve of blood, but C is obtained by putting together observations made over a range of PO_2's.

This angle does give some suggestion of a reality to the constant C used in presenting responses to hypoxia: it is the difference between the easily measured P_AO_2 or P_aO_2 and the inaccessible P_tO_2 in the carotid body. Blood flow may be huge through the CB —its own volume every 3 sec— but still P_tO_2 is less than P_aO_2 by a very definite amount. Also, it is interesting that C for discharge and C for ventilation are similar; which suggests that the ventilation in l/min, produced by chemoreceptor discharge, is linearly related to the frequency of the discharge in impulses/min.

2.3. Carbon Dioxide

If the PO_2 is held steady whilst the PCO_2 is varied over a moderate range, the response increases linearly with PCO_2, and if the response line is extrapolated to lower PCO_2^s, it cuts the PCO_2 axis well below a resting PCO_2. At a lower, steady PO_2 the response is greater, as has already been said, and a change of PCO_2 has a greater effect upon it: the response line becomes steeper as PO_2 is lowered (Fig 5) and it cuts the PCO_2 axis at a lower PCO_2 (Fitzgerald & Parks, 1971). A set of CO_2 response lines determined at various PO_2^s, extrapolates to meet below the PCO_2 axis at PCO_2 only a little above zero. The threshold for CO_2 of the fibre is of course given by where a CO_2 response line cuts the PCO_2 axis. The PCO_2 threshold is lower, the lower the PO_2, and the relation between PO_2 and PCO_2 at threshold is not far from linear except at a high PO_2. The point of convergence of the CO_2 response lines is some 20 Torr or more below a resting PCO_2 and is below the PCO_2 axis. That is in great contrast to the ventilation lines in man. Ventilation CO_2 response lines radiate from a point on the PCO_2 axis which is only 2–3 Torr below a

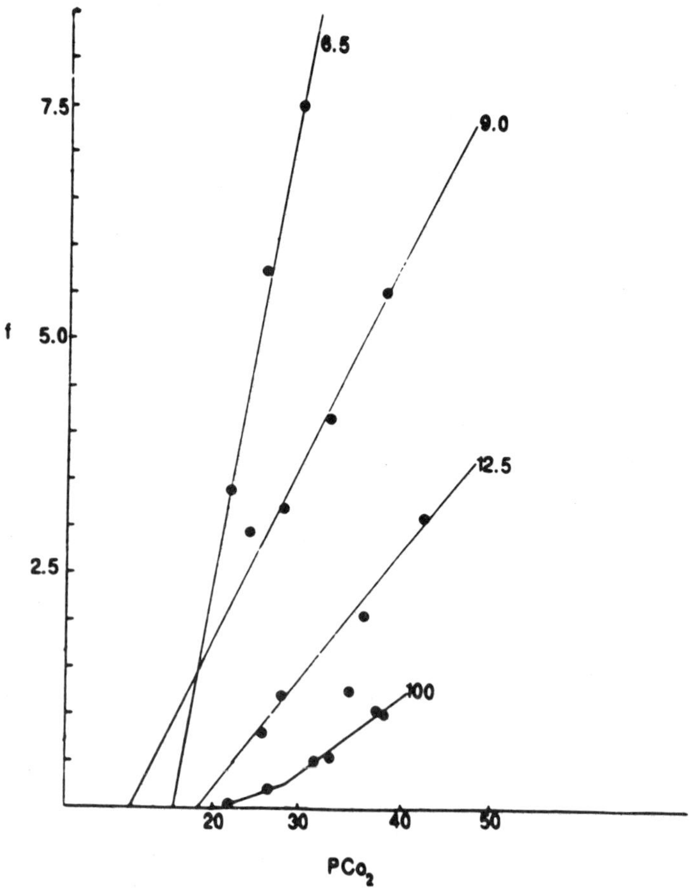

Figure 5. Effect of alveolar PCO_2 (Torr) upon steady discharge (impulses/sec), of a single carotid chemoreceptor fibre at four different levels of O_2 (labelled as F_{LT}% and equal to PO_2^s of about 45, 65, 90 and 700 Torr. (Hayes, 1974).

resting value of P_ACO_2. Put otherwise, increasing P_ACO_2 by 1 Torr from a resting value increases chemoreceptor discharge by about 5%. It increases breathing by about 50%, a huge effect which cannot conceivably be attributed to the change that CO_2 produces in the peripheral chemoreceptor discharge.

2.4. High PCO_2

If P_aCO_2 is raised very high, the response line suddenly bends over and becomes parallel to the PCO_2 axis. The PCO_2 at which this happens is lower at low PO_2 but the intensity of the discharge at the bend over varies little with PO_2. There is a limit to the intensity that is maintained by a chemoreceptor, even though that limit may transiently be much exceeded at a sudden increase in P_aCO_2. The receptor adapts down to discharge at an intensity that is independent both of PCO_2 and of PO_2. This is the limiting discharge described by Paintal (1967).

3. TRANSIENT RESPONSES

The response of chemoreceptors to a rise of stimulus takes some time to reach a peak and it may then adapt. The time course of the response depends on which stimulus, PO_2 or PCO_2, is changed.

3.1. Development of the CO_2 Response

The response to CO_2 is faster than the response to hypoxia, and the fastest response is produced by injecting quickly a slug, or small volume, of saline of high PCO_2 into the carotid sinus of a cat through a cannula tied into the external carotid artery with the common carotid open (Hanson et al, 1981): that response starts in about 100 msec and is near to its peak after a further 100 msec. But if instead the stimulus is altered by altering gas tensions in the lungs, there is, in addition, a circulatory delay from the lungs to the carotid sinus. In a cat (Kumar et al, 1988) that response starts after about 1.5 sec from the change in the lungs and builds up more slowly over about 1 sec, a difference in build up that must at least in part be due to the dispersion in time of the step in the stimulus as it is carried in the blood from the lungs to the carotid body.

Clearly the CO_2 stimulus must get into the carotid body tissue quickly from the carotid sinus and also the delay from the lungs may seem surprisingly short: about one breath. But those observations were made on the cat and one must bear in mind that times in the body vary with body weight, W, and are proportional to $W^{0.25}$ and so in man they are longer : about 2.5 times as great in a man as in a 2 kg cat. But the length of the respiratory cycle varies similarly with body size and so observations on the phase relations of variables to ventilation are transferable between animals of very different sizes, even though the time relations are not. This is an important point in the study of transmission of the respiratory oscillations in alveolar gas tensions to the carotid body and of the resulting oscillations in its discharge. A change in the alveolar stimulus produced by one inspiration can alter the next inspiration reflexly (Paterson & Nye, 1995).

The response to a sudden increase of PCO_2 (Fig 6a) rises from control. A, to a rather rounded maximum, B, and then it declines exponentially with a time constant of 5–10 sec to settle at a new steady level, C, above that of the control period, A. It undershoots, D, at the "off". This transient response to CO_2 can be presented (Fig 6b) in relation to a steady

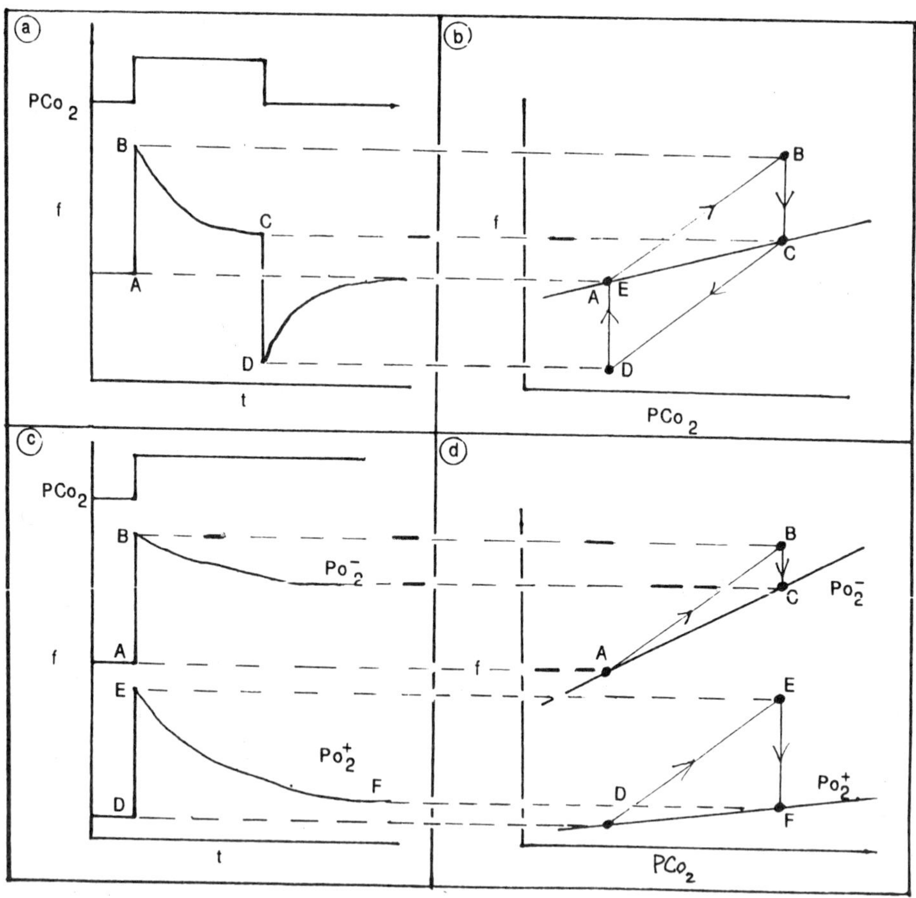

Figure 6. (a) Time course of development and adaptation of the "on" and "off" responses of a chemoreceptor to a step up and then down of PCO_2. (b) Data of Figure 6a plotted onto one steady state and two transient CO_2 response lines. (c & d) As for Figure 6a & b at two different levels of hypoxia and with only the "on" responses plotted. This illustrates that the size of the initial increase in response at the "on" in independent of PO_2 but that adaptation is greater in normoxia than in hypoxia, and that gives a steeper steady state response line in hypoxia than in normoxia even though the transient response lines are parallel whatever the PO_2.

state CO_2 response line, AC. The control, A, and the final adapted point, C, both lie on the steady state line, but the peak during the transient, B, lies above that line. B can be thought of as being on a transient response line, AB, which joins the initial point, A on the steady state line, to the early point, B to which the discharge immediately moves. The transient line is steeper than the steady state line. At the off of the stimulus, a different transient line, CD, is followed. It is the one through C for full adaptation to the higher PCO_2 of the stimulus. The sequence is C to D and then back up to A.

Thus one must think of a steep transient line passing through every point on a steady state line and of the transient line giving the immediate change in response for any sudden change in the stimulus away from a steady level.

One also has to think of every point on either side of a steady state line, *i.e,* every unsteady state point, having one of these transient lines passing through it, and of discharge at a change of stimulus behaving as if the receptor is fully adapted to the stimulus intensity at the point where that transient line crosses the steady state line. This is what happens if a receptor is exposed to a stimulus of an intensity to which it is not fully adapted and the intensity of the stimulus changes. And it must be considered because an entirely steady stimulus is a fiction of the laboratory: in life, the respiratory gas stimuli are always going up and down in the alveoli at the frequency of respiration and the response to them is moving up and down a steep transient line. That is why the oscillations in discharge that result have a much greater amplitude than a steady state line would predict.

3.2. Transients to O_2

The response to hypoxia at a fixed PCO_2 develops rather more slowly than does the response to CO_2 (Kumar et al, 1988). It starts at 2–3 sec from a sharp fall of P_AO_2, and takes longer than a second to reach a peak. It usually adapts little when hypoxia is made more intense but when it is again made less intense, the response not uncommonly undershoots and then recovers to a new steady level. Adaptation and undershoot are most prominent when hypoxia is severe, and at zero PO_2, the response may even adapt to silence, but adaptation then might well be due to failure of the receptor mechanism from O_2 lack and the undershoot to its gradual recovery.

The time course of the response to hypoxia can be changed. Recently Iturriaga (1993) has shown that the development of the response is very much slowed in a perfused carotid body if CO_2-HCO_3^- buffer is entirely omitted from the perfusate, but the off of the response is little slowed. Something like this may account for the slow response to hypoxia seen by Black et al (1971), for when they studied the effect of changing hypoxia, they held PCO_2 very low by hyperventilation in the belief that the response of the carotid body would then be one to hypoxia only. And similarly, when studying the effect of CO_2, they held O_2 very high, again in the belief that the response would be a pure one, this time to CO_2 only. But it is now recognised that that was a vain hope: if there is any response to hypoxia, it can be reduced or abolished by lowering PCO_2. There is not some PCO_2 below which there is a response to hypoxia which is not affected by CO_2. In this respect, the discharge of chemoreceptors is unlike the ventilation of man in marked hypoxia (Paterson & Nye, 1995): below some PCO_2, ventilation is little reduced by reducing PCO_2 further, a characteristic that is called the “Dog Leg” phenomenon.

3.3. Summary of Transient Responses

At any moment, one can state the PCO_2 to which a chemoreceptor is exposed and the PCO_2 to which it is fully adapted. And with the oscillating stimuli typical of normal life, these two PCO_2s are very unlikely to be equal. For if PCO_2 is changing, and the rate of discharge at some moment is plotted against the PCO_2 at that moment, the point that results is very unlikely to be on the steady state CO_2 response line. Rather, it will be above the line if PCO_2 has recently increased, or below it if PCO_2 has decreased. A single transient response line can be drawn through that point and it is the transient line of the receptor when it is fully adapted to the PCO_2 where the transient line cuts the steady state line.

When there is a step increase in the PCO_2 from a steady control level, the immediate response is along the line for full adaptation of the receptor to the control PCO_2. And then, as adaptation develops and discharge falls, the response lies successively on transient lines for adaptation to successively higher PCO_2s until eventually it is on the line for the new higher steady PCO_2 at the point where that line cuts the steady state line.

3.4. The Problem in Life

An experiment of Kumar (1986) illustrates this point well (Fig 7). The sophisticated ventilator of Kumar et al (1988) was used to make PCO_2 vary over a repeated 75 sec cycle in which P_ACO_2 was held steady for the first 45 sec of the cycle at a modest level, and then, in the next 30 sec, it was made to alternate five times between two higher levels, one of the levels being 10 Torr above control and the other 55 Torr above. Chemoreceptor discharge was steady late in the control half of the cycle. During each alternation, it rose quickly to a peak and then it fell, also quickly, to a trough, but the heights of the peaks and of the troughs of response fell successively throughout the first part of the alternation. Then they held steady. The amplitude of the alternation of the discharge did not change much throughout the half cycle. When the stimulus became steady at a low level at the beginning of the next cycle, the discharge immediately fell below the level at the end of the first half of the cycle and then it rose exponentially back up to that level. Many cycles of discharge were summed to bring out this time course of the response. If the instantaneous discharge is plotted against PCO_2 for the various stages of the response, the points at the peaks and the troughs of the alternations can have lines drawn through them which suggest transient lines moving initially to the right. That is, they indicate increasing adaptation to the increased mean PCO_2. But by the last alternation, adaptation had become steady.

The sort of change of stimulus that was used in this experiment is comparable with the changes in pH that Wolff (1992) has shown to take place in the arterial blood at the start of exercise. Over that period, the blood changes can be followed, and Wolff has done that, but the discharge cannot yet be recorded. Some system for deriving the likely discharge of arterial chemoreceptors from the course of their stimuli in the blood or in the alveoli would be valuable. But first a point must be made about lack of effect of PO_2 on the slopes of the transient CO_2 response lines.

3.5. Transient Response Lines to CO_2 Are Parallel

The steady state CO_2 response lines at various levels of PO_2 form a fan: at any given PCO_2, their slope is higher, the more intense the hypoxia. But the slopes of the transient response lines cutting the lines of the fan at that given PCO_2 are independent of PO_2: they are parallel. It will become apparent that this is a very important point.

That the transient lines are parallel was first suggested by the old observation (Goodman et al, 1974) that the respiratory oscillations in chemoreceptor discharge, which are believed to be due mainly to oscillations in PCO_2, have an amplitude that is little de-

Figure 7. Effect of a regularly varying CO_2 stimulus on the response of chemoreceptors (Kumar, 1986). Traces from above: 1) Time course of one cycle of the CO_2 stimulus in tracheal gas during ventilation at 2/sec. Inspired PCO_2 could be changed breath by breath. Except during the five increases of the stimulus, $P_{EI}CO_2$ is given by the upper level of the PCO_2 oscillation. During the increases, CO_2 is taken into the cat, and so, transiently $P_{ET}CO_2$ is less than inspired PCO_2 and is at the lower level of the oscillation. 2) Responses of a multifibre preparation of carotid chemoreceptors to a single cycle of the CO_2 stimulus. 3) Average of many cycles of 2). Heavy line: a running bin length of 600 msec. Light line: using a longer running bin length of 6 sec, the length of one CO_2 cycle, in order to smooth out the oscillations in discharge and to show more clearly the course of adaptation. 4) Data for peaks and troughs of heavy line of 3) plotted as in Figure 6 against the instantaneous CO_2 stimulus to give a single thick steady state line and to suggest a sequence of thin transient lines which initially shift downwards with adaptation and then hold steady.

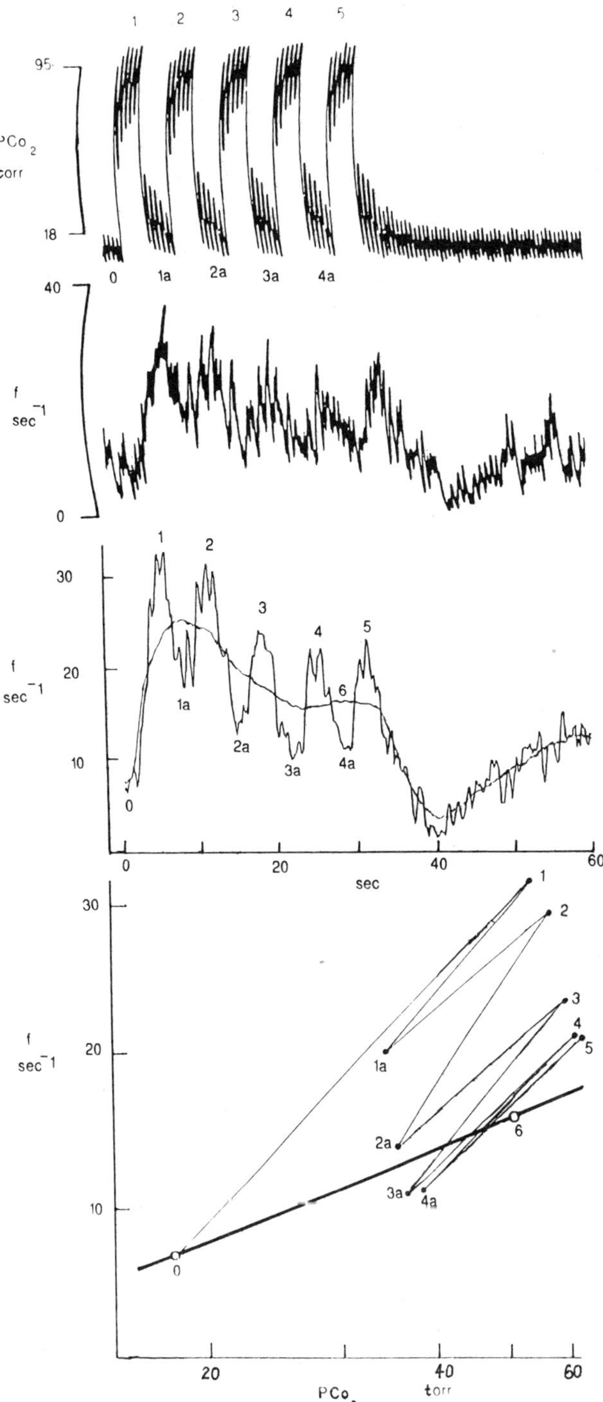
1
2
3
4
5
95
PCo2
torr
18
0
1a
2a
3a
4a
40
f
sec⁻¹
0
30
20
10
6
0
20
40
60
sec
PCo2
torr

pendent on PO_2. More recently, Kumar et al (1988) have made this point more definitely by alternating the alveolar PCO_2 between two levels with the PO_2 held at various steady levels: the amplitude of the oscillation in output was independent of PO_2 and that means that the transient lines are parallel.

If

1. the transient lines are indeed parallel;

but

2. the steady state lines are a fan;

then

3. the degree of adaptation at a change of PCO_2 is greater, the higher the PO_2.

The first two of these statements imply the third that adaptation is PO_2 dependent. The three of them together also imply that the process that gives adaptation is the only process that is affected by hypoxia.

3.6. The Discharge of an Adapting Receptor

It has been remarked that the stimuli to chemoreceptors in the blood rise and fall within each breath at rest, let alone with changes in the intensity of exercise and other such things. And the receptors do follow these changes in their stimuli with swings in discharge that are greater than the slope of the steady state lines would suggest. So consider now how one might obtain some estimate of the discharge of an adapting chemoreceptor when the stimuli to it are changing and can be measured, but the discharge from it cannot be recorded.

At any moment, the discharge at a steady PO_2 but a changing PCO_2:

1. changes at a rate proportional to the rate of change of the stimulus, *i.e.*, $dR/dt_1 = b\, dS/dt$, where: S = excess of stimulus over threshold; R = response; b = slope of transient response line.

The discharge also:

2. decays exponentially with time constant, T, from what it is, R, towards the value it would have in the steady state at the PCO_2 existing at that moment, aS. *i.e.*, $dR/dt_2 = -(R-aS)/T$, where a= slope of steady state response line.

Overall,

$$dR/dt = dR/dt_1 + dR/dt_2 = b\, dS/dt - (R-aS)/T.$$

Such a differential equation for the rate of change of the response could be used to develop a method that would give the output of the chemoreceptors over a period in which the PCO_2 stimulus is altering, and it would give the output much better than would simply reading off the response at successive moments from a fan of steady state response lines because it considers adaptation. The PO_2 could be brought in by using the finding of Kumar et al (1988) that the change in the response when both PO_2 and PCO_2 are varying is equal to the sum of the changes when each of them is varying separately, and simply using the steady state line to get the PO_2 component of the response since the PO_2 response adapts much less than does the response to PCO_2.

In dealing with a series of PO_2 and PCO_2 values varying with time, one would have to start from some imagined initial response, obtained by supposing, for example, that the initial response is that given by a fan of steady state response lines at the initial PO_2 and PCO_2. After a period equal to a few time constants, what was assumed for the initial discharge would matter little.

3.7. Respiratory Oscillations in Discharge

It has long been known that PO_2 and PCO_2 in alveolar gas vary with respiration, the PO_2 being raised and the PCO_2 lowered by the fresh air reaching the alveoli in inspiration and changing in the opposite directions in expiration. These gas tension changes are carried to the carotid body in the blood and cause its output to oscillate at the frequency of respiration. Because of the random timing of impulses in a single chemoreceptor fibre, this oscillation of discharge is best studied by summing the discharge of a single fibre over many respiratory cycles (Goodman et al, 1974). The cycle of discharge in the cat lags by a circulation time of about 2 sec behind the cycle in the alveolar gas that gives rise to it. The fall in discharge caused by inspiration is usually the quickest change and then the discharge builds up again, initially linearly, but if respiration is slow, the discharge then tends to a plateau, in part because the alveolar gas tensions tend to those of the venous blood but also because of adaptation of the receptor's response to CO_2. The course of discharge can be altered by altering the rate at which a given volume of air is driven into the lungs in inspiration. Also, if the throughput of CO_2 in a cat is doubled by gut-loading, the amplitude of the oscillation is doubled: CO_2 is important in causing the oscillation (Nye & Marsh, 1982).

Nevertheless, the respiratory oscillations of P_ACO_2 in a quietly breathing animal are only about 2–3 Torr in amplitude and a receptor following a typical steady state response line to CO_2 with a typical intercept on the PCO_2 axis at 20 Torr or more below a resting PCO_2, would have an oscillation in its discharge with an amplitude of only 10–15% of the mean and that would be less than doubled if O_2 were considered as well. But the respiratory oscillations observed in discharge are commonly 60% of the mean and may even be 100% or more. Adaptation can account for this, for, in the cat breathing slowly with a breath length of 4 sec, inspiration and expiration each last about 2 sec and that is less than half of the time constant of adaptation. So the response follows a steep transient line rather than a shallower steady state one. It would have a time course similar to the input in that case. But if the cycle of the stimulus were much longer than the time constant, adaptation would be greater and the gain for the output would tend to that of the steady state line and so would be much less.

In responding to respiratory oscillations in its stimuli, the receptor behaves as a proportional receptor unless the respiration is very slow. If the output of a receptor in response to a varying stimulus simply follows a single response line, it is said to be a proportional receptor, but if the output differs from that of a proportional receptor, the difference in its response is referred to as its dynamic response, and it is often supposed that, if there is any dynamic component of the response, then that part of the response is a differential one, related strictly to the rate of change of the stimulus, dS/dt. But as has just been said, a difference may also arise because the receptor adapts, to use a physiological term, or because it behaves as a "lead network".

A test between these two possibilities has been made by exposing a receptor to a symmetrical sawtooth CO_2 stimulus of a standard amplitude but of a fourfold range of frequencies so that the rate of change of the stimulus changed over a fourfold range (Kumar et al, 1994). It was found that the amplitude of the output oscillation it gave rise to decreased somewhat towards the higher frequencies, whereas it would have increased had the receptor been a rate receptor. Also, the output was a sawtooth like the input, and it did not alternate between two levels as it would have done had the response been a true rate response to the sawtooth input. This conclusion is supported by another experiment (Torrance et al, 1994). In a regularly ventilated cat, delaying or advancing the end of an expiration increased or decreased respectively the amplitude of the rise in chemoreceptor discharge caused by that expiration but it did not alter the rate of change of the stimulus. Such an increase in discharge after delaying an inspiration would occur, for example, after swallowing and it would tend to compensate for the loss of ventilation during the swallow by increasing reflexly the depth of the next breath. It would do that well because the later stage of an inspiratory phrenic nerve activity is the part that is most increased by a sudden rise in chemoreceptor input.

Kumar et al (1988) set up oscillations of P_AO_2 and of P_ACO_2 alone or of both together. An oscillation of P_AO_2 of any amplitude was more effective in hypoxia as might be expected from the PO_2 response line. O_2 contributes to the respiratory oscillation except at a high PO_2.

4. THE MECHANISM OF THE RESPONSE TO CO_2

The response of chemoreceptors to a sudden change of CO_2 provides a useful access to the mechanisms of their response. It has two components and each can give a way into the receptor mechanism.

1. Firstly, there is an "on" step up of the response which is quick and its height varies with the size of the increase in the stimulus, PCO_2, but the height of the step is independent of PO_2.
2. Secondly, there is an exponential decline, or adaptation, of the response and the degree of adaptation is very dependent on PO_2.

This relation that the degree of adaptation is less if the hypoxia is more intense, is very important: adaptation in chemoreceptors is not just one of those things that happens, "más o menos", in all receptors. A sudden CO_2 stimulus separates out in time, a quick, purely CO_2 response from a slower, O_2 dependent one, and the latter appears as adaptation.

4.1. The "on" of the Response and Carbonic Anhydrase

Consider first the "on". It is produced by CO_2. CO_2 does of course hydrate spontaneously to carbonic acid, but, in the body, the reaction is usually accelerated by carbonic anhydrase (CA). Lee & Mattenheimer (1964) found that CA activity in the CB is high at about 1/3 of that in the kidneys tubules. So when Black et al (1971) found that the response to CO_2 is fast, they investigated the importance of CA in the speed of the response by poisoning the CA of the CB with acetazolamide and then suddenly perfusing it with blood of a high PCO_2 that had not been poisoned and so could still give off CO_2 quickly and quickly raise the PCO_2 of the CB tissue. The response of the CB to CO_2 was greatly slowed by poisoning and there was no overshoot of the response. It appeared, then, that for CO_2 to excite normally, it has first to be hydrated to carbonic acid in some space in the carotid body that contains CA. Molecular CO_2 has no effect.

Acetazolamide also alters the steady state responses of the CB: it reduces them (Hayes et al, 1976). The slope of the CO_2 response line at any PO_2 is reduced by it and so the fan of PCO_2 lines for various PO_2s is closed up downwards. A reduction in discharge by CA inhibition in the steady state, as against the transient, can be accounted for if it is supposed that there is steady active transport in the CB as in the kidney tubule, and CA inhibition in the CB causes a disequilibrium pH as it does in the kidney. In the CB, it could affect pH in the space in which CO_2 is hydrated by CA before it acts, and inhibition of that CA would cause a change of pH in the space. The change could be compared to the disequilibrium pH towards acidity that develops in the lumen of the proximal tubule of the kidney after CA poisoning. There, acid is still secreted into the tubule but CO_2 does not escape freely from the HCO_3 buffer in the lumen when there is no tubular surface luminal CA to dehydrate H_2CO_3. But in the CB, it is acidity that excites, and inhibition of CA reduces excitation; and presumably inhibition of CA does so by increasing alkalinity. It was therefore suggested that movement of acid in the carotid body is the reverse of that in the kidney tubule: acid is secreted out of the space in which CA acts, not into it, and so the secretion tends to reduce excitation of the receptor. If CA is inhibited, an alkaline disequilibrium pH develops and so excitation is even less. Of course, "H^+ out" and "OH^- in" are tantamount to each other, and "OH^- in", like "H^+ out", would have its effect reduced by CA inhibition since CO_2 escape would be slowed. But if it were quite strictly HCO_3^- that is moved, the reverse would be true of the effect of CA inhibition. For if HCO_3^- were pushed into a buffered space, CA inhibition would delay the escape of CO_2, and the pH would therefore become more acid and excitation would become greater.

This line of thought suggests a model of the receptor region of the CB in which CO_2 is hydrated by CA in a space in which pH is constantly being driven towards alkalinity by the pumping of H^+ or OH^-, rather than of HCO_3^-.

4.2. An Extracellular or an Intracellular pH?

Initially it was supposed that the space is an extracellular space (Torrance, 1976), in imitation of ideas about the central CO_2 receptors which were then firmly believed to be excited by the pH of the extracellular space of the medulla in which they lie. Such an idea raised problems with the CB, for in the CB, the extracellular space leaks heavily to the plasma as had been shown by the penetration of peroxidase into it (Woods, 1975). That meant that the space had to be thought of as being pushed to the alkaline side of the already alkaline plasma pH from a relaxed pH equal to plasma pH.

The alternative was to suppose that it is an intracellular pH, pH_i, that sets off impulses; and that idea had the merit that pH_i in cells in general tends towards acidity at a relaxed pH of pH 6.2 if pH_i control mechanisms fail, and such a pH would excite the CB.

To choose between the alternatives of an intracellular and an extracellular site for the hydration of CO_2 by CA, two inhibitors of CA were compared (Hanson et al, 1981). One acetazolamide, penetrates cells easily and so should inhibit the CA of an intracellular space or of an extracellular one but the other, benzolamide, penetrates cells only slowly and so it should act early only on an extracellular CA. Benzolamide had a much slower effect than acetazolamide on excitation of chemoreceptors by CO_2 so it was suggested that it is hydration of CO_2 to change an intracellular pH that is the important action of CA in the CB. Impulses are set off when that intracellular pH, pH_i, goes acid. And for maximum simplicity, the response to that pH_i was supposed to be instant, linear, and without adaptation. And now Iturriaga (1996) has found that adding acetate/acetic acid buffer to the perfusate of his CB preparation without changing perfusate pH, increases the CB responses. That also points to an intracellular pH, as he says, since the fat soluble, unionised, acetic acid enters cells, and then lowers their pH_i by ionising, even when the acetate buffer added is not allowed to alter the cells' external pH, pH_0. CO_2 excites by lowering an intracellular pH.

4.3. Adaptation and PO_2

After the immediate step up of the response to CO_2, the response adapts exponentially and the degree of adaptation depends on PO_2. There is an immediate response to CO_2 and then it declines, or is switched off, to an extent that is PO_2 dependent (Fig 6c,d). The degree of switch off is PO_2 dependent. And that is all that O_2 ever does: it reduces the size of the response that CO_2 would otherwise be producing. And applying the CO_2 stimulus quickly makes it possible to separate out in time an immediate response to CO_2 and a later PO_2 dependent reduction or adaptation of that response.

4.4. The Bicarbonate Hypothesis

If adaptation is looked at in this way, the obvious suggestion to make about its mechanism is that the immediate change of pH_i that CO_2 produces is actively reduced by a mechanism of pH_i control. That reduces the response; it gives adaptation. But since adaptation is PO_2 dependent, so also must that pH_i control be. And if one supposes that the whole of adaptation of discharge takes place because of a process of pH_i control, then the whole of the effect of PO_2 on discharge, the whole of the PO_2 sensitivity of the CB, is due to an effect on pH_i control. If PO_2 alone changes, it alters the degree to which the response to an unchanged CO_2 stimulus is adapted (Hanson et al, 1981). This is the pH_i control idea of how chemoreceptors work, and it has come to be called the Bicarbonate Hypothesis (Torrance et al, 1993).

4.5. What Alternatives Are Possible?

If there is no mechanism of PO_2 dependent pH_i control, we do still have a pH_i that is altered by CO_2 and there is a mechanism for responding to it. Also the steady state effects of inhibition of CA suggest that there is manipulation of pH_i. But this manipulation could be quite independent of PO_2 and so be the mechanism of a pH_i control which, like that in other cells, is independent of PO_2. It keeps pH_i near to neutral and away from a relaxed value around pH 6.2.

The obvious alternative to pH_i control is in the world of membrane conductances. When, for example, a mechanoreceptor adapts, adaptation arises either in the development of a generator potential at the nerve ending, or in the response of the initial segment of the afferent fibre, the regenerative region, to the generator potential. Somehow a stimulus causes depolarisation of a membrane and that depolarisation stimulates an adjacent bit of membrane to fire off nerve impulses repetitively, just as in the classical example of this, a crab nerve fibre. The response of that fibre to a sustained electrical stimulus at a point on it comes quickly to a peak and then decays exponentially over seconds (Hodgkin, 1947), with the extent of the decay varying from fibre to fibre and being partial or complete. That is the sort of thing that a CB afferent fibre does. The sequence from a graded local depolarisation to a declining train of all or nothing nerve impulses has been analysed in mechanoreceptors (Eyzaguirre & Kuffler, 1955) and the speed and degree of decline in them may be the same as in chemoreceptors. Those declines could both result from an exponential increase in the number of membrane stabilising channels that are open in the regenerative region.

But the mechanism of adaptation is PO_2 dependent in chemoreceptors. Therefore we come to the idea that adaptation is due to the recruitment of membrane channels that tend to stabilise a membrane potential, E_m, in the face of things such as a generator potential that tend to shift it, and that after the initial response to a CO_2 stimulus these channels are activated by the depolarisation that the generator potential has produced. But the degree to which they are activated is affected by PO_2. Put otherwise, the probability that a channel will open is increased by depolarisation of the membrane in which it lies, and is also increased by a high CO_2 and decreased by a low one. It is not necessary to regard this effect of PO_2 as an effect merely on adaptation. It can be looked at it in another way. The response to CO_2 is fast. The response to O_2 is slower, and it is a mechanism that reduces the response to CO_2. It does so to a degree that is greater when the PO_2 is higher, and is zero when it is low.

4.6. Allosterism

Suppose that PCO_2 is held constant but PO_2 is changed. Initially there is a steady state in which the number of adaptation producing channels counters the number of pH_i dependent depolarising channels. Then, when PO_2 changes but pH_i does not change, the number of excitatory pH_i dependent channels open does not change. But the adaptation producing channels are E_m dependent and PO_2 dependent also. They respond slowly and their new equilibrium state is approached exponentially. But adaptation is slower than the response to O_2. That could be because O_2 and E_m affect the channels at different speeds. And that could be because they act at different points on the channel. Hb is the original allosteric molecule and, if one is naive enough, it is easy to imagine that a haem group has been stuck onto an E_m sensitive channel. If O_2 binds to the haem, the probability of the channel opening is increased. E_m acts elsewhere on the channel to increase opening, but the effects of the two stimuli, PO_2 and E_m, do not necessarily develop at the same rate.

The response to PO_2 is rather slower than the response to PCO_2 but it is distinctly faster than adaptation. These times of response are principally determined, on the present idea, by the time for the channel in the membrane to alter. For when a channel does alter, this membrane, like other membranes, comes quickly, in msec, to the appropriate E_m for the new pattern of ion conductances, irrespective of whether they have changed by O_2 or E_m or pH_i or whatever. The slow time course of adaptation of sec comes from slow reactions of channels and not from a slow passage of ions through them. And their reaction to PO_2 is faster than their reaction to E_m.

4.7. Times with the Bicarbonate Hypothesis

In contrast in the pH_i control hypothesis, one supposes that the rate of pumping of H^+/OH^- changes quickly in response to a change of pH_i or of PO_2 and that the speed of the change that results in pH_i, and so in discharge, derives from the speed of pumping H^+, the cell volume and the size of its leak away. The time taken to alter pH_i throughout a finite space, the cell cytoplasm, can be very different from the time needed to build up very local ionic concentrations at a cell membrane to change E_m. *In vitro*, the rate of change of pH_i in isolated cells when they are controlling pH_i is slow for accounting for adaptation and very slow for accounting for the response to PO_2. Also one would expect the half time of build up of pH_i within a cell to be independent of whether a change in the rate of pumping of H^+/OH^- is evoked by PO_2 or by E_m. But the observation is that the half time of the response to PO_2 is much less than the half time of adaptation. The speed for pH_i is very much a matter of the surface area to volume ratio of the cell, an $r^2:r^3$ problem; and a fine nerve ending or a wide but thin *en calyce* ending would raise that problem less acutely than would a spherical Type I cell.

When it was supposed that pH in the very narrow extracellular spaces of the carotid body, pH_o, rather than pH in its cells, pH_i, excited the nerve endings, there was not much of a problem in thinking that pH in so small a volume with so large a surface area might change quickly. There was no problem in accounting for the speed of the responses. And Hanson et al (1981) did find some effect of the slowly penetrating benzolamide on responses, but after it had produced its full effect, there was still a lot left for acetazolamide to do: there may be some CA in an extracellular space in which changes in pH affect discharge.

If adaptation is the result of pH_i control in a CB cell, then it should be affected by an appropriate inhibitor of H^+ transport. The Type I cell has at least two pH_i control mechanisms, and each of them has its own ionic requirements and inhibitor sensitivities (Peers & Buckler, 1995).

The dependence of the speed of the "hypoxia on" response upon the presence of HCO_3^- buffer (Iturriaga, 1993) has an explanation that adaptation and the "hypoxia on" response depend on an H^+ channel that requires HCO_3^-, and such channels have been found in the Type I cell *in vitro*. But the speed of the "hypoxia off" response depends little on HCO_3^-, another Iturriaga (1993) finding, and that could be because it is produced by another H^+ channel that does not depend on HCO_3^-. But there is an alternative explanation that Iturriaga himself favours: without HCO_3^-, the pH_i of the Type I cell, *in vitro* at least, is very alkaline, and the cell may not respond properly *in vivo* to hypoxia unless its pH_i is near to normal.

Several papers have described attempts to detect pH_i changes in the CB in response to hypoxia but nothing much has been found (Iturriaga, 1993). The Type I cell seems striking for lacking pH_i control mechanisms rather than for having extraordinarily refined ones. pH_i varies a lot when the external pH, pH_o, varies. But if pH_i is somehow pushed away from its normal steady value for the existing pH_o, control mechanisms bring it back (Peers & Buckler, 1995). Such a Type I cell could well give the responses of the CB to CO_2, and the basic mechanism of the responses to hypoxia could be O_2 sensitive membrane channels such as have just been discussed, rather than an O_2 sensitive control of pH_i.

A perfused preparation of the CB is needed that shows adaptation to a CO_2 stimulus. Gray (1971) has a brief remark that his preparation shows adaptation to CO_2 if the perfusate contains a second buffer in addition to HCO_3^- buffer, and Iturriaga's (1993) preparation adapts to CO_2 if HEPES is in the perfusate. Those are very important findings. For a basic message of this review is that adaptation to a sharp change of PCO_2 and the response to PO_2 are very much interrelated, and their study provides a way into the problem of chemoreception. A good perfusion preparation would be valuable for doing this, but many seem to fail after a short period without blood. Also, if the transient of a response is to be studied, a change of stimulus in the perfusate must be made to reach quickly the origin of the CB artery from the carotid sinus by somehow reducing the dead space delay before the change arrives at the CB. Ideally, a perfused CB should follow oscillations in its stimulus at the frequency of respiration as well as does the blood perfused CB of the intact animal. Adding CA to a perfusate containing a second buffer would make it give off CO_2 more rapidly.

4.8. Where Do Things Happen?

We have to work out where: 1) CO_2 produces the change in pH_i that sets off nerve impulses, and where: 2) that nerve response is reduced, either by altering the pH_i change itself or by changing its effect on an excitable membrane. If O_2 and adaptation join in to alter the response to CO_2 by altering pH_i, then the whole process of sensing both CO_2 and O_2 must take place in the same cell. But if O_2 and adaptation involve alterations in an excitable membrane, that membrane need not necessarily be in the cell in which CO_2 changes pH_i. pH_i in one cell could set off a transmitter action onto another cell, and O_2 and adaptation could alter the reaction of the second cell to a graded transmitter action from the first. And there are several other ways in which O_2 and CO_2 might converge to excite the same afferent fibre: a dozen or more of them (Torrance, 1977).

4.9. Structures Involved

This discussion has so far been an almost abstract one of unidentified spaces. What is the model of structure and function to which it must be related? The carotid body has a recurring structure of a glomerulus which is made up of a group of about six Type I cells enveloped by Type II cells, and with sensory nerve fibres and nerve endings within the spaces between the cells. There are many capillary blood vessels. De Castro's original model (De Castro & Rubio, 1968) of function is that the Type I cells taste the blood, he supposes both for CO_2 and for O_2, and then they excite the nerve endings. The model raises the problem of synaptic transmission, and it emerged in the 1930s when it was being established that transmission may be chemical. It would be valuable if the relations between all the cells of a whole glomerulus were worked out in more detail, perhaps in a serial section study with the extracellular spaces defined with peroxidase (Woods, 1975).

De Castro involved all the elements of the CB in his original model of function, and, if we accept his model, we have to consider how the Type I cell excites the nerve ending. At the most classical, the cell develops action potentials in response to CO_2 making its pH_i more acid, and hypoxia comes in, either by increasing the swing of pH_i, or else by increasing the action that pH_i has at the membrane of the Type I cell by some effect on membrane excitation. The action potentials of the Type I cell then make it release a transmitter which gives all or nothing impulses in the afferent nerve fibre.

It is often said in teaching that chemical transmission across a synapse allows the presynaptic element to be much smaller than the postsynaptic element that it excites. Think of the diminutive motor nerve ending that excites a massive striated muscle fibre with a tiny squirt of ACh. In the CB, the geometry is more nearly symmetrical across the synaptic cleft and approximates rather to the synapse of the chick ciliary ganglion which also has large, *en calyce*, nerve endings and can transmit impulses electrically in either direction (Martin & Pilar, 1963). Does the CB synapse "need" to employ a chemical transmitter?

Consider now the setting up of nerve impulses in the afferent fibre. So far as the membrane area is concerned, a problem arises. The geometry of the nerve endings is like the relation between a nerve cell body and the nerve fibre arising from it in which impulses are set up. The *en calyce*, or cup-like, nerve ending has the appearance of a punctured tennis ball: it has a membrane capacity as if it were a punctured nerve cell. For a nerve cell to set off impulses in the nerve fibre arising from it, there are conditions of the relative areas of the nerve cell body and of the nerve fibre arising from it. It is like the old problem of the critical length of a nerve fibre that has to be depolarised to set off a nerve impulse propagating along it. The same problem must arise in all receptors, but the way of accumulating an adequate area of membrane to set off the nerve fibre is not always the same. In baroreceptors, it is accumulated by repeated branching of the fibre into many fine endings. In contrast are the *en calyce* endings of the chemoreceptors: very few of those large nerve endings have to be connected to a nerve fibre for them to be able to set it off.

This difference should emerge in a section of the CB. If nerve impulses are indeed set up by many fine nerve endings, as Biscoe (1971) once thought, the sum of their perimeters in cross-section must be as great as that sum for a similarly effective, and so less numerous, set of much larger en calyce endings. There would have to be very many fine endings if that were the way the CA works, and they would not be anywhere near as elusive as Biscoe (1971) found them to be when he was searching for more of them after de Kock and Dunn (1968) had stumbled on a few rather by chance. It was all a bit like Bessie Bighead, hired help in Salt Lake Farm in Dylan Thomas' Under Milk Wood, dreaming of Gomer Owen "who kissed her once by the pigsty when she wasn't looking and never kissed her again although she was looking all the time".

And so, either 1) the nerve ending comes in merely by responding to a transmitter action of the Type I cell and there are no direct effects of PO_2 or pH_i upon the ending itself, O_2 and PCO_2 being worked out completely in the Type I cell; or else, 2) only CO_2 acts upon the Type I cell and the transmitter action of the Type I cell on the nerve ending is affected by an action of PO_2 on the ending. Donnelly (1995) seems to make it necessary to consider the second possibility, and to do so, the endings themselves would have to be studied. It is fortunate that Eyzaguirre (Hayashida et al, 1980) has shown that intracellular recordings can be made from nerve fibres and nerve endings within the carotid body in his *in vitro* preparation.

5. SOME RANDOM EPILEGOMENA

5.1. Electrical Transmission?

Transmission could be electrical rather than chemical. This was not a plausible suggestion so long as the Type I cell had not been shown to produce action potentials, APs, but since the late 1980s, it has been found in several laboratories that an isolated Type I cell can be got to give a short burst of APs if first it has had its membrane electrically clamped for some time to prime it, and then it is left free. And now Buckler (Peers & Buckler, 1995) has managed the difficult, and much more conclusively relevant, experiment of eliciting a well sustained train of APs from a Type I cell that has not been primed, a condition Buckler now refers to as "zero current clamp". This means that the possibility of electrical transmission has now simply got to be considered. The geometry is appropriate for electrical transmission and the enveloping Type II cells might focus the Type I cells' APs onto the large, *en calyce*, nerve endings. Type I cells are electrically connected to one another but not, it seems, to the nerve endings (but see Kondo and Iwasa, this volume).

5.2. The Rejected Transmitters

I now arrive at transmitters, and that really is the end of my remit. But just one or two comments upon them. The classical model of transmission in the CB, and the blindingly obvious one, comes from De Castro; the Type I cell tastes the blood and passes its message on to the nerve ending by releasing a chemical transmitter (De Castro & Rubio, 1968). It was WW Douglas (1952) who stopped it all being quite so simple. Samson Wright had sloshed acetylcholine at the carotid body and it had excited it. So cholinergic transmission in the CB was born. But Douglas showed that you can block the action of injected ACh on the CB without blocking natural stimuli. And that sort of experiment has been a recurring problem for candidate transmitters. But there are alternative possibilities, as has been hinted.

There have been so many candidate transmitters that have not made the grade that I wonder what their status now can be. Once they were cherished because they excited, or were present in the CB, or did something else that was transmitter-like, but now they are forgotten. But they would not have excited, had there not been a membrane receptor that responded to them. And they would not have been found in the carotid body, had they not been synthesised there, or at least had a mechanism that took them in from the blood and stored them. Perhaps it is that the carotid body is derived from cells of the neural crest that once were totipotential cells for transmission, and that the cells retain a slight suspicion still within them of each of the quite different things they might have become had they been moved, early on, or bit further up, or a bit further down, the neural crest. And since the carotid body has not really got a phasic transmitter at all, the fantastically sensitive methods we now have for the study of transmitters are revealing no more than traces of the might have beens. Now I had better back to physiology.

5.3. Fine Nerve Endings?

But there has always been another possibility: only the nerve ending is phasically active at each afferent nerve impulse, a possibility that was prominent around 1970 (Biscoe, 1971). The Type I cell is, of course, needed for chemoreception, and it somehow gives the nerve fibre its specificity, as Dinger et al (1984) have so elegantly shown by re-innervating the carotid body with glossopharyngeal taste fibres which then become chemoreceptors. The Type I cell might give the ending its own complete phasic sensitivity without the Type I cell itself being phasically active. There is space enough in the *en calyce* ending to accommodate the sort of membrane mechanisms that have earlier been considered responsible for the reactions of the Type I cell to CO_2 and O_2: and if they are in the ending rather than in the cell, no problem of synaptic transmission arises. This problem came alive in 1968 when efferent effects of glossopharyngeal fibres on the CB were being actively discussed. Out of this, Biscoe (1971) proposed two things: that a set of fine nerve endings are themselves sensitive to respiratory gases, and that the *en calyce* endings are efferent. Hess and Zapata (1972) instantly disposed of the second proposal, but the first remains, though not for the fine nerve endings that Biscoe had hoped would be discovered, but rather for the large, *en calyce* endings.

5.4. Extracellular Ionic Concentrations

There are reports of measuring extracellular concentrations of ions in the CB which are different from those of the plasma and are sustained. But it must be relevant that the extracellular spaces of the CB are penetrated by peroxidase from the blood (Woods, 1975); and that K^+ enters the spaces quickly from the blood and depolarises the Type I cells but is then quickly washed away (Goodman & McCloskey, 1972). And many drugs build up transient concentrations from the blood but are soon washed away if one may judge by the time course of the nerve response to them. Are there reserves enough of an ion such as K^+ within the CB for its concentration to be made higher than in the blood for more than a very short time in so open an extracellular space? There might, nevertheless, be some extracellular space of the CB that cannot be entered by non-fat-soluble substances from the blood and has its composition actively controlled by the cells surrounding it, rather as Eyzaguirre once suggested (Eyzaguirre & Zapata, 1968) when he was considering the access of inhibitors from the blood to a part of the cholinesterase of the CB. Or might such a transcellular space be manufactured by an electrode that is blocking a vessel?

5.5. Arteriovenous Anastomoses

The a-v anastomoses of the CB have long been a mystery but there is one interesting consequence of their large blood flow in parallel with the nutritive capillary flow. It may not itself supply the cells of the CB, but it does ensure that the dead space of the CB artery is quickly washed through. That, combined with the fact that the origin of the CB artery from the carotid sinus is hit by the fast axial flow of blood along the centre of the common carotid artery, must contribute to the surprisingly short latency of less than 2 sec in a cat, corresponding to 5 sec in a man, with which a change in a gas tension in the lung may reach the CB and change its discharge.

5.6. Arterial Chemoreceptors of Man

Do the chemoreceptors of man respond like those of the cat? Cunningham has often said that they do not, asserting in particular that their fan of CO_2 response lines intersects on the PCO_2 axis at a very few Torr, about 2 Torr, below a resting PCO_2. Also, mathematical modellers of the system of respiratory control have not yet taken on board fully that the responses of CB chemoreceptors to CO_2 adapt even though they accept that the receptors respond to the small respiratory oscillations in gas stimuli in the arterial blood with a wide oscillation in discharge (Cunningham et al, 1986). Swanson and Bellville (1974) found that the relative effectiveness of CO_2 and O_2 as stimuli to ventilation in hypoxia and in mild hypercapnia is 1:2.9 in man, and that is exactly the figure found by Kumar et al (1988) at similar gas tensions for discharge in the cat. The figure is determined by the steepness of the transient CO_2 response line and its intercept on the PCO_2 axis. If it is at all possible to record the discharge of chemoreceptors directly, that should be done to get an idea of their behaviour. Trying to derive their behaviour by interpreting their reflex effects is rather like looking at them backwards way down the distorting spectacles of the central nervous system.

5.7. Biochemistry and the Metabolic Hypothesis

The Metabolic Hypothesis, that a fall in [ATP] somewhere within the carotid body sets off discharge, now looks very uncertain. Once, many papers and even a whole book were devoted to it, but the uncoupler, DNP, has now been shown to excite the CB without changing [ATP] in it, a death knell for the metabolic hypothesis perhaps, but without its death (Peers & Buckler, 1955) it can hardly be said that hypoxia affects discharge because O_2 can react directly with a K^+ channel, an idea which does not have any problems in accounting for the speed of the response to hypoxia. A pity. The metabolic hypothesis did seem to tie in the whole oxidative biochemistry with excitation of the carotid body. It was built upon the excitatory effects of a whole array of wonderfully specific metabolic inhibitors. And those effects must still have some explanation.

6. ENVOI

The carotid body is not a dreary little CO_2 receptor that is brought to life by hypoxia: it is a very excitable CO_2 receptor that is calmed down by oxygen.

7. REFERENCES

Biscoe TJ (1971) Carotid body: structure and function. Physiol Rev 51: 427–495

Black AMS, McCloskey DI & Torrance RW (1971) The responses of carotid body chemoreceptors in the cat to sudden changes in hypercapnic and hypoxic stimuli. Respir Physiol 13: 36–49

Black AMS & Torrance RW (1971) Respiratory oscillations in chemoreceptor discharge in the control of breathing. Respir Physiol 13: 221–237

Cunningham DJC, Robbins PA & Wolff CB (1986) Integration of respiratory responses to changes in alveolar partial pressures of CO_2 and O_2 in arterial pH. In: Handbook of Physiology, sect 3: Respiratory System, vol 2: Control of Breathing (Cherniack NS & Widdicombe JG, eds). Bethesda, Md: Amer Physiol Soc. pp 475–528

de Castro F & Rubio M (1968) The anatomy and innervation of the blood vessels of the carotid body and the role of chemoreceptive reactions in the autoregulation of the blood flow. In: Torrance RW (ed) Arterial Chemoreceptors. Oxford: Blackwell. pp 267–277

Dejours P (1966) Respiration. New York: Oxford University Press

de Kock LL & Dunn AEG (1966) An electron microscopic study of the carotid body. Acta Anat 64: 163–173

Dinger BG, Stensaas LJ & Fidone SJ (1984) Chemosensory end-organs re-innervated by normal and foreign nerves. In: Pallot DJ (ed) The Peripheral Arterial Chemoreceptors. London: Croom Helm. pp 225–234

Donnelly DF (1995) Modulation of glomus cell membrane currents of intact rat carotid body. J Physiol, London 489: 677–688

Douglas CG, Haldane JS, Henderson Y & Schneider EC (1913) Physiological observations made on Pike's Peak, Colorado, with special reference to adaptation to low barometric pressures. Phil Trans Roy Soc, London 203B: 185–318

Douglas WW (1952) The effect of a ganglion-blocking drug, hexamethonium, on the response of the cat's carotid body to various stimuli. J Physiol, London 118: 373–383

Euler US von, Liljestrand G & Zotterman Y (1939) The excitation mechanism of the chemoreceptors of the carotid body. Skand Arch Physiol 83: 132–152

Eyzaguirre C & Kuffler SW (1955) Processes of excitation in the dendrites and in the soma of single, isolated nerve cells of the lobster and crayfish. J Gen Physiol 39: 87–119

Eyzaguirre C & Zapata P (1968) A discussion of possible transmitter or generator substances in carotid body chemoreceptors. In: Torrance RW (ed) Arterial Chemoreceptors. Oxford: Blackwell. pp 213–251

FitzGerald MP (1913) The changes in the breathing and the blood at various high altitudes. Phil Trans Roy Soc, London 203B: 351–371

Fitzgerald RS & Parks C (1971) Effect of hypoxia on carotid chemoreceptor response to carbon dioxide in cats. Respir Physiol 12: 218–229

Gonzalez C, Lopez-Lopez JR, Obeso A, Perez-Garcia MT & Rocher A (1995) Cellular mechanisms of oxygen chemoreception in the carotid body. Respir Physiol 102: 137–147

Goodman NW (1974) Some observations on the homogeneity of response of single chemoreceptor fibres. Respir Physiol 20: 271–281

Goodman NW & McCloskey DI (1972) Intracellular potentials in the carotid body. Brain Res 39: 501–504

Goodman NW, Nail BS & Torrance RW (1974) Oscillations in the discharge of single carotid chemoreceptor fibres of the cat. Respir Physiol 20: 251–269

Gray BA (1971) On the speed of the carotid body response in relation to CO_2 hydration. Respir Physiol 11: 235–246

Hanson MA, Nye PCG & Torrance RW (1981) The exodus of an extracellular bicarbonate theory of chemoreception and the genesis of an intracellular one. In: Belmonte C, Pallot DJ, Acker H & Fidone S (eds) Arterial Chemoreceptors. Leicester: Leicester University Press. pp 403–416

Hayashida Y, Koyano H & Eyzaguirre C (1980) An intracellular study of chemosensory fibres and endings. J Neurophysiol 44: 1077–1088

Hayes MW (1974) The mechanism of initiation of impulses in arterial chemoreceptors. MSc Thesis. Oxford University

Hayes MW, Maini BK & Torrance RW (1976) Reduction of the responses of carotid chemoreceptors by acetazolamide. In: Paintal AS (ed) Morphology and Mechanisms of Chemoreceptors. Delhi: Vallabhbhai Patel Chest Institute. pp 36–45

Hess A & Zapata P (1972) Innervation of the cat carotid body: normal and experimental studies. Fed Proc 31: 1365–1382

Heymans C & Neil E (1958) Reflexogenic Areas of the Cardiovascular System. London: Churchill

Hodgkin AL (1948) The local electric changes associated with repetitive action in a non-medullated axon. J Physiol, London 107: 165–181

Iturriaga R (1993) Carotid body chemoreception: the importance of CO_2-HCO_3^- and carbonic anhydrase. Biol Res 26: 319–329

Kumar P (1986) Oscillations in the discharge of arterial chemoreceptors: their origin and some reflex effects. D Phil Thesis, Oxford University

Kumar P, Nye PCG & Torrance RW (1988) Do oxygen tension variations contribute to the respiratory oscillations of chemoreceptor discharge in the cat? J Physiol, London 395: 531–552

Kumar P, Nye PCG & Torrance RW (1994) Proportional sensitivity of arterial chemoreceptors to CO_2. Adv Exp Med Biol 360: 237–239

Lee KD & Mattenheimer H (1964) The biochemistry of the carotid body. Enzymol Biol Clin 4: 199–216

Lloyd BB, Jukes MGM & Cunningham DJC (1958) The relation between alveolar oxygen pressure and the respiratory response to carbon dioxide in man. Quart J Exp Physiol 43: 214–227

Martin AR & Pilar G (1963) Dual mode of synaptic transmission in the avian ciliary ganglion. J Physiol, London 168: 443–463

Nye PCG & Marsh J (1982) Ventilation and carotid chemoreceptor discharge during venous CO_2 loading via the gut. Respir Physiol 50: 335–350

Paintal AS (1967) Mechanism of stimulation of aortic chemoreceptors by natural stimuli and chemical substances. J Physiol, London 189: 63–84

Paterson DJ & Nye PCG (1994) Reflexes arising from the arterial chemoreceptors. Adv Exp Med Biol 360: 71–86

Peers C & Buckler KJ (1995) Transduction of chemostimuli by the Type I carotid body cell. J Membr Biol 144: 1–9

Silk N (1967) Mechanism of excitation of chemoreceptors. B Sc Thesis. Oxford University

Stein RB (1968) Some implications of the variability in chemoreceptor discharge. In: Torrance RW (ed) Arterial Chemoreceptors. Oxford: Blackwell. pp 205–212

Swanson GD & Bellville JW (1974) Hypoxic-hypercapnic interactions in human respiratory control. J Appl Physiol 36: 480–487

Torrance RW (1976) A new version of the acid receptor hypothesis of carotid chemoreceptors. In: Paintal AS (ed) Morphology and Mechanisms of Chemoreceptors. Delhi: Vallabhbhai Patel Chest Institute. pp 131–137

Torrance RW (1977) Convergence of stimuli in arterial chemoreceptors. Adv Exp Med Biol 78: 203–207

Torrance RW, Bartels EM & McLaren AJ (1993) Update on the bicarbonate hypothesis. Adv Exp Med Biol 337: 241–250

Torrance RW, Iturriaga R & Zapata P (1994) Effect of expiratory duration on chemoreceptor oscillations. Adv Exp Med Biol 360: 241–243

Whalen WJ & Nair P (1977) Tissue PO_2 in the cat carotid body and related functions. Adv Exp Med Biol 78: 225–232

Wolff CB (1992) The physiological control of respiration. Molec Aspects Med 13: 445–567 (Fig 6)

Woods RI (1975) Penetration of horseradish peroxidase between all elements of the carotid body. In: Purves MJ (ed) The Peripheral Arterial Chemoreceptors. London: Cambridge University Press. pp 195–205

3

DANIEL J. C. CUNNINGHAM*

Oration at His Funeral Service†

Brian B. Lloyd

Oxford, United Kingdom

With over a hundred publications to his name, Dan Cunningham achieved important advances in respiratory physiology.

A year before the 2nd World War, he won a Nuffield Medical Exhibition from Loretto, in Edinburgh, to Worcester College, Oxford, where, in passing the preclinical examinations for the BM BCh degrees, he won the Theodore Williams Scholarships, open to the whole University, in both Physiology and Anatomy. He did his clinical course in Edinburgh in six months fewer than usual by redrafting, with his colleagues Gus Born and David Clark, the established course.

After being house physician to Sir Stanley Davidson at the Royal Infirmary, he joined the RAMC and the third Parachute Regiment, working throughout the campaign in Europe, and in the landing at Arnhem. After the war Dr HM Sinclair, recalling Dan's spectacular achievements in First BM, got him seconded, as Major Cunningham, to the leadership of the main nutrition survey team in Düsseldorf, which he took over with tact and effectiveness. Through no fault of his own, he was unable to complete his interesting work on the discovery of normal plasma protein concentrations in hunger oedema in the German population, then on restricted rations.

Returning to Oxford, he got a first in Physiology in 1947, having been tutored by Geoffrey Dawes, and then succeeded Robert Thompson as Radcliffe Medical Fellow of University College, Oxford, retiring in 1987 into an Emeritus Fellowship. He also held the Schorstein Research Fellowship in Medical Science, after which he was appointed to a permanent Lectureship in the University Laboratory of Physiology in 1952, by which time he had proved to be a devoted tutor and an excellent lecturer and research worker.

---

* Daniel John Chapman Cunningham. Born Kasauli, India, 21st October 1919. Died Oxford, UK, 26th February 1996. Married (1947) to Judith Hill, violinist; one son: John, MD; one daughter: Jane, PhD in Art History; 3 grandsons. Studies at Loretto School, Edinburgh; Worcester College, Oxford; Edinburgh University. Served at Royal Infirmary, Edinburgh; RAMC. Radcliffe Medical Fellow, University College, Oxford; Lecturer, Laboratory of Physiology, Oxford University. Emeritus Fellow (1987), University College, Oxford.

† Stanton St John Church; 1st March 1996.

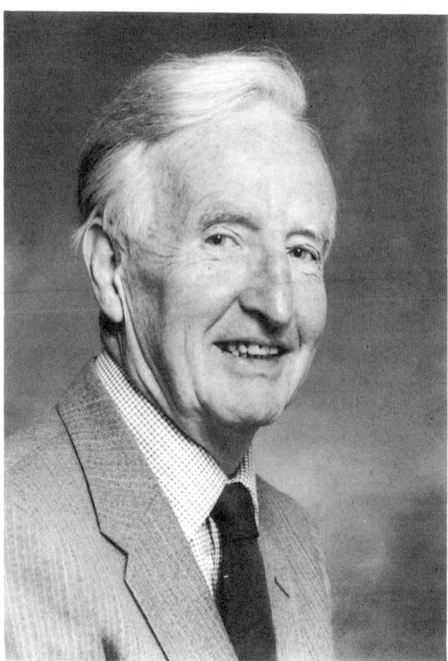

Figure 1. Daniel JC Cunningham.

His experience in nutrition brought him towards respiration and metabolism, in which CG Douglas was the departmental leader. Douglas was the last survivor of the important school of respiratory physiology set up by JS Haldane, whom Dan claimed as his scientific hero, and his papers with Douglas and Roger Bannister were based on Roger‡ and others, such as Jeffrey Archer,° running with or without oxygen supplementation on a treadmill built in the department and later run on by Ed Hillary.+ After his work with Bannister, Dan decided to follow up the Danish work of Nielsen and Smith with a direct investigation of the effect of carbon dioxide (CO_2) on the response to reduced oxygen, and to challenge the linear-additive theory of JS Gray. He showed with Cormack and Gee that the response to oxygen lack was hyperbolic and multiplicative rather than linear and additive, as Gray thought. He then went on with other colleagues to see the effect of various stimuli such as acid-base changes, noradrenaline infusion and raised body temperature on the ventilation, CO_2, oxygen relationship, an approach that proved fruitful. Dan thus demonstrated that the separation of factors so successful in the physical sciences could be applied in human physiology, and even applied, by means of breath holding, to the investigation of willpower. Having made important contributions to the science of steady-state respiration, Dan moved to transient phenomena, one of his recent collaborators being Peter Robbins, who is now carrying on the Oxford tradition of respiratory physiology.

‡ Roger Bannister, first four-minute miler.

° Now Lord Archer. Distinguished sprinter and gymnast while studying at Oxford University (Athletics blues 1963–65; Gymnastics blue 1965; Oxford 100-yard sprint record, 1966), career politician (formerly Member of the House of Commons; Life Peer UK, 1992) and prolific author (*Shall We Tell the President?, Kane and Abel, First Among Equals, Beyond Reasonable Doubt*).

+ Edmund Hillary, first conqueror of Mount Everest.

Dan's success in respiration, which was recognised worldwide, was based on the various excellences of his personality. First and foremost he had a very good brain, capable of holding complex and disparate ideas simultaneously, and of having bright ideas. This is exemplified in the following bit of discussion, which took place at the "International Cerebrospinal Fluid Symposium" in New York in April 1964, after a paper by John Pappenheimer. Dan said: "I think Dr Pappenheimer's difficulty may be that he can't see any teleology behind the superficial receptors. I think I might be able to supply it because I don't work in this field". This was greeted with laughter, which Dan intended, and to which he responded with: "I think the point would be that if you had cells whose activity is increased by CO_2 detecting the CO_2 concentration in their own locality, you would have a positive feedback system which would be undesirable in this situation". This caused a long silence, the audience being **dumbfounded**. Dan's next question, "Was that plain?", was followed by **quiet** laughter. I remember that dumbfounded silence very well. Everyone seemed to know that Dan had raised a fundamental point of general physiological interest, but few were shrewd enough to grasp it. The Chairman's comment that "You have created a silence" released tension into an explosion of **loud** laughter. The Chairman then attributed the silence to low blood sugar, but the real culprit was not hypoglycaemia, but the quick profundity of Dan's thinking, of which I became aware again in discussing some of the obscurer factors in respiration when I was about to take over his course of lectures for a few years.

Any collaborator of Dan's enjoyed life in the laboratory to the full. A given experiment could last for 4 or 5 hours, and inevitably involved a team of people, working in solemn silence, as talking disturbed the responses of the subject, usually a male undergraduate, who inevitably produced anomalous readings when a pair of high heels tripped down the hard floor of the corridor outside the lab. Fragmentary results emerged as the experiment proceeded but the full picture only after hours of calculation and exhilarating discussions round the blackboard, at which Dan, as often as not, had the last word.

Dan's point in New York arose out of his wisdom, and that wisdom gave him sapiential authority in a life in which his formal structural authority scarcely altered, though he was certainly offered chairs in some half-dozen other universities. When the Dr Sinclair I have already mentioned found himself in trouble over some building work he was alleged to have commissioned in the name of the University, one of its boards was asked to assess the matter: a bright spark suggested a subcommittee, and Dan was nominated as its first member. The then Professor of Physiology, Pat Liddell, drily commented that the smallest committees were the best, and that Dan should act alone. The board, knowing Dan, accepted this, and Dan then had some gruelling weeks unearthing the facts and making his report, which was greatly appreciated.

Dan's friends, and many in the US have already expressed their deep sorrow, may know how much they have lost in losing Dan; but this is a small proportion of the great loss suffered by his family, his wife Judy and his children Jane, and John with his wife Debbie and the three grandsons, and his sister Mary. Dan was particularly grateful and explicit about what a very good wife Judy had been to him, in their lives and their last days together. I think that if he had known Dan, Geoffrey Chaucer would have had him in mind when he wrote these lines:

> He loved chivalry,
> Truth and honour, freedom and courtesy.
> He was a very perfect gentle knight.

SELECTED REFERENCES ON RESPIRATORY REGULATION

Bannister RG & Cunningham DJC (1954) The effects on the respiration and performance during exercise of adding oxygen to the inspired air. J Physiol, London 125: 118–137

Bascom DA, Clements ID, Cunningham DA, Painter R & Robbins PA (1990) Changes in peripheral chemoreflex sensitivity during sustained isocapnic hypoxia. Respir Physiol 62: 161–176

Bhattacharyya NK, Cunningham DJC, Goode RC, Howson MG & Lloyd BB (1970) Hypoxia, ventilation, PCO_2 and exercise. Respir Physiol 9: 329–347

Cormack RS, Cunningham DJC & Gee JBL (1957) The effect of carbon dioxide on the respiratory response to want of oxygen in man. Quart J Exp Physiol 42: 303–319

Cunningham DJC (1963) Some quantitative aspects of the regulation of human respiration in exercise. Brit Med Bull 19: 25–30

Cunningham DJC (1967) Regulation of breathing in exercise. Circ Res 20/21 (suppl 1): 122–131

Cunningham DJC (1974) The control system regulating breathing in man. Quart Rev Biophys 6: 433–483

Cunningham DJC (1974) Integrative aspects of the regulation of breathing: a personal view. In: International Review of Science, sect 1: Physiology, vol 2: Respiration (Widdicombe JG, ed). London: Butterworths. pp 303–369

Cunningham DJC (1975) A model illustrating the importance of timing in the regulation of breathing. Nature 253: 440–442

Cunningham DJC (1983) Introductory remarks. Some problems in respiratory physiology. In: Whipp BJ & Wiberg DM (eds) Modelling and Control of Breathing. New York: Elsevier. pp 3–19

Cunningham DJC (1987) Studies on arterial chemoreceptors in man. J Physiol, London 384: 1–26

Cunningham DJC & Lloyd BB (eds) (1963) The Regulation of Human Respiration. Oxford: Blackwell

Cunningham DJC & O'Riordan JLH (1957) The effect of a rise in the temperature of the body on the respiratory response to carbon dioxide at rest. Quart J Exp Physiol 42: 329–345

Cunningham DJC, Hey EN & Lloyd BB (1958) The effect of intravenous infusion of noradrenaline on the respiratory response to carbon dioxide in man. Quart J Exp Physiol 43: 394–399

Cunningham DJC, Shaw DG, Lahiri S & Lloyd BB (1961) The effect of maintained ammonium chloride acidosis on the relation between pulmonary ventilation and alveolar oxygen and carbon dioxide in man. Quart J Exp Physiol 46: 323–334

Cunningham DJC, Hey EN, Patrick JM & Lloyd BB (1963) The effect of noradrenaline infusion on the relation between pulmonary ventilation and the alveolar PO_2 and PCO_2 in man. Ann N Y Acad Sci 109: 756–770

Cunningham DJC, Patrick JM & Lloyd BB (1964) The respiratory response of man to hypoxia. In: Dickens F & Neil E (eds) Oxygen in the Animal Organisms. Oxford: Pergamon. pp 277–291

Cunningham DJC, Elliott DH, Lloyd BB, Miller JP & Young JM (1965) A comparison of the effects of oscillating and steady alveolar partial pressures of oxygen and carbon dioxide on the pulmonary ventilation. J Physiol, London 179: 498–508

Cunningham DJC, Spurr D & Lloyd BB (1968) The drive to ventilation from arterial chemoreceptors in hypoxic exercise. In: Torrance RW (ed) Arterial Chemoreceptors. Oxford: Blackwell. pp 301–323

Cunningham DJC, Howson MG & Pearson SB (1973) The respiratory effects in man of altering the time profile of alveolar CO_2 and O_2 within each respiratory cycle. J Physiol, London 234: 1–28

Cunningham DJC, Drysdale DB, Gardner WN, Jensen JI, Petersen ES & Whipp BJ (1977) Very small, very short-latency changes in human breathing induced by step changes in alveolar gas composition. J Physiol 266: 411–421

Cunningham DJC, Metias EF, Howson MG & Petersen ES (1983) Patterns of reflex responses to dynamic stimulation of the human respiratory system. In: Schlaefke ME, Koepchen HP & See WR (eds) Central Neurone Environment. Heidelberg: Springer-Verlag. pp 116–123

Cunningham DJC, Howson MG, Metias EF & Petersen ES (1986) Patterns of breathing in response to alternating alveolar patterns of PCO_2 in man. J Physiol, London 376: 31–45

Cunningham DJC, Robbins PA & Wolff CB (1986) Integration of respiratory responses to changes in alveolar partial pressures of CO_2 and O_2 and in arterial pH. In: Handbook of Physiology, sect 3: The Respiratory System, vol 2: Control of Breathing (Cherniack NS & Widdicombe JG, eds). Bethesda, Md: Am Physiol Soc. pp 475–528

Drysdale DB, Jensen JI & Cunningham DJC (1981) The short-latency respiratory response to sudden withdrawal of hypercapnia and hypoxia in man. Quart J Exp Physiol 66: 203–210

Goode RC, Brown EB Jr, Howson MG & Cunningham DJC (1969) Respiratory effects of breathing down a tube. Respir Physiol 6: 343–359

Hey EN, Lloyd BB, Cunningham DJC, Jukes MGM & Bolton DPG (1966) Effects of various respiratory stimuli on the depth and frequency of breathing in man. Respir Physiol 1: 193–205

Lloyd BB & Cunningham DJC (1963) Quantitative approach to the regulation of human respiration. In: Cunningham DJC & Lloyd BB (eds) The Regulation of Human Respiration. Oxford: Blackwell. pp 331–349

Lloyd BB, Jukes MGM & Cunningham DJC (1958) The relation between alveolar oxygen pressure and the respiratory response to carbon dioxide in man. Quart J Exp Physiol 43: 214–227

Lloyd BB, Cunningham DJC & Goode RC (1968) Depression of hypoxic hyperventilation in man by sudden inspiration of carbon monoxide. In: Torrance RW (ed) Arterial Chemoreceptors. Oxford: Blackwell. pp 145–148

Marsh RHK, Lyen KR, McPherson GAD, Pearson SB & Cunningham DJC (1973) Breath-by-breath effects of imposed alternate-breath oscillations of alveolar CO_2. Respir Physiol 18: 80–91

Metias EF, Cunningham DJC, Howson MG, Petersen ES & Wolff CB (1981) Reflex effects on human breathing of breath-by-breath changes of the time profile of alveolar PCO_2 during steady hypoxia. Pflügers Arch 389: 243–250

Miller JP, Cunningham DJC, Lloyd BB & Young JM (1974) The transient respiratory effects in man of sudden changes in alveolar CO_2 in hypoxia and in high oxygen. Respir Physiol 20: 17–31

Pearson SB & Cunningham DJC (1973) Some observations on the relation between ventilation, tidal volume and frequency in man in various steady and transient states. Acta Neurobiol Exp 33: 177–188

Ward SA, Drysdale DB, Cunningham DJC & Petersen ES (1979) Inspiratory-expiratory responses to alternate-breath oscillation of PA,CO_2 and PA,O_2. Respir Physiol 36: 311–325

4

RE-EXAMINATION OF THE CAROTID BODY ULTRASTRUCTURE WITH SPECIAL ATTENTION TO INTERCELLULAR MEMBRANE APPOSITIONS

Hisatake Kondo and Hiroo Iwasa

Department of Anatomy
School of Medicine
Tohoku University
Sendai 980, Japan

1. SUMMARY

Ultrathin sections of the carotid body of adult rats, processed through freeze-substitution after aldehyde-prefixation, showed a substantial number of presumed gap junctions between two adjacent chief cells, between chief and sustentacular cells, and between chief cells and carotid nerve terminals. The junctions showed a very narrow intercellular space of 2 nm and ranged in length from 200 nm to 1 μm. They may form the morphological substrate for electrical coupling between cells, the occurrence of which has been demonstrated by electrophysiology. Further studies using freeze-fracture and immunocytochemistry for connexins are necessary to confirm this possibility. In addition, small tight junctions are present between chief and sustentacular cells, and between adjacent sustentacular cells.

2. INTRODUCTION

The carotid body is mainly composed of chief (glomus, type I) cells and sustentacular cells and it detects chemical changes in the blood such as PO_2, PCO_2 and pH. Although the exact mechanisms of chemosensory transduction are not completely understood, it is generally agreed that the chief cells are the primary transducer elements. They also are secretory elements releasing ACh, catecholamines and neuropeptides. The released chemicals may exert synaptic or paracrine effects on the carotid nerve terminals and adjacent chief cells and this is accompanied by increased sensory discharges in the carotid nerve. The secretion increases during physiological stimulation (Fidone & González, 1986).

Frontiers in Arterial Chemoreception, edited by Zapata *et al.*
Plenum Press, New York, 1996

Previous electrophysiological studies have demonstrated dye- and electrotonic coupling between the chief cells. Stimulation by hypoxia and acidity increase the coupling resistance (Baron & Eyzaguirre, 1977; Monti-Bloch et al, 1993; Abudara & Eyzaguirre, 1994). In relation to these electrophysiological findings, the presence of a few and small sites of close membrane appositions with intercellular spaces of about 2 nm between the chief cells has been reported by electron microscopy, suggesting the presence of gap junction (McDonald, 1981). However, the occurrence (2–3%) and size (up to 200 nm in length) of such appositions were too small to be compatible with the rather frequent occurrence of the electrotonic coupling.

To resolve this discrepancy, we have reexamined the ultrastructure of the carotid body using aldehyde-prefixed and freeze-substitution electron microscopy. This approach (rather than conventional electron microscopy) has been considered to produce ultrastructural images closer to what occurs in the living cells (Chan et al, 1993).

3. MATERIALS AND METHODS

The carotid bifurcations were excised from young adult rats under pentobarbital (40 mg/kg body weight) anesthesia and the carotid bodies were isolated from the bifurcation and placed in an aerated bicarbonate buffer solution. As a control, and to see whether freeze-substitution preserves tissues well, the kidney was also excised and trimmed into small pieces by razor blades and placed in the buffer. The tissues were subsequently immersed in 2.5% glutaraldehyde / 2% paraformaldehyde containing 0.5% tannic acid in 0.1 M sodium cacodylate buffer for 2 h at 4°C. After overnight immersion in 40% glycerin at 4°C, tissue blocks were frozen in liquid nitrogen and immediately dipped into 4% OsO_4 in absolute acetone containing 0.5% uranyl acetate which had been pre-cooled at -80°C. The tissue blocks were maintained for 48 h at -80°C, 24 h at -20°C, 12 h at -4°C, and 12 h at 4°C. They were brought to room temperature for 2 h and rinsed several times in fresh absolute acetone for 20 min. They were then embedded in Epon.

4. RESULTS

Control renal tissues as well as the carotid bodies showed fairly good tissue preservation. A reticulated appearance, characteristic of ice-crystal formation, was not obvious in any portion of the cytoplasm and nucleus. Also, the trilaminar structure of the plasma membranes and intracellular membranes was evident at higher magnification (Fig 1).

The ultrastructure of the kidney also presented an example of good tissue preservation. The basement membrane of the renal glomeruli consists of a uniform lamina densa in contact with the plasma membranes of the podocyte pedicles and of the endothelial cells without intervening lamina lucidae (data not shown). This feature represents a major characteristic in the ultrastructure of renal glomeruli by the freeze-substitution either following rapid freezing without chemical fixation or following aldehyde-prefixation (Chan et al, 1993; Kondo, 1995). Therefore, freeze substitution following aldehyde-prefixation, is regarded as a reliable method to produce ultrastructural images closer to what occurs in the living state, rather than conventional electron microscopy.

Apposed plasma membranes of adjacent chief and sustentacular cells are separated in large areas by an intercellular space of 15–20 nm (Figs 1, 2, 3). However, careful examination of the plasma membranes at higher magnification showed that every chief cell

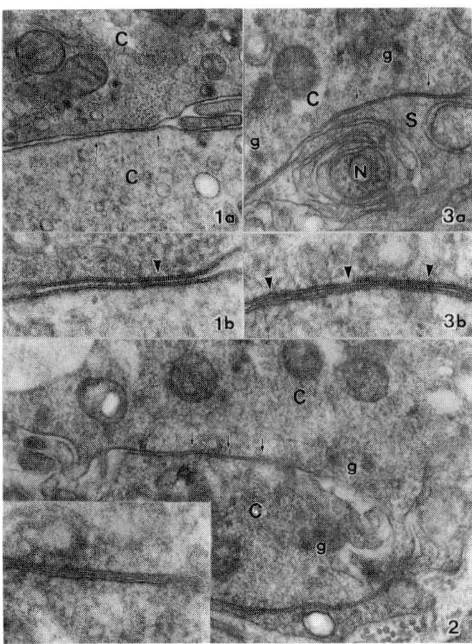

Figure 1. a. Simple apposition between two adjacent chief cells (C). X: 46,000. **b.** A portion of the apposition marked with arrows at higher magnification. Note a distinct intercellular space of about 20 nm between apposed membranes (arrowhead). X: 150,000.

Figure 2. Presumed gap junction between two adjacent chief cells (C) characterized by granular vesicles (g). Inset shows a portion of the junction marked with arrows at higher magnification. Note a uniform gap of 2 nm, a thickness similar to one leaflet of the membrane, resulting in appearance of evenly seven-lamination of the apposed membranes. X: 46,000; 150,000 (inset).

Figure 3. a. Presumed gap junction between a chief cell (C) containing granular vesicles (g) and a sustentacular cell (S) enclosing a thin axon (N). **b.** Portion of the junction at higher magnification. Note a seven-lamination of the apposed membranes. X: 46,000 (a); 150,000 (b).

contained sites of close membrane appositions. These appositions did not occur infrequently: one to four sites in a section area of 60,000 μm^2, which is reported to contain about 20 sensory synapses (Kondo, 1976). Such close apposition sites were variable in size, ranging from 200 nm to 1 µm. Some of them had uniform intercellular spaces of 4 to 5 nm, whereas in others uniform intercellular spaces of 2 nm were found (Figs 1, 2). Since each leaflet of the trilaminar plasma membrane is approximately 2 nm in thickness, the appositions appeared as even seven-lamination structures. Most of the seven-laminated appositions were seen not only between chief cells, but also between chief and sustentacular cells, although the latter were smaller and occurred less frequently (Fig 3). Furthermore, close appositions with seven-laminations were occasionally found between chief cells and carotid nerve terminals (Fig 4). These were small, 150 to 200 nm in length, and appeared next to the sensory synaptic junctions which are characterized by accumulation of granular vesicles inside the cells.

In addition, tight junctions were also found between chief and sustentacular cells and between sustentacular cells. They were small (100 nm in size) and appeared as a five-lamination structure (Fig 5). Tight junctions occurred with a frequency of 5–10 in a section area of 60,000 μm^2.

Concerning adhering junctions, associated with cytoplasmic dense materials including the synaptic junctions, their ultrastructure and frequency of occurrence were not dif-

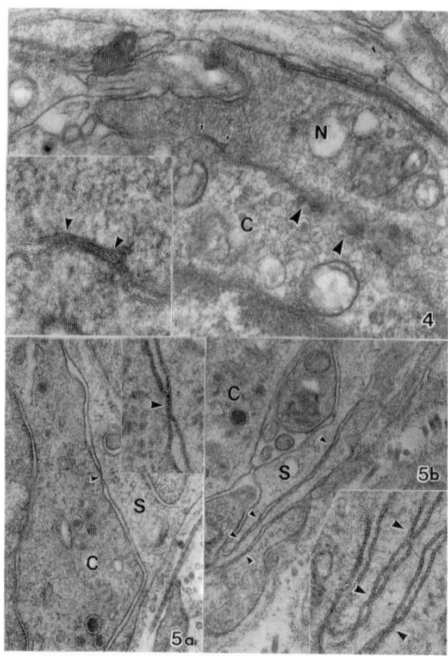

Figure 4. Presumed gap junction (arrows) between a chief cell (C) and a nerve terminal (N). The junction and sensory or afferent synapses (large arrowheads), characterized by accumulation of granular vesicles inside the chief cell, are located next to each other. Inset shows the gap junction (small arrowheads) at higher magnification. X: 46,000; 150,000 (inset).

Figure 5. Small tight junctions (arrowheads) between **(a)** a chief cell (C) and a sustentacular cell (S) and **(b)** between sustentacular cells. Inset, junction at higher magnification. A five-lamination of the junction is evident. X: 46,000; 180,000 (inset).

ferent from what has been previously published (Kondo, 1971; McDonald & Mitchell, 1975; Fidone & González, 1986), and no details are presented here.

5. DISCUSSION

This is the first report describing seven-laminated membrane appositions of substantial length and frequency between carotid body chief cells. According to a previous study (McDonald, 1981), the only one clearly describing the presence of close membrane appositions between chief cells, these occurred very infrequently (about two or three junctions per 100 chief cells) in single sections.

Several explanations are possible for this discrepancy in occurrence frequency. One, and plausible explanation, is due to differences in specimen preparation, that is, freeze-substitution *vs.* conventional fixation. As seen in the present study using freeze-substitution, the basement membrane of renal glomeruli appeared as a uniform lamina without laminae lucidae whether we employed direct rapid-freezing or aldehyde-prefixation. By contrast and using the conventional electron microscope, one sees three laminae —a lamina densa sandwitched by two laminae lucidae. This suggests that conventional specimen preparation for electron microscopy, especially fixation by OsO_4 and ethanol dehydration at above 0°C, may produce images inconsistent with what occurs in the living cell. This interpretation could be applied to the intercellular spaces and close appositions in living cells that may have been split more widely when using conventional fixation for electron microscopy. Alternatively, the possibility exists that freezing, through ice-crystal formation and invisible in the specimens, might make two apposed membranes with 15–20 nm gaps to appear much closer than what happens in the living cells. Thus, it is necessary to re-examine the intercellular spaces in various tissues by freeze-substitution and compared them with conventionally prepared specimens.

Considering their substantial length along the surface of chief cells and their frequency of occurrence, the seven-laminated membrane appositions could act as gap junctions mediating electrical and dye coupling between chief cells, as shown by Eyzaguirre and his group (Baron & Eyzaguirre, 1977; Monti-Bloch et al, 1993; Abudara & Eyzaguirre, 1994). To confirm this possibility, it is crucial to find the characteristic gap junction clusters of intramembranous protein particles by freeze-fracture, and to demonstrate the presence and chemical identity of connexons by immunohistochemistry and molecular biotechnology. Previous freeze-fracture studies failed to detect such clusters of membrane particles (Kondo, 1981, 1993).

With regard to connexons, each one having six connexins subunits, several connexin molecules have been identified in other cells. Connexins 26, 32 and 43 are well known. C-26 predominates in liver cells, C-32 in neurons, and C-43 in cardiac muscle cells (Dermietzel & Spray, 1993). Immunohistochemical identification of C-26 and C-43 in the carotid body has not been successful in our preliminary study. Identification of C-32 has not been tried. It is also possible that new, yet unidentified connexin molecules comprise the connexons in the carotid body.

If the seven-laminated membrane appositions are the true gap junctions in the carotid body, the present findings suggest that adjacent chief cells can be electrically coupled. Furthermore, coupling may also involve multiple chief cells with surrounding sustentacular cells through gap junctions. This suggestion leads us to think that a certain number of chief and sustentacular cells form a functional unit and that multiple units of such cellular compositions comprise the carotid body. This idea has already been proposed by our previous study in which thin and wide sheaths of perineurial cells were shown to enclose individual cellular units, though incompletely (Kondo, 1993).

The detection of seven-laminated junctions next to sensory synapses implies the involvement of electrical as well as chemical transmission between chief cells and carotid nerves. Since chemicals released from the chief cells affect the chemosensory discharge (Fidone & González, 1986), the responsiveness of the chemoreceptors to physiological stimuli is expected to be affected by selective antagonists of the released chemicals. However, the available evidence has been conflicting (McQueen & Evrard, 1990). These conflicting findings may be explained by the presence of gap junctions between carotid nerves and chief cells.

6. REFERENCES

Abudara V & Eyzaguirre C (1994) Electrical coupling between cultured glomus cells of the rat carotid body: Observations with current and voltage clamping. Brain Res 664: 257–265

Baron M & Eyzaguirre C (1977) Effects of temperature on some membrane characteristics of carotid body cells. Am J Physiol 233: C35-C46

Chan FL, Inoue S & Leblond CP (1983) The basement membranes of cryofixed, freeze substituted tissues are composed of a lamina densa with no lamina lucida. Cell Tiss Res 273: 41–52

Dermietzel R & Spray DC (1993) Gap junctions in the brain: where, what type, how many and why? Trends Neurosci 16: 186–192

Fidone SJ & González C (1986) Initiation and control of chemoreceptor activity in the carotid body. In: Handbook of Physiology, sect 3: The Respiratory System, vol II: Control of Breathing (Cherniack NS & Widdicombe JG, eds). Bethesda, MD: American Physiological Society. pp 247–312

Kondo H (1971) An electron microscopic study on innervation of the carotid body of guinea pig. J Ultrastr Res 37: 544–562

Kondo H (1976) An electron microscopic study on the development of synapses in the rat carotid body. Neurosci Lett 3: 197–200

Kondo H (1981) Evidence for the secretion of chief cells in the carotid body. In: Belmonte C, Pallot, DJ, Acker H & Fidone S (eds) Arterial Chemoreceptors. Leicester: Leicester Univ Press. pp 45–53

Kondo H & Yamamoto M (1993) Multi-unit compartmentation of the carotid body chemoreceptor by perineurial cell sheaths: Immunohistochemistry and freeze-fracture study. Adv Exp Med Biol 337: 61–66

Kondo H (1995) On the trilaminar structure of the basal membrane of the renal glomerulus. Acta Anat Nippon 70: 502

McDonald DM (1981) Peripheral chemoreceptors: structure-function relationships of the carotid body. In: Lung Biology in Health and Disease, vol 17: Regulation of Breathing (Hornbein TF, ed). New York: Marcel Dekker. pp 105–320

McDonald DM & Mitchell RA (1975) The innervation of glomus cells, ganglion cells and blood vessels in the rat carotid body: a quantitative ultrastructural analysis. J Neurocytol 4: 177–230

McQueen DS & Evrard Y (1990) Use of selective antagonists for studying the role of putative transmitters in chemoreception. In: Eyzaguirre C, Fidone SJ, Fitzgerald RS, Lahiri S & McDonald DM (eds) Arterial Chemoreception. New York: Springer-Verlag. pp 186–194

Monti-Bloch L, Abudara V & Eyzaguirre C (1993) Electrical communication between glomus cells of the rat carotid body. Brain Res 622: 119–131

5

TWO MORPHOLOGICAL TYPES OF CHEMORECEPTOR AFFERENTS INNERVATE THE RABBIT CAROTID BODY

Fernando Torrealba

Departamento de Ciencias Fisiológicas
Facultad de Ciencias Biológicas
Pontificia Universidad Católica de Chile
Santiago, Chile
Department of Anatomy
University of Leicester
Leicester, United Kingdom

1. INTRODUCTION

Electrophysiological (Fidone & Sato, 1969; Donoghue et al, 1984) and morphological (Torrealba & Alcayaga, 1986) studies have shown that both A- (myelinated) and C- (unmyelinated) afferent fibers from the carotid nerve, innervate the carotid body of the cat. To elucidate whether the existence of two classes of chemoreceptors is of a more general validity, I decided to study in rabbits the structure of the terminal arborization, within the carotid body, of axons forming the carotid nerve, so as to compare these axonal patterns to those already described in cats (Torrealba & Alcayaga, 1986). To this end, I labeled a small number of carotid nerve axons, by way of the intra axonal diffusion of horseradish peroxidase (HRP). This technique allows the complete tracing of axons or neuronal cell bodies, in a Golgi stain-like fashion, up to 3 or 4 mm from the injection site.

2. METHODS

Four adult white New Zealand rabbits received intramuscular injections of ketamine (15 mg/kg) to allow endotracheal intubation and halothane anesthesia. Surgery was done under sterile conditions on animals in supine position. A midline neck incision permitted bilateral access to the carotid bifurcation. The carotid nerves were exposed and HRP crystals pushed into a nerve filament with the help of fine forceps. The animals recovered from the anesthesia, and after 20 h were anesthetized with pentobarbital (50 mg/kg) and perfused through the abdominal aorta with 2% paraformaldehyde, 2% glutaraldehyde in

Frontiers in Arterial Chemoreception, edited by Zapata *et al.*
Plenum Press, New York, 1996

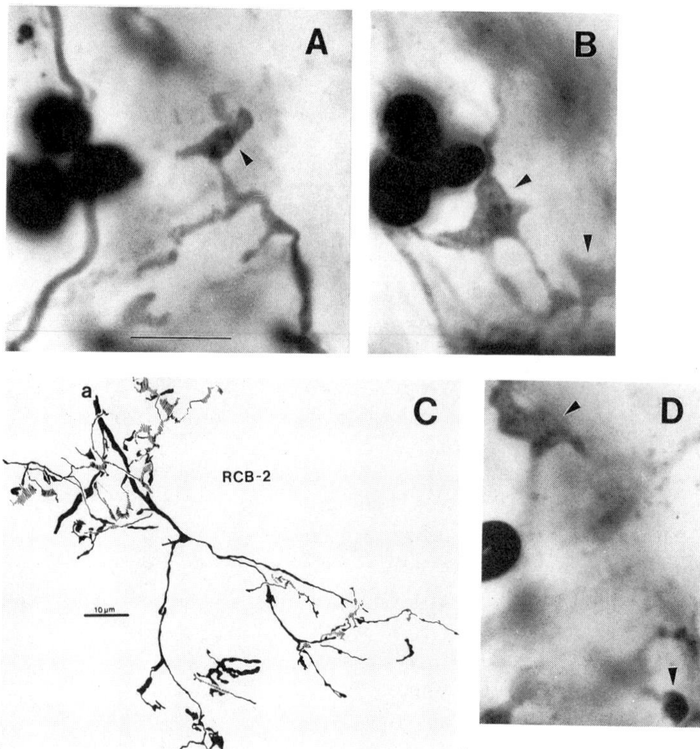

Figure 1. Terminal arborizations from two myelinated afferents into the rabbit carotid body. *In vivo* axonal labeling with HRP. **A, B & D**. Through focus series of the same cluster of terminals (indicated by arrowheads). Three red blood cells serve as landmark. **C**. Camera lucida drawing of a typical myelinated chemoreceptor afferent, having three clusters of terminals. The axon is indicated by the (a). Bars, 10 μm.

0.1 M phosphate buffer, pH 7.3, at room temperature. The carotid bodies were removed, embedded in agar and cut with a Vibratome into 80 μm sections. The sections, cut in a plane parallel to that of the carotid arteries, were processed with 0.05% diaminobenzidine, 0.02% cobalt chloride and 0.01% hydrogen peroxide in 0.1 M phosphate buffer for 20 min. The sections were counterstained with cresyl violet, mounted on subbed slides, dehydrated and coverslipped with Permount.

3. RESULTS

Several bundles of HRP labeled axons could be seen entering the carotid body from the neural pole. A variable number of terminal arborizations were present throughout the carotid body parenchyma. The most prominent type of axonal arborization (Fig 1) consisted of a relatively thick axon that gave off one to three clusters of large and small swellings embedded within a glomoid. Each of the sets of terminals stemming from these thick afferents formed a three dimensional domain having the size and shape of a single glomoid (Fig 1 A, B, D). The largest terminals present in these clusters corresponded to the classic calyces (arrowheads in Fig 1A, B) that wrap around individual glomus cells (Nishi & Stensaas, 1974), but also smaller boutons were present in these arborizations.

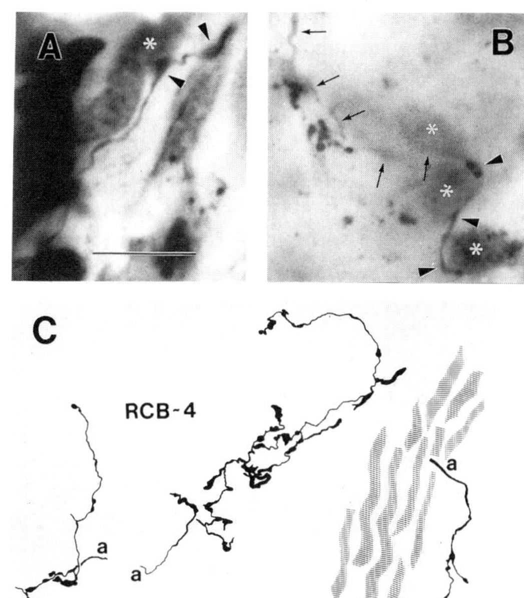

Figure 2. Terminal arborizations from five unmyelinated afferents to the rabbit carotid body. *In vivo* axonal labeling with HRP. **A** & **B**. Photomicrographs of two axons (arrows in B) and their boutons (arrowheads) in the vicinity of glomus cells (asterisks). **C**. Three terminal arborizations stemming from thin, unmyelinated axons (a). The axon at the right emerges from a bundle of labeled fibers (hatched) within the carotid body. Magnifications as in Figure 1.

The second type of axonal arborization was less visible, and consisted of very thin axons having mainly small *en passant* and terminal swellings (Fig 2). The number of axonal swellings of a single unmyelinated, sparsely branched afferent was much lower (see Fig 2C) than the number of swellings and calyces arising from one myelinated afferent (see Fig 1C).

4. DISCUSSION

It is well established that the carotid nerve of carnivores, and rodents contains myelinated and unmyelinated chemoreceptor axons (Kondo & Yamamoto, 1988; Kummer et al, 1989; Torrealba, 1992) that innervate the carotid body. Also in the rabbit carotid body one can find myelinated and unmyelinated axons (Verna, 1979), though it has not been shown if both types originate from the carotid nerve. However, only in cats electrophysiological studies have been conducted to characterize the physiological properties of the A- and C-fiber chemoreceptors. Fidone & Sato (1969) found that chemoreceptor A-fibers have lower thresholds, shorter response latencies, more rapid acceleration of discharge and higher discharge rates than chemoreceptor C-fibers. We have proposed that the response properties that distinguish A- and C-fiber chemoreceptors can be explained by the much larger terminal arborization, and the more numerous swellings of A-fibers within the carotid body (Torrealba & Alcayaga, 1986), as well as by the fact that C-fibers do not directly contact glomus cells (Torrealba & Correa, 1995). On the other hand, there are indications that the central projections of A- and C-fibers differ. The thinner axons from the glossopharyngeal nerve, originating from the smaller petrosal ganglion cells project bilaterally to the medial regions (Claps et al, 1989) of the nucleus of the solitary tract (NTS). In agreement with this general pattern, C-fiber chemoreceptors terminate in the medial NTS (Donoghue et al, 1984). In contrast, the thicker glossopharyngeal nerve axons project ipsilaterally to the lateral regions of the NTS (Claps et al, 1989). Since lateral and medial NTS subnuclei have different patterns of connections within the central nervous system (Loewy & Burton 1978; Ricardo & Koh, 1978), it is likely that chemoreceptor A- and C-fibers participate in different central circuits involved in autonomic regulation.

The present findings in the rabbit concerning the existence of two morphological classes of terminal arborizations from carotid nerve axons, suggest that the two types of chemoreceptor fibers found in the cat, and described using several experimental approaches, may also be present in lagomorphs. Further studies, in particular those emphasizing the physiological and innervating properties of A- and C-fibers are needed to test the validity of this classification.

5. ACKNOWLEDGMENTS

I thank Dr David Pallot for the use of his facilities at the Department of Anatomy, University of Leicester.

Financed by grant 1940652 from FONDECYT (National Fund for Scientific and Technological Development, Chile).

6. REFERENCES

Claps A, Calderón F & Torrealba F (1989) Segregation of coarse and fine glossopharyngeal axons in the visceral nucleus of the tractus solitarius of the cat. Brain Res 489: 80–92

Donoghue S, Felder RB, Jordan D & Spyer KM (1984) The central projections of baroreceptors and chemoreceptors in the cat: a neurophysiological study. J Physiol, London 347: 397–409

Fidone SJ & Sato A (1969) A study of chemoreceptor and baroreceptor A and C-fibres in the cat carotid nerve. J Physiol, London 205: 527–548

Kondo H & Yamamoto M (1988) Occurrence, ontogeny, ultrastructure and some plasticity of CGRP (calcitonin gene-related peptide)- immunoreactive nerves in the carotid body of rats. Brain Res 473: 283–293

Kummer W, Fischer A & Heym C (1989) Ultrastructure of calcitonin gene-related peptide- and substance P-like immunoreactive nerve fibres in the carotid body and carotid sinus of the Guinea pig. Histochemistry 92: 433–439

Loewy AD & Burton H (1978) Nuclei of the solitary tract: efferent projections to the lower brain stem and spinal cord of the cat. J Comp Neurol 421–450

Nishi K & Stensaas LJ (1974) The ultrastructure and source of nerve endings in the carotid body. Cell Tiss Res 154: 303–319

Ricardo JA & Koh ET (1978) Anatomical evidence of direct projections from the nucleus of the solitary tract to the hypothalamus, amygdala and other forebrain structures. Brain Res 153: 1–26

Torrealba F (1992) Calcitonin gene-related peptide immunoreactivity in the nucleus of the tractus solitarius and the carotid receptors originates from peripheral afferents. Neuroscience 47: 165–173

Torrealba F & Alcayaga J (1986) Nerve branching and terminal arborizations in the carotid body of the cat. A light microscopic study following anterograde injury filling of carotid nerve axons with horseradish peroxidase. Neuroscience 19: 581–595

Torrealba F & Correa R (1995) Ultrastructure of calcitonin gene-related peptide-immunoreactive, unmyelinated afferents to the cat carotid body: a case of volume transmission. Neuroscience 64: 777–785

Verna A (1979) Ultrastructure of the carotid body in mammals. Intl Rev Cytol 60: 271–330

6

MITOCHONDRIAL DIVISION, BLOOD VESSEL DILATION, AND LARGE INTERCELLULAR SPACE EXPANSION OF GOAT CAROTID BODY DURING HYPOXIA

Dahai Xue, Ingegerd M. Keith, Melinda R. Dwinell, and Gerald E. Bisgard

Department of Comparative Biosciences
University of Wisconsin
Madison, Wisconsin 53706

1. INTRODUCTION

The increased sensitivity of the carotid bodies (CB) of different animals and humans to hypoxia is a well documented mechanism contributing to ventilatory acclimatization to hypoxia. The goat CB is special in that it increases its sensitivity to hypoxia in merely 4 h (Bisgard, 1994), which is compared with that of the rat, cat or humans which need longer periods of hypoxia to reach the peak of their increased sensitivity to hypoxia. The underlying mechanisms accounting for increased CB sensitivity to hypoxia is unknown. The objectives of this study were to define the morphology of the goat CB and to determine if structural changes could be detected associated with a change in the hypoxic sensitivity of the goat CB.

2. MATERIALS AND METHODS

The animals were initially anesthetized with pentothal sodium (15–20 mg/kg, iv), followed by slow infusion of chloralose at the rate of 25–100 mg/kg/h to maintain a surgical plane of anesthesia. Tracheal cannulation was used and the animals were artificially ventilated for 4 h. A cannula was placed in the femoral artery for the monitoring of blood pressure and sampling for blood gases. A femoral vein was cannulated for the infusion of sodium bicarbonate solution if needed to maintain acid-base balance. Heparin was infused iv prior to the removal of the carotid bifurcation to prevent clotting and facilitate the flush of the CB and perfusion fixation in later steps. The blood gas, acid-base balance and blood pressure were monitored frequently. After the cannulation, the operation for exposing the carotid bifurcation and the carotid sinus nerves generally was carried out while maintaining arterial blood gases according to the following protocols.

Frontiers in Arterial Chemoreception, edited by Zapata *et al.*
Plenum Press, New York, 1996

Fifteen mixed-bred goats were randomly divided into three groups: (1) Control (n = 5): The blood gas of the animals was kept at normoxic level (PaO_2 = 100 Torr, $PaCO_2$ Torr) for the 4 h; (2) short term hypoxia (n = 5): The blood gas was first kept at normoxic level as above and at the last 30 min prior to the removal of the carotid bifurcation, the PaO_2 was lowered to the hypoxic level of 40 Torr with the $PaCO_2$ kept at 40 Torr; (3) long term hypoxia (n = 5): The blood gas was kept at the above hypoxic level throughout the 4 h period.

The carotid arteries were reached via a midline ventral cervical incision and the carotid bifurcation areas were exposed and dissected in order to locate the CB. The animals were given heparin (10,000 units iv) to prevent clotting. A cannula was put into the common carotid artery with the opening towards the carotid bifurcation. Other carotid artery branches were then tied off, and 200 ml heparinized saline was injected through the cannulation to flush the CB which still had the outlet via occipital artery. The occipital artery was then clamped, and the vascular bifurcation and sinus nerve were rapidly excised and placed in cold saline. The bifurcation was then flushed with 500 ml cold (4° C) saline at the pressure of 120 mm Hg, and then perfused at the same pressure with 300 ml cold Bouin's fixative for one of the CBs and Karnovsky's fixative for the other. There was a 3–5 min lapse between the termination of the blood flow and the induction of the fixatives to the CB. The CBs were immediately dissected out and immersed in the same fixative for two hours at 4° C, and then moved to 0.1 M phosphate buffer saline pH 7.4 with 0.05 M sucrose at 4° C overnight.

The CB fixed in Bouin's fixative was embedded in paraffin. Serial sections of 5 μm were cut throughout the CB, every 20th section was mounted on poly L-lysine coated slides, and stained with hematoxylin and eosin. This preparation was for general observations and the measurement of the total CB volume. The CB fixed in Karnovsky's fixative was post fixed with OsO_4 and embedded in Araldite resin. 0.5 μm semi-thin sections were cut and stained with toluidine blue. This preparation was for light microscopical (LM) quantitation of blood vessels (BV) and the large intercellular spaces (LICS). The quantitation under LM was performed on randomized microimages at a total of 1,000 x magnification with Gundersen's square lattice test grid superimposed on the image, and the grid was calibrated with a stage micrometer. Sixty nm thick sections were cut and stained with uranyl acetate and lead citrate, observed under electron microscope (EM), and quantitation of mitochondria was done on enlarged micrographs (72,000 x final magnification) with superimposed grid calibrated with a carbon replica of 2160 lines per mm.

The stereological method applied was summarized by Weibel et al (1969, 1979), and modified for the study of CB (Xue et al, 1991, 1992). Point counting was carried out using the Gundersen's square lattice test grid (Gundersen et al, 1988a,b) using randomized sampling. Student's *t* test was used for statistical analysis, with Cochran's formula for calculation of the standard deviation for the estimation of a ratio (Cochran, 1977). $P \leq 0.05$ was considered significant.

3. RESULTS

The general architecture of the goat CB was similar to that found previously (Heath et al, 1989a,b) except that the goat CB parenchyma was embedded in thick layers of dense connective tissue. Like the CBs of other animals, there were abundant BV in the goat CB and mitochondria in their type I cell cytoplasm. A finding apparently unique to the goat was that LICS were found in all CBs studied, among type-I cells and between type-I cells and other structures such as type II cells, nerve endings, or endothelial cells. The LICS were irregular shaped intercellular spaces mostly having the diameter of 1–20 μm, compared with 10–20 nm intercellular spaces usually found at the place. They were walled by the plasma membrane of the structures around it. There were active exocytoses from the type I cells to the LICS. The matrix of the LICS was relatively electron dense, and sometimes contained deteriorating membrane structures resembling exocytotic vesicles.

The total volume of the goat CB ranged from 0.26 to 1.06 mm^3, with the mean of 0.64 ± 0.04 mm^3 taking account of all three groups. There was no significant difference detected between the 3 groups. Data with various treatments are presented in Table 1.

Hypoxia (both 30 min and 4 h) increased percentage volume of BV in the parenchyma as well as the total volume of BV in each CB. The increased vessel volume was due to dilation since there was no significant increase of wall area and the ratio of BV's wall surface area to its volume decreased accordingly. LICS doubled their percentage volume in the parenchyma and in the type I and type II cell clusters, as well as their total volume in each CB, starting at 30 min hypoxia. The number of mitochondria in each type I cells ranged from 82 to 379 in the control group. The average number of mitochondria in each type I cell and the total number in each CB increased in the first 30 min of hypoxia and significantly increased further after 4 h of hypoxia. Meanwhile the average volume of individual mitochondria in type-I cells decreased after 30 min hypoxia and remained at the low level after 4 h of hypoxia. These data suggest that mitochondria underwent division during hypoxia which may be time-dependent. The total volume of mitochondria in a CB remained constant suggesting the lack of accumulation of substances for mitochondrial construction in the short time period. The surface/volume ratio of the mitochondria did not change after hypoxia suggesting that the mitochondria did not significantly change their shape.

4. DISCUSSION

The change of BV may be related to the dilation of arterioles which could increase the blood flow. The carotid body has complex vasculature and huge blood flow in the normoxic condition (MacDonald, 1989; Clarke et al, 1986; Hilman et at, 1987). It is consid-

Table 1. Quantitative changes in goat carotid bodies after hypoxia exposure (means ± SEM's)

	Control	30 min hypoxia	4 h hypoxia
BV % volume (in the parenchyma)	15.6 ± 1.0	20.5 ± 1.0*	19.2 ± 1.4*
BV total volume (mm^3/CB)	0.039 ± 0.002	0.069 ± 0.001*	0.060 ± 0.003*
BV surface volume ratio ($\mu m^2/\mu m^3$)	0.80 ± 0.06	0.59 ± 0.02*	0.54 ± 0.03*
LICS % volume (in parenchyma)	5.55 ± 0.72	8.41 ± 0.89*	8.65 ± 0.74*
LICS % volume (in cell clusters)	13.69 ± 1.31	24.47 ± 1.84*	25.97 ± 1.66*
LICS total volume in each CB (mm^3/CB)	0.0346 ± 0.003	0.0821 ± 0.002*	0.0813 ± 0.004*
MIT % volume (in the cytoplasm)	9.9 ± 0.3	9.7 ± 0.6	10.9 ± 0.3
MIT number per type I cell	283.0 ± 39.2	446.8 ± 21.6*	546.2 ± 51.0**
MIT total number (million/CB)	38.6 ± 5.4	71.9 ± 8.1*	95.8 ± 6.9**
MIT average volume (mm^3)	0.13 ± 0.010	0.07 ± 0.002*	0.06 ± 0.003*
MIT surface volume ratio ($\mu m^2/\mu m^3$)	14.8 ± 0.28	15.7 ± 0.69	15.5 ± 0.21

* $P < 0.05$ *vs* control group.
** $P < 0.05$ *vs* both control and 30 min hypoxia groups.
BV: blood vessels; LICS: large intercellular spaces; MIT: mitochondria.

ered that this is closely related to the chemoreception function (Sherpa et al, 1989) although another viewpoint suggested that the dilation of the blood vessels was a non-specific reaction to hypoxia (Laidler et al, 1975a,b). The division of the mitochondria may be associated with an increased oxygen consumption, but it may also be related to the increased sensitivity of CB to hypoxia, since mitochondria are one of the candidates for the place where O_2 sensing molecules reside (Mills & Jobsis, 1972; Wilson et al, 1994). LICS appear to be real structures on the basis of finding no evidence of cell degeneration, or edema. However, the possibility that they may be some artifact of tissue handling cannot be completely ruled out. Assuming these are real structures, the expansion of LICS may be as a storage pool for the endocrine functions of the type I cells, and may also be related to CB function after hypoxic challenge.

5. REFERENCES

Bisgard GE (1994) The role of arterial chemoreceptors in ventilatory acclimatization to hypoxia. Adv Exp Biol Med 360: 109–122

Clarke JA, de Burgh-Daly M & Ead HW (1986) Dimensions and volume of the carotid body in the adult cat, and their relation to the specific blood flow through the organ. A histological and morphometric study. Acta Anat 126: 84–86

Cochran WG (1977) Sampling Techniques. New York: John Wiley & Sons. p 33

Gundersen HJ, Bagger P, Bendtsen TF, Evans SM, Korbo L, Marcussen N, Moller A, Nielsen K, Nyengaard JR & Pakkenberg B (1988a) The new stereological tools: Dissector, fractionator, nucleator and point sampled intercepts and their use in pathological research and diagnosis. Acta Pathol Microbiol Immunol Scand 96: 857–881

Gundersen HJ, Bendtsen TF, Korbo L, Marcussen N, Moller A, Nielsen K, Nyengaard JR, Pakkenberg B, Sorensen FBM & Vesterby A (1988b) Some new, simple and efficient stereological methods and their use in pathological research and diagnosis. Acta Pathol Microbiol Immunol Scand 96: 379–394

Heath D & Williams DR (1989a) High Altitude Medicine and Pathology. London: Butterworth. pp 74–87

Heath D & Williams DR (1989b) High Altitude Medicine and Pathology. London: Butterworth. pp 223–231

Hilsman J, Degner F & Acker H (1987) Local flow velocities in the cat carotid body tissue. Eur J Physiol 410: 204–211

Laidler P & Kay JM (1975a) The effect of chronic hypoxia on the number and nuclear diameter of type I cells in the carotid bodies of rats. Am J Pathol 79: 311–320

Laidler P & Kay JM (1975b) A quantitative morphological study of the carotid bodies of rats living at a simulated altitude of 4,300 metres. J Pathol 117: 183–191

MacDonald DM (1989) Routes for blood flow through the rat carotid body. In: Lahiri S, Forster RE, Davies RO & Pack AI (eds) Chemoreceptors and Reflexes in Breathing - Cellular and Molecular Aspects. New York: Oxford Univ Press. pp 5–12

Mills E & Jobsis FF (1972) Mitochondrial respiratory chain of carotid body and chemoreceptor to changes in oxygen tension. J Neurophysiol 35: 405–428

Sherpa AK, Albertine KH, Denney DG, Thompkins B & Lahiri S (1989) Chronic CO exposure stimulates erythropoiesis but not glomus cell growth. J Appl Physiol 67: 1383–1387

Weibel ER (1969) Stereological principles for morphometry in electron microscopic cytology. Intl Rev Cytol 26: 235–302

Weibel ER (1979) Stereological methods. Vol 1. Practical Methods for Biological Morphometry. London: Academic Press

Wilson DF, Mokashi A, Chugh D, Vinogradov S, Osanai S, Lahiri S (1994) The primary oxygen sensor of the cat carotid body is cytochrome a_3 of the mitochondrial respiratory chain. FEBS Lett 351: 370–4

Xue DH (1992) Morphometry application to the study of the carotid body. Acta Academiae Medicinae Qinghai (China) 13: 148–153

Xue DH, Yang FX (1991) A simple correction in calculating the numerical density of particles. In: Proc Symp of Anatomy Assoc Chinese Northwest Region (Yinchuan, China). p 86

7

PO_2 AFFINITIES, HEME PROTEINS, AND REACTIVE OXYGEN INTERMEDIATES INVOLVED IN INTRACELLULAR SIGNAL CASCADES FOR SENSING OXYGEN

Helmut Acker

Max Planck Institut für molekulare Physiologie
44139 Dortmund, Germany

1. SUMMARY

The oxygen partial pressure field in different organs ranging from 0 to 100 Torr is likely to be a mirror of oxygen sensitive intracellular signal cascades determining ion channel open probability, metabolic pathway activities and gene expression. High or low PO_2 affinities of the particular signal cascade optimize the oxygen sensitive cellular response for adapting organ functions to variations of the oxygen supply conditions. The signal cascades are triggered by an oxygen sensor which is believed to be a heme protein. In some cases reactive oxygen intermediates (ROI) are acting as second messengers revealing these signal cascades as an evolutionary highly conserved principle first described in bacteria.

2. THE OXYGEN SENSITIVE RESPONSE

To assert a constant oxygen supply to different organs and herewith a constant energy supply maintaining highly specialized organ functions, cells able to sense oxygen levels in the tissue are situated at different locations in the body stimulating various reflex pathways. This oxygen sensing process comprises a sensor protein which undergoes conformational changes in dependence on oxygen and a signal cascade, which transfers the message stimulated by the sensor to ion channels, metabolic pathways or specific gene regions (for review see Acker, 1994). For the last pathway numerous examples are given in the literature like the $CoCl_2$ impedible induction of phosphoenolpyruvate carboxykinase (PCK) by glucagon in hepatocytes (Kietzmann, 1992), the regulation of the glutathione peroxidase content in cardiomyocytes (Cowan et al, 1993), the gene expression for tyrosine hydroxylase in carotid body type I - and PC12 - cells (Czyzyk-Krzeska et al, 1994),

Frontiers in Arterial Chemoreception, edited by Zapata *et al.*
Plenum Press, New York, 1996

the regulation of the bovine endothelial constitutive nitric oxide synthase (Liao et al, 1995) or the production of erythropoietin, vascular endothelial growth factor, platelet-derived growth factor A and B chains, placental growth factor and transforming growth factor in various cell lines (Gleadle et al, 1995; Goldberg et al, 1994). Metabolic pathways comprise the lactate dehydrogenase activity (Marti et al, 1994), the mitochondrial manganese-containing superoxide dismutase (MnSOD) activity of the lung (Russel et al, 1995) or the pregnenolone and aldosterone synthesis (Raff & Jankowski, 1995). Well known examples for the participation of ion channels in the oxygen sensing process are oxygen sensitive potassium channels of type I cells of the carotid body (Ureña et al, 1994), of cells of neuroepithelial bodies in the lung (Youngson et al, 1993), of smooth muscle cells of the lung vasculature (Weir et al, 1995) or of central neurons (Jiang & Haddad, 1994). Oxygen sensitive calcium channels are described for peripheral vascular smooth muscles (Franco-Obregón et al, 1995) as well as for rabbit carotid body type I cells (Montoro et al, 1996).

3. PO_2 AFFINITIES

The oxygen level in the tissue of different organs is determined by the oxygen partial pressure and the O_2 transport capacity of the blood as well as by the vascular structure, blood flow, oxygen consumption and diffusion conditions of each particular organ. Characteristically the different organs have a frequency distribution of oxygen partial pressure values ranging from about 0 to 100 Torr with mean values between 20 and 50 Torr (Acker, 1994). While in former times the meaning of this PO_2 distribution was mainly discussed for its importance for energy supply under normoxic and hypoxic conditions, it is obvious now that the PO_2 distribution expresses the different oxygen sensitivities of the above mentioned ion channels, metabolic pathway activities and gene regions. Low as well as high PO_2 values have distinct influences. Low PO_2 is accompanied by an enhanced production of erythropoietin, vascular endothelial growth factor platelet-derived growth factor A and B chains, placental growth factor and transforming growth factor (Gleadle et al, 1995, Goldberg et al, 1994), or tyrosine hydroxylase (TH) (Czyzyk-Krzeska et al, 1994) peaking between 1% and 3% O_2 whereas high PO_2 incites a higher production of glutathione peroxidase (Cowan et al, 1993) or of phosphoenolpyruvate carboxykinase (Kietzmann et al, 1992) and an enhanced activity of the endothelial constitutive nitric oxide synthase (Lioa et al, 1995). Lactate dehydrogenase activity is increased (Marti et al, 1994) whereas MnSOD activity is decreased under low oxygen levels (Russel et al, 1995). In contrast pregnenolone and aldosterone synthesis is enhanced under high oxygen levels (Raff & Jankowski, 1995). The potassium channels decrease their open probability under hypoxia leading to membrane potential depolarisation and opening of voltage sensitive calcium channels with a subsequent increase of the intracellular calcium level inducing neurotransmitter release (Ureña et al, 1994, Youngson et al, 1993) or smooth muscle contraction (Weir et al, 1995). For the carotid body two different PO_2 affinities are described: the 40 pS potassium channel of rabbit carotid body type I cells closing at PO_2 values of about 80 Torr (López-Barneo, 1993) and the 240 pS potassium channel of the rat carotid body starting to get inhibited at PO_2 values below 20 Torr (Wyatt et al, 1995). Central neurons silence under hypoxia mediated by the oxygen sensitive potassium channel (Jiang & Haddad, 1994). The calcium channels decrease their open probability under low oxygen levels, too, leading to peripheral vasodilatation under hypoxia due to an impaired calcium influx (Franco-Obregón et al, 1995). The average hypoxic inhibition of the calcium current of the rabbit carotid body type I cells is 30% at a membrane potential of -20 mV but only 2% at +30 mV. The differential inhibition of potassium and calcium channels of this cell type leads under exposure to low PO_2 to a rise of the cytosolic calcium with two distinguishable peaks: an initial period at PO_2 values between 150 and 70 Torr during which the increase of cytosolic calcium is very small and a second phase with PO_2 values below 70 Torr, characterized by a sharp rise of the calcium level accompanied by transmitter release (Montoro et al, 1996). The described ion channels, metabolic pathways and gene expressions with their different PO_2 affinities reveal the PO_2 frequency distribution as a trigger field for various cellular activities either to optimize living conditions or to protect against hypoxic and hyperoxic damages.

4. Heme Proteins and Reactive Oxygen Intermediates

Whereas the oxygen responsive elements of the genes encoding the different proteins have been partly identified (Cowan et al, 1993; Gleadle et al, 1995; Goldberg et al, 1994), the nature of the oxygen sensing protein influencing ion channel activity, metabolic pathway activities and gene expression is still unclear in mammalian cells. However, studies on bacteria could describe signal cascades influencing gene expression under hypoxic as well as hyperoxic conditions. Activation of the nitrogen fixation gene in *Rhizobium meliloti* under hypoxia is mediated by a cell membrane located heme-based sensor which phosphorylates a transcription factor for facilitating its DNA binding (Gilles-González & González, 1993). *Escherichia coli* contains the SoxR protein which, activated by oxidative stress like hyperoxia through a variable redox state of its FeS cluster, induces transcription of the SoxS gene, which in turn increases expression of defensive genes such as Mn-containing superoxide dismutase (Hidalgo & Demple, 1994). The involvement of a heme-type PO_2 sensor protein has been suggested for explaining the molecular mechanism of the inhibitory effect of low PO_2 on potassium-channel conductivity of carotid body, neuroepithelial bodies and smooth musculature of lung vasculature (Acker 1994; Youngson et al, 1993; Weir et al 1995). Cross et al (1990) as well as Acker & Xue (1995) carried out a detailed photometric analysis of the rat carotid body to gain more information about heme protein characteristics in this tissue. They detected beside typical absorption peaks of the different cytochromes of the respiratory chain, a measurable heme signal with absorbance maxima at 558 nm, 518 nm and 425 nm suggesting the presence of a b-type cytochrome. This was confirmed by pyridine hemochrome and CO spectra. This heme protein is capable of H_2O_2 formation and seems to possess, therefore, similarities with flavocytochrome b_{558} of the NAD(P)H oxidase in neutrophils. $p22_{phox}$, $gp91_{phox}$, $p47_{phox}$ and $p67_{phox}$ the typical components of the NAD(P)H oxidase (Bokoch, 1993) could be identified immunohistochemically in type I cells of the human, rat and guinea pig carotid body by Kummer & Acker (1995) as well as by Youngson et al (1993) in neuroepithelial bodies of the lung highlighting the probability of the involvement of an NAD(P)H oxidase or a related isoform in the cellular oxygen sensing in these cell types using ROI as second messengers. ROI comprise oxygen radicals, hydrogen peroxide, hydroxyl radicals as well as peroxynitrite, which is formed by oxygen radicals and NO (Khan & Wilson, 1995). NO which is synthesized in carotid body nerve fibers (Wang et al, 1993) might therefore mediate its inhibitory action on carotid body sensory discharge not only via cGMP (Prabhakar et al, 1993) but also by ROI effects.

Of special interest in this context are findings as published by López-López & González (1992) showing that the hypoxia induced decrease of the activity of potassium channels of type I cells can be inhibited by CO. This might be interpreted as due to CO inducing an oxidation of a heme protein which interacts with potassium channels in the cell membrane of type I cells. A hydrogen peroxide generating oxidase, which was characterized as an NADH oxidoreductase by Kamal et al (1994), seems to be involved in the control of the open probability of potassium channels in the smooth musculature of lung vessels (Weir et al, 1995). McCormack & McCormack (1994) identified the *Shaker* potassium channel ß subunits as belonging to an NAD(P)H dependent oxidoreductase superfamily which highlights a possible molecular mechanism of the oxygen sensitive potassium channels. Instead of a heme protein a nonheme iron containing protein is likely to be responsible for oxygen sensing in central neurons (Jiang & Haddad, 1994). It has been shown that hypoxia induced Epo production of HepG2 cells is mediated by a non respiratory heme protein acting as an oxygen sensor which was proposed to be similar to the NAD(P)H oxidase described above (Görlach et al, 1993). This oxidase has a declining H_2O_2 formation in HepG2 cells under hypoxia which might be due to a changed redox state of the cells promoting the binding of transcription factors to the oxygen responsive element of the Epo gene (Fandrey et al, 1994). Gleadle et al (1995a) underlined the importance of a flavoprotein oxidoreductase as an oxygen sensor by inhibiting the hypoxia induced gene expression of five genes by means of diphenylene iodonium, an inhibitor of the neutrophile NAD(P)H oxidase. According to Bastian & Hibbs (1994), this oxidase might be termed a low output form with respect to the rate of H_2O_2 production. This is in contrast to the stimulus-dependent respiratory burst-like activity of the high output oxidase in leucocyte defense mechanisms having an about 95% higher production rate than the low output form (Jones et al, 1995). The specificity of the low output form as a putative oxygen sensor is substantiated by findings of Wenger et al (1996) showing an unimpaired oxygen sensing mechanism of $p22_{phox}$ and gp91 deficient B lymphocytes of chronic granulomatous disease patients unable to generate respiratory burst activity. Instead, it is consistent with continuous enzyme activity related to continuous on-line monitoring of oxygen supply for regulating erythropoietin production. In the case of hyperoxia induced aldosterone production, the oxygen sensitive side is likely to be located in the mitochondrial aldosterone synthase enzyme complex (Raff & Jankowski, 1995). No heme-protein seems to be involved in this oxygen sensing process.

5. CONCLUSION

It might therefore be concluded that hypoxia and hyperoxia could be sensed by different mechanisms in mammalian cells as is likely to be the case in bacteria. This oxygen sensing process might be a highly conserved evolutionary principle by which organisms adapting from anaerobic to aerobic environmental conditions learned to record the availability of oxygen as well as to cope with reactive oxygen intermediates (Pahl & Baeuerle, 1994). Lack of energy or impairment of mitochondrial respiration, however, seem not to be involved in all the cases so far described of oxygen sensing, underlining the significance of the critical mitochondrial PO_2 value below 1 Torr for securing a constant energy supply in all cells located at different spots in the PO_2 field.

6. REFERENCES

Acker H (1994) Mechanisms and meaning of cellular oxygen sensing in the organism. Respir Physiol 95: 1–10

Acker H & Xue D (1995) Mechanisms of oxygen sensing in the carotid body in comparison to other oxygen sensing cells. News Physiol Sci 10: 211–217

Bastian NR, Hibbs JB Jr (1994) Assembly and regulation of NADPH oxidase and nitric oxide synthase. Curr Opin Immunol 6: 131–139

Bokoch GM (1993) Biology of the Rap proteins, members of the ras superfamily of GTP-binding proteins. Biochem J 289: 17–24

Cowan DB, Weisel RD, Williams WG & Mickle DAG (1993) Identification of oxygen responsive elements in the 5′flanking region of the human glutathion peroxidase gene. J Biol Chem 268: 26904–26910

Cross AR, Henderson L, Jones OTG, Delpiano MA, Hentschel J & Acker H (1990) Involvement of an NAD(P)H oxidase as a PO_2 sensor protein in the rat carotid body. Biochem J 272: 743–747

Czyzyk-Krzeska M, Furnari BA, Lawson EE & Millhorn DE (1994) Hypoxia increases rate of transcription and stability of tyrosine hydroxylase mRNA in pheochromocytoma (PC12) cells. J Biol Chem 7: 760–764

Fandrey J, Frede S & Jelkmann W (1994) Role of hydrogen-peroxide in hypoxia-induced erythropoietin production. Biochem J 303: 507–510

Franco-Obregón A, Ureña J & López-Barneo J (1995) Oxygen-sensitive calcium channels in vascular smooth muscle and their possible role in hypoxic arterial relaxation. Proc Natl Acad Sci USA 92: 4715–4719

Gilles-González MA & González G (1993) Regulation of the kinase activity of heme protein FixL from the two-component system FixL/FixJ of *Rhizobium meliloti*. J Biol Chem 268: 16293–16297

Gleadle JM, Ebert BL, Firth JD & Ratcliffe PJ (1995) Regulation of angiogenic growth factor expression by hypoxia, transition metals and chelating agents. Am J Physiol 268: C1362-C1368

Gleadle JM, Ebert BL & Ratcliffe PJ (1995a) Diphenylene iodonium inhibits the induction of erythropoietin and other mammalian genes by hypoxia-implications for the mechanism of oxygen sensing. Eur J Biochem 234: 92–99

Goldberg MA & Schneider ThJ (1994) Similarities between the oxygen sensing mechanisms regulating the expression of vascular endothelial growth factor and erythropoietin. J Biol Chem 269: 4355–4359

Görlach A, Holtermann G, Jellkmann W, Hancock JT, Jones SA, Jones OTG & Acker H (1993) Photometric characteristics of haem proteins in erythropoietin producing hepatoma cells (HepG2). Biochem J 290: 771–776

Hidalgo E & Demple B (1994) An iron-sulfur center essential for transcriptional activation by the redox-sensing SoxR protein. EMBO J 13: 138–146

Jiang Ch & Haddad GG (1994) A direct mechanism for sensing low oxygen levels by central neurons. Proc Natl Acad Sci USA 91: 7198–7201

Jones OTG, Jones SA & Wood JD (1995) Expression of components of the superoxide generating NAD(P)H oxidase by human leucocytes and other cells. Protoplasma 184: 79–85

Kamal M, Mohazzab H & Wolin MS (1994) Sites of superoxide anion production detected by lucigenin in calf pulmonary artery smooth muscle. Am J Physiol 267: L815-L822

Khan AU & Wilson Th (1995) Reactive oxygen species as cellular messengers. Chemistry & Biology 2: 437–445

Kietzmann Th, Schmidt H, Probst I & Jungermann K (1992) Modulation of the glucagon-dependent activation of the phosphoenolpyruvate carboxykinase gene by oxygen in rat hepatocyte cultures. FEBS Lett 311: 251–255

Kummer W & Acker H (1995) Immunohistochemical demonstration of 4 subunits of neutrophil NAD(P)H oxidase in type I cells of carotid body. J Appl Physiol 78: 1904–1909

Lioa JK, Zulueta JJ, Yu FSh, Peng HB, Cote CG & Hassoun PM (1995) Regulation of bovine endothelial constitutive nitric oxide synthase by oxygen. J Clin Invest 96: 2661–2666

López-Barneo J, Benot AR & Ureña J (1993) Oxygen sensing and the electrophysiology of arterial chemoreceptor cells. News Physiol Sci 8: 191–195

López-López JR & González C (1992) Time course of K^+ current inhibition by low oxygen in chemoreceptor cells of adult rabbit carotid body. Effects of carbon monoxide. FEBS Lett 299: 251–254

Marti HH, Jung HH, Pfeilschifter J & Bauer C (1994) Hypoxia and cobalt stimulate lactate dehydrogenase (LDH) activity in vascular smooth muscle cells. Pflügers Arch 429: 216–222

McCormack I & McCormack K (1994) *Shaker* K^+ channel ß subunits belong to an NAD(P)H-dependent oxidoreductase superfamily. Cell 79: 133–1135

Montoro RJ, Ureña J, Fernández-Chacón R, Alvarez de Toledo G & López-Barneo J (1996) Oxygen sensing by ion channels and chemotransduction in single glomus cells. J Gen Physiol 107: 133–143

Pahl HL & Baeuerle PA (1994) Oxygen and the control of gene expression. BioEssays 16: 497–502

Prabhakar NR, Kumar GK, Chang ChH, Agani FH & Haxhiu MA (1993) Nitric oxide in the sensory function of the carotid body. Brain Res 625: 16–22

Raff H & Jankowski B (1995) O_2 dependence of pregnenolone and aldosterone synthesis in mitochondria from bovine zona glomerulosa cells. J Appl Physiol 78: 1625–1628

Russel WJ, Ho YS, Parish G & Jackson RM (1995) Effects of hypoxia on MnSOD expression in mouse lung. Am J Physiol 269: L221-L226

Ureña J, Fernández-Chacón R, Benot AR, Alvarez de Toledo G & López-Barneo J (1994) Hypoxia induces voltage-dependent Ca^{2+} entry and quantal dopamine secretion in carotid body glomus cells. Proc Natl Acad Sci USA 91: 10208–10211

Wang ZZ, Bredt DS, Fidone SJ & Stensaas LJ (1993) Neurons synthesizing nitric oxide innervate the mammalian carotid body. J Comp Neurol 336: 419–432

Weir EK & Archer StL (1995) The mechanism of acute hypoxic pulmonary vasoconstriction: the tale of two channels. FASEB J 9: 183–189

Wyatt CN, Wright C, Bee D & Peers C (1995) O_2-sensitive K^+ currents in carotid body chemoreceptor cells from normoxic and chronically hypoxic rats and their roles in hypoxic chemotransduction. Proc Natl Acad Sci USA 92: 295–299

Youngson Ch, Nurse C, Yeger H & Cutz E (1993) Oxygen sensing in airway chemoreceptors. Nature 365: 153–155

8

PHOTOCHEMICAL ACTION SPECTRA, NOT ABSORPTION SPECTRA, ALLOW IDENTIFICATION OF THE OXYGEN SENSOR IN THE CAROTID BODY

S. Lahiri,[1] D. F. Wilson,[2] S. Osanai,[1] A. Mokashi,[1] and D. G. Buerk[1]

[1] Department of Physiology
[2] Biochemistry and Biophysics
University of Pennsylvania School of Medicine
Philadelphia, Pennsylvania 19104–6085

1. INTRODUCTION

Carbon monoxide competitively inhibits reactions of many heme proteins with oxygen, including mitochondrial cytochrome oxidase, by forming a heme CO complex which can be dissociated with light. This results in an inhibition of O_2 consumption in the dark which is reversed by light. This light-induced reversal of respiratory inhibition is dependent on the wavelength of irradiating light because the amount of light absorbed by the CO complex depends on the absorption coefficient of the complex at each wavelength (photochemical action spectrum). This property was originally used to identify the mitochondrial oxidase (Kubowitz & Haas, 1932; Melnick, 1942; Warburg & Negelein, 1928; Warburg, 1949). In measurements of the oxygen sensory activity of the isolated, perfused-superfused carotid body, CO was observed to be competitive with respect to oxygen, an effect reversed by light. The dependence of the photo-reversal of the CO effect on the wavelength of light has been measured and shown to be characteristic of mitochondrial cytochrome oxidase (Wilson et al, 1994). Since the carotid body chemoreceptors show O_2-CO_2 interaction in which the hypoxic response is enhanced by CO_2, it is reasonable to expect that CO sensitivity would also show a similar interaction with CO_2. These characteristics of the cat carotid chemosensory fibers were examined and are presented in this paper.

2. METHODS

The activity of the chemosensory fibers was recorded from a perfused/superfused cat carotid body as described previously (Lahiri et al, 1995). All the perfusate and super-

Frontiers in Arterial Chemoreception, edited by Zapata *et al.*
Plenum Press, New York, 1996

fusate Tyrode's solution containing CO_2-HCO_3^- were equilibrated with appropriate gases (CO, O_2, CO_2 and N_2). The solutions were mixed in 50 ml syringes and were delivered to the carotid body by pumps. Carotid body tissue PO_2 was measured by microelectrodes (Buerk et al, 1989). All perfusate/superfusate contained PO_2 of about 100 Torr, and initial pH was 7.39 at PCO_2 of 32 Torr at 36.5°C. Three types of protocols were followed: (a) Carotid body tissue PO_2 and chemosensory discharge with and without PCO of >500 Torr. After measuring the initial responses with and without light, the flow to the carotid was interrupted and the measurements continued in the dark interrupted with light. (b) Carotid chemosensory discharges were measured with and without bright light, and with various monochromatic light from wavelengths of 400 nm to 630 nm. (c) PCO-PCO_2 interaction of chemosensory discharge to various PCO of 150 Torr to >500 Torr at PCO_2 16 Torr to 60 Torr was also measured.

3. RESULTS

3.1. CO Diminished O_2 Consumption of Carotid Body in the Dark

Figure 1 shows the effect of CO with and without light on flow interruption. Control data are shown on left-hand panels. On flow interruption, the tissue PO_2 began to fall with

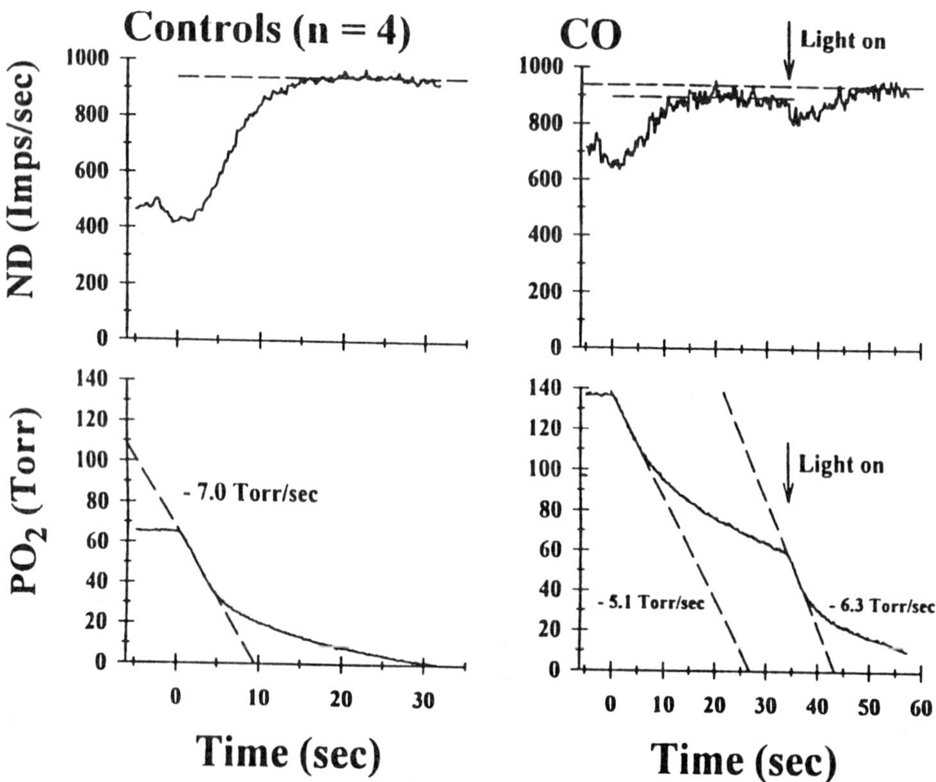

Figure 1. Simultaneous measurement of tissue PO_2 and chemosensory neural discharge (ND) of carotid body in presence (left-hand panels) and absence (right-hand panels) of CO. Perfusate flow interrupted at zero time.

the increase of chemosensory discharge until zero PO_2 was reached. The slope of dPO_2/dt gave the measure of O_2 consumption, and the chemoreceptor activity was related to this. In the right-hand panel, the carotid body was perfused with CO. The initial PO_2 was higher because O_2 consumption was lowered, and the chemoreceptor activity was greater. On interruption of perfusate in the dark, the tissue PO_2 began to fall but at a distinctly slower rate and sensory discharge increased to near maximum. Exposure to light restored the dPO_2/dt and showed a slight decrease in the discharge rate which was restored because of a decrease in tissue PO_2. Thus CO increased the chemosensory discharge rate and caused photoreversible decrease in O_2 consumption.

3.2. The Photochemical Action Spectrum of O_2 Sensing

Figure 2 shows the light wavelength dependence of chemosensory discharge corrected to the relative quantum intensity (taken from Wilson et al, 1994). The perfusion medium was changed from control solution to a medium equilibrated with CO. The chemosensory activity increased approximately 20-fold. The carotid body was subjected to 6-s periods of illumination using monochromatic light of the indicated wavelengths, separated by brief recovery periods in the dark. A given response at 432 nm required 6–7 times less light than that at 590 nm, indicating that the absorption of the CO-compound was 6–7 times greater at 432 nm than at 590 nm. The positions of the maxima were more accurately determined using small (2 nm) changes in wavelengths of illumination. These values are characteristic of the photochemical action spectrum of the CO complex of cytochrome a_3 (Warburg & Negelein, 1928; Kubowitz & Haas, 1932; Melnick, 1942; Caster & Chance, 1955), as shown in Figure 3.

3.3. PCO-PCO_2 Interaction

The steady states of carotid chemosensory activities are shown at PCO of 150 Torr and 500 Torr at various levels PCO_2 in the dark (Fig 4). The response to PCO_2 was enhanced by PCO (Osanai et al, 1996). This resembled the PO_2-PCO_2 interaction in the chemosensory discharge (Lahiri & Delaney, 1975). Decreasing PCO would diminish the PCO/PO_2 ratio. However, PCO of 150 Torr was sufficient to stimulate maximally the chemoreceptor (Osanai et al, 1996).

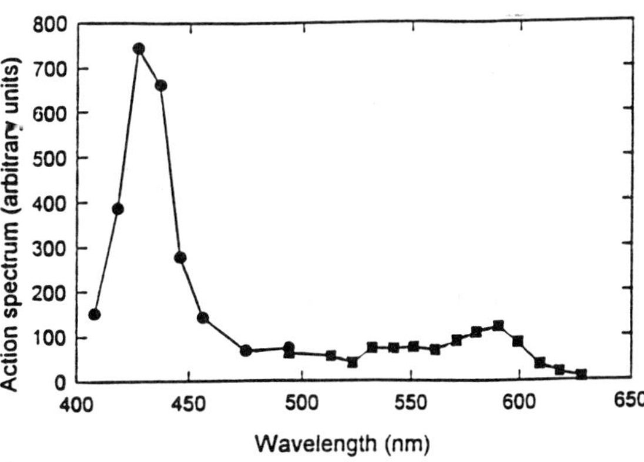

Figure 2. Photochemical action spectrum of cat carotid body treated with 67% CO, 23% O_2 and 5% CO_2, and then subjected to 6–8 periods of monochromatic illumination. Spectrum plotted against light wavelength after correction for same energy. (Reproduced from Wilson et al, 1994, by permission of the publishers).

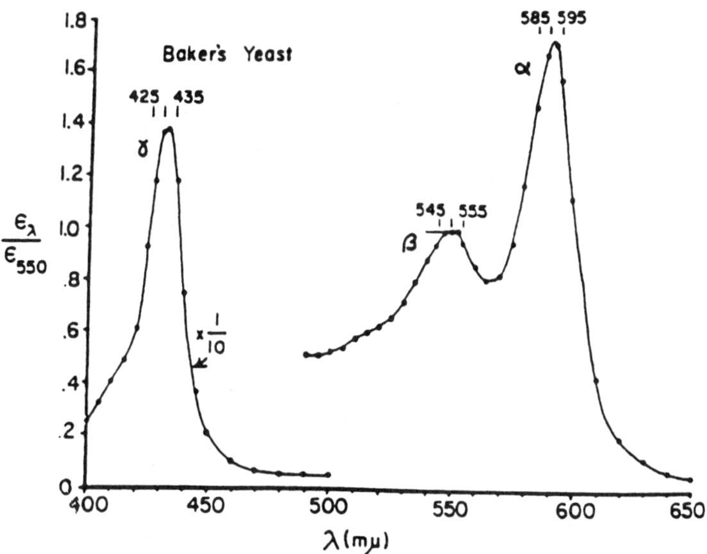

Figure 3. The photochemical action spectrum of bakers' yeast. Index of O_2 consumption plotted against light wavelength. Soret's band on the left depressed by a factor of 10. (Reproduced from Caster & Chance, 1955, by permission of the authors and publishers).

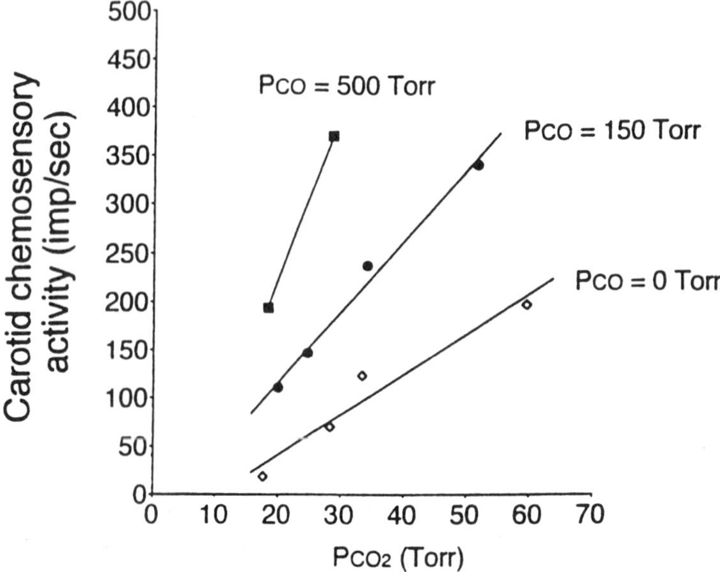

Figure 4. PCO-PCO_2 interaction. Chemosensory activity plotted against PCO_2 at three different PCO's (0, 150 and 500 Torr). (Reproduced from Osanai et al, 1996, by permission of the publishers).

4. DISCUSSION

Evidence has been presented that CO causes photoreversible decrease of O_2 consumption and enhances oxygen chemosensory excitation of the carotid body (Lahiri et al, 1995). The photo-reversal of the CO excitation is dependent on the wavelength of light. Maximal responses were observed at 432 nm and 590 nm, with a response ratio of 6.0 - 6.5 (Wilson et al, 1994). Also, characteristically, PCO interacted with PCO_2 in the same manner as PO_2 interacts with PCO_2 (Lahiri & Delaney, 1975). These are all consistent with the observations of Mulligan et al (1981) and Duchen & Biscoe (1992).

Carbon monoxide functions as a very specific metabolic inhibitor by binding with enzymes which react with O_2 (Warburg & Negelein, 1928; Melnick, 1942; Caster & Chance, 1955; Keilin, 1970). This property and thereby the photochemical action spectra have been invaluable assets in the studies of cellular respiration. It is impossible to accurately measure the absorption spectra of carotid body due to its small size, light scattering by the tissue and several pigments with overlapping absorption spectra. Even if accurate absorption spectra could be measured, this could not distinguish the particular component responsible for O_2 sensing from the other pigments of the carotid body. The photochemical action spectrum is, in contrast, highly specific for the oxygen sensor when the carotid body response is used to measure the photochemical action spectrum, *i.e.*, its oxygen pressure dependent chemosensory discharge is used as the measure of the photo-response. These light-induced changes are not affected by other tissue pigments, even those which bind CO but are not involved in generating the neural signal, or by light scattering by the tissue. The measured action spectrum showed no contribution, for example, due to other heme-CO components such as cytochrome P_{450} (maximum at 558 nm), which were possible oxygen sensors. The photochemical action spectrum is not affected by the many pigments of the tissue which do not contribute to the CO/O_2 induced changes in sensory discharge and their reversal by light.

Acker and Xue (1995) failed to find any indication of an absorption change in the carotid body corresponding to the white light effect of sensory discharge in the CO-treated aerobic carotid body. This is not surprising, because the reported signal to noise would have made it difficult to observe the absorption change induced by 100% formation of the cytochrome a_3-CO compound, and in the aerobic steady state the amount of CO-compound present would have been at most a few percent. As a result, the light induced absorption change would have been much too small to be detected by direct absorption measurements. Thus, the measuring of the photochemical action spectrum is the only available approach by which the spectrum of the oxygen sensor can be measured and the role of mitochondrial cytochrome oxidase in oxygen sensing established.

The maximal increase in chemosensory activity induced by CO at moderate PO_2 is 80% of that induced by interruption of perfusate flow. The increase in activity by CO is accompanied by 30% reduction of O_2 consumption and is fully reversed by light (Lahiri et al, 1995). Thus, mitochondrial cytochrome oxidase and thereby oxidative phosphorylation is responsible for most of the oxygen chemosensory activity. Other mechanisms of inhibition of oxygen sensing by CO, such as that of the hypoxic response of glomus cell K^+ current (López-López & González, 1992), and of hypoxic chemosensory discharge (Lahiri et al, 1993; Prabhakar et al, 1995), may contribute to the oxygen sensory response, but only a small fraction of that of cytochrome oxidase. Mitochondrial cytochrome a_3 is the primary oxygen sensor in the carotid body.

That high CO behaves like hypoxia is also evident in the manifestation of PCO-PCO_2 interaction which mimics the PO_2-PCO_2 interaction, although the mechanism of the interaction between the two sensory systems remains unknown.

The currently available data indicate that CO reacts with mitochondrial cytochrome oxidase, decreasing the capacity of the mitochondria to maintain the cellular metabolic energy level. The resulting decrease in energy level may trigger increased permeability of the plasma membrane to Ca^{2+} and the resulting increased intracellular Ca^{2+} then increases neurotransmitter release and neural discharge. Photodissociation of the CO complex reverses the inhibition of cellular energy metabolism, resulting in Ca^{2+} extrusion and suppression of neural activity.

5. PERSPECTIVES

There are several competing hypotheses of O_2 chemoreception in the carotid body. The membrane hypothesis, as presented in summary by López-Barneo (1996), states that hypoxia causes suppression of K^+ and Ca^{2+} currents which set off the membrane depolarization. But the PO_2's at which the suppression of ion currents was observed were higher than those at which normal chemosensitivity occurs. In addition, the resting membrane potential is more negative than the reported PO_2 threshold of the I-V curve. Acker & Xue (1995) proposed that decrease of NADPH-oxidase activity during hypoxia decreases H_2O_2 production and increases GSH/GSSG. This alters the redox state of membrane channels and thereby causes excitation of chemoreceptor cells. This hypothesis is difficult to test because no one knows about H_2O_2 production in glomus cell during hypoxia, nor the redox state and its effect on the membrane channels. One possible test would be to determine if chemoreception is depressed in granulomatous disease affecting NADPH-oxidase (Dinauer, 1993). It will be interesting to examine the oxygen sensory activity in instances where chemosensory function to hypoxia but not to hypercapnia is blunted (Lahiri et al, 1990). What is the basis for the blunted response? Is it specific for chemoreceptor cells alone? What channels and intracellular organelles are involved which are unique in these cells?

6. ACKNOWLEDGMENTS

We are grateful to Mary Pili for her secretarial assistance. Supported in part by HL-43413–06 and HL-50180–03 grants.

7. REFERENCES

Acker H & Xue D (1995) Mechanisms of O_2 sensing in the carotid body in comparison with other O_2-sensing cells. News Physiol Sci 10: 211–216

Buerk DG, Nair PK & Whalen WJ (1989) Two-cytochrome model for carotid body $P_{ti}O_2$ and chemosensitivity changes after hemorrhage. J Appl Physiol 67: 60–67

Caster LN & Chance B (1955) Photochemical action spectra of carbon monoxide-inhibited respiration. J Biol Chem 217: 453–464

Dinauer MC (1993) The respiratory burst oxidase and the molecular genetics of chronic granulomatous disease. Crit Revs Clin Lab Sci 30: 329–369

Duchen MR & Biscoe TJ (1992) Mitochondrial function in Type I cells isolated from rabbit arterial chemoreceptors. J Physiol, London 450: 13–31

Keilin D (1970) The History of Cell Respiration and Cytochrome. London: Cambridge Univ Press. pp 221–327

Kubowitz F & Haas E (1932) Ausbau der photochemische Methoden zur Untersuchung des sauerstoffübertrgenden Ferments. Biochem Z 255: 247–277

Lahiri S & Delaney RG (1975) Stimulus interaction in the responses of carotid body chemoreceptor single afferent fibers. Respir Physiol 24: 249–266

Lahiri S, Iturriaga R, Mokashi A, Ray DK & Chugh D (1993) CO reveals dual mechanisms of O_2 chemoreception in the cat carotid body. Respir Physiol 94: 227–240

Lahiri S, Buerk DG, Chugh DK, Osanai S & Mokashi A (1995) Reciprocal photolabile O_2 consumption and chemoreceptor excitation by carbon monoxide in the cat carotid body: evidence for cytochrome a_3 as the primary O_2 sensor. Brain Res 684: 194–200

López-Barneo J (1996) O_2 sensing by ion channels and the regulation of cellular function. Trends Neurosci (in press)

López-López JR & González C (1992) Time course of K^+ current initiation by low oxygen in the chemoreceptor cells of adult rabbit carotid body. FEBS Lett 299: 251–254

Melnick JL (1942) The photochemical action spectrum of cytochrome oxidase. J Biol Chem 146: 385–390

Mulligan E, Lahiri S & Storey BT (1981) Carotid body O_2 chemoreception and mitochondrial oxidative phosphorylation. J Appl Physiol 51: 438–446

Osanai S, Chugh DK, Mokashi A & Lahiri S (1996) Stimulus interaction between CO and CO_2 in the cat carotid body chemoreception. Brain Res 711: 56–63

Prabhakar NR, Dinerman JL, Agani FH & Snyder SH (1995) Carbon monoxide: a role in carotid body chemoreception. Proc Natl Acad Sci USA 92: 1994–1997

Warburg O (1949) Heavy Metals Prosthetic Group and Enzyme Action. Translated by A Lawson. Oxford: Clarendon Press

Warburg O & Negelein E (1928) Über die photochemische dissoziation bei intermittierender Bleichtung und das absolute Absorptionsspektrum des atmungsferments. Biochem Z 202: 202–228

Wilson DF, Mokashi A, Chugh D, Vinogradov S, Osanai S & Lahiri S (1994) The primary oxygen sensor of the cat carotid body is cytochrome a_3 of the mitochondrial respiratory chain. FEBS Lett 351: 370–374

9

MECHANISMS OF CAROTID CHEMORECEPTOR RESETTING AFTER BIRTH

In Vitro Studies

John L. Carroll,[1] Laura M. Sterni,[1] Owen S. Bamford,[1] and Marshall H. Montrose[2]

[1] Department of Pediatrics
Division of Pediatric Respiratory Sciences
The Johns Hopkins Children's Center
[2] Department of Medicine
Division of Pediatric Gastroenterology
The Johns Hopkins School of Medicine
Baltimore, Maryland

1. CAROTID CHEMORECEPTOR RESETTING AND POSTNATAL MATURATION

The carotid chemoreceptors are important in the neonate for maturation of normal cardiorespiratory control and for survival of the neonatal period. Critically important features of normal respiratory control —such as recovery from apnea, ventilatory defense during hypoxic stress, arousal from sleep during hypoxemia or upper airway obstruction, and development of normal breathing patterns during postnatal maturation— all depend on the carotid chemoreceptors. Current evidence suggests involvement of the carotid chemoreceptors in a variety of neonatal disorders including high mortality rates in infants with bronchopulmonary dysplasia, severe bradycardia during hypoxemia, and the sudden infant death syndrome (SIDS).

The critical importance of carotid chemoreceptor function during infancy has been demonstrated by experiments in which the carotid sinus nerves are severed just after birth. Although adults survive bilateral carotid denervation, this intervention in newborns results in hypoventilation, more and longer central apnea, abnormal breathing pattern development, and mortality rates as high as 66% in the neonatal period (Bureau et al, 1985; Hofer, 1986; Donnelly & Haddad, 1990). Bureau's group found that 43% of newborn lambs carotid denervated at 1–2 days of age died suddenly and unexpectedly between 4–5 weeks of age, which is reminiscent of the SIDS and suggests that the carotid chemoreceptors become important for survival within a particular age range during development (Bureau et al, 1985).

Frontiers in Arterial Chemoreception, edited by Zapata *et al.*
Plenum Press, New York, 1996

In every species studied to date, the ventilatory response to hypoxia increases with age during infancy, due in part to maturation of carotid chemoreceptor function. Although the ventilatory response to hypoxia in neonates is complex, involving CNS inhibition (Lawson & Long, 1983; Martin-Body, 1988) and hypoxic hypometabolism in some species (Mortola et al, 1989; Frappell et al, 1991), the importance of the carotid chemoreceptors is clear.

The fetal carotid chemoreceptors are adapted to a baseline PaO_2 of ~23 mm Hg as 'normoxia' and respond to lowering of PaO_2 below that level (Blanco et al, 1984). At birth, air breathing begins and within minutes there is a 3–4 fold increase in arterial PaO_2, sufficient to silence the carotid chemoreceptors. In the relative hyperoxia of the extrauterine environment, no carotid sinus nerve activity can be elicited. However, by 2–3 days after birth the carotid chemoreceptors again show tonic activity and a brisk response to hypoxia, except that the range of O_2 sensitivity has shifted to the right (more sensitive) compared to the fetal response. The PaO_2 of ~23 mm Hg that was seen as 'normoxia' by the fetal carotid chemoreceptors elicits a vigorous response in the 2–3 day old lamb and is sensed by the chemoreceptors as severe hypoxia. This rightward shifting of the O_2 response range at birth is "resetting" of the arterial chemoreceptors, and it occurs in both the carotid and aortic chemoreceptors (Kumar & Hanson, 1989).

Our studies in cats and those of others using neural recording techniques have shown a slower phase of carotid chemoreceptor maturation, with O_2 sensitivity increasing slowly over weeks or months (cat, rat, swine) (Mulligan, 1991; Kholwadwala & Donnelly, 1992; Marchal et al, 1992; Carroll et al, 1993; Tomares et al, 1994). At the present time it is unclear whether resetting right after birth and the slower maturation phase of chemoreceptor development occur by the same or different mechanisms.

It is widely accepted that the rise in oxygen tension at birth is the major factor leading to carotid chemoreceptor resetting. The conclusion that resetting is modulated mainly by O_2 tension is supported by several lines of evidence: a) raising the PaO_2 of the near-term sheep fetus initiates carotid chemoreceptor resetting *in utero* (Blanco et al, 1988); b) chronic hypoxia from birth delays resetting of arterial chemoreflexes (Eden & Hanson, 1987; Hanson et al, 1989; Hertzberg et al, 1992); and c) after delay of chemoreflex development by chronic hypoxia, restoring to normoxia then initiates resetting (Hertzberg et al, 1992). The mechanism(s) by which O_2 tension modulates carotid chemoreceptor resetting are not known.

2. TYPE-I CELL DEVELOPMENT AT THE CELLULAR LEVEL

Until recently, it was unknown whether the oxygen sensitivity of the type-I cell itself changes after birth. Using Fura-2 to measure intracellular calcium ($[Ca^{2+}]_i$), we recently reported that isolated type-I cells of the newborn rabbit, free from influences of blood flow, oxygen delivery, or neural and humoral modulation, clearly show smaller $[Ca^{2+}]_i$ responses to hypoxia compared to cells isolated from adults and studied under identical conditions (Sterni et al, 1995). $[Ca^{2+}]_i$ responses of glomus cells to hypoxia were 3–5 fold larger in cells from adults compared to newborns. In addition, the response of newborn rabbit cells to sudden challenge with hypoxic buffered salt solution was slow in onset and without overshoot (Sterni et al, 1995). In marked contrast, carotid chemoreceptor cells from adult rabbits demonstrated a large initial peak and subsequent adaptation when challenged with hypoxic perfusate (Sterni et al, 1995). Thus not only was the response magnitude much larger in glomus cells from adults compared with newborns, but the response profile also changed with age. These data provided the first support for the hypothesis that carotid chemoreceptor cell sensitivity to hypoxia depends on the level of postnatal maturity.

3. AN *IN VITRO* MODEL OF TYPE-I CELL RESETTING

Recent work in our laboratory examines whether rat glomus cell oxygen sensitivity also depends on the level of postnatal maturity and whether resetting of type-I cell O_2 sensitivity is modulated by oxygen tension. Because O_2 tension is believed to be a major determinant of glomus cell resetting, we hypothesized that after harvesting glomus cells from newborn rats, exposure to ambient O_2 tension (~ 150 mm Hg) would result in "resetting" of glomus cell O_2 sensitivity in culture. In addition, we hypothesized that keeping the cells under hypoxic conditions in culture would prevent resetting of oxygen sensitivity.

The methods used were as follows: carotid chemoreceptor type-I cells were isolated from < 24 hour old newborn rats and studied a) freshly isolated, b) after 72 hours in culture in air, and c) after 72 hours in culture in 1.5% O_2. The same protocol was followed with carotid chemoreceptor cells from 2 week old rats. Cells were loaded with Fura-2, superfused at 35°C with balanced salt solution equilibrated with 5% CO_2, and $[Ca^{2+}]_i$ responses to 3 minute anoxia challenges (using sodium dithionite) were measured using a digital imaging microscope. The fluorescence intensity ratio was used to calculate $[Ca^{2+}]_i$, as previously reported (Sterni et al, 1995).

Preliminary results indicate that, as in glomus cells from rabbits, the $[Ca^{2+}]_i$ response of newborn rat glomus cells to anoxic challenge is small compared to responses of cells from 2 week old rats (Fig 1). Data obtained to date suggest that the magnitude of the $[Ca^{2+}]_i$ response to anoxia of freshly isolated cells from 2 week old rats may be as much as 5 fold larger compared to cells from newborns. Also similar to the rabbit, the $[Ca^{2+}]_i$ response profile to anoxia of freshly isolated cells from newborns is nearly flat, in marked contrast to the response profile of glomus cells from 2 week old rats, which shows a large, rapid-onset, initial overshoot and subsequent adaptation (Fig 1).

In sharp contrast to the small $[Ca^{2+}]_i$ responses to anoxia of freshly isolated cells from newborns, preliminary data suggest that newborn glomus cell peak $[Ca^{2+}]_i$ responses

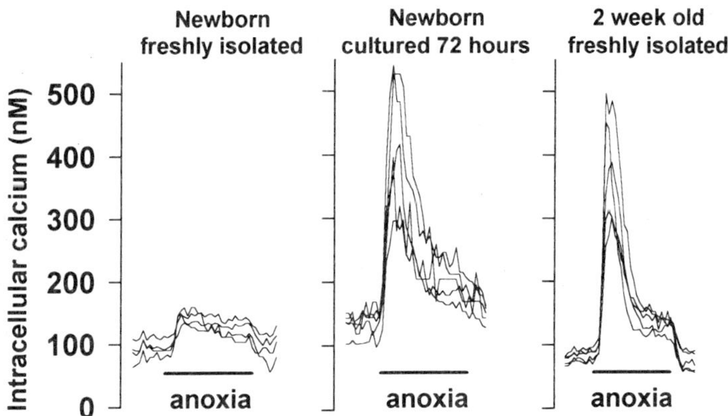

Figure 1. Typical $[Ca^{2+}]_i$ responses to anoxia of type-I cells obtained from rat carotid bodies. Each line represents response of one carotid chemoreceptor cell.

to anoxia increase more than 5 fold after 72 hours in culture (Fig 1). In addition, the $[Ca^{2+}]_i$ response profile changes from the flatter "immature" shape to the typical "mature" response profile characteristic of cells from older rats (Fig 1) and adult rabbits (Sterni et al, 1995). Identical studies on carotid chemoreceptor cells harvested from 2 week old rats demonstrate that the magnitude and shape of $[Ca^{2+}]_i$ responses to anoxia in freshly isolated cells are of adult type, with no change after 72 hours in culture. The data obtained to date are consistent with the hypothesis that newborn type-I cells may 'reset' their O_2 sensitivity after exposure to ambient oxygen tension for 72 hours. Although further work is needed, additional preliminary results indicate that culturing newborn cells under hypoxic conditions (1.5% O_2) prevented resetting of the $[Ca^{2+}]_i$ response to anoxia observed under ambient O_2 culture conditions (Fig 1).

4. SUMMARY

The results of these studies are consistent with the hypothesis that carotid chemoreceptor type-I cell resetting occurs, at least in part, at the level of the type-I cell. Furthermore, we have developed an *in vitro* model of newborn type-I cell resetting, in which freshly isolated glomus cells from newborns exhibit small, immature $[Ca^{2+}]_i$ response to anoxia, but —after 72 hours in culture— $[Ca^{2+}]_i$ responses convert to adult magnitude and profile. Finally, work so far suggests that glomus cell resetting in this model is modulated by oxygen tension. The mechanisms of glomus cell resetting remain unknown. Resetting of O_2 sensitivity could result from withdrawal of tonic inhibitory influences present *in vivo*, changes in the oxygen sensor itself, changes in ion channel expression, modulation, and function, or other mechanisms occurring around the time of birth. Additional work is needed to determine the mechanisms of glomus cell resetting at the cellular level, and the role of O_2 tension and other potential modulators of resetting.

5. REFERENCES

Blanco CE, Dawes GS, Hanson MA & McCooke HB (1984) The response to hypoxia of arterial chemoreceptors in fetal sheep and newborn lambs. J Physiol, London 351: 25–37

Blanco CE, Hanson MA & McCooke HB (1988) Effects on carotid chemoreceptor resetting of pulmonary ventilation in the fetal lamb in utero. J Dev Physiol 10: 167–174

Bureau MA, Lamarche J, Foulon P & Dalle D (1985) Postnatal maturation of respiration in intact and carotid body-chemodenervated lambs. J Appl Physiol 59: 869–874

Carroll JL, Bamford OS & Fitzgerald RS (1993) Postnatal maturation of carotid chemoreceptor responses to O_2 and CO_2 in the cat. J Appl Physiol 75: 2383–2391

Donnelly DF & Haddad GG (1990) Prolonged apnea and impaired survival in piglets after sinus and aortic nerve section. J Appl Physiol 68: 1048–1052

Eden GJ & Hanson MA (1987) Effects of chronic hypoxia from birth on the ventilatory response to acute hypoxia in the newborn rat. J Physiol, London 392: 11–19

Frappell P, Saiki C & Mortola JP (1991) Metabolism during normoxia, hypoxia and recovery in the newborn kitten. Respir Physiol 86: 115–124

Hanson MA, Kumar P & Williams BA (1989) The effect of chronic hypoxia upon the development of respiratory chemoreflexes in the newborn kitten. J Physiol, London 411: 563–574

Hertzberg T, Hellström S, Holgert H, Lagercrantz H & Pequignot JM (1992) Ventilatory response to hyperoxia in newborn rats born in hypoxia — possible relationship to carotid body dopamine. J Physiol, London 456: 645–654

Hofer MA (1986) Role of carotid sinus and aortic nerves in respiratory control of infant rats. Am J Physiol 251: R811-R817

Kholwadwala D & Donnelly DF (1992) Maturation of carotid chemoreceptor sensitivity to hypoxia: *in vitro* studies in the newborn rat. J Physiol, London 453: 461–473

Kumar P & Hanson MA (1989) Re-setting of the hypoxic sensitivity of aortic chemoreceptors in the new-born lamb. J Dev Physiol 11: 199–206

Lawson EE & Long WA (1983) Central origin of biphasic breathing pattern during hypoxia in newborns. J Appl Physiol 55: 483–488

Marchal F, Bairam A, Haouzi P, Crance JP, Di-Giulio C, Vert P & Lahiri S (1992) Carotid chemoreceptor response to natural stimuli in the newborn kitten. Respir Physiol 87: 183–193

Martin-Body RL (1988) Brain transections demonstrate the central origin of hypoxic ventilatory depression in carotid body-denervated rats. J Physiol, London 407: 41–52

Mortola JP, Rezzonico R & Lanthier C (1989) Ventilation and oxygen consumption during acute hypoxia in newborn mammals: a comparative analysis. Respir Physiol 78: 31–43

Mulligan EM (1991). Discharge properties of carotid bodies: Developmental aspects. In: Haddad GG & Farber JP (eds) Developmental Neurobiology of Breathing. New York: Marcel Dekker. pp 321–340

Sterni LM, Bamford OS, Tomares SM, Montrose MH & Carroll JL (1995) Developmental changes in intracellular Ca^{2+} response of carotid chemoreceptor cells to hypoxia. Am J Physiol 268: L801-L808

Tomares SM, Bamford OS, Sterni LM, Fitzgerald RS & Carroll JL (1994) Effects of domperidone on neonatal and adult carotid chemoreceptors in the cat. J Appl Physiol 77: 1274–1280

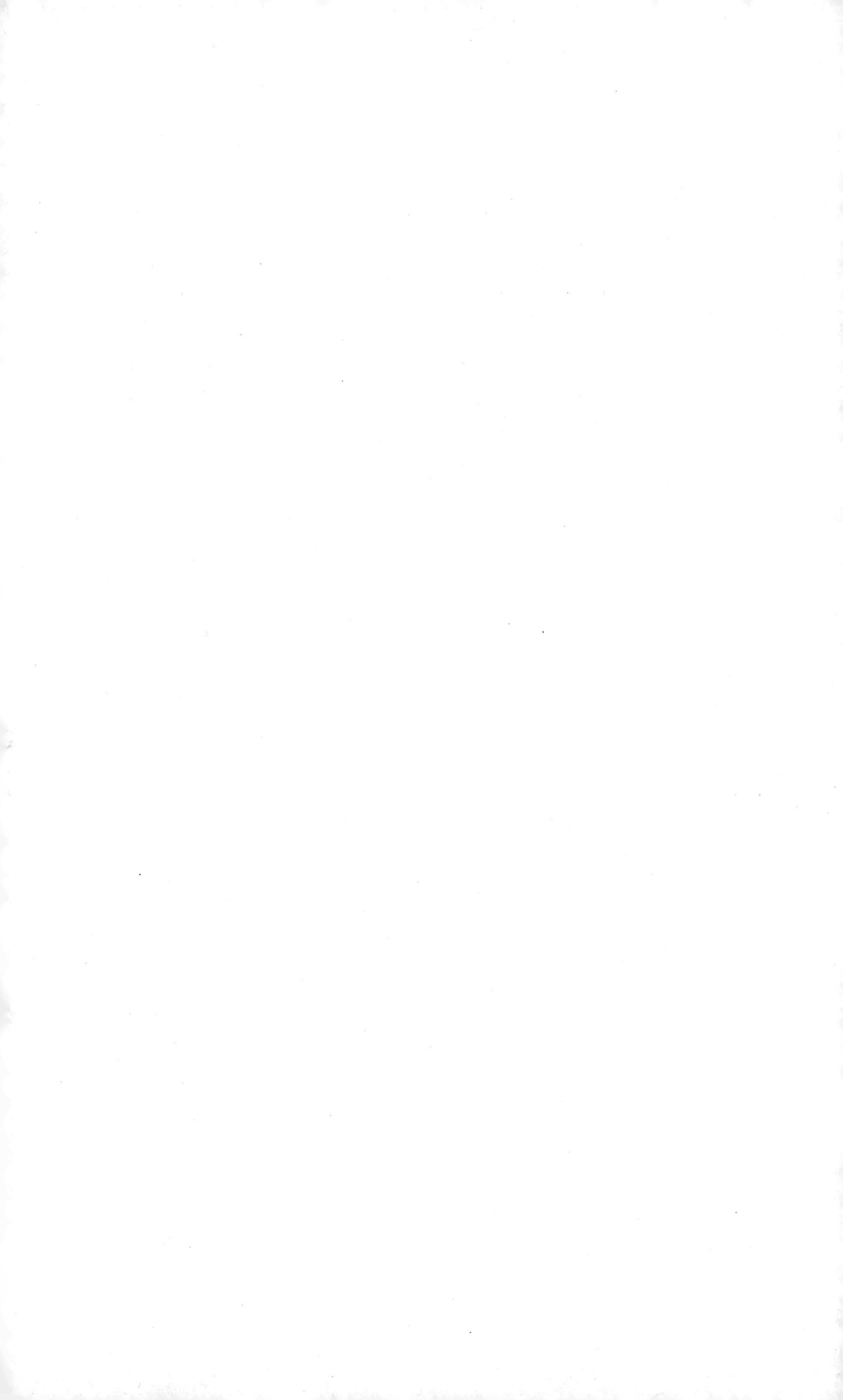

10

CAROTID CHEMOSENSORY RESPONSE TO CAFFEINE IN DEVELOPING CATS

A. Bairam,[1] P. De Grandpré,[1] C. Dauphin,[1] and F. Marchal[2]

[1] Laboratoire de Néonatologie
Centre Hospitalier Universitaire de Québec
Centre de Recherche, Pavillon SFA
Québec, PQ, Canada
[2] Laboratoire de Physiologie
Faculté de Médecine de Nancy
Nancy, France

1. INTRODUCTION

It has been suggested that the increase of ventilation with methylxanthines (caffeine, theophylline and aminophylline) is mainly due to a stimulation of respiratory centers in adult subjects (Sawynok, 1995). However, methylxanthines seem to act also on carotid chemoreceptors in newborns since caffeine failed to increase ventilation in chronically chemodenervated lambs (Blanchard et al, 1986). Also, aminophylline did not prevent the ventilatory depression elicited by hypoxia in chemodenervated piglets (Cattarossi et al, 1995). Indeed, aminophylline has been shown to enhance the ventilatory chemoreflex response to hyperoxia in newborn infants (Cattarossi, 1993). Despite the frequent use of caffeine in the treatment of neonatal apnea (Sawynok, 1995; Bairam et al, 1987), the magnitude of its effects on carotid chemosensory activity is still unclear. In the majority of studies, ventilation has been measured in order to evaluate the effects of methylxanthines on the peripheral chemoreceptors. The aims of the present study were to determine the effects of caffeine on the carotid sinus nerve chemosensory activity (CSNA) and on its response to hypoxia in newborn and adult cats.

2. MATERIALS AND METHODS

The effects of iv bolus injection of caffeine 10 mg/kg on CSNA were studied in 6 kittens aged 17 to 21 days and in 3 adult cats. Animals were anesthetized with pentobarbitone sodium, 35 mg/kg ip in kittens and iv in cats, ventilated artificially with a respiratory pump and paralyzed with doxacuronium chloride (1 mg/kg, iv). A femoral artery was cannulated to

Frontiers in Arterial Chemoreception, edited by Zapata *et al.*
Plenum Press, New York, 1996

measure continuously the arterial blood pressure (ABP). The two femoral veins were also cannulated, and one was used to infuse the maintenance dose of anesthesia (pentobarbitone sodium, 3 to 5 mg/kg/h) while the second served for drug administration. Rectal temperature was maintained between 37°C and 38°C with a regulated heating pad. Under surgical microscope, one carotid sinus nerve was dissected, desheathed and cut near the petrosal ganglion. The details of the surgical procedure and the technique for recording the discharge of a few chemosensory fibers of the carotid sinus nerve were similar to those described previously by Marchal et al (1992). The signals were amplified, band-pass filtered, fed to a window discriminator and to an audio amplifier and displayed on an oscilloscope and a chart recorder. The activity was also displayed as impulse/sec. The same chemosensory preparation, free of baroreceptor discharge, was used throughout a given animal.

Caffeine was administered in normoxia and the immediate CSNA and ABP responses were evaluated within 1 min of each injection. The steady-state response was studied by averaging the activity over a period of 1 min, 5 and 15 min after caffeine in normoxia. The hypoxic response was evaluated by changing the inspired gas from air to hypoxia (8% O_2 in N_2) then to hyperoxia (100% O_2) before and at 10 min of caffeine injection. The steady-state activity was averaged over 1 min in normoxia, hypoxia and hyperoxia. Caffeine plasma level was assessed before and at 15 min of caffeine injection by an HPLC method.

Data were compared using two-way ANOVA for repeated measurements and expressed as a mean ± SEM. A difference was considered as statistically significant at $p < 0.05$.

3. RESULTS

3.1. Effects of Caffeine on CSNA in Normoxia

In all kittens and cats studied, the injection of caffeine produced an immediate but transient increase in CSNA associated with a decrease in ABP. In kittens, the mean CSNA increased from 4.1 ± 0.6 to 8.1 ± 1.0 imp/sec, $p < 0.001$; and ABP decreased from 49.5 ± 5.0 to 38.0 ± 3.0 mm Hg, $p < 0.001$. In cats, the CSNA increased from 2.9 ± 0.1 to 7.9 ± 1.0 imp/sec while the ABP decreased from 114.9 ± 14.1 to 93.3 ± 11.7 mm Hg (n = 3). The mean steady-state CSNA and ABP were comparable to control values at 1, 5, 10 and 15 min of caffeine injection in kittens and cats. However, during the control period, caffeine plasma concentration was not detectable and was 54.3 ± 2.8 μmol/l in kittens and 76.6± 6.7 μmol/l in cats at 15 min of caffeine injection.

3.2. Effect of Caffeine on Carotid Chemosensory Response to Hypoxia

Before caffeine, the steady-state CSNA increased significantly in response to hypoxia from 4.2 ± 0.9 imp/sec to 36.8 ± 7.4 imp/sec in kittens; $p < 0.001$, and from 4.9 ± 0.4 imp/sec to 39.9 ± 5.8 imp/sec in cats (n = 3). After caffeine, the CSNA in hypoxia was not different from control, *i.e.*, 36.4 ± 8.0 imp/sec in kittens and 39.7 ± 2.0 imp/sec in cats. Caffeine did not influence the CSNA in hyperoxia either.

4. DISCUSSION

This study demonstrates that the bolus injection of caffeine regularly induced a short-lasting excitation of the CSNA in normoxia in kittens and cats. The carotid chemoreceptor response to natural stimuli is known to mature with age (Marchal et al, 1992; Carroll et al, 1993), but this does not seem to account for the transient stimulatory effect of caffeine in kittens since a similar pattern of response was observed in cats. The transient increase in CSNA may not be related to a direct effect of caffeine but may be due to the decrease in ABP to which it was closely associated. Indeed, the fall in ABP may in turn produce a transient fall in carotid body blood flow large enough to stimulate the chemosensory activity. It has been shown that steady-state chemosensory activity increases dramatically when blood pressure is gradually lowered to less than 60 mm Hg in cats (Lahiri et al, 1980) and less than 30 mm Hg in kittens (Bairam et al, 1994). The effect of a sudden drop in ABP may be more effective in activating CSNA, thus occurring at higher mean blood pressure.

Methylxanthines are known to have a long-lasting stimulatory effect on ventilation, an action which is dose-dependent and mostly explained by a direct stimulation of the respiratory neurons (Sawynok, 1995). However, a contribution of the peripheral chemoreceptors has also been suggested (Blanchard et al, 1986; Cattarossi et al, 1993; 1995). In this study, the steady-state chemosensory activity in normoxia, hypoxia and hyperoxia was not influenced by caffeine. Thus, the carotid chemoreceptors may not play a determinant role in the ventilatory effect of caffeine, a result which is at variance with the study by Blanchard et al (1986) who showed that 10 mg/kg caffeine failed to stimulate ventilation in lambs aged 82 ± 11 days which were chemodenervated at birth. In these animals, it is difficult to relate the lack of effect of caffeine on ventilation to the absence of chemoreceptors, since it has been shown that chronic chemodenervation alters the respiratory behavior and exposes the animals to sudden death (Donnelly & Haddad, 1990).

In conclusion, caffeine transiently stimulates the CSNA and this may be explained by an indirect effect of caffeine on carotid body perfusion. Since caffeine has no long-term effect on the CSNA discharge in air or in response to hypoxia, its short-lasting action may not account for the known sustained stimulation of ventilation induced by caffeine.

5. ACKNOWLEDGMENTS

Study supported by CRM and APQ.

6. REFERENCES

Bairam A, Boutroy MJ, Badonnel Y, Vert P (1987) Theophylline versus caffeine: comparative effects in treatment of idiopathic apnea in the preterm infant. J Pediatr 110: 636–639

Bairam A, Hannahart B & Marchal F (1994) Effects of haemorrhagic hypotension on carotid chemosensory discharge in the kitten. Acta Paediatr 83: 236–240

Blanchard PW, Côté A, Hobbs S, Foulon P, Aranda JV & Bureau M (1986) Abolition of ventilatory response to caffeine in chemodenervated lambs. J Appl Physiol 61: 133–137

Carroll JL, Bamford OS & Fitzgerald RS (1993) Postnatal maturation of carotid chemoreceptor responses to O_2 and CO_2 in the cat. J Appl Physiol 75: 2383–2391

Cattarossi L, Rubini S, Macagno F (1993) Aminophylline and increased activity of peripheral chemoreceptors in newborn infants. Arch Dis Child 69: 52–54

Cattarossi L, Haxhiu-Poskurica B, Haxhiu MA, Litmanovitz I, Martin RJ & Carlo WA (1995) Carotid bodies and ventilatory response to hypoxia in aminophylline-treated piglets. Pediatr Pulmonol 20: 94–10

Donnelly DF & Haddad GG (1990) Prolonged apnea and impaired survival in piglets after sinus and aortic nerve section. J Appl Physiol 68: 1048–1052

Lahiri S, Nishino T, Mokashi A & Mulligan E (1980) Relative responses of aortic body and carotid body chemoreceptors to hypotension. J Appl Physiol 48: 781–788

Marchal F, Bairam A, Haouzi P, Crance JP, Di Giulio C, Vert P & Lahiri S (1992) Carotid chemoreceptor response to natural stimuli in the newborn kitten. Resp Physiol 87: 183–193

Sawynok J (1995) Pharmacological rationale for the clinical use of caffeine. Drugs 49: 37 - 50

11

ROLE OF POTASSIUM CHANNELS IN HYPOXIC CHEMORECEPTION IN RAT CAROTID BODY TYPE-I CELLS

K. J. Buckler

University Laboratory of Physiology
Parks Road, Oxford, UK

1. INTRODUCTION

It has been proposed that the modulation of potassium channel activity by hypoxia plays a key role in oxygen sensing by the type-I cells of the carotid body. To date, two main types of oxygen-sensitive K-channels have been characterised in type-I cells. These are a high conductance (190 pS) calcium activated potassium channel (BK_{Ca}) found in rat type-I cells (Wyatt & Peers, 1995), and lower conductance (40 pS) calcium insensitive channel (termed the K_{O2}-channel) found in rabbit type-I cells (Ganfornina & Lopez-Barneo, 1991). It has been suggested that inhibition of these channels by hypoxia is responsible for membrane depolarisation which in turn induces voltage-gated calcium entry and neurosecretion.

This model of oxygen chemoreception has been called into question by the observation that pharmacological compounds which also inhibit these oxygen sensitive K^+-channels (*e.g.*, TEA, 4-AP and charybdotoxin) fail to excite the intact carotid body under normoxic conditions (Donnelly, 1995; Pepper et al, 1995). Indeed the spectacular failure of these experiments could imply that the events seen in isolated cells (*i.e.*, depolarisation and elevation of $[Ca^{2+}]_i$) have little to do with O_2-transduction in the intact organ. An alternative interpretation, however, is that these experiments highlight a weakness in the fundamental assumption that the modulation of voltage-gated K-channels will result in significant changes to the cells resting potential (approximately -50 mV). If this latter interpretation is correct, then an alternative explanation must be found for the membrane depolarisation that is observed in hypoxia.

This paper presents the results of experiments designed to test the role of BK_{Ca} and K_{O2}-channels in setting the resting potential of neonatal rat type-I cells and examines the cause of the depolarisation seen in hypoxia.

Frontiers in Arterial Chemoreception, edited by Zapata *et al.*
Plenum Press, New York, 1996

2. METHODS

The methods for cell isolation have been described previously (Buckler & Vaughan-Jones, 1993). Briefly, 11–16 day old Sprague-Dawley rat pups were anaesthetized with 4% halothane and their carotid bodies excised and stored in cold phosphate buffered saline. Type-I cells were isolated by a mixture of enzymic treatment (collagenase/trypsin) and mechanical dispersion, plated onto poly-*d*-lysine coated coverslips and kept in Hams-F12 culture medium until use (3–12 h).

$[Ca^{2+}]_i$ was measured using Indo-1, as previously described (Buckler & Vaughan-Jones, 1993). Cells were loaded with Indo-1 by incubation in a 2.5 μM solution of Indo-1-AM in Hams F-12 culture medium for 1 h at room temperature. Indo-1 fluorescence was excited at 340 nm and measured at 405 and 495 nm.

Voltage and clamp recordings were performed using the perforated-patch, whole-cell recording technique. Electrodes were fabricated from thick-walled borosilicate glass tubing and were fire polished before use. The internal filling solution contained (in mM), 55 K_2SO_4, 30 KCl, 20 HEPES, 1 EGTA and 5 $MgCl_2$, adjusted to pH 7.2 at 37°C with NaOH. To this solution was added 240 μg/ml amphotericin B (prepared as a stock solution of 60 mg/ml DMSO).

The standard extracellular solution contained (in mM) NaCl 117, KCl 4.5, $NaHCO_3$ 23, $MgCl_2$ 1.0, $CaCl_2$ 2.5, glucose 11 and was equilibrated with 5% CO_2/95% air, pH at 37°C was 7.4–7.45. Hypoxic solutions were equilibrated with 5% CO_2, 95% N_2, (P_{O2} 5–10 Torr). Anoxia was produced by equilibrating solutions with 5% CO_2/95% N_2 plus the addition of 100–500 μM $Na_2S_2O_4$. All experiments were conducted at 35–37°C.

3. RESULTS

The effects of several K-channel inhibitors were tested on cells which responded to either hypoxia or anoxia with a large, rapid, rise in $[Ca^{2+}]_i$. These included 20 nM charybdotoxin, an inhibitor of BK_{Ca}-channels, 10 mM TEA a potent inhibitor of BK_{Ca}, K_{O2} (Ganfornina & Lopez-Barneo, 1991), and other K-channels; 1 and 5 mM 4-AP, an inhibitor of K_{O2} and other K-channels. None of these inhibitors evoked a significant rise in $[Ca^{2+}]_i$ (Fig 1).

These data suggest that the inhibition of maxi-K^+, and other voltage-gated K^+ channels may be unable to evoke a significant depolarisation of type-I cells. In order to confirm this, the effects of a combination of 10 mM TEA and 5 mM 4-AP upon type-I cell membrane potential was studied directly using the perforated patch whole cell recording technique. The combined application of both TEA and 4-AP failed to evoke a significant depolarisation of type-I cells (control = -58 ± 3.5 mV; plus TEA and 4-AP = -60 ± 2.4 mV; n = 6; ns). The presence of these agents did not, however, prevent membrane depolarisation in response to hypoxia (E_m = -37.5 ± 6.0 mV; P< 0.01). Thus, neither BK_{Ca} channels nor any other TEA or 4-AP sensitive K^+-channels make a significant contribution to the control of the resting membrane potential under normoxic conditions in these cells. Consequently inhibition of any such channels cannot account for the depolarisation seen in hypoxia.

We have previously reported that, in cells voltage clamped close to their normal resting potential, anoxia evokes a small inward shift in holding current of a few pA (Buckler & Vaughan-Jones, 1994; see also Fig 2A). Given the high input impedance of type-I cells, this current is sufficient to cause a substantial depolarisation. To gain further insight into the possible origin of this current, I determined the current-voltage (I/V) relation for

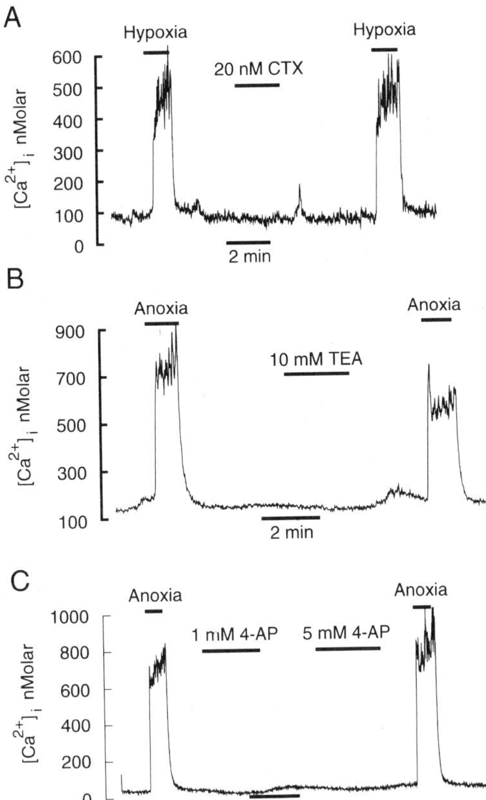

Figure 1. Effects of K-channel inhibitors on intracellular calcium in neonatal rat type-I cells. **A**. Effects of 20 nM charybdotoxin; similar results obtained in 4 other cells. **B**. 20 mM tetraethylammonium; similar results seen in 4 other cells. **C**. 1 and 5 mM 4-aminopyridine; similar results in 4 other cells.

type-I cells over a limited range of potentials from -90 to -30 mV. I/V relations were determined by averaging 10 to 20 individual current records obtained in response to a ramp depolarisation both under control and anoxic conditions. Anoxia was observed to caused a marked flattening of the cell's current voltage relation (Fig 2B). The mean membrane resistance, measured from -50 to -60 mV, was 3.1 ± 0.5 GΩ under normoxic conditions, and 7.6 ± 2.2 GΩ under anoxic conditions (n = 5; P<0.05). This decrease in membrane conductance suggested that anoxia might be inhibiting an outward current. The I/V relation of this oxygen-sensitive resting current (given as the difference control-anoxia; Fig 2B) shows a reversal potential of about -90 mV in normal extracellular $[K^+]_o$ further suggesting that this current might be carried by potassium ions (theoretical reversal potential for K-current under these conditions: E_K = -91 mV). In order to confirm the role of K^+-ions in mediating this current, a second I/V relation was constructed at 20 mM extracellular K^+. This second I/V relation shows a marked positive shift in the reversal potential of the anoxia sensitive current to -51 mV (E_K = -52 mV). These results confirm that this oxygen-sensitive current is indeed carried by K^+ ions.

4. DISCUSSION

The data presented in this paper clearly shows that, in isolated rat type-I cells, TEA, 4-AP and charybdotoxin are unable to evoke a significant rise in intracellular calcium or

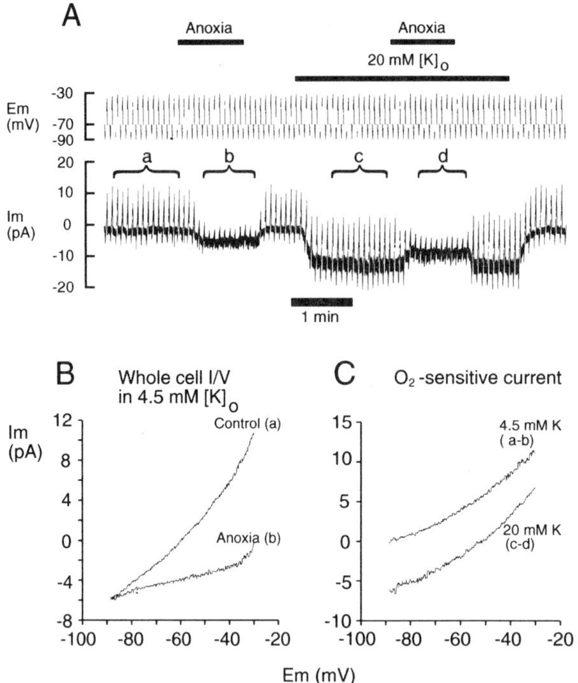

Figure 2. Effects of anoxia on type-I cells resting membrane conductance. **A.** Perforated patch recording of membrane current in an isolated neonatal rat type-I cell subjected to repetitive voltage ramps from -90 to -30 mV; holding potential = -70 mV. During first half of recording, cell bathed in normal bicarbonate Tyrode containing 4.5 mM $[K^+]_o$. In second half of recording, $[K^+]_o$ increased to 20 mM. Note that anoxia induces an inward shift in holding current in 4.5 mM $[K^+]_o$, but an outward shift at 20 mM $[K^+]_o$. **B.** Averaged ramp I/V curve constructed from data obtained during normoxia (period a) and anoxia (period b). Note that anoxia substantially decreases the cells resting conductance. **C.** O_2-sensitive difference currents obtained in 4.5 mM $[K^+]_o$ (a-b) and 20 mM $[K^+]_o$ (c-d).

membrane depolarisation. These results cast serious doubt upon the proposed role of BK_{Ca} channels, or indeed any other TEA, 4-AP or CTx sensitive K-channels in initiating the membrane depolarisation seen in hypoxia. These results are not entirely surprising, in view of the fact that in many cell types BK_{Ca} channels require either a strong depolarisation and/or a rise in $[Ca^{2+}]_i$ in order to be activated. Moreover, these observations are consistent with reports that TEA also fails to excite the intact rat carotid body (Donnelly, 1995).

Despite the above observations, the hypoxic receptor potential (depolarisation of type-I cells) results primarily from the inhibition of a resting potassium conductance. This potassium current however is insensitive to both TEA and 4-AP, and shows little voltage sensitivity (Buckler, 1996). It is therefore a new O_2-sensitive K^+-current, clearly distinct from both the BK_{Ca} or K_{O2}-channels.

In summary, these investigations have shed new light on the role of K^+ channels in O_2-chemoreception, in that it is now clear that the response to hypoxia cannot be explained by the inhibition of large voltage-gated K^+-conductances alone. Instead, it is proposed that the initial depolarisation, or receptor potential, is mediated via the inhibition of a small resting K^+ conductance. This will probably serve to initiate electrical activity and Ca^{2+} influx, which could then be further controlled by the modulation of voltage-gated/Ca^{2+}-dependent K^+ channels. Although such a role for BK_{Ca} channels remains to be formally proven, it has recently been reported that charybdotoxin, although not excitatory under normoxic conditions, can potentiate the effects of moderate hypoxia. In any event, since the receptor potential is primarily responsible for initiating electrical activity and/or Ca-influx, it is apparent that the O_2-sensitive resting K^+ current plays a major role in oxygen chemoreception in these cells.

5. ACKNOWLEDGMENTS

This work was supported by the MRC and the Wellcome Trust.

6. REFERENCES

Buckler KJ (1996) Effects of hypoxia on resting (leak) potassium conductance in carotid body type-I cells of the neonatal rat. J Physiol, London (in press)

Buckler KJ & Vaughan-Jones RD (1993) Effects of acidic stimuli on intracellular calcium in type-I cells of the neonatal rat carotid body. Pflügers Arch 425: 22–27

Buckler KJ & Vaughan-Jones RD (1994) Effects of hypoxia on membrane potential and intracellular calcium in rat neonatal carotid body type-I cells. J Physiol, London 476: 423–428

Donnelly DF (1995) Modulation of glomus cell membrane currents of intact rat carotid body. J Physiol, London 489: 677–688

Ganfornina MD & Lopez-Barneo J (1991) Single K^+ channels in membrane patches of arterial chemoreceptor cells are modulated by O_2 tension. Proc Natl Acad Sci USA 88: 2927–2930

Pepper DR, Landauer RC & Kumar P (1995) Effect of charybdotoxin on hypoxic chemosensitivity in the adult rat carotid body, in vitro. J Physiol, London 487: 177P

Wyatt CN & Peers C (1995) Ca^{2+}-activated K^+ channels in isolated type I cells of the neonatal rat carotid body. J Physiol, London 483: 559–565

12

IS CYTOCHROME P-450 INVOLVED IN HYPOXIC INHIBITION OF K^+ CURRENTS IN RAT TYPE I CAROTID BODY CELLS?

Christopher J. Hatton and Chris Peers

Institute for Cardiovascular Research
Leeds University
Leeds LS2 9JT, United Kingdom

1. INTRODUCTION

Patch-clamp studies of isolated type I carotid body cells have revealed that hypoxia inhibits K^+ channels (reviewed in Peers & Buckler, 1995). In cells isolated from young (*ca.* 10 days old) rats, hypoxia predominantly inhibits high conductance Ca^{2+}-activated K^+ (K_{Ca}) channels (Peers, 1990; Wyatt & Peers, 1995), an effect which leads to cell depolarization sufficient to open voltage-gated Ca^{2+} channels (Wyatt & Peers, 1995) and hence trigger Ca^{2+} influx (Buckler & Vaughan-Jones, 1994), which is necessary for initiation of transmitter release. Hypoxic inhibition of K_{Ca} channels is not a membrane-delimited effect, but requires undefined cytosolic factors (Wyatt & Peers, 1995).

In this study we investigated a possible involvement of cytochrome P-450, since pharmacological P-450 inhibitors mimic the inhibitory actions of hypoxia on K^+ currents in smooth muscle cells of the pulmonary vasculature (Yuan et al, 1995).

2. METHODS

Isolated type I cells were prepared by enzymatic digestion of carotid bodies taken from halothane-anaesthetized rat pups, as previously described (Wyatt & Peers, 1995).

Outward K^+ currents were recorded using whole-cell patch clamp techniques, whilst cells were perfused and dialysed with HEPES-buffered solutions of compositions described elsewhere (Peers, 1990; Peers & Green, 1991). Drugs were applied either by bath application during recordings or, in some cases, by incubation of cells for 1 h in a static solution containing the drug (see Results). Ca^{2+} channel currents were recorded using solutions designed to block outward K^+ currents and with 10 mM Ba^{2+} as charge carrier (see Peers & Green, 1991, for further details). All currents were evoked from a holding potential of -70 mV using 50 ms step depolarizations, and all experiments were conducted at

Frontiers in Arterial Chemoreception, edited by Zapata *et al.*
Plenum Press, New York, 1996

room temperature (21–24°C). Currents were filtered at 1 kHz and digitised at 2–5 kHz for off-line measurement of amplitude using pClamp software (Axon Instruments).

3. RESULTS

Bath application of the imidazole antimycotic P-450 inhibitors miconazole or clotrimazole caused time-dependent, poorly reversible inhibitions of K^+ currents in type I cells. For example, currents were inhibited by 70.1 ± 4.8% with 3 μM miconazole ($p < 0.005$, paired Student's *t*-test) after 3 min application (*e.g.*, Fig 1A). Miconazole also irreversibly inhibited Ca^{2+} currents, by 38.6 ± 4.6% (3 μM, 3 min application, $p < 0.01$, *e.g.*, Fig 1B). By contrast, acute (3 min) application of the suicide substrate P-450 inhibitor 1-aminobenzotriazole (1-ABT) was without effect on K^+ (Fig 1C) or Ca^{2+} current amplitudes (Fig 1D).

Hypoxia (PO_2 16–23 Torr) reversibly inhibited K^+ currents in type I cells by 30.5 ± 4.4% (n = 16, $p < 0.01$), and under hypoxic conditions miconazole (3 μM) was without significant further effect (n = 6 cells; *e.g.*, Fig 2A). Furthermore, as illustrated in Figure

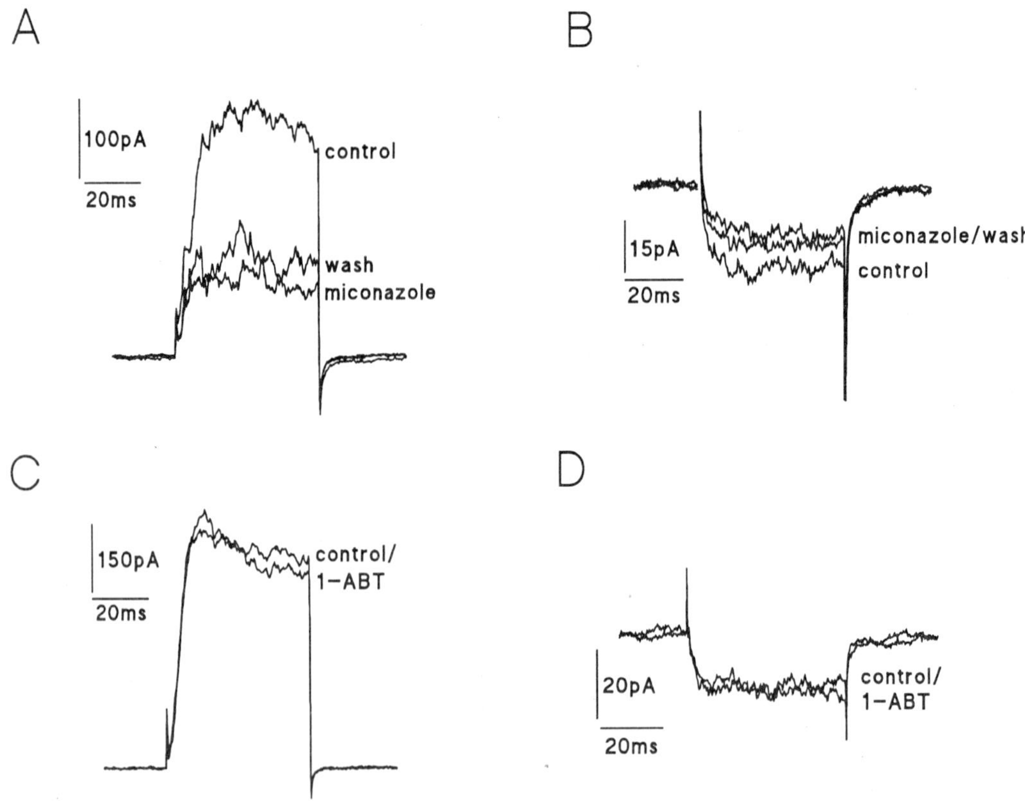

Figure 1. (**A**) K^+ currents evoked in a type I cell by step depolarizations from -70 mV to +20 mV before, during and after bath application of 3 μM miconazole, as indicated. (**B**) Ca^{2+} channel currents recorded in another type I cell by step depolarizations from -70 mV to 0 mV before, during and after bath application of 3 μM miconazole, as indicated. (**C**) K^+ currents recorded as in A, except that 3 mM 1-ABT was applied to the cell as indicated. (**D**) Ca^{2+} currents recorded as in B, except that 3 mM 1-ABT was applied to the cell, as indicated.

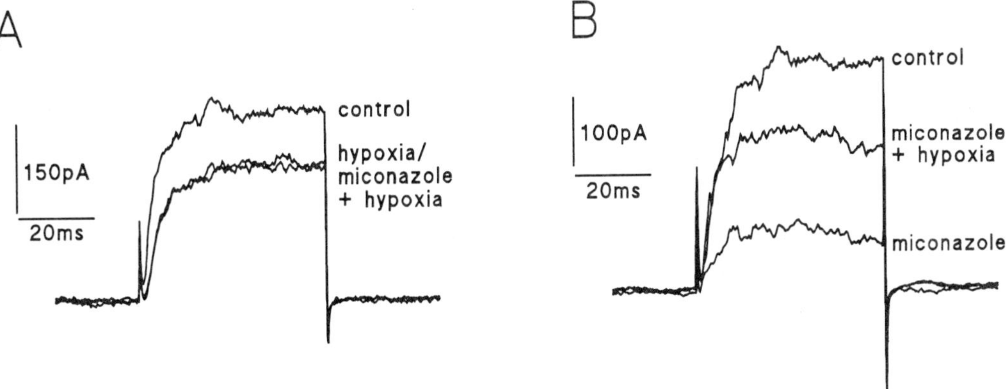

Figure 2. **(A)** K^+ currents recorded in a type I cell by step depolarizations from -70 mV to +20 mV before and during hypoxia (PO_2 ~ 20 Torr) as indicated, then following application of 3 μM miconazole in the continued presence of hypoxia. **(B)** K^+ currents evoked in another type I cell by step depolarizations from -70 mV to +20 mV before and during application of miconazole, then after lowering PO_2 to ~ 20 Torr in the continued presence of 3 μM miconazole, as indicated.

2B, hypoxia caused partial reversal of the inhibition caused by miconazole, a result consistently seen in 5 cells. Although 1-ABT was without effect when applied acutely (Fig 1C), we found that when cells were incubated in its presence for 1 h, these cells had a significantly ($p < 0.02$ unpaired Student's *t*-test) smaller response to hypoxia in terms of K^+ current inhibition (11.3 ± 2.9% inhibition, *e.g.*, Fig 3, representative of 6 cells studied) than cells which were not pre-incubated with 1-ABT.

4. DISCUSSION

Our results indicate that imidazole antimycotic P-450 inhibitors block ionic currents in type I cells non-selectively (Fig 1A, B), a finding which is distinct from the selective action of hypoxia on K_{Ca} channels (Wyatt & Peers, 1995). However, we also found that hypoxia prevented the inhibitory actions of miconazole, and indeed could reverse miconazole's inhibitory action when applied in normoxia (Fig 2). Hepatic P-450 activity is altered in hypoxia (Woodrooffe et al, 1995), and it is possible that hypoxia alters P-450 in type I cells in such a way as to prevent or at least reduce the effectiveness of miconazole. This tentative suggestion implies that P-450 is involved in the coupling of hypoxia to K^+ channel activity, and results obtained using 1-ABT further support this idea: 1-ABT is structurally and mechanistically distinct from miconazole, and did not affect K^+ or Ca^{2+}

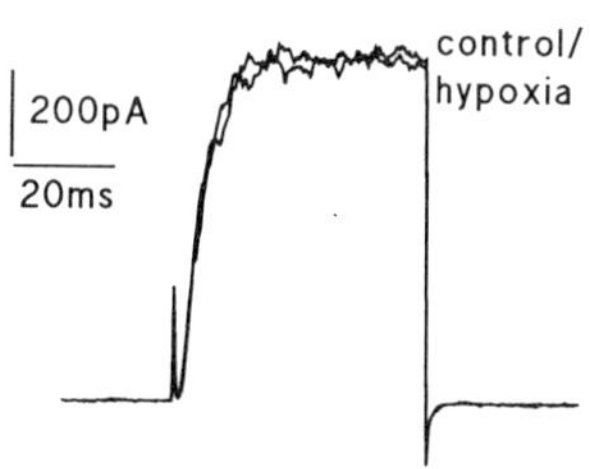

Figure 3. K^+ currents recorded in a type I cell using step depolarizations from -70 mV to +20 mV before and during exposure to hypoxic solution (PO_2 ~ 20 Torr). This cell had previously been incubated for 1 h with 3 mM 1-ABT. Note the reduced effect of hypoxia as compared with untreated cells (Fig 2A).

currents when applied acutely. However, after 1 h incubation with 1-ABT, hypoxia was found to be far less effective in suppressing K^+ currents (Fig 3).

The above findings suggest (on the assumption that the P-450 inhibitors used are selective agents) that P-450 may be involved in hypoxic inhibition of K^+ currents in type I cells.

5. ACKNOWLEDGMENTS

This work was supported by the British Heart Foundation. CJH is a B.H.F. PhD Student and CP is a B.H.F. Lecturer.

6. REFERENCES

Buckler KJ, Vaughan-Jones RD (1994) Effects of hypoxia on membrane potential and intracellular calcium in rat neonatal carotid body type I cells. J Physiol, London 476: 423–428

Peers C (1990) Hypoxic suppression of K^+ currents in type I carotid body cells: selective effect on the Ca^{2+}-activated K^+ current. Neurosci Lett 119: 253–256

Peers C & Green FK (1991) Intracellular acidosis inhibits Ca^{2+}-activated K^+ currents in isolated type I cells of the neonatal rat carotid body. J Physiol, London 437: 589–602

Peers C & Buckler KJ (1995) Transduction of chemostimuli by the type I carotid body cell. J Memb Biol 144: 1–9

Woodrooffe AJM, Bayliss MK & Park GR (1995) The effects of hypoxia on drug-metabolizing enzymes. Drug Metab Rev 27: 471–495

Wyatt CN & Peers C (1995) Ca^{2+}-activated K^+ channels in isolated type I cells of the neonatal rat carotid body. J Physiol, London 483: 559–565

Yuan X-J, Tod ML, Rubin LJ & Blaustein MP (1995) Inhibition of cytochrome P-450 reduces voltage-gated K^+ currents in pulmonary arterial myocytes. Am J Physiol 268: C259-C270

13

CYCLIC NUCLEOTIDE ANALOGS DO NOT INTERFERE WITH HYPOXIC INHIBITION OF K^+ CURRENTS IN ISOLATED RAT TYPE I CAROTID BODY CELLS

C. J. Hatton and C. Peers

Institute for Cardiovascular Research
Leeds University
Leeds LS2 9JT, United Kingdom

1. INTRODUCTION

Numerous reports have provided evidence to suggest that chemotransduction in the type I carotid body cell involves hypoxic inhibition of K^+ channels, which leads to cell depolarization, opening of voltage-gated Ca^{2+} channels and the consequent influx of Ca^{2+}, which triggers neurosecretion (González et al, 1994; Peers & Buckler, 1995). In adult rabbit type I cells, hypoxia inhibits K^+ channels in a membrane-delimited, possibly direct manner (Ganfornina & López-Barneo, 1991). However, in type I cells of young (approximately 10 days old) rats, hypoxia inhibits K^+ channels via a mechanism which involves an as yet unidentified cytosolic factor (Wyatt & Peers, 1995).

A series of independent reports have recently indicated that cyclic nucleotide levels in type I cells are influenced by hypoxia (Wang et al, 1989; Pérez-García et al, 1990; Delpiano & Acker, 1991): cyclic AMP (cAMP) levels are known to rise with lowered PO_2, whilst cyclic GMP (cGMP) levels fall, the latter being associated with reduced nitric oxide synthase activity which is located primarily in the endings of nerves closely associated with type I cells (see Prabhakar, 1994). In this study, we have investigated whether cAMP or cGMP can modulate K^+ currents as measured using whole-cell patch clamp techniques in young rat type I cells. Furthermore, we have investigated whether hypoxic inhibition of K^+ currents can be influenced by agents which alter intracellular cyclic nucleotide levels.

2. METHODS

Type I cells were isolated from rat pups using mechanical and enzymatic methods as previously described (Wyatt & Peers, 1995), and maintained in culture for up to 48 h. For

Frontiers in Arterial Chemoreception, edited by Zapata *et al.*
Plenum Press, New York, 1996

electrophysiological studies, cells were transferred to a perfused recording chamber. The perfusate was of composition (in mM): NaCl 135, KCl 5, $MgSO_4$ 1.2, $CaCl_2$ 2.5, HEPES 5, glucose 10 (pH 7.4, 21–24°C). Whole-cell patch-clamp recordings were made using pipettes (4–8 MΩ resistance) filled with (in mM): KCl 117, $CaCl_2$ 1, $MgSO_4$ 2, NaCl 10, EGTA 11, HEPES 11, ATP 2 (pH 7.2). Cells were voltage-clamped at -70 mV and step depolarized to various test potentials for 50 ms every 5 s. Evoked currents were filtered at 1–2 kHz and digitised at 2–5 kHz before being stored on computer for off-line analysis. All currents were measured for amplitude over the last 10–15 ms of a step depolarization or, if they displayed partial inactivation, at their peak. The various drugs tested (see Results) were bath applied either alone or, if they were not designed to be resistant to endogenous phosphodiesterases, in the presence of 0.5 mM isobutylmethylxanthine (IBMX). The effects of drugs and/or hypoxia are expressed as a percentage of the control (pre-drug or pre-hypoxia) current amplitude measured in the same cell before exposure to drug and/or hypoxia.

3. RESULTS

To investigate possible modulation of K^+ currents in type I cells by cyclic nucleotides, we bath-applied membrane permeable analogs of these messengers during whole-cell patch clamp recordings. Figure 1 illustrates the lack of effect of one such analog, Sp-cAMPS. Indeed, as summarized in Table 1, we tested the effects of four cAMP analogs, two cGMP analogs and the nitric oxide (NO) donor S-nitroso-N-acetylpenicillamine (SNAP). In short, none of the test compounds produced significant modulation of K^+ current amplitudes. Such results lead us to conclude that cyclic nucleotides do not appear to influence K^+ channel activity in type I cells under normoxic conditions.

We next investigated whether these compounds could in any way influence hypoxic inhibition of K^+ currents in type I cells. Figure 2 shows an example of such experiments. Hypoxia (PO_2 16–23 Torr) reversibly reduced K^+ current amplitudes in all cells studied, and application of either cAMP inhibitors or cGMP analogs or SNAP, failed to significantly alter the degree of hypoxic inhibition of K^+ currents. These findings are summarised in Table 2.

4. DISCUSSION

There is compelling evidence that cyclic nucleotide levels within type I cells are altered in hypoxia, and that pharmacological modulators of cyclic nucleotide levels can

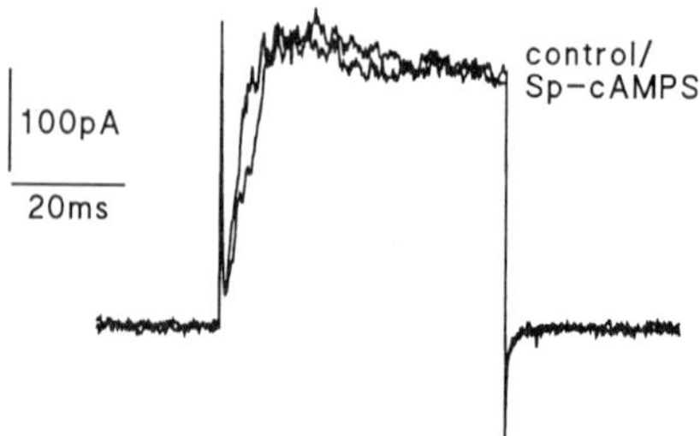

Figure 1. Outward K^+ currents recorded in a type I cell by step depolarizations from -70 mV to +20 mV before and during bath application of Sp-cAMPS (50 μM), as indicated.

Table 1. Effects of cyclic nucleotide analogs and SNAP on K^+ currents in type I cells

Analog	Concentration mM	% of control K^+ current amplitude	n
8-Br-cAMP*	2	91.6 ± 9.9	6
db-cAMP*	5	93.7 ± 4.5	4
Sp-cAMPS	0.05	93.9 ± 19.9	7
Sp-8-Br-cAMPS	0.05	90.1 ± 6.5	5
8-Br-cGMP*	2	102.9 ± 5.5	6
PET-cGMP	0.1	102.0 ± 7.3	10
SNAP	0.5	95.2 ± 5.2	4

*All currents were evoked by step depolarizations from -70 mV to +20 mV. Analogs marked * were applied in the presence of 0.5 mM IBMX to prevent degradation by phosphodiesterases.

strongly influence intact carotid body responses to hypoxia (see Introduction). These findings, coupled with our observation that hypoxic inhibition of K^+ currents in type I cells requires cytosolic factors, prompted us to investigate cAMP and cGMP as candidate mediators for the actions of hypoxia on K^+ channels in type I cells. Our results indicate that K^+ channel activity and its modulation by hypoxia is not affected by cAMP or by cGMP. These findings contrast with those of López-López et al (1993) who found cAMP to inhibit K^+ currents in rabbit type I cells. Since the analogs we used were highly active in other systems (we found them to fully relax Guinea pig basilar artery rings which had been pre-constricted with 20 mM K^+), the lack of cyclic nucleotide involvement in K^+ channel regulation in our rat type I cells may potentially indicate another species difference between rat and rabbit carotid body functioning.

In summary, our findings suggest that cyclic nucleotides are not involved in one of the early steps of type I cell hypoxic chemotransduction, namely the inhibition of K^+ channels. Obviously, there are numerous other steps within the chemotransductive pathway which lead to release of transmitters from type I cells, and many of these could provide target sites for the actions of cyclic nucleotides.

5. ACKNOWLEDGMENT

This work was supported by The British Heart Foundation.

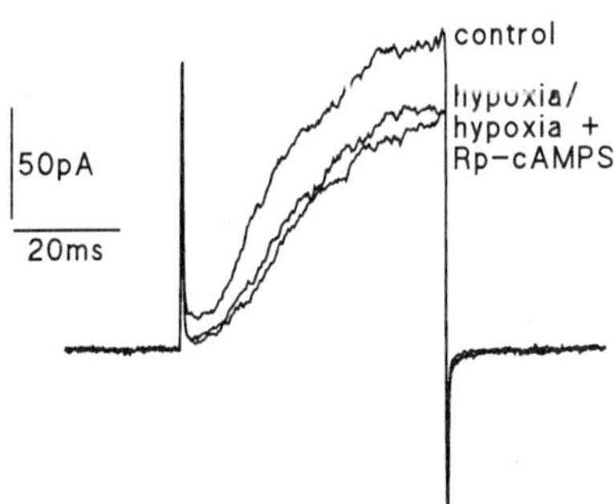

Figure 2. Outward K^+ currents recorded in a type I cell by step depolarizations from -70 mV to +20 mV before and during exposure to hypoxia (PO_2 ~ 20 Torr), and then during exposure to Rp-cAMPS in the continued presence of hypoxia.

Table 2. Effects of protein kinase A inhibitors, cGMP analogs and SNAP on the inhibition of K^+ currents by hypoxia

Agent used	Concentration mM	% K^+ current remaining in hypoxia	n
No added agent		69.5 ± 4.4	16
Rp-cAMPS	0.05	64.3 ± 6.0	6
Rp-8-Br-cAMPS	0.2	66.4 ± 6.4	4
8-Br-cGMP	2	73.2 ± 3.4	5
PET-cGMP	0.1	58.9 ± 12.3	3
SNAP	0.5	79.3 ± 5.5	6

All currents were evoked by step depolarizations from -70 mV to +20 mV. 8-Br-cGMP was applied in the presence of 0.5 mM IBMX. Hypoxic solutions were of PO_2 values between 16 and 23 Torr.

6. REFERENCES

Delpiano MA & Acker H (1991) Hypoxia increases the cyclic AMP content of the cat carotid body. J Neurochem 57: 291–297

Ganfornina MD & López-Barneo J (1991) Single K^+ channels in membrane patches of arterial chemoreceptor cells are modulated by O_2 tension. Proc Natl Acad Sci USA 88: 2927–2930

González C, Almaraz L, Obeso A & Rigual R (1994) Carotid body chemoreceptors: from natural stimuli to sensory discharges. Physiol Rev 74: 829–898

López-López JR, De Luis DA & González C (1993) Properties of a transient K^+ current in chemoreceptor cells of rabbit carotid body. J Physiol, London 460: 15–32

Peers C & Buckler KJ (1995) Transduction of chemostimuli by the type I carotid body cell. J Memb Biol 144: 1–9

Pérez-García MT, Almaraz L & González C (1990) Effects of different types of stimulation on cyclic AMP content in the rabbit carotid body: functional significance. J Neurochem 55: 1287–1293

Prabhakar NR (1994) Neurotransmitters in the carotid body. Adv Exp Med Biol 360: 57–70

Wang W-J, Cheng G-F, Dinger BG, Fidone SJ (1989) Effects of hypoxia on cyclic nucleotide formation in rabbit carotid body *in vitro*. Neurosci Lett 105: 164–168

Wyatt CN & Peers C (1995) Ca^{2+}-activated K^+ channels in isolated type I cells of the neonatal rat carotid body. J Physiol, London 483: 559–565

MODULATION OF VOLTAGE-GATED Ca^{2+} CHANNELS BY O_2 TENSION

Significance for Arterial Oxygen Chemoreception

Alfredo Franco-Obregón, Rafael Montoro, Juan Ureña, and
José López-Barneo

Departamento de Fisiología Médica y Biofísica
Facultad de Medicina
Universidad de Sevilla
E-41009 Sevilla, Spain

1. INTRODUCTION

Physiological adaptations to changes in oxygen availability are expressed in several tissues, which facilitate survival in situations of oxygen rarity, or hypoxia. These physiological responses to hypoxia are mediated by the arterial chemoreceptors which have classically been treated as synonymous with the carotid bodies (for a review see González et al, 1992) but which, in a broader sense, should also include the arterial smooth muscle cell layer (Sparks, 1980; Wadsworth, 1994). Among the acute responses to hypoxia are hyperventilation and active changes in vascular resistance controlling local circulation. Combined these physiological responses to hypoxia act to increase the uptake and ventilation of oxygen within the lungs, as well as, to better irrigate hypoxic regions of the body. Hyperventilation ensues from the activity of peripheral chemoreceptors located in the carotid and aortic bodies which transduce changes in blood oxygen content into neurosecretory activity. Chemotransduction in the carotid body has been attributed, among other factors, to the existence in glomus cells of K^+ channels regulated by blood PO_2 (López-Barneo et al, 1988; Delpiano & Hescheler, 1989). Thus, similar O_2-modulated ion channels may also be present in other tissues responsive to alterations in PO_2. We have recently demonstrated the existence of O_2-modulated Ca^{2+} channels in vascular smooth muscle cells where they may play a key role in the vasomotor responses to hypoxia (Franco-Obregón et al, 1995; Franco-Obregón & López-Barneo, 1996). A similar effect of PO_2 on the voltage-gated Ca^{2+} channels of the chemoreceptive cells of the rabbit carotid body has also been recently found (Montoro et al, 1996). Since in both preparations (glomus cells and vascular smooth muscle) the transduction of the hypoxic stimulus requires the modulation of cytosolic Ca^{2+} levels, the O_2-sensitive Ca^{2+} channels described here are well suited to confer chemoreceptive properties to these tissues.

Frontiers in Arterial Chemoreception, edited by Zapata *et al.*
Plenum Press, New York, 1996

2. O_2-SENSITIVITY OF Ca^{2+} CHANNELS IN VASCULAR SMOOTH MUSCLE AND VASOMOTOR RESPONSES TO LOW PO_2

Blood oxygen content is a key determinant in the local regulation of circulation (Sparks, 1980; Wadsworth, 1994). The systemic circulation is largely characterized by a vasodilatory response to regional decreases in PO_2 (Hellstrand et al, 1977; Detar, 1980; Marriot & Marshall, 1990). This systemic response acts to increase the perfusion of blood to oxygen deprived regions of the body. Although there is evidence implicating the endothelium in the elaboration of the hypoxic-vasomotor responses (Fredricks et al, 1994; Pittman, 1981), a considerable amount of work also suggests that these responses may be inherent to the arterial smooth muscle; for example, hypoxic vasodilatation has been observed in arteries denuded of the endothelium (Leach et al, 1994; Yuan et al, 1990) and in isolated arterial myocytes (Madden et al, 1992). Recently it was shown that Fura 2-loaded arterial myocytes exhibit spontaneous oscillations of cytosolic Ca^{2+}, or Ca^{2+} spikes (Fig 1; see also Franco-Obregón et al, 1995), much like those previously described in other cell

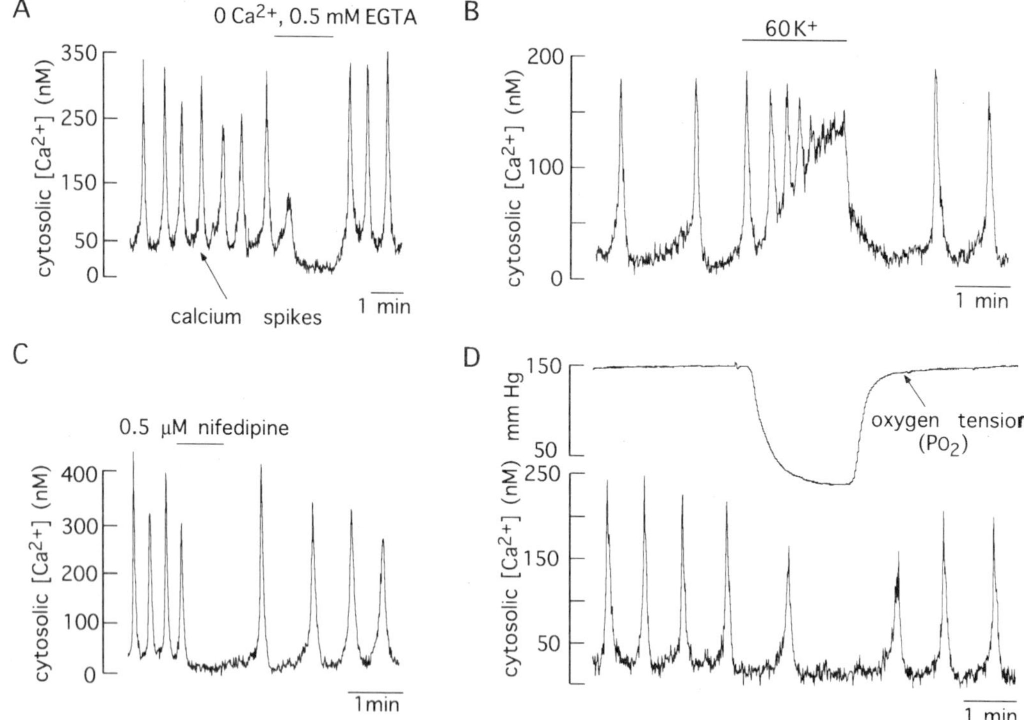

Figure 1. Oscillations of cytosolic $[Ca^{2+}]$ in arterial myocytes and their regulation by Ca^{2+} influx and ambient oxygen tension (PO_2). **A**. Suppression of the Ca^{2+} spikes after briefly removing external Ca^{2+}. **B**. Reversible increase of Ca^{2+} spike frequency in response to membrane depolarization with 60 mM extracellular K^+. **C**. Blocking the activity of voltage-dependent, L-type, Ca^{2+} channels with nifedipine also reversibly interrupts the Ca^{2+} spikes. **D**. Parallel recordings of bathing PO_2 and intracellular $[Ca^{2+}]$ in a fura-2-loaded myocyte illustrating the reversible inhibition of the Ca^{2+} oscillations (spikes) in response to hypoxia. Note that the spikes are reversibly suppressed upon reaching extreme low PO_2 levels (~20 mm Hg) as indicated from the signal from the oxygen-sensing electrode placed in the vicinity of the cell and shown above on the corresponding time base. The application of the different test solutions is indicated by the horizontal bars (Adapted from Franco-Obregón et al, 1995).

types (Girard & Clapham, 1993; Berridge, 1993) including vascular smooth muscle cells (Weissberg et al, 1989; Blatter & Weir, 1992). It can be shown that the Ca^{2+} spikes require the presence of extracellular Ca^{2+} for their generation as removing extracellular Ca^{2+} reversibly abolishes the spikes (Fig 1A). The pathway for Ca^{2+} entry into vascular smooth muscle appears to be voltage-gated, L-type, Ca^{2+} channels since depolarizing myocytes with elevated extracellular K^+ increases spike frequency (Fig 1B) while blocking the activity of L-type Ca^{2+} channels interferes with the generation of the Ca^{2+} spikes (Fig 1C). Interestingly, hypoxia also inhibits the generation of the Ca^{2+} spikes suggesting that low PO_2 may be attenuating the entry of extracellular Ca^{2+} through L-type Ca^{2+} channels (Fig 1D). These results are also in agreement with previous observations indicating that low PO_2 attenuates Ca^{2+} entry in arterial bath preparations (Ebeigbe et al, 1980; Marriott & Marshall, 1990; Pearce et al, 1992) as well as decreases cytosolic Ca^{2+} in arterial myocytes (Vadula et al, 1993).

Consistent with our intracellular Ca^{2+} measurements we found that the macroscopic Ca^{2+} current of systemic arterial myocytes is reversibly inhibited by low PO_2 (Fig 2). In the left set of current traces (recorded from a dispersed celiac myocyte) we examine the effect of hypoxia (h) on the Ca^{2+} current generated over a range of membrane potentials. For comparison we also include the current traces obtained in normoxia both before exposure to hypoxia (n) and following recovery (r). The extent of current inhibition (downward arrows) or potentiation (upward arrows) induced by hypoxia is shown next to their respective current traces. It is apparent that the effect of hypoxia on the whole-cell Ca^{2+} current is strongly voltage-dependent producing a marked inhibition of the current generated with moderate depolarizations while having very little effect, or even potentiating, the current

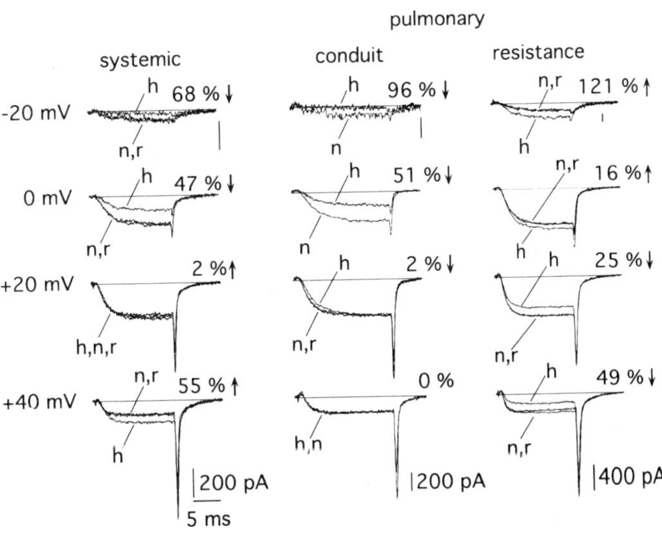

Figure 2. Differential O_2-sensitivity of Ca^{2+} channels in the systemic and pulmonary vasculature. Current traces demonstrating the effect of hypoxia (h) on the calcium currents elicited by voltage pulses to -20, 0, +20 and +40 mV (holding potential = -80 mV) in systemic (left), pulmonary conduit (middle) and pulmonary resistance (right) arterial myocytes. Control (n) and recovery (r) traces are shown superimposed. The changes in peak current amplitude expressed as percentage of the control values are given in each case near the set of traces. Upward arrows indicating potentiation and downward arrows indicating inhibition. In the recordings obtained at -20 mV (top) the vertical scale bars correspond to 100 pA (Adapted from Franco-Obregón & López-Barneo, 1996).

amplitude at strongly depolarized membrane potentials. Since it is well established that cytosolic [Ca^{2+}] is the variable that determines smooth muscle contractility (van Breemen & Saida, 1989) and that L-type Ca^{2+} channels are major regulators of smooth muscle tension (Nelson et al, 1990), it is reasonable to presume that the O_2-sensitive Ca^{2+} channels studied here directly contribute to the regulation of cytosolic Ca^{2+} and hence arterial tone.

The vasomotor responses of the pulmonary artery are somewhat more elaborated than those expressed by systemic arteries. As in systemic arteries, the main trunk and the large branches of the pulmonary artery vasodilate in response to alveolar hypoxia (Fishman, 1976). On the other hand, hypoxic vasoconstriction has been described for the finer more distal branches of the pulmonary artery (see, for example, Madden et al, 1992). The combination of these two responses divert pulmonary circulation to better ventilated alveolar regions of the lung. The middle and rightmost set of current traces in Figure 2 demonstrate the voltage-dependent effect of hypoxia on the Ca^{2+} currents recorded from conduit (main trunk; middle) and resistance (distal branches; right) regions of the pulmonary arterial tree. In myocytes isolated from the pulmonary main trunk (conduit) hypoxia exerts an effect much like that previously described in systemic myocytes; inhibition of current amplitude at negative membrane potentials while having little effect at more depolarized membrane potentials (Fig 2; middle). By contrast, an opposed voltage-dependence is observed in pulmonary myocytes isolated from the distal branches where low PO_2 can be shown to augment Ca^{2+} entry through L-type Ca^{2+} channels at negative membrane potentials (Fig 2; right). Therefore, over the range of membrane potentials normally experienced by vascular smooth muscle hypoxia would decrease resting Ca^{2+} entry in systemic and main pulmonary arteries while potentiate resting Ca^{2+} entry in resistance pulmonary myocytes.

3. DIFFERENTIAL O_2-SENSITIVITY OF Ca^{2+} AND K^+ CHANNELS AND CHEMOTRANSDUCTION IN THE CAROTID BODY

The carotid bodies respond to reductions in blood PO_2 with the release of neurotransmitters onto sensory afferents of the sinus nerve projecting to brain stem centers controlling breath rate; as a result they mediate reflexive hyperventilation in response to hypoxia. Rabbit glomus cells, the main elements in the carotid body, have been shown to be electrically excitable and are able to generate repetitive action potentials. Thus, it has been suggested that chemotransduction in the carotid body is conferred by a class of K^+ channel present in glomus cells whose activity is inhibited in response to a reduction of PO_2 (López-Barneo et al, 1988; González et al, 1992; Lopez-Barneo et al, 1993). Based on these findings a model was proposed whereby hypoxia, through its effect on O_2-regulated K^+ channels, depolarizes the cell, opening voltage-dependent Ca^{2+} channels and ultimately leading to neurosecretory activity (for reviews see González et al, 1992; López-Barneo et al, 1993).

Figure 3A illustrates the response of K^+ channels to low PO_2. With voltage-pulses to +20 mV (holding potential = -80 mV) the macroscopic K^+ current is reversibly inhibited by low PO_2 while the macroscopic Ca^{2+} current remains unaltered. Figure 3B, on the other hand, demonstrates that the Ca^{2+} currents of glomus cells is influenced by PO_2 but, as in vascular smooth muscle, the effect is markedly voltage-dependent. With voltage-pulses to 0 mV hypoxia produced a clear and reversible inhibition of the macroscopic Ca^{2+} current (Fig 3B; top). However, no effect of hypoxia was observed with voltage-pulses to +20 mV accounting for the previously undetected sensitivity of the Ca^{2+} current to low PO_2 at posi-

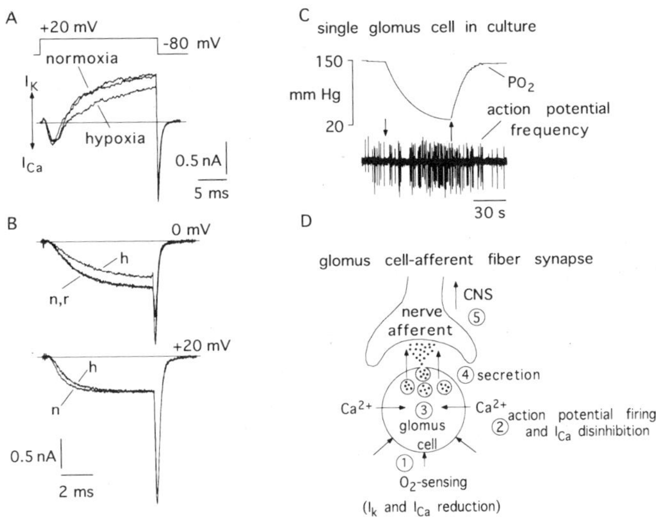

Figure 3. Chemotransduction in the mammalian carotid body and the differential regulation of K^+ and Ca^{2+} channels of glomus cells by PO_2. **A.** Differential effect of low PO_2 on the macroscopic K^+ and Ca^{2+} currents recorded simultaneously with voltage-pulses to +20 mV from the holding potential of -80 mV. The current traces while under normoxic conditions were recorded before the application of low PO_2 and following recovery of the current amplitude. With this voltage-pulse protocol low PO_2 selectively and reversibly inhibited the outward K^+ current without altering the inward Ca^{2+} current. **B.** Voltage-dependent inhibition of the Ca^{2+} current by hypoxia. Ca^{2+} currents were generated with voltage-pulses to the indicated membrane potentials from the holding potential of -80 mV. **C.** Reversible increase in action potential firing frequency (recording action currents with a cell-attached pipette) during exposure of a glomus cell in culture to low PO_2. The signal from the oxygen-sensing electrode placed in the vicinity of the cell is shown above for reference. **D.** Schematic diagram of the major steps in chemosensory transduction in glomus cells as described in the text. Panels A, B, C adapted from Montoro et al, 1996.

tive membrane potentials (compare with Fig 3A). The strong voltage-dependence of hypoxia on the Ca^{2+} currents could act as a molecular switch in the chemotransduction process of glomus cells. In this respect, mild hypoxia would initially prevent Ca^{2+} entry as a result of the inhibition of the Ca^{2+} current. However, at more extreme levels of hypoxia the K^+ current would also become strongly inhibited, depolarizing the cell and leading to an increase in action potential frequency. The resulting voltage-dependent disinhibition of the Ca^{2+} current would then allow Ca^{2+} entry into the cell and the subsequent liberation of neurotransmitters (see Montoro et al, 1996). Hypoxia can be shown to augment action potential frequency in spontaneously active individual glomus cells maintained in culture indicating that they possess similar properties as the entire carotid body (Fig 3C). Thus, O_2-sensitive ion channels seem to have a major role in the sensory function of the carotid body. Their contribution to chemotransduction in this organ can be explained by the simplified scheme shown in Figure 3D which qualitatively works as follows. Reductions of O_2 tension are detected by both voltage-dependent K^+ and Ca^{2+} channels (1); however, unlike the K^+ channels, the Ca^{2+} channels are totally released from the hypoxic inhibition at positive membrane potentials. The reduction of the K^+ conductance by hypoxia depolarizes the cell, increasing the frequency of action potentials which subsequently releases the Ca^{2+} channels from inhibition (2). The influx of Ca^{2+} through the channels raises cytosolic $[Ca^{2+}]$ (3), which, after reaching a threshold level, triggers transmitter release (4). Glomus cells are known to contain catecholamines and numerous neuropeptides; however, the transmitter that presumably activates the afferent fibers of the sinus nerve (5) is still unknown. Since the O_2-sensitive channels are voltage-dependent, this model implies that quiescent glomus cells will exhibit little sensitivity to PO_2 changes and that those glomus cells firing action potentials in normoxia are the most capable of transducing reductions of PO_2 into secretory signals.

4. CONCLUDING REMARKS

Here we describe the existence of voltage-dependent Ca^{2+} channels whose activity is regulated by PO_2. These channels are ubiquitous (López-Barneo, 1994), being observed in such diverse species as rabbit, rat and pig and in distinct tissues including the coronary, celiac, middle cerebral, femoral, mesenteric and pulmonary arteries, as well as in glomus cells of the carotid body. In vascular smooth muscle, where there is predominantly L-type Ca^{2+} channels, the effect of hypoxia appears to be specific for the L-type Ca^{2+} channels (Franco-Obregón et al, 1995). An additional level of specificity is demonstrated by the fact that low PO_2 inhibits the Ca^{2+} current of glomus cells and vascular smooth muscle of systemic and main pulmonary arteries while augmenting Ca^{2+} entry in resistance pulmonary myocytes. Furthermore, as the effect of hypoxia on the Ca^{2+} current occurs within a few seconds of lowering PO_2 and is unchanged following intracellular dialysis with either fluoride or GTP-g-S, agents known to irreversibly activate G-proteins, it appears that hypoxia acts via a membrane delimited mechanism without the involvement of soluble cytosolic mediators. Since both the hypoxic-vasomotor responses and chemotransduction in the carotid body require modifications of cytosolic Ca^{2+} concentrations, it is reasonable to presume that the O_2-sensitive Ca^{2+} channels described here help confer chemoreceptive properties to these tissues. Furthermore, the future identification of the molecular motifs conferring O_2-sensitivity will surely stimulate the design of pharmacological agents of use against systemic and pulmonary hypertension.

5. ACKNOWLEDGMENTS

This work was supported with grants from the *Dirección General de Investigación Científica y Técnica* (DGICYT) of the Spanish Ministry of Science and Education and the European Community (DGXII). Alfredo Franco-Obregón is a NSF-NATO Postdoctoral Fellow.

6. REFERENCES

Berridge MJ (1993) Inositol triphosphate and calcium signalling. Nature 361: 315–325

Blatter LA & Wier WG (1992) Agonist-induced $[Ca^{2+}]_i$ waves and Ca^{2+}-induced Ca^{2+} release in mammalian vascular smooth muscle cells. Am J Physiol 263: H576–586

Delpiano MA & Hescheler J (1989) Evidence for a PO_2-sensitive K^+ channel in the type I cell of the carotid body. FEBS Lett 249: 195–198

Detar R (1980) Mechanism of physiological hypoxia-induced depression of vascular smooth muscle contraction. Am J Physiol 238: H761-H769

Ebeigbe AB, Pickard JD & Jennett S (1980) Responses of systemic vascular smooth muscle to hypoxia. Quart J Exp Physiol 65: 273–292

Fishman AP (1976) Hypoxia on the pulmonary circulation: how and where it acts. Circ Res 38: 221–231

Franco-Obregón A & López-Barneo J (1996) Differential oxygen sensitivity of calcium channels in rabbit smooth muscle cells of conduit and resistance pulmonary arteries. J Physiol, London 491: 511–518

Franco-Obregón A, Ureña J & López-Barneo J (1995) Oxygen-sensitive calcium channels in vascular smooth muscle and their possible role in hypoxic arterial relaxation. Proc Natl Acad Sci USA 92: 4715–4719

Fredricks KT, Liu Y & Lombard JH (1994) Response of extraparenchymal resistance arteries of rat skeletal muscle to reduced PO_2. Am J Physiol 267: H706-H715

Girad S & Clapham D (1993) Acceleration of intracellular calcium waves in xenopus by calcium influx. Science 260: 229–232

González C, Almaraz L, Obeso A & Rigual R (1992) Oxygen and acid chemoreception in the carotid body chemoreceptors. Trends Neurosci 4: 146–153

Hellstrand P, Johansson B & Norberg K (1977) Mechanical, electrical and biochemical effects of hypoxia and substrate removal on spontaneously active vascular smooth muscle. Acta Physiol Scand 100: 69–83

Leach RM, Robertson TP, Twort CHC & Ward JPT (1994) Hypoxic vasoconstriction in rat pulmonary and mesenteric arteries. Am J Physiol 266: L223-L231

López-Barneo J (1994) Oxygen-sensitive ion channels: how ubiquitous are they? Trends Neurosci 17: 133–135

López-Barneo J, López-López JR, Ureña J & González C (1988) Chemotransduction in the carotid body: K^+ current modulated by PO_2 in type I chemoreceptor cells. Science 242: 580–582

López-Barneo J, Benot AR & Ureña J (1993) Oxygen sensing and the electrophysiology of arterial chemoreceptor cells. News Physiol Sci 8: 191–195

Madden JA, Vadula MS & Kurup VP (1992) Effects of hypoxia and other vasoactive agents on pulmonary and cerebral artery smooth muscle cells. Am J Physiol 263: L384-L393

Marriott JF & Marshall JM (1990) Differential effects of hypoxia upon contractions evoked by potassium and noradrenaline in rabbit arteries *in vitro*. J Physiol, London 422: 1–13

Montoro RJ, Ureña J, Fernández-Chacón R, Alvarez de Toledo G & López-Barneo J (1996) Oxygen sensing by ion channels and chemoreception in single glomus cell. J Gen Physiol 107: 133–143

Nelson MT, Patlak JB, Worley JF & Standen NB (1990) Calcium channels, potassium channels and voltage-dependence of arterial smooth muscle tone. Am J Physiol 259: C3-C18

Pearce WJ, Ashwal S, Long DL & Cuevas J (1992) Hypoxia inhibits calcium influx in rabbit basilar and carotid arteries. Am J Physiol 262: H106-H113

Pittman RN (1981) Influence of O_2 lack on smooth muscle contraction. In: Vanhoutte PM & Leusen I (eds) Vasodilatation. New York: Raven Press. pp 181–191

Sparks H (1980) Effect of local metabolic factors on vascular smooth muscle. In: Handbook of Physiology, sect 3: The Cardiovascular System, vol II: Vascular Smooth Muscle (Bohr DF, Somlyo AP & Sparks HV, eds). Bethesda, MD: American Physiological Society. pp 475–513

Vadula MS, Kleinman JG & Madden JA (1993) Effect of hypoxia and norepinephrine on cytoplasmic free Ca^{2+} in pulmonary and cerebral arterial myocytes. Am J Physiol 256: L591-L597

van Breemen C & Saida K (1989) Cellular mechanisms regulating $[Ca^{2+}]_i$ in smooth muscle. Annu Rev Physiol 51: 315–329

Wadsworth RM (1994) Vasoconstriction and vasodilator effects of hypoxia. Trends Physiol Sci 15: 47–53

Weissberg PL, Little PJ & Bobik A (1989) Spontaneous oscillations in cytoplasmic calcium concentration in vascular smooth muscle. Am J Physiol 256: C951-C957

Yuan X, Tod ML, Rubin LJ & Blaustein MP (1990) Contrasting effects of hypoxia on tension in rat pulmonary and mesenteric arteries. Am J Physiol 259: H281-H289

Ca^{2+} CHANNEL CURRENTS IN TYPE I CAROTID BODY CELLS FROM NORMOXIC AND CHRONICALLY HYPOXIC RATS

E. Carpenter,[1] C. N. Wyatt,[2] C. J. Hatton,[1] D. Bee,[3] and C. Peers[1]

[1] Institute for Cardiovascular Research
Leeds University
Leeds LS2 9JT, UK
[2] Department of Pharmacology
Royal Free Hospital Medical School
London, United Kingdom
[3] Department of Medicine
Royal Hallamshire Hospital
Sheffield, United Kingdom

1. INTRODUCTION

Rats born and reared under chronically hypoxic (10% O_2) conditions do not respond to acute hypoxia with an increased ventilation. Their carotid bodies undergo hyperplasia and hypertrophy and we have recently shown that K^+ channels recorded in type I carotid body cells isolated from normal and chronically hypoxic (CH) rats show marked differences (Wyatt et al, 1995): normoxic type I cells express Ca^{2+}-activated K^+ (K_{Ca}) channels which are inhibited by acute hypoxia, leading to cell depolarization, opening of voltage-gated Ca^{2+} channels (VGCCs) and the consequent influx of Ca^{2+} to trigger neurotransmitter release (Peers & Buckler, 1995). In type I cells from CH rats, there is far less expression of K_{Ca} channels, and, whilst the remaining K^+ channels are inhibited by hypoxia, this does not lead to cell depolarization, which may explain the lack of ventilatory response to acutely inspired hypoxia in intact CH rats (Wyatt et al, 1995). An important factor in the response of normal type I cells to hypoxia is the activation of VGCCs, of which numerous sub-types exist in various tissues. It is known that L-type VGCCs are involved in hypoxic chemotransduction (Buckler & Vaughan-Jones, 1994), but very little is known about the possible presence of other VGCCs, whether they may be involved in chemotransduction, and whether they are affected by chronic hypoxia. We have therefore compared the properties of VGCCs in type I carotid body cells isolated from normoxically-reared and CH rats.

Frontiers in Arterial Chemoreception, edited by Zapata *et al.*
Plenum Press, New York, 1996

2. METHODS

Type I cells were enzymatically isolated from carotid bodies of young (*ca.* 10 days) rats reared normally or in a 10% O_2 chamber, as previously described (Wyatt & Peers, 1995). Whole-cell Ca^{2+} channel currents were recorded from individual type I cells using patch pipettes filled with (in mM): CsCl 130, EGTA 1.1, $MgCl_2$ 2, $CaCl_2$ 0.1, NaCl 10, HEPES 10, ATP 2 (pH 7.2), and cells were perfused with a solution of (in mM): NaCl 110, CsCl 5, $MgCl_2$ 0.6, $BaCl_2$ 10, HEPES 5, glucose 10, tetraethylammonium 20 (pH 7.4, 21–24°C). Cells were voltage-clamped usually at -70 mV and step depolarized to various test potentials for 50 ms at a frequency of 0.2 Hz. Evoked currents were filtered (1–2 kHz) and digitised at 5 kHz for off-line analysis of amplitudes using the pClamp software suite (Axon Instruments), following leak subtraction which was achieved by the subtraction of appropriately scaled average currents evoked by small (≤30 mV) depolarizing and hyperpolarizing steps.

3. RESULTS

In both control and CH type I cells, step depolarizations activated VGCCs at -40 mV and more positive potentials. Our first aims were to investigate the pharmacological properties of these currents, and we found that bath application of the L-type Ca^{2+} channel agonist Bay K 8644 always (n = 6 control and 6 CH cells) enhanced current amplitudes (*e.g.*, Fig 1A), indicating that L-type channels were always present in both populations of cells. A supramaximal concentration (5 μM) of the antagonist nifedipine was also tested, and again always partially reduced current amplitudes in both control and CH cells (*e.g.*, Fig 1B). The degree of inhibition was variable from cell to cell (ranging from 28% to 83% inhibition), suggesting that channels other than L-type were also present in these cells. To investigate the presence of N-type channels we tested the effects of 1 μM ω-conotoxin GVIA (ω-CgTx). In 3 of 12 control cells and 2 of 15 CH cells, ω-CgTx caused partial, irreversible current inhibition but in the remaining cells of each population the toxin was without effect (Fig 2). These findings suggest a heterogeneous distribution of N-type Ca^{2+} channels in type I cells.

Although the voltage-dependence of Ca^{2+} channel currents appeared indistinguishable between the two cell types studied, we noted that Ca^{2+} current amplitudes were greater in CH cells (Fig 3A). This does not appear, however, to be a specialised adaptive

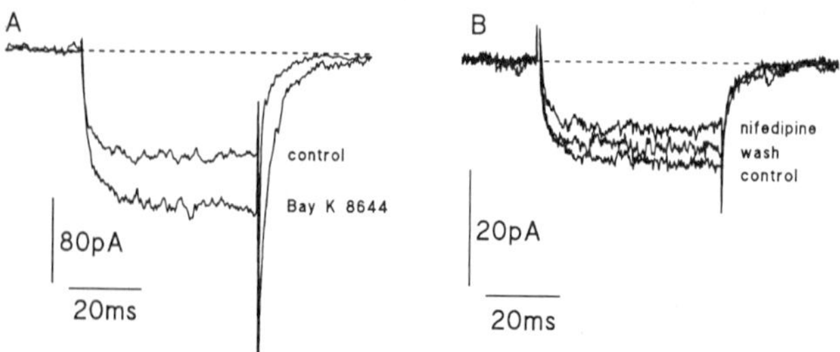

Figure 1. Ca^{2+} channel currents evoked in type I cells by step depolarizations to 0 mV from -70 mV before and during bath application of 2 μM Bay K 8644 (A, CH cell) or 5 μM nifedipine (B, normoxic cell). Similar results were obtained in both normoxic and CH type I cells with both drugs.

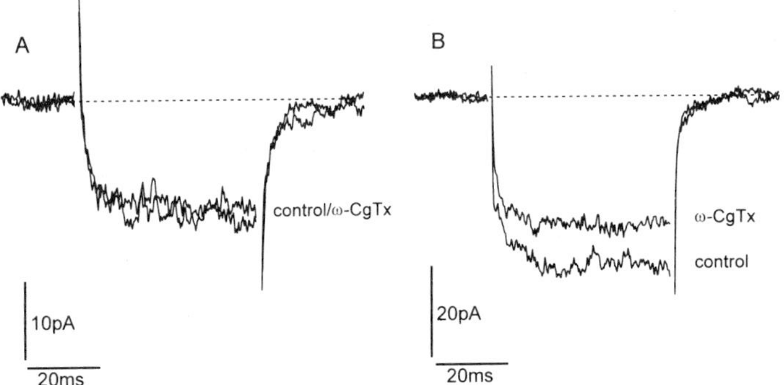

Figure 2. Example Ca^{2+} channel currents (evoked by step depolarizations from -70 mV to 0 mV) before and during application of 1 μM ω-CgTx. In most cells (*e.g.* A, normoxic cell) ω-CgTx was without effect but in some cells ω-CgTx caused irreversible, partial current inhibition (*eg.* B, normoxic cell). Similar results were obtained in CH type I cells.

change because when corrected for cell size — CH type I cells being larger than control cells (Wyatt et al, 1995) — current density was not significantly different between the two cell types, being ~ 10 pA/pF at a test potential of 0 mV. Steady-state inactivation curves (Fig 3C) also failed to distinguish between the two cell types. Boltzmann fits to the two sets of data yielded $V_{1/2}$ and slope factors of -36 mV and 10 mV for control and -34 mV and 11 mV for CH cells.

4. DISCUSSION

Our studies have revealed that all type I cells from young rats possess L-type Ca^{2+} channels, and that other channel types also exist. In the minority of cells, N-type Ca^{2+} channels appear to be present, a finding consistent with the observations of Fieber & McCleskey (1993). A recent study in adult rat type I cells (e Silva & Lewis, 1995) indi-

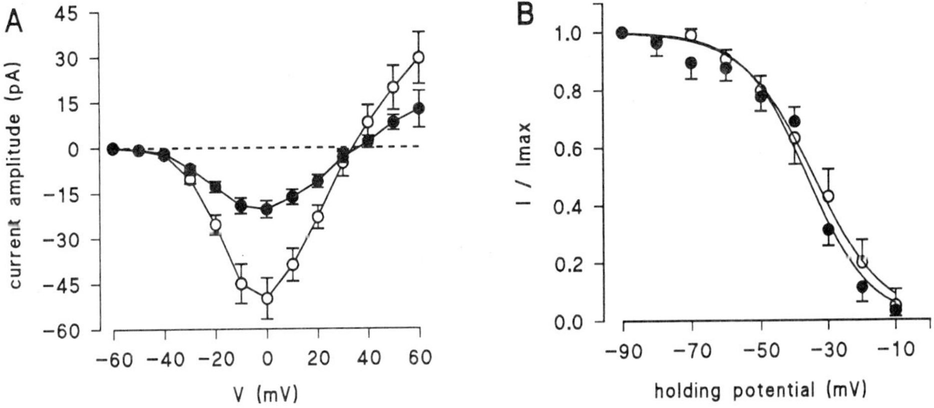

Figure 3. (A) Mean (± SEM) Ca^{2+} current voltage relationships obtained from 14 normoxic type I cells (filled circles) and 19 CH type I cells (open circles). Holding potential -70 mV. (B) Steady state inactivation curves obtained by step depolarizations to 0 mV from various holding potentials. Current amplitudes were normalized to those obtained from -90 mV. Control cells (filled circles) (n = 5), CH cells (open circles) (n = 7).

cates that N-type channels are always present, which could imply that our type I cells are not fully mature in terms of expression of N-type Ca^{2+} channels. Hypoxia elevates $[Ca^{2+}]_i$ in these young rat cells by stimulating influx of Ca^{2+} via VGCCs and this influx cannot be fully abolished even using 10 μM nicardipine (Buckler & Vaughan-Jones, 1994), suggesting even at this age that VGCCs other than L-type may have a role to play in hypoxic chemotransduction. It is noteworthy that in the present study nifedipine never fully abolished current amplitudes, and ω-gTx was only effective in some cells; taken together, these findings indicate the likely presence of other sub-types of VGCCs in these cells.

Ca^{2+} channel currents recorded from CH type I cells were very similar to those recorded in normoxic cells, except that current amplitudes were larger. The increased amplitude was accounted for by increased cell size (Wyatt et al, 1995), indicating that no specific adaptive changes were detected in Ca^{2+} currents which could be attributed to chronically hypoxic conditions: in both cell types, evidence for L- and N-type (and other) channels was found, and since the cells have very similar resting potentials (*ca.* -40 to -45 mV) (Wyatt et al, 1995), in both cases the majority of Ca^{2+} channels are available for activation upon cell depolarization (Fig 3B). It thus appears that the effects of chronic hypoxia on K^+ currents (Wyatt et al, 1995) is a selective adaptive effect, and Ca^{2+} channel currents are not modulated by prolonged hypoxic conditions.

5. ACKNOWLEDGMENTS

This work was supported by The Wellcome Trust.

6. REFERENCES

Buckler KJ & Vaughan-Jones RD (1994) Effects of hypoxia on membrane potential and intracellular calcium in rat neonatal carotid body type I cells. J Physiol, London 476: 423–428

Fieber LA & McCleskey EW (1993) L-type Ca^{2+} channels in type I cells of the rat carotid body. J Neurophysiol 70: 1378–1384

Peers C & Buckler KJ (1995) Transduction of chemostimuli by the type I carotid body cell. J Memb Biol 144: 1–9

e Silva MJM & Lewis DL (1995) L- and N-type Ca^{2+} channels in adult rat carotid body chemoreceptor type I cells. J Physiol, London 489: 689–699

Wyatt CN & Peers C (1995) Ca^{2+}-activated K^+ channels in isolated type I cells of the neonatal rat carotid body. J Physiol, London 483: 559–565

Wyatt CN, Wright C, Bee D & Peers C (1995) O_2-sensitive K^+ currents in carotid body chemoreceptor cells from normoxic and chronically hypoxic rats and their roles in hypoxic chemotransduction. Proc Natl Acad Sci USA 92: 295–299

METABOLIC INHIBITORS AFFECT THE CONDUCTANCE OF LOW VOLTAGE-ACTIVATED CALCIUM CHANNELS IN BRAIN CAPILLARY ENDOTHELIAL CELLS

M. A. Delpiano

Max-Planck-Institut für Molekulare Physiology
Dortmund, Germany

1. INTRODUCTION

The brain capillary endothelium plays an essential role in the preservation of the blood-brain barrier and in the control of blood microcirculation. Since hypoxia (Po_2: 20 Torr) increases K^+ conductance in brain capillary endothelial cells (BCECs) (Delpiano, 1994), the question arises whether chemical agents that impair cell metabolism may produce similar changes in Ca^{2+} conductance. To better understand the signal transduction mechanism that operates on BCECs during hypoxia and which may be of physiological relevance for the control of brain blood flow microcirculation, these cells were investigated in voltage-clamp experiments using the perforated nystatin patch-clamp technique (Horn & Marty, 1988).

2. MATERIAL AND METHODS

"Pure" inward Ca^{2+} currents on BCECs were obtained by superfusing cells with an extracellular solution composed of (in mM): N–methyl-D–glucamine 145, $CaCl_2$ 10, $MgCl_2$ 1.2, HEPES 10, and glucose 5.5, adjusted with HCl to a pH of 7.4 and with sucrose to 300 mOsm. The tip of fire-polished borosilicate pipettes, of 3 mΩ resistance, was filled with an intracellular solution composed of (in mM): CsCl 50, Cs_2SO_4 70, $MgCl_2$ 1.2, HEPES 10, glucose 10, adjusted with CsOH to a pH of 7.28 and with sucrose to 290 mOsm. Immediately before each cell recording, pipettes were back-filled with the same intracellular solution sonicated with 200 µg/ml nystatin (stock solution 60 mg/ml in dimethylsulfoxide). Fresh dissociated BCECs resuspended on a glass cover-slip and continuously superfused in a small chamber (400 µl) were recorded at room temperature (21–24°C). After formation of a gigaohm seal (5–10 GΩ), the progressive perforation of

Frontiers in Arterial Chemoreception, edited by Zapata *et al.*
Plenum Press, New York, 1996

cell membrane by nystatin was monitored by measuring series resistance with an EPC-7 patch preamplifier (HEKA Elektronik, Germany), until a whole-cell recording was achieved. Pulse protocols and data sampling were controlled using an HP microcomputer with a CED 1401 interface and software (Cambridge Instruments, UK). Different agents like sodium cyanide (NaCN), 4–dinitrophenol (DNP), acid stimuli (external solution adjusted with propionic acid) and low Po_2 were applied directly to the cells through a superfusion device connected to separated reservoirs, that allowed fast solution exchange (0.5 s). The Po_2 in the superfusion was monitored with a catheter electrode, as described elsewhere (Hescheler et al, 1989).

3. RESULTS AND DISCUSSION

BCECs clamped at a holding potential of –80 mV, under the recording conditions mentioned above (see Methods), exhibited inward currents of fast inactivation and low voltage-activation (LVA), when tested by depolarizing pulses (Fig 1A). These inward currents were not TTX (5 μM) sensitive, neither affected by replacing the external Na^+ ions, nor by dihydropyridine derivative, but affected by amiloride (50 μM) and Ni^{2+} (40 μM), as previously characterized (Delpiano & Cavalié, 1993). They represented LVA Ca^{2+} currents (T–type). As illustrated in the current-voltage (I-V) relationship of Figure 1B, LVA Ca^{2+} currents in BCECs exhibited a threshold for activation at a membrane potential of –60 mV, with a peak maximum of about 200 pAmp at a membrane potential of –25 mV. Although such voltage-activated Ca^{2+} channels have been considered absent in endothelial cells of large vessels, it seems that they are expressed in microvessels as shown herein, and in agreement with findings in endothelial cells of bovine adrenal medulla (Bossu et al, 1989).

Hypoxia and metabolic inhibitors (DNP and NaCN) activated the K^+ conductance in BCECs (Delpiano, 1994, 1996) in a similar mode as already found with Ca^{2+}-sensitive K^+ channels in smooth muscle cells (Gebremedhin et al, 1994; Miller et al, 1993). Since BCECs contain Ca^{2+}-sensitive K^+ channels, and they could be reversibly inhibited by 30 nM charybdotoxin (Delpiano, 1996), the question arose as whether the changes in the K^+

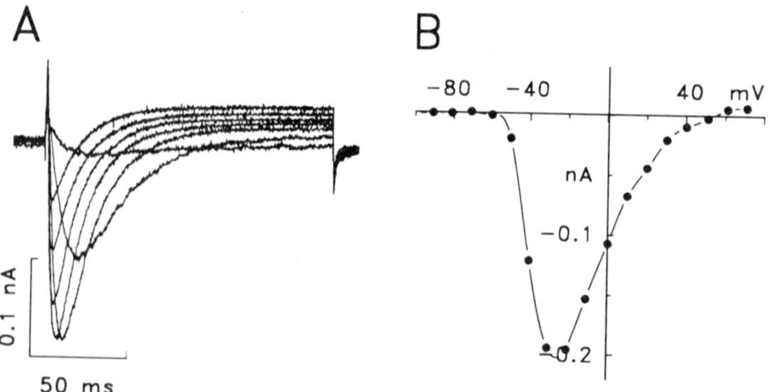

Figure 1. Ca^{2+} currents and current-voltage (I–V) relationship in BCECs. **A.** Original traces of voltage-activated Ca^{2+} elicited from a holding potential of –80 mV by depolarizing test pulses of 150 ms duration. Note fast inactivation. **B.** I–V relationship of Ca^{2+} currents in **A**, plotted from peak current *vs* membrane potential.

conductance produced by these agents could be indirectly ascribed to changes in Ca^{2+} influx by activation of Ca^{2+} channels. When experiments were initiated, the classical dialyzed whole-cell technique was used and the responsiveness of the Ca^{2+} channel was tested by low external pH, as LVA channels in BCECs are very sensitive to pH changes, as well as temperature (unpublished). As illustrated in Figure 2A (first response), when cells were exposed to a decrease of external pH of 1 unit (from pH 7.4 to 6.4), the Ca^{2+} current was reversibly depressed by about 43%. Under these recording conditions, knowing the viability of the channel, applying DNP at concentrations of 300 and 700 µM did not notably affect the current (second and thirst response). However, when the perforated nystatin whole-cell technique was used, as shown in Figure 2B, the Ca^{2+} current was depressed with increasing DNP concentrations of 100, 200 and 600 µM, by 80, 91 and 96%, respectively. This demonstrated, on the one side, that an intact cell structure was pre-condition to reveal the DNP effect and, on the other, that the above mentioned activation of the K^+ current observed with DNP (Delpiano, 1996) could not be ascribed, at least, to Ca^{2+} influx through LVA channels, although the participation of high voltage-activated (HVA) Ca^{2+} channels (L–type) can not be ruled out. It is worth to be mentioned that the necessity of an intact cell structure to reveal this effect of DNP pointed out to the requirement of essential intracellular compounds (phosphorylation, second messengers, high energy substrates) for the functional integrity of the Ca^{2+} channel-coupling. In this context, it was

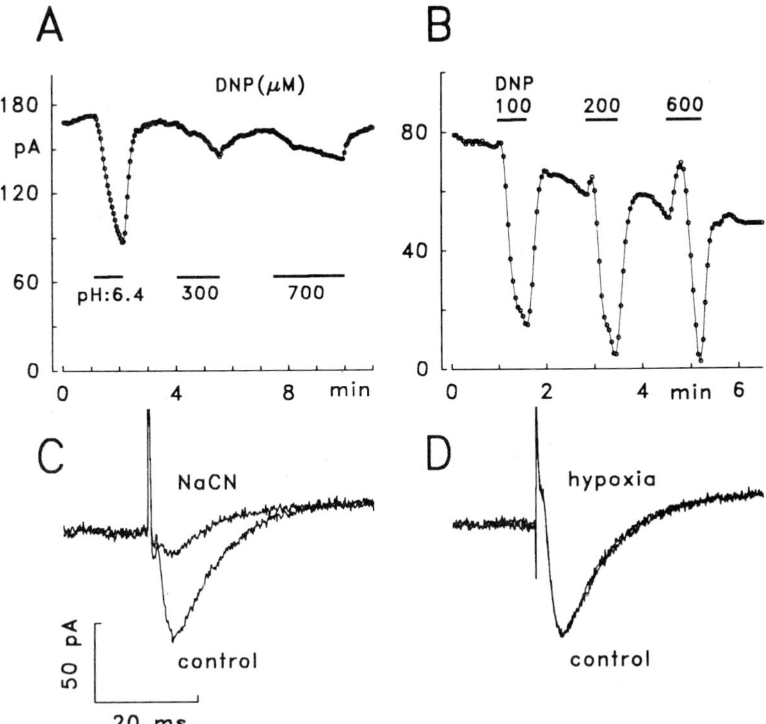

Figure 2. Effect of DNP, NaCN and hypoxia on low voltage-activated Ca^{2+} currents of BCECs. **A.** Effect of low pH and DNP on the peak current amplitude of a single current elicited by single test pulses to –25 mV at a holding potential of –80 mV. **B.** Similar experiment as in **A**, but using the perforated nystatin whole-cell technique. **C.** Effect of NaCN on single Ca^{2+} currents stimulated with a pulse protocol as in **A. D.** Effect of low Po_2 (12 Torr) on Ca^{2+} currents elicited as in **C.**

interesting to find out that an in initial Ca^{2+} current activation transiently appeared when the DNP concentration was step wise increased (Fig 2B). Since activation of T–type Ca^{2+} channels in adrenal glomerulosa cells required energy dependent processes (Lu et al, 1994), in analogy, one can speculate that this initial activation might be linked to an initial increase in cell metabolism produced by DNP, probably due through its uncoupler property. When the DNP concentration increased further, this initial uncoupler effect could be overcame through its protonophore property leading to cytosolic acidification and thereby to a breakdown of energy metabolism, the cause of the LVA channel inactivation, as reflected by the inward Ca^{2+} current (Fig 2B).

When BCECs were exposed to NaCN (2 mM), a blocker of the mitochondrial respiratory chain and therefore of the energy production, the Ca^{2+} current was reversibly depressed (Fig 2C), in a similar form as found with high DNP concentrations (Fig 2B). In contrast, hypoxia (Po_2: 12 Torr) did not affect the LVA Ca^{2+} current in BCECs (Fig 2D). This last result should be apparently in contradiction with the common targeting site for these stimuli, namely the impairment of the substrate-dependent energy production. A possible explanation for the lack of hypoxic effect could be either: 1) that LVA (T–type) Ca^{2+} channels are not involved in this transductory process, as presumed in smooth muscle cells (Franco-Obregón et al, 1995); or 2) that the Ca^{2+} channel, as in smooth muscle and glomus type I cells (Franco-Obregón et al, 1995; Montoro et al, 1996), underlies a strong voltage-dependent Po_2 regulation. According to this second possibility, which in BCECs needs further elucidation, an effect could be only revealed if during hypoxia the Ca^{2+} channel should not be maximal activated, *i. e.*, only depolarized to lower membrane potentials. In previous studies on glomus cells, no changes in the Ca^{2+} current were also found (López-Barneo et al, 1988; Hescheler et al, 1989). However, recent studies proved the opposite (Montoro et al, 1996). The effect in the Ca^{2+} conductance produced by DNP and NaCN in this study are in agreement with the observed hyperpolarization that these metabolic inhibitors, as well as hypoxia, induced in BCECs (Delpiano, 1996), and supports the idea that the transduction mechanism of the endothelium-dependent vasodilation, observed in systemic and brain vessels (Busse et al, 1983; Bereczki et al, 1993), should be closely mediated by these metabolic-regulated channels.

4. REFERENCES

Bereczki D, Wei L, Otsuka V, Acuff K, Pettigrew C & Fenstermacher J (1993) Hypoxia increases velocity of blood flow through parenchymal microvascular system in brain. J Cereb Blood Flow Metab 13: 465–486

Bossu JL, Feltz A, Rodeau JL & Tanzi F (1989) Voltage-dependent transient calcium currents in freshly dissociated capillary endothelial cells. FEBS Lett 255: 377–380

Busse R, Pohl U, Kellner C & Klemm U (1983) Endothelial cells are involved in the vasodilatory response to hypoxia. Pflügers Arch 397: 78–80

Delpiano MA (1994) Ionic currents on endothelial cells of rat brain capillaries. Adv Exp Med Biol 360: 183–186

Delpiano MA (1996) Transmembrane currents on endothelial cells from rat brain capillaries: Effect of hypoxia and inhibitors of cell metabolism. Am J Physiol (submitted)

Delpiano MA & Cavalié A (1993) Evidence for low-activated calcium channels on endothelial cells from rat brain capillaries. Eur J Neurosci, suppl 6: 949

Franco-Obregón A, Ureña J & López-Barneo L (1995) Oxygen-sensitive calcium channels in vascular smooth-muscle and their possible role in hypoxia. Proc Natl Acad Sci USA 92: 4715–4719

Gebremedhin D, Bonnet P, Greene AS, England SK, Rush NJ, Lombard JH & Harder DR (1994) Hypoxia increases the activity of Ca^{2+}-sensitive K^+ channels in cat cerebral arterial muscle cell membranes. Pflügers Arch 428: 621–630

Horn R & Marty A (1988) Muscarinic activation of ionic currents measured by a new whole-cell recording method. J Gen Physiol 92: 145–159

Hescheler J, Delpiano MA, Acker H & Pietruschka F (1989) Ionic currents on type-I cells of the rabbit carotid body measured by voltage-clamp experiments and the effect of hypoxia. Brain Res 486: 79–88

López-Barneo J, López-López JR, Ureña J & Gonzalez C (1988) Chemotransduction in the carotid body: K+ currents modulated by $P0_2$ in type I chemoreceptor cells. Science 241: 580–582

Lu HK, Fern RJ, Nee JJ & Barret PQ (1994) Ca^{2+}-dependent activation of T–type Ca^{2+}-channels by calmodulin-dependent protein kinase II. Am J Physiol 267: F183-F189

Miller AL, Morales E, Leblanc NR & Cole WC (1993) Metabolic inhibition enhances Ca^{2+}-activated K^+-current in smooth muscle cells of rabbit portal vein. Am J Physiol 265: H2184-H2195

Montoro RJ, Ureña J, Fernández-Chacón, Alvarez de Toledo G & López-Barneo J (1996) Oxygen sensing by ionic channels and chemotransduction in single glomus cells. J Gen Physiol 107: 133–143

TRANSMEMBRANE CURRENTS IN CAPILLARY ENDOTHELIAL CELLS ARE MODULATED BY EXTERNAL Mg^{2+} IONS

M. A. Delpiano[1] and Burton M. Altura[2]

[1] Max-Planck-Institut für molekulare Physiology
Dortmund, Germany
[2] Departments of Physiology and Medicine
State University of New York
Health Science Center at Brooklyn
New York, New York 11203

1. INTRODUCTION

The capillary endothelium of the brain is involved essentially in the preservation of the blood-brain barrier and in the regulation of brain microcirculation. As a biological membrane lining the inner wall of blood vessels, the endothelium is exposed to many environmental alterations of the blood composition. In this context, it is known that changes in the concentration of extracellular magnesium ions ($[Mg^{2+}]_o$) play important roles in the control of vascular reactivity, by modulating the myogenic tone and the contractile response of vascular smooth muscle cells to various physiological and pharmacological stimuli (Altura & Altura, 1981). Recent studies on endothelial cells demonstrate that changes in $[Mg^{2+}]_o$ can modify the state of the cytosolic free calcium (Zhang et al, 1993). The aim of the present study was, therefore, to investigate whether in fact this modulatory effect of Mg^{2+} could be ascribed to some effect on the excitability of the cell membrane of endothelial cells. For this purpose, transmembrane currents of rat brain capillary endothelial cells (BCECs) were investigated in whole-cell experiments with the patch-clamp technique (Hamill et al, 1981).

2. MATERIAL AND METHODS

Voltage-clamp experiments were performed on BCECs attached to a glass cover-slip and superfused in a polycarbonate chamber with an extracellular solution consisting of (in mM): NaCl 135, KCl 5.6, $CaCl_2$ 2.5, $MgCl_2$ 1.2, glucose 5.5, HEPES 10, adjusted to pH 7.4 with NaOH. Patch electrodes were prepared from borosilicate glass (Science Products,

Frontiers in Arterial Chemoreception, edited by Zapata *et al.*
Plenum Press, New York, 1996

Germany) and had a resistance of about 3 MΩ when filled with an intracellular solution consisting of (in mM): K^+-aspartate 80, KCl 50, $MgCl_2$ 1.2, EGTA 10, HEPES 10, pH: 7.28. All solutions had an osmotic pressure of 300 mOsm. To obtain inward Ca^{2+} currents without contaminating outward and inward components, the Na^+ and K^+ ions of the extra- and intracellular solutions were replaced by N–methyl-D–glucamine (NMDG) and the external Ca^{2+} concentration increased to 10 mM. Under voltage-clamp conditions, BCECs were clamped at a holding potential of –60 or –80 mV to record K^+ or Ca^{2+} currents, respectively. Currents were recorded during 150 ms test pulses to various membrane potentials to determine the current-voltage (I–V) relationship. The steady-state inactivation of the Ca^{2+} current was measured using a 50 ms test pulse to –20 mV from a holding potential of –90 mV, preceded by conditioning prepulses of 150 ms duration and starting from different holding potentials (range: –90 to –10 mV). The inactivation curve was fitted to the Boltzmann equation; $I/Imax = 1/\{1+\exp[-(CP-V_{0.5})/k]\}$, where CP is the amplitude of a conditioning prepulse, $V_{0.5}$ equals the half-maximal inactivation voltage and k is the inactivation slope. Pulse protocol and data acquisition were done as described elsewhere (Delpiano, 1996).

3. RESULTS AND DISCUSSION

When the $[Mg^{2+}]_o$ was increased from 1.2 (control) to 4.8 mM, the outward K^+ current was depressed by about 20% in a reversible form. The I–V curve in Figure 1A illustrates that this effect occurred at all activating potentials. This change could be observed in all experiments.

Since Mg^{2+}, as well known, is a mild blocker of Ca^{2+} channels (Altura & Altura, 1981), its depressing effect on low voltage-activated (LVA) Ca^{2+} currents of BCECs (Fig 1B) may be the cause for the K^+ current inactivation, taking into account that this current may be carried by Ca^{2+}-activated K^+ currents, which as previously demonstrated are present in BCECs (Delpiano, 1996). Herein, the property of high Mg^{2+} of preventing blood vessels tone (Turlapaty & Altura, 1978) should be closely related to its depressing action on this K^+ conductance, as demonstrated in this study.

When BCECs were exposed to a low $[Mg^{2+}]_o$ of 0.3 mM, unexpectedly, both the K^+ and Ca^{2+} current were mildly activated and depressed, respectively. The original traces of Figure 1C illustrate this effect on both currents when they were simultaneously elicited by clamping BCECs at a holding potential of –80 mV and stimulating them by depolarizing pulses. Since LVA Ca^{2+} currents, which predominate in BCECs, have a more negative threshold for activation (–50mV) than outward K^+ currents (–30mV), the differential effect of low Mg^{2+} on these currents could be revealed, as shown in Figure 1C. BCECs do not express Na^+ currents (Delpiano, unpublished observations). The effect of low Mg^{2+} on the Ca^{2+} current elicited by a pulse to –25 mV of Figure 1C is shown in more detail in Figure 1D. However, since this depressing effect of low Mg^{2+} on LVA currents contradicted its blocking property at high concentration (Fig 1B), a kind of negative screening was assumed rather than a true inhibition, *i. e.*, reduction of positive charges on the surface potential of the membrane. Therefore, the steady-state inactivation for the Ca^{2+} current under control and low Mg^{2+} was investigated.

Figure 2A shows the original Ca^{2+} currents elicited by a single depolarizing test pulse to –20 mV and 50 ms duration (**b**, inset of Fig 2A), from different holding potentials (**a**, inset of Fig 2A). In the lower panel of Figure 2A, it can be seen that the Ca^{2+} currents elicited under low Mg^{2+} exhibited a reduced activation compared to controls (upper panel). Such effect is

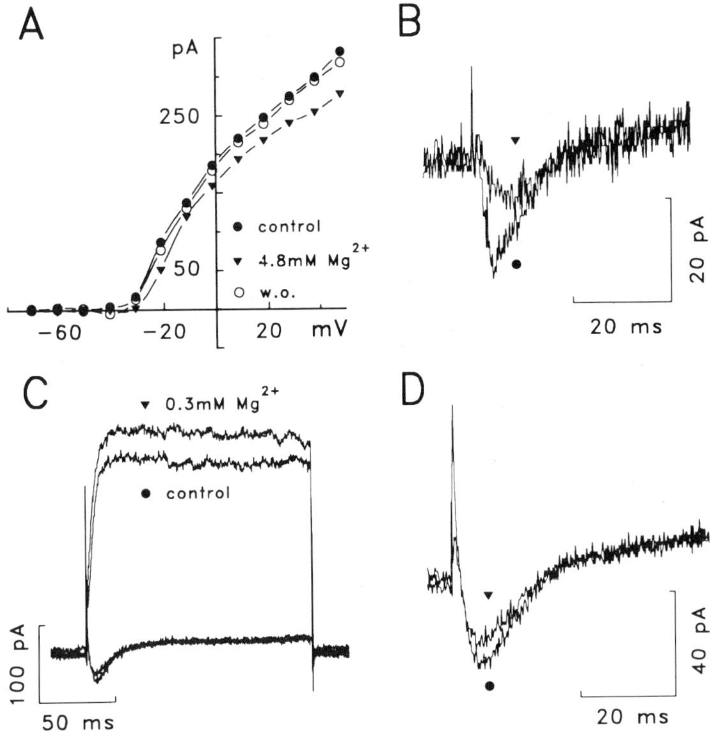

Figure 1. Effect of extracellular Mg^{2+} on K^+ and Ca^{2+} currents of BCECs. **A.** I–V curve of K^+ currents illustrates the inhibitory effect of high Mg^{2+} (4.8 mM). Note the threshold for activation at –30 mV and a clear outward rectification. **B.** Original traces of voltage-activated Ca^{2+} currents, elicited from a holding potential of –80 mV and pulse to –20 mV, during control condition (1.2 mM Mg^{2+}, filled circle) and high Mg^{2+} (4.8 mM, open circle). **C.** Original outward K^+ and inward Ca^{2+} currents stimulated from a holding potential of –80 mV and test pulses to +50 and –25 mV, respectively. **D.** Magnified Ca^{2+} current of **C**, to show the apparent inhibition produced by low Mg^{2+}.

more clearly illustrated in Figure 2B, where inward currents measured during the test pulse (**b**) were normalized to the maximal current and plotted against the different holding potentials (**a**). It is clearly shown that low $[Mg^{2+}]_o$ shifted by about 6 mV the half-maximal voltage ($V_{0.5}$) of the steady-state inactivation to more hyperpolarizing potentials.

The above results support the contention that extracellular Mg^{2+} affected both the activation and inactivation of the Ca^{2+} channel in endothelial cells of brain microvessels and, therefore, the contractility of blood vessels. Since the membrane potential in BCECs is primarily controlled by K^+ ions, one can expect that elevation of extracellular Mg^{2+} should depolarize BCECs by depressing K^+ channels (Fig 1A) and the opposite should occur with low $[Mg^{2+}]_o$.

As the concentration of Mg^{2+} has been shown recently to influence endothelial-derived relaxant factors (EDRF) (Ku & Ann, 1991); and nitric oxide (NO) generation (Howard et al, 1995), it is distinctly possible that the electrophysiological actions shown here may be pivotal in elaboration of EDRF and NO. It may be of more than passing interest to note here that a low $[Mg^{2+}]_o$ of 0.3 mM, as used, here has been found recently to be present in the serum of some patients with ischemic heart disease and stroke (Altura & Altura, 1995).

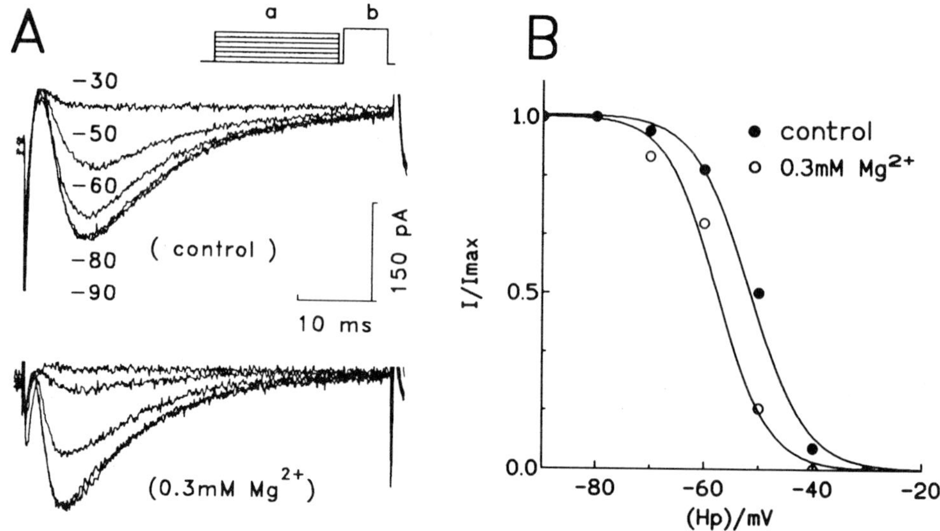

Figure 2. Steady-state inactivation of LVA Ca^{2+} currents of BCECs. **A**. Original traces of Ca^{2+} currents stimulated from different holding potentials (indicated by superposed values) and test pulses to −20 mV, under control conditions (1.2 mM Mg^{2+}, upper panel) and low Mg^{2+} concentration (0.3 mM, lower panel). Inset: pulse protocol for steady-state inactivation (see Methods). **B**. Curve of the steady-state inactivation (I/Imax) plotted by normalizing current amplitude to the maximal current *vs* the corresponding holding potentials (Hp/mV).

4. REFERENCES

Altura BM & Altura BT (1981) Magnesium ions and contraction of vascular smooth muscle: relationship to some vascular diseases. Fed Proc 40: 2672–2679

Altura BM & Altura BT (1995) Magnesium and cardiovascular biology - an important link between cardiovascular risk factors and atherogenesis. Cell Mol Biol Res 41: 347–359

Delpiano MA (1996) Metabolic inhibitors affect the conductance of low voltage-activated calcium channels in brain capillary endothelial cells. Adv Exp Med Biol 410:109–113

Hamill OP, Marty A, Neher E, Sakmann E & Sigworth FJ (1981) Improved patch-clamp technique for high-resolution current recordings from cells and cell-free membrane patches. Pflügers Arch 391: 85–100

Howard AB, Alexander RW & Taylor WR (1995) Effects of magnesium on nitric oxide synthase activity in endothelial cells. Am J Physiol 269: C612-C618

Ku DD & Ann HS (1991) Differential effects of magnesium on basal and agonist-induced EDRF relaxation in canine coronary arteries. J Cardiovasc Physiol 17: 999–1006

Turlapaty PDMV & Altura BM (1978) Extracellular magnesium ions control calcium exchange and content of vascular smooth muscle. Eur J Pharmacol 52: 421–423

Zhang A, Cheng TP, Altura BT & Altura BM (1993) Mg^{2+} and caffeine-induced intracellular Ca^{2+} release in human vascular endothelial cells. Br J Pharmacol 109: 291–292

18

EVALUATION OF GENE EXPRESSION IN THE RAT CAROTID BODY USING THE DIFFERENTIAL DISPLAY TECHNIQUE

J. Chen,[1] J. Swensen,[2] B. Dinger,[1] and S. Fidone[1]

[1] Department of Physiology
[2] Department of Medical Informatics
University of Utah School of Medicine
Salt Lake City, Utah 84108

1. INTRODUCTION

A fundamental doctrine of biology holds that cell- and tissue-specific functions are guided by selective gene expression. Thus, in the developing carotid body it is expected that the emergence of unique chemoreceptor function is directed by mRNA transcripts which convey specific sensitivities to hypoxia, hypercapnia, etc. In addition, altered gene expression likely contributes to the important morphological changes and physiological adjustments which occur in the carotid body during exposure to chronic hypoxia. Unfortunately, previous attempts to identify these important genes using conventional molecular biological techniques (*i.e*, RNA blotting and probing) have been hampered by the requirement of relatively large tissue samples for nucleic acid extraction. Furthermore, these methods do not allow assessment of the multitude (~15,000) of transcripts usually expressed in eukaryotic cells, nor do they reveal unknown genes which may be crucial to specific functions and adaptations.

The objective of the present study was to develop an efficient experimental strategy for detecting changes in gene expression and for identifying differentially expressed mRNA transcripts in the carotid body. We have based our approach on the differential display technique (Liang & Pardee, 1992), an mRNA fingerprinting method which facilitates the side-by-side comparison of specific transcripts obtained from tissues exposed to differing physiological or pathological conditions. The application of this recently developed technology to various tissues obtained from chronically hypoxic rats has suggested that low O_2 exposure alters the expression of many more transcripts in the carotid body, for example, than in the superior cervical ganglia. Further study of selected transcripts has also shown that adaptation to chronic hypoxia involves gene products with important regulatory functions.

Frontiers in Arterial Chemoreception, edited by Zapata *et al.*
Plenum Press, New York, 1996

2. METHODS

Young adult male rats (180–200 g) were exposed to hypoxia in a hypobaric chamber at a barometric pressure of 350 Torr (approx. 5500 m). The pressure was reduced incrementally from the ambient pressure over a four-day period and then maintained for 10 or 11 additional days. Other age-matched male rats were exposed immediately to 350 Torr and maintained at that pressure for three or four days. Fresh food, water and litter were provided every three days. Normoxic control rats were kept in identical cages at ambient pressure. Following exposure the carotid bodies and superior cervical ganglia (SCG) were surgically removed from both experimental and control rats under pentobarbital anesthesia (40 mg/kg). The tissues were quickly frozen on dry ice and total RNA was extracted using the guanidinium-thiocyanate-phenol-chloroform method (Chomczynski & Sacchi, 1987). Following two precipitations of the RNA in ethanol, the samples were treated with DNase (RNase-free) to remove any contaminating DNA (Liang et al, 1993). The samples were again extracted in phenol/chloroform (1:1), precipitated in ethanol (2X) and evaporated to dryness.

Differential display (DD) was performed in accord with instructions provided by GenHunter Corporation (Brookline, MA, USA; Liang et al, 1994) in a kit containing buffer, MMLV reverse transcriptase, anchored primers ($T_{11}G$; $T_{11}A$; $T_{11}C$) and arbitrary primers (13-mers). PCR was carried out in the presence of $\alpha[^{35}S]dATP$ (> 1000 Ci/mmol; 1 μl in each 20 μl reaction). Bands of interest (identified on the autoradiogram) were excised from the gel, reamplified using the same primer set, and the DNA was sequenced (chain termination method; cycle-sequencing).

Changes in transcript level indicated by DD were confirmed with a competitive PCR technique which utilizes neutral mimic DNA molecules as an internal standard in the reaction mix (Clontech, Palo Alto, CA). Mimic and target DNA share identical priming sites but differ slightly in size so that they can be separated on an agarose gel for analysis (Siebert & Kellogg, 1995).

3. RESULTS

A DD autoradiogram is shown in Figure 1. The data represent PCR products ranging in size from approximately 250 to 500 base pairs which were generated by the $T_{11}C$ 3'-primer combined with the HAP-2 13-mer (GenHunter Corporation). The three columns on the left are products from carotid bodies exposed to 0, 3 or 14 days of hypoxia. Data for superior cervical ganglia (SCG) are represented by the three columns to the right. Visual examination of the autoradiogram suggests that the level of expression of multiple specific transcripts in the carotid body is either increased or decreased by chronic hypoxia; the expression of other transcripts remained stable. In contrast to this dynamic effect of chronic hypoxia on carotid body gene expression, the expression of only a few transcripts in the SCG appear to be influenced by the chronic hypoxic stimulation. The banding pattern present in the autoradiogram (Fig 1) was reproducible when the PCR was repeated using the same batch of cDNA, and importantly, when the entire experiment was repeated with a different group of animals.

Figure 2 shows densitometer scans of the autoradiogram from Figure 1. Arrowheads indicate peaks (transcripts) which are regulated by chronic hypoxia. It is evident that some transcripts are upregulated, while the expression of others is decreased substantially. A highly regulated transcript is indicated by the PCR product at ~320 bp, which was present

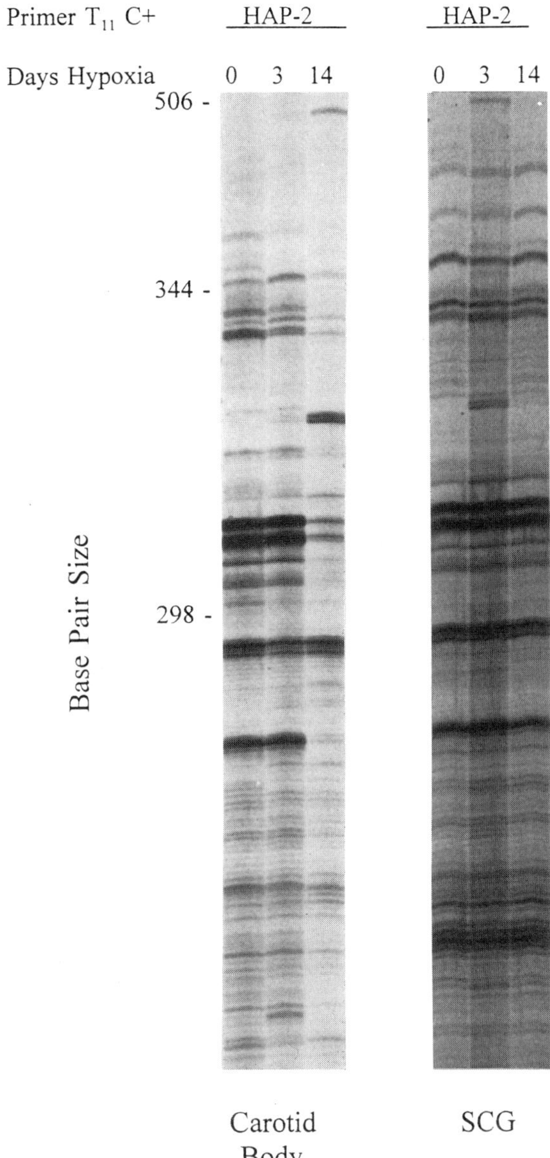

Figure 1. Differential display of mRNA from normal and chronically hypoxic rat carotid bodies and superior cervical ganglia (SCG). Primer combinations and the duration of hypoxic exposure are shown at the top of the columns.

after 14 days of hypoxia but was not detectable in normal animals. A survey of similar densitometer scans generated from six different primer sets revealed that the incidence of altered transcript expression evoked by chronic hypoxia is approximately three-fold greater in the carotid body than in the SCG.

A subset of seven bands from another primer set (T_{11}A + HAP-3) were selected for further study, based upon autoradiographies which indicated substantial changes in the level of transcript expression. Of these, four were successfully reamplified and the DNA was sequenced for comparison with available sequence databases. Two of the hypoxia-regulated mRNAs share extensive sequence homology (> 90%) with rat transcripts which

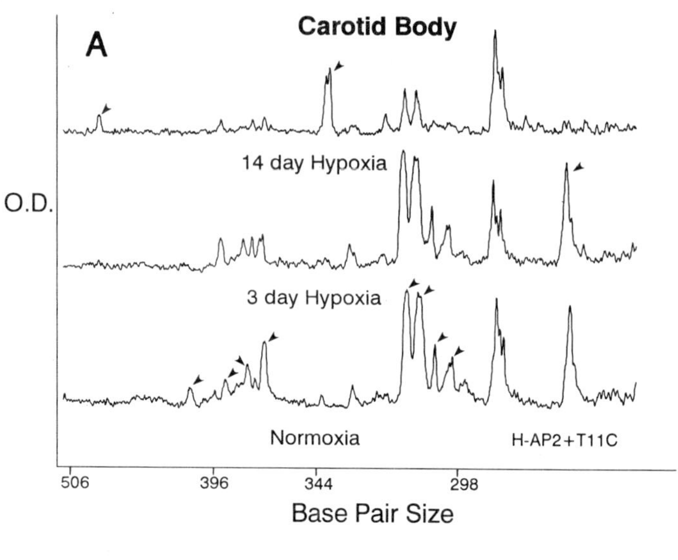

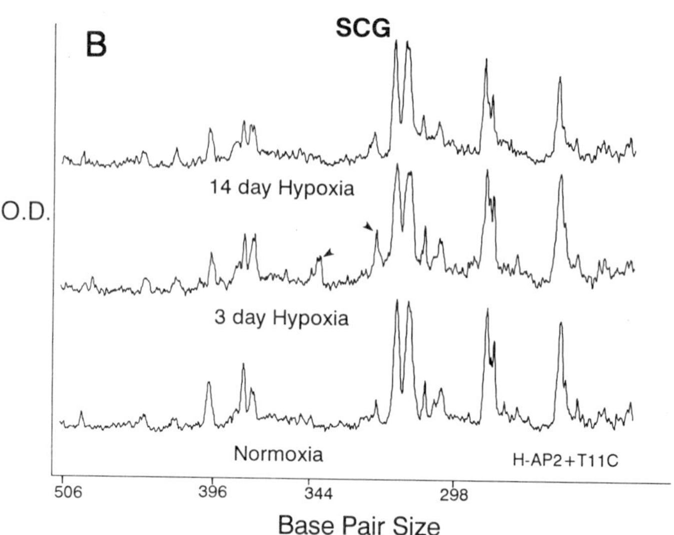

Figure 2. Densitometer scans of autoradiography from Figure 1. Peaks showing substantially altered band intensity are indicated by arrowheads for A, carotid body and, B, superior cervical ganglion.

code for ribosomal proteins (GeneBank accession nos. X53504 and X52733), a third transcript shared 85.7% homology with a mouse sequence coding for a putative calcium binding protein (accession no. X14938), and the fourth sequence was not matched by available coding regions for vertebrate proteins.

The 3'-PCR product for this lattermost gene, detected with the $T_{11}A$ + HAP-3 primer set, was estimated to be 363 bp on the DD. In normal animals, this gene produced only a faint band on the autoradiogram, but after four days of hypobaric hypoxia the signal was greatly intensified and this apparent high level of expression was maintained throughout the 15 days of chronic hypoxic exposure. Although DD is a highly reproducible technique,

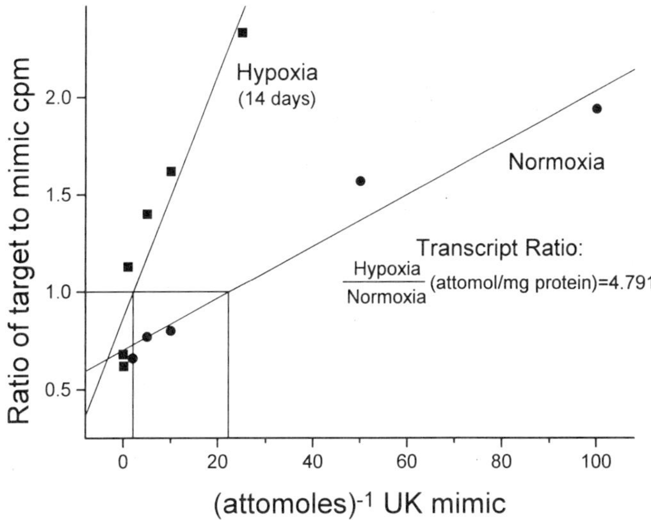

Figure 3. Competitive PCR results for an unidentified 366 base pair transcript (UK) which appeared to intensify on the differential display following hypoxia (4 and 15 days). Data indicate nearly a 4.8-fold increase in UK transcript following 14 days of hypobaric hypoxia. See text for details.

false-positive or artifactual results have also been reported. For this reason, we have adopted a competitive PCR technique in order to confirm DD results of selected transcripts. This method utilizes a neutral mimic DNA molecule which contains incorporated priming sites identical to the target, but with a non-identical intervening sequence of somewhat different size. After harvesting total RNA and completing reverse transcription, multiple cDNA samples containing equal concentrations of the target sequence are spiked with measured amounts of the mimic at different concentrations. Following PCR in the presence of a radiolabeled primer, the samples are electrophoresed on an agarose gel and visualized bands are extracted for determination of radioactivity. Figure 3 shows results for the 363 bp unknown transcript. The x-axis plots the reciprocal of the amount of mimic DNA added to each sample, and the y-axis the ratio of target-to-mimic dpm. A ratio of one theoretically indicates an equal concentration of target and mimic in the reaction mix, and the corresponding x-intercept estimates the number of target molecules present. Data for the unidentified transcript presented in Figure 3 indicates an increase of approximately one order of magnitude for the expression of this gene in carotid bodies taken from 14 day chronically hypoxic rats. Because these chronically hypoxic carotid bodies are significantly enlarged (2–5 fold) over normoxic control organs, the data are also expressed per mg protein, which results in an approximately 4.79-fold increase in transcript expression following chronic hypoxic stimulation. Assessments of other genes which did not reveal differential expression on the DD following hypoxia, likewise in competitive PCR experiments yielded hypoxia/normoxia transcript ratios near unity.

4. DISCUSSION

In the present study, we have used a combination of modern molecular biological techniques to evaluate changes in gene expression in the rat carotid body and superior cervical ganglion. In our experiments, the total RNA extracted from six carotid bodies provided an adequate sample for DD. Sample preparation included treatment with DNase in order to eliminate DNA contamination. The small size of the rat carotid body hampers the use of conventional blotting and hybridization assays (*i.e*, Northern blots; nuclease protection assays) to confirm evidence of altered gene expression. We therefore adopted a quantitative PCR method which involves competition for specific primers between target and neutral mimic molecules (Siebert & Kellogg, 1995). This procedure, including the incorporation of specific priming sites, subsequent amplification of mimic molecules, competitive PCR, gel electrophoresis and determination of radioactivity, can be completed in three days or less.

Our results from DD using only six of the possible 240 primer combinations (three anchored primers; 80 arbitrary 13-mers) suggest that chronic hypoxia evokes changes in the expression of multiple transcripts in the carotid body and SCG. These findings are consistent with the well-documented changes in morphology and physiology of the carotid body which occur during prolonged hypoxia (see McDonald, 1981; and Fidone et al, 1996, for review). They further suggest that adjustment to chronic chemoreceptor stimulation involves a complex array of cellular events, some of which are derived from altered gene expression. Our experimental assessments indicate that these changes may include the transcription of previously unexpressed genes, and the down regulation of other genes. We observed similar qualitative changes in the pattern of gene expression in the SCG; however, fewer transcripts appear to be affected by chronic stimulation of this tissue. Chronic hypoxic stress elevates impulse traffic in the sympathetic nervous system, and thus changes in gene expression might be expected to occur in this ganglion, including the trans-synaptic induction of catecholaminergic synthetic enzymes (Black et al, 1985; Cooper et al, 1986).

In summary, the application of DNA amplification techniques including DD and competitive PCR, appears to provide a powerful and efficient strategy for the detection and identification of gene expression in the rat carotid body. Multiple changes in transcript levels are induced by chronic stimulation, and the data suggest therefore that many of the observed morphological and physiological adjustments to chronic hypoxia are initiated by altered gene expression. We anticipate that future attempts to understand the cellular events which occur in the chronically hypoxic and developing carotid bodies will be facilitated by the identification (and localization) of specific transcripts which code for regulatory proteins capable of influencing chemoreceptor transduction pathways and/or growth related processes.

5. ACKNOWLEDGMENTS

Supported by USPHS Grants NS12636 and NS07938.

6. REFERENCES

Black IB, Chikaraishi DM & Lewis EJ (1985) Trans-synaptic increase in RNA coding for tyrosine hydroxylase in a rat sympathetic ganglion. Brain Res 339: 151–153

Chomczynski P & Sacchi N (1987) Single-step method of RNA isolation by acid guanidinium thiocyanate-phenol-chloroform extraction. Analyt Biochem 162: 156–159

Cooper JR, Bloom FE & Roth RH (1986) The Biochemical Basis of Neuropharmacology. NY, Oxford: Oxford University Press

Fidone SJ, Gonzalez C, Almaraz L & Dinger B (1996) Cellular mechanisms of peripheral chemoreceptor function. In: RG Crystal, JB West, E Weibel & PJ Barnes (eds) The Lung: Scientific Foundations. Philadelphia: Lippincott-Raven Publishers. pp 128.1–128.22

Liang P & Pardee AB (1992) Differential display of eukaryotic messenger RNA by means of the polymerase chain reaction. Science 257: 967–971

Liang P, Averboukh L & Pardee AB (1993) Distribution and cloning of eukaryotic mRNAs by means of differential display: refinements and optimization. Nucleic Acids Res 21: 3269–3275

Liang P, Zhu W, Zhang X, Guo Z, O'Connell RP, Averboukh L, Want F & Pardee AB (1994) Differential display using one-base anchored oligo-dT primers. Nucleic Acids Res 22: 5763–5764

McDonald DM (1981) Peripheral chemoreceptors: Structure-function relationships of the carotid body. In: TF Hornbein (ed) Regulation of Breathing, Part I. NY, Basel: Marcel Dekker. pp 105–319

Siebert PD & Kellogg DE (1995) PCR mimics: Competitive DNA fragments for use in quantitative PCR. In: MJ McPherson, BD Hames & GR Taylor (eds) PCR 2: A Practical Approach. NY, Oxford: Oxford University Press. pp 135–148

19

INDUCTION OF IMMEDIATE EARLY RESPONSE GENES BY HYPOXIA

Possible Molecular Bases for Systems Adaptation to Low pO_2

N. S. Cherniack, P. C. Shenoy, R. Mishra, M. Simonson, and N. R. Prabhakar

Case Western Reserve University
Cleveland, Ohio
New Jersey Medical School
Newark, New Jersey

1. INTRODUCTION

One of the distinguishing characteristics of living organisms is their ability to compensate for stresses in the environment, such as hypoxia, which disturb homeostasis. Homeostasis is preserved mainly by control systems, which maintain levels of crucial chemicals in the body such as oxygen within acceptable limits. These control systems operate largely through negative feedback of signals from sensory receptors like the peripheral chemoreceptors (Longobardo & Cherniack, 1986). Over the years much has been learned about the operation of biological control systems using the same techniques employed to analyze man-made control systems. Both types of systems can be considered to consist of a controller (the brain and the chemoreceptors in the case of O_2 control), and the plant (the O_2 stored in the blood and in the lungs), which the controller manipulates by producing changes in ventilation and blood flow. The response characteristics of each of these components is studied in isolation and while connected; and these relationships are expressed quantitatively so that the overall function of the system is described by a set of mathematical equations. This kind of analysis assumes that the properties of the components, both static and dynamic are fixed. Although important gaps in our knowledge remain, this approach has been quite successful in predicting ventilatory changes during acute hypoxia (Yang & Khoo, 1994). However, the changes in system responses that occur as the time of hypoxic exposure lengthens suggest that the properties of the control system itself are not fixed and even may be subject to some higher order regulation.

It is now recognized that environmental stimuli can activate genetic mechanisms and produce phenotypic changes. It has been suggested that these genetic mechanisms not infrequently involve the activation of immediate early response genes (IERG) that encode proteins which in turn affect specific target genes. IERG, which can be divided into several super families, can be activated within minutes by a stimulus (Morgan & Curran, 1991).

Frontiers in Arterial Chemoreception, edited by Zapata *et al.*
Plenum Press, New York, 1996

The most extensively studied of the IERG are members of the fos-jun family (c-fos, Fos B, Fra-1, Fra-2, c jun, jun B, and jun D). These genes form transacting proteins which bind at AP-1 sites in the promoter region of target genes increasing their transcriptional activity. The transacting proteins are either homodimers of Jun proteins or heterodimers of Fos and Jun. Post transcriptional processes can affect the stability of the RNA messages while post translational effects can modify the ability of Fos and Jun to bind to DNA and to enhance transcription. For example, phosphorylations of Fos and Jun protein affect their binding ability to target genes, while the binding of these proteins is tighter when the cysteine in the AP-1 protein complex is in the reduced state (Xanthoudakis et al, 1992). In addition, the protein products themselves can link to the promoter areas of the genes which encoded them and depending on binding site can enhance or suppress the activity of the parent gene (Angel et al, 1988). The effects of Fos and Jun can be modified by products of other IERG. For example, by complexing with proteins encoded by the ATF/CRE super family of IERG, Fos and Jun proteins can bind at CREB sites in promoter regions (Hait & Curran, 1991). Because of the diversity of the factors that can influence the effects of the IERG on specific target gene transcription, and the potential regulation of IERG themselves by feedback from protein end products and by hypoxia, IERG activity may be able to fine tune adjustments to different types of hypoxic environment.

IERG triggering has been demonstrated in intact animals during nerve stimulation, osmotic stress, convulsive activity, and ischemia by the appearance of Fos protein at one or more sites in the central nervous system (Morgan & Curran, 1991). In anesthetized animals exposed to hypercapnia or hypoxia, or carotid sinus nerve stimulation Fos protein can be demonstrated in the ventral and dorsal medulla, and to a lesser extent in the brain stem, and even in the cortex (Erickson & Millhorn, 1991; Haxhiu et al, 1995). In general, the appearance of Fos is limited to sensory and second order neurons and appears rarely if at all in motor neurons. It is of interest that the magnitude of IERG activation by hypoxia changes over time. For example, exposure of unanesthetized rats to hypoxia for one to four hours significantly enhances the expression of Fos-like immunoreactive protein in the nucleus tractus solitarius (NTS) as well as other regions of the brain. However, if hypoxic exposure is continued for 7 days, the number of cells expressing Fos in the NTS decreases although remaining higher than in control rats (Haxhiu MA, Eroku B & Cherniack NS, in preparation). The reduction in Fos at one week is not due to some change that interferes generally with c-fos activation, because when the rats are exposed to 15% CO_2 in 21% O_2 after 7 days of hypoxia there is a further increase in Fos labeling.

Since many different stimuli, nonspecific stresses, as well as trans-synaptic activity produce the appearance of Fos in intact animals, the chain of events by which hypoxia activates IERG is difficult to determine.

The object of the studies that will be described are to develop a cell model in which the effects of hypoxia on IERG expression can be examined and then to use this model to determine sites of O_2 sensitivity. From a more long range view point, these are the initial investigations of a possible second layer of control operating at the genetic level which preserves O_2 homeostasis.

2. METHODS AND RESULTS

In these studies we used PC-12 cells and compared results obtained in these cells to those obtained in neuroblastoma and other cells. Pheochromocytoma cells-12 (PC-12), developed from rat adrenal medullary tumor cells, resemble glomus cells of the carotid body in several ways. Both are of neural crest origin. Dopamine is released by hypoxia from type I cells, and, as shown by the following study, so do PC-12 cells (Kumar & Prabhakar, 1995). PC-12 cells were raised in growth medium (RPMI; GIBCO) supplemented with 5% horse serum, 10% fetal calf serum and antibiotics in a humidified CO_2 incubator. After cells reached 90% confluence, they were plated at a density of 10^6 cells in tissue culture flasks containing serum free medium. Cells were exposed for 15 min to three levels of pO_2: 145, 70, and 40 Torr. Following the hypoxic challenge, the dopamine content of the medium was analyzed by HPLC combined with an ECD detection method. These experiments showed that hypoxia results in enhanced release of dopamine. The effects of low pO_2 on dopamine release from PC-12 cells were reduced to 70% in presence of nitrendipine (10 μM), suggesting that an increase in intracellular calcium and the involvement of L-type voltage gated calcium channels may be necessary for hypoxia-induced dopamine release. Hypoxia increases intracellular calcium in many type I cells (Agani et al, 1993). Increases in intracellular Ca^{++} cells with hypoxia also occur in PC-12 cells and can be detected by fluorescent imaging using the dye Fura-2. An elevation of $[Ca^{++}]_i$ was seen immediately after the onset of hypoxia in PC-12 cells and persisted during the entire period of hypoxia. In contrast, vascular smooth muscle cells (A7r5) responded with a slow increase in calcium only when they were exposed to 30 min of hypoxia and calcium levels remained elevated even after termination of the stimulus. Thus in both PC-12 and type I cells, hypoxia increases intracellular calcium and causes dopamine release.

We next studied the effects of hypoxia on c-fos, jun-B, jun-c, jun-D mRNA expression in PC-12 cells (Prabhakar et al, 1995). Cells were maintained in cultures as described above, and were exposed either to normoxia (pO_2 =149 Torr; pCO_2 = 40 Torr) or to hypoxia (pO_2 = 33 Torr; pCO_2 = 42 Torr) for one hour and processed for RNA extraction and northern blot analysis. Although hypoxia stimulated mRNA expression of c-fos, jun B, jun C, jun D, relative increases amongst IERG's varied considerably. For instance, c-fos expression increased by 12 fold, whereas elevation of Jun B, C, D ranged between 1.5 to 3 fold (Fig 1).

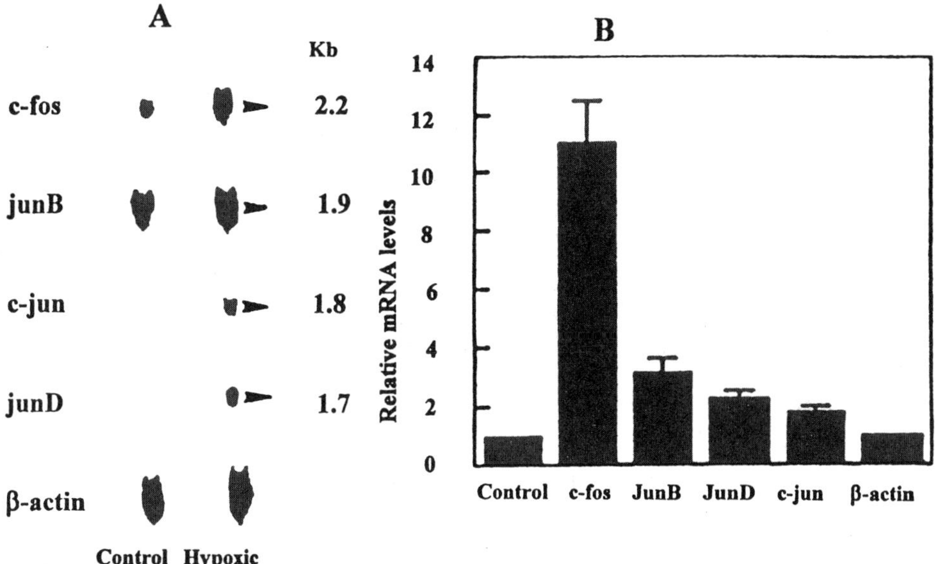

Figure 1. Effect of hypoxia on the expression of different IERGs in PC-12 Cells. (From Prabhakar et al, 1995).

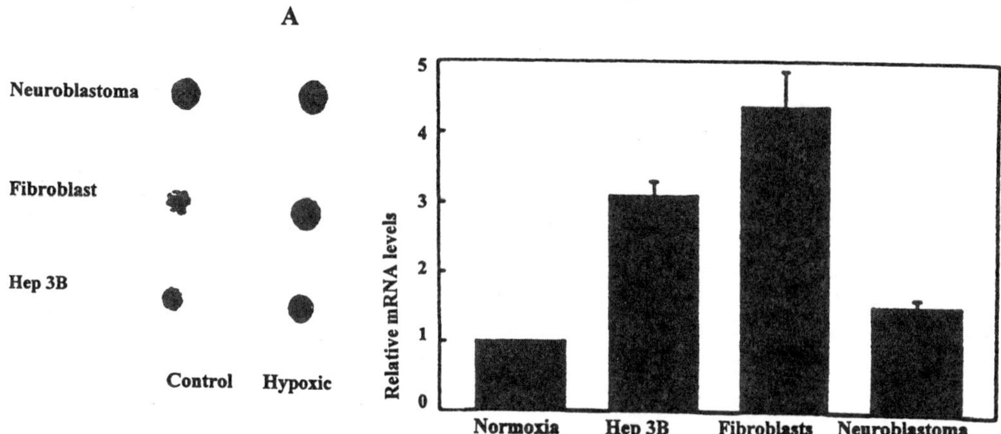

Figure 2. Effect of hypoxia on c-fos expression in different cell lines. (From Prabhakar et al, 1995).

The effects of hypoxia could be seen with low pO_2 exposure as short as 15 min, and mNRA levels were greater at one compared to 10 h of hypoxia. In other preparations such as propagating neuroblastoma, myeloma, Hep-3B and fibroblast cell lines, the effects of hypoxia on IERG varied as shown in Figure 2. Neuroblastoma and myeloma cells, for example, showed no expression of c-fos mRNA, while hypoxia induced c-fos mRNA expression in fibroblasts and Hep-3B cells, even though the magnitude was 6 times less than PC-12 cells.

We also found that hypoxia can affect levels of second messengers in type I cells. In a series of experiments, we examined the effects of hypoxia on cyclic nucleotide levels in PC-12 cells. The cells were exposed to hypoxia (5% O_2) for one hour, followed by homogenization in a buffer. The homogenate was centrifuged and cAMP and cGMP levels were analyzed by radio immunoassay in the supernatant fraction. Hypoxia increased cAMP and cGMP levels in PC-12 cells. Levels of cyclic nucleotides in turn could affect c-fos since

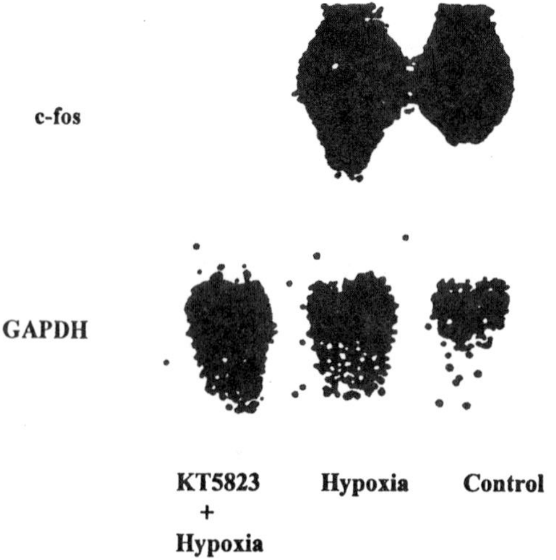

Figure 3. Inhibition of hypoxia-Induced c-fos expression by a cGMP kinase inhibitor.

prior treatment of PC-12 cells with KT-5823 (2 μM), a cGMP kinase inhibitor markedly attenuated the hypoxia-induced increase in c-fos mRNA but did not affect other genes as shown in Figure 3 (Morgan & Curran, 1991). We have as not yet examined the effect of cAMP inhibition.

Hypoxia may increase mRNA of IERG by enhancing transcription or by increasing the stability of the mRNA. In further experiments we asked whether hypoxia stimulates transcription of the c-fos IERG. We transiently transfected PC-12 cells with a CAT (chloramphenicol acetyl transferase) reporter containing 356 bp of the murine c-fos promoter. After 24 h, cells were exposed to normoxia, hypoxia, or normoxia and fetal bovine serum (20% FBS), a well-characterized stimulus to the c-fos promoter. Following a 12 h incubation, the cells were lysed and CAT activity was measured. Hypoxia stimulated a 3.1-fold increase in CAT activity in PC-12 cells compared to normoxic controls, and was even greater than stimulation by FBS. On the other hand, FBS, but not hypoxia, increased CAT activity in neuroblastoma cells. These results demonstrate that in susceptible cells the hypoxia-responsive elements are contained within the 5'356 upstream nucleotides of the promoter.

Since the c-fos promoter contains AP-1 sites, we also compared the effects of hypoxia on AP-1 transcription factor activity in PC-12 cells and neuroblastoma cells using a luciferase and β-galactosidase assay systems. Luciferase was used to assess transcription activity and β-galactosidase to evaluate transfection efficiency. A plasmid containing two AP-1 sequences linked to luciferase reporter gene was obtained from MG Rosenfeld (see Nelson et al, 1988). In this construct, two AP-1 consensus sequences with minimal prolactin promoter are tagged to the 5' side of the luciferase gene. Cells were challenged with 3% O_2 for 1, 2, 8, and 18 h. No increase in luciferase activity was seen after 1 h of exposure to hypoxia with either cell type. However AP-1 activity increased progressively over 18 h in PC-12 cells but not in neuroblastoma cells as shown in Figure 4. This supports the idea that the effects of hypoxia involve changes in AP-1 activity.

Hypoxia induces expression of several target genes including tyrosine hydroxylase (TH), which contain AP-1 binding sites in their promoter regions. It is possible that hypoxia-induced expression of TH may in part depend on the formation of the AP-1 protein complexes. The following preliminary studies were performed on PC-12 cells to test this possibility. Cells were transiently transfected with 4 μg TH gene promoter constructs linked to CAT and 1 μg of RSV β-galactosidase (β-gal) plasmid. Twenty-four hours after transfection, cells were placed in serum free medium for an additional 16 h. Following which, they were exposed either to normoxia (21% O_2) or to hypoxia (5% O_2, for 12 h). Subsequently, cells were lysed and assayed for CAT and β-galactosidase activity. As can be seen from Figure 5, TH expression increased by nearly 100% in response to hypoxia in cells transfected with wild type TH promoter (TH HYP). In contrast, cells transfected with point mutated AP-1 site in the TH promoter (AP1MUT HYPO), TH expression by hypoxia was increased only by 20%. These observations suggest that the AP-1 site plays an important role in hypoxia-induced TH expression.

3. DISCUSSION

The summarized studies demonstrate that IERG of the fos-jun superfamily can be activated by hypoxia but only in certain cell types. For example, distinct differences were demonstrated in the response of PC-12 and neuroblastoma cells. Even relatively brief exposure to moderate hypoxia increased gene transcription, formation of AP-1 protein com-

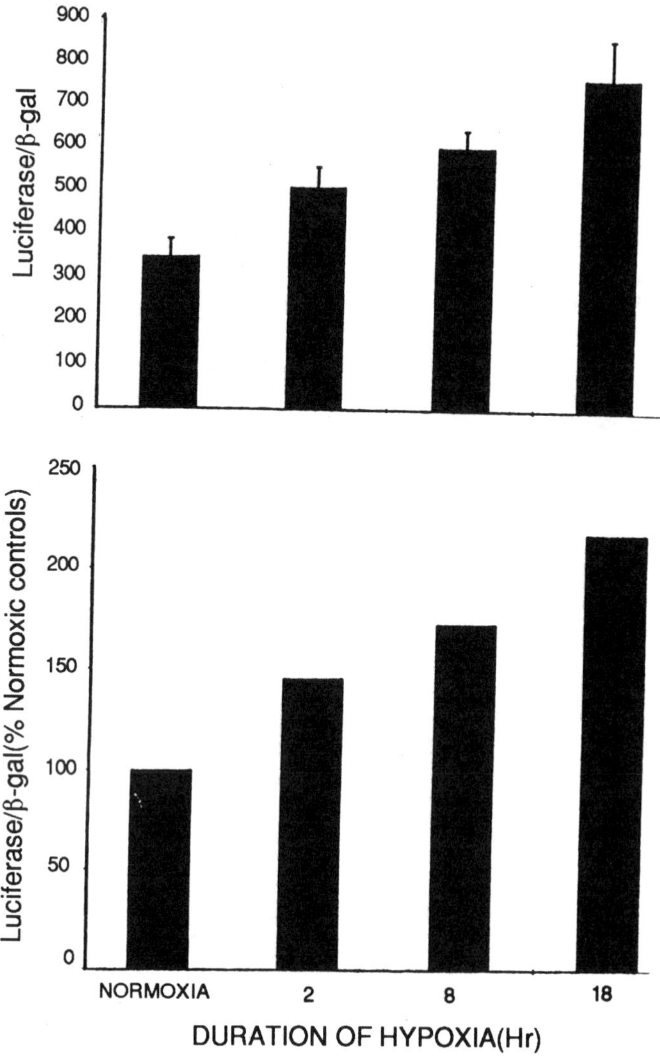

Figure 4. Effect of hypoxia on activator protein-1 transcription factor activity in PC-12 cells.

plexes, and AP-1 activity in PC-12 cells but not in neuroblastoma cells. One important region of O_2 sensitivity seems to be the AP-1 binding site and mutations at this site reduce the effects of hypoxia on the TH gene activation (an important enzyme in the carotid body). Hypoxia can also increase the stability of TH mRNA (Czyzyk-Krzeska et al, 1994).

Genes responding to hypoxia can have important adaptive effects and have been identified even in yeasts and bacteria. Hypoxia has also been reported to increase the transcriptional activity of genes encoding TH erythropoietin, and to activate glycolytic enzymes involved in anaerobic metabolism (Semenza et al, 1994; Norris & Millhorn, 1996). These responses at the gene level enhance the ability of cells to survive during prolonged hypoxia.

The genes which are activated by hypoxia can vary in different cell types. All the effects of hypoxia may not be mediated by IERG, but may include direct effect on target

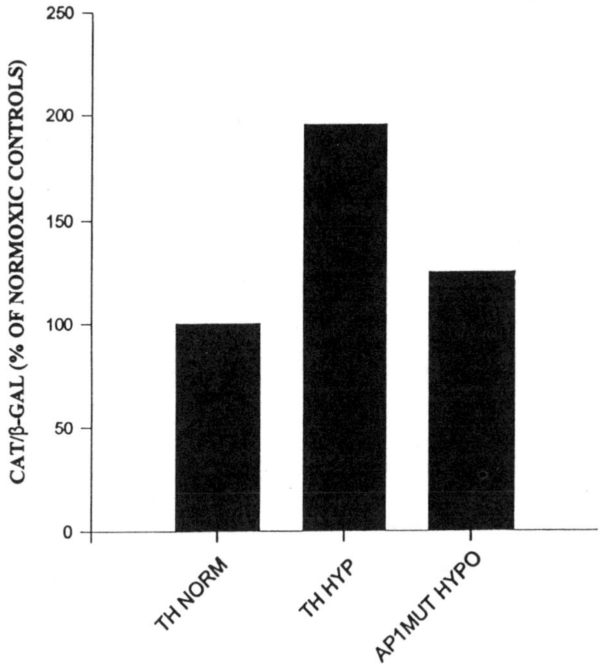

Figure 5. Effect of hypoxia on the wild type and a mutated AP-1 element of the tyrosine hydroxylase gene.

genes. Additionally, hypoxia may have effects at the cell membrane as well as the nucleus and mitochondria. This diversity of action of hypoxia might allow the cell to respond precisely to different levels of severity of hypoxia alone or in combination with other stresses. These cellular actions of hypoxia, which also could greatly increase the range of biological adaptation, may themselves be regulated. This is suggested by our observations that IERG activation is transient, and confined to certain cell types.

4. REFERENCES

Agani F, Hague U, Bright G & Prabhakar NR (1993) Hypoxia and intracellular calcium changes in PC-12 cells: Comparison with carotid body cells. FASEB J 7: A398.

Angel P, Hattori K, Smeal T & Karin M (1988) The jun proto-oncogene is positively autoregulated by its products. Cell 55: 875–885

Czyzyk-Krzeska MF, Furnari BA, Lawson EE & Millhorn DE (1994) Hypoxia increases rate of transcription and stability of tyrosine hydroxylase mRNA in pheochromocytoma CPC-12 Cell. J Biol Chem 269: 760–764

Erickson JT & Millhorn DE (1991) Fos-like protein is induced in neurons of the medulla oblongata after stimulation of the carotid sinus nerve in awake and anesthetized rats. Brain Res 567: 11–24

Hait T & Curran T (1991) Cross-Family dimerization of transcription factors Fos/Jun and ATF/CREB alters DNA binding specificity. Proc Natl Acad Sci USA 88: 3720–3724

Haxhiu MA, Strohl KP & Cherniack NS (1995) The N-methyl-D-aspartate receptor pathway is involved in hypoxia-induced c-fos protein expression in the rat nucleus of the solitary tract. J Auton Nerv Syst 55: 65–68

Kumar GK & Prabhakar NR (1995) Hypoxia stimulates dopamine release in pheochromocytoma cells. FASEB J 9: A650

Longobardo GS & Cherniack NS (1986) Abnormalities in respiratory rhythm. In: Cherniack NS & Widdicombe JG (eds) Handbook of Physiology, vol 2, part II, section 3. Bethesda, MD: Amer Physiol Soc. pp 729–750

Morgan JI & Curran T (1991) Stimulus-transcription coupling in the nervous system: Involvement of the inducible proto-oncogenes fos and jun. Annu Rev Neurosci 14: 421–451

Nelson C, Alberti VR, Elsholtz HP, Lu LIW & Rosenfeld MG (1988) Activation of cell-specific expression of rat growth hormone and prolactin genes by a common transcription factor. Science 239: 1400–1405

Norris ML & Millhorn DE (1996) Hypoxia-induced protein binding to O_2-responsive sequences on the tyrosine hydroxylase gene. J Biol Chem 270: 23774–23779

Prabhakar NR, Shenoy BC, Simonson MS & Cherniack NS (1995) Cell selective induction and transcriptional activation of immediate early genes by hypoxia. Brain Res 697: 266–270

Semenza GL, Roth PH, Fang HM & Wang GI (1994) Transcriptional regulation of gene coding glycolytic enzymes by hypoxia-inducible factor I. J Biol Chem 269: 23757–23763

Xanthoudakis S, Miao G, Wang F, Pan E YC & Curran T (1992) Redox activation of fos-jun DNA binding activity is mediated by a DNA repair enzyme. EMBO J 11: 3323–3335

Yang F & Khoo M (1994) Ventilatory response to randomly modulated hypercapnia and hypoxia in humans. J Appl Physiol 76: 2216–2223

20

REGULATION OF IONIC CONDUCTANCES AND GENE EXPRESSION BY HYPOXIA IN AN OXYGEN SENSITIVE CELL LINE

David E. Millhorn, Laura Conforti, Dana Beitner-Johnson, Wylie Zhu, Richard Raymond, Theresa Filisko, Shuichi Kobayashi, Mei Peng, and Mary-Beth Genter

Department of Molecular and Cellular Physiology
College of Medicine, University of Cincinnati
Cincinnati, Ohio

1. INTRODUCTION

Oxygen is the final acceptor of electrons in the synthesis of ATP by the mitochondrial respiratory chain and is therefore an obligatory substrate for energy transformation in most biological systems. A reduction in O_2 tension severely limits the ability of cells to perform energy-dependent functions and, if the hypoxia is severe enough, it can be life threatening. It is therefore not surprising that an elaborate control system has evolved in most species for optimizing the delivery of O_2 to cells. In mammals, an essential component of this system is the carotid body; a small organ that is located bilaterally at the bifurcation of the carotid artery. The carotid body contains O_2-sensitive (type I) cells that are stimulated by reduced O_2 tension. The type I cells transmit information concerning the O_2 status of arterial blood to closely situated primary sensory afferent fibers by release of neurotransmitter. A major problem confronting contemporary biology is identification of the molecular and cellular mechanisms that couple environmental stimuli with changes in cell phenotype and function. However, after several decades of intense investigations, the mechanisms by which type I cells detect changes in O_2 tension and transduce this signal into an increase in neurotransmitter synthesis and release remain unknown.

2. STIMULATION OF TYROSINE HYDROXYLASE GENE EXPRESSION BY HYPOXIA

The catecholamine neurotransmitter dopamine is synthesized and released from type I cells during hypoxia (Fidone et al, 1982; Obeso et al, 1992). Recent findings from our

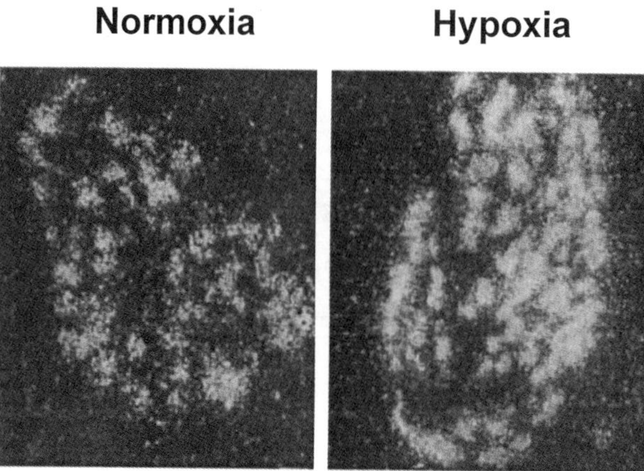

Figure 1. Effect of hypoxia on TH gene expression in the rat carotid body. Dark field photomicrographs showing silver grains from *in situ* hybridization of TH mRNA on sections from carotid bodies exposed to either normoxia (21% O_2) or hypoxia (10% O_2) for 6 h.

laboratory revealed that gene expression for tyrosine hydroxylase (TH; *EC 1.14.16.2*), the rate-limiting enzyme in the biosynthesis of dopamine, is stimulated by hypoxia in type I cells (Czyzyk-Krzeska et al, 1992). *In situ* hybridization experiments were performed to measure the effect of hypoxia on TH mRNA level in carotid bodies of rats exposed to hypoxia. Figure 1 shows that the level of TH mRNA (silver grain density) in carotid bodies from rats exposed to hypoxia (10% O_2) was markedly increased over the level measured in a carotid body exposed to normoxia (21% O_2) for the same period (6 h). It is important to note that after just 1 h of exposure to 10% O_2, TH gene expression is doubled (not shown) and that peak expression occurred after just 6 h of exposure to hypoxia. Importantly, expression remained elevated well above the control level during 24 h exposure to hypoxia.

We have used the dopaminergic PC12 cell line to investigate the molecular mechanisms that regulate gene expression during hypoxia. We first showed that PC12 cells express an O_2-sensitive K channel that is inhibited by reduced O_2 (Fig 2). Inhibition of the O_2-sensitive K current leads to membrane depolarization, an increase in cytosolic Ca^{2+}, and dopamine release during hypoxia (Fig 3). Thus, PC12 cells respond to reduced O_2 tension in a manner that is similar to the carotid body type I cells.

Experiments were performed to determine if TH gene expression is regulated in PC12 cells by physiological levels of hypoxia. In one series of experiments, PC12 cells were exposed to 5% O_2 for 1–12 h and TH mRNA level measured with Northern blot analysis (Fig 4A). The level of TH mRNA was increased at 1 h, reached a peak at 6 h and remained elevated above the initial control level at 12 h. We also examine the effect of graded hypoxia on TH gene expression in PC12 cells (Fig 4B). We found that a reduction in O_2 from 21 to 15% was sufficient to increase significantly TH gene expression and more severe levels of hypoxia led to further increases in TH mRNA. Thus, TH gene ex-

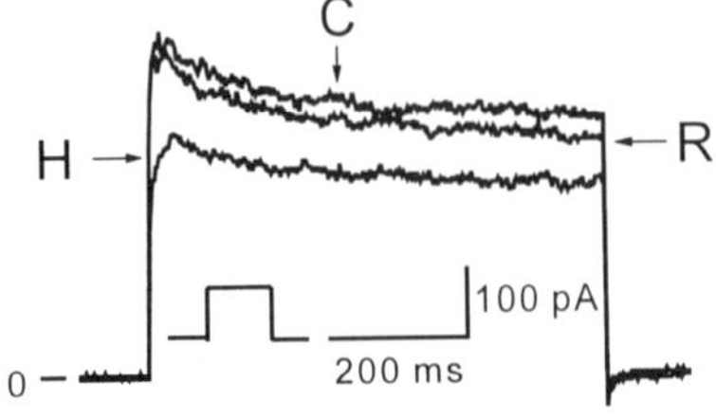

Figure 2. Effect of hypoxia on voltage-dependent outward current in PC12 cells. Superimposed current traces recorded during control (C, normoxia), after steady-state inhibition by hypoxia (H), and after returning to normoxic conditions (R). Currents recorded at +50 mV for 800 ms, from a hyperpolarizing potential of -90 mV. Standard pipette and bath solutions were used.

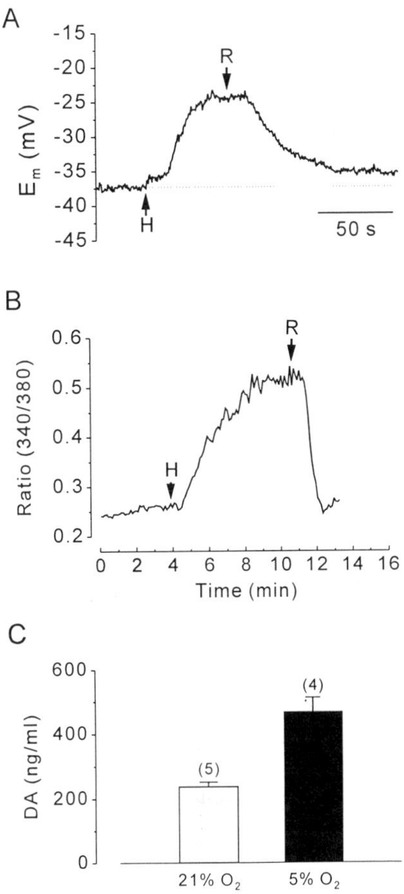

Figure 3. Effects of hypoxia on resting membrane potential, intracellular free calcium concentration and dopamine release in PC12 cells. **A.** Membrane depolarization produced by hypoxia in normal Ca^{2+} (normal pipette and external solution) conditions. Membrane potential recorded in current-clamp mode. Broken line, resting potential. **B.** Increase in cytosolic Ca^{2+} during hypoxia. Fura-2 loaded cells were imaged using 340:380 ratio method. Data are expressed as fluorescence ratio and represent the average results from 15 cells. Arrows, points of introduction of hypoxia (H) and return to control conditions (normoxia, R, 150 Torr). **C.** Spontaneous release of dopamine from PC12 cells during exposure to 21 and 5 % O_2. Numbers above bars, numbers of independent experiments. Dopamine release measured with HPLC.

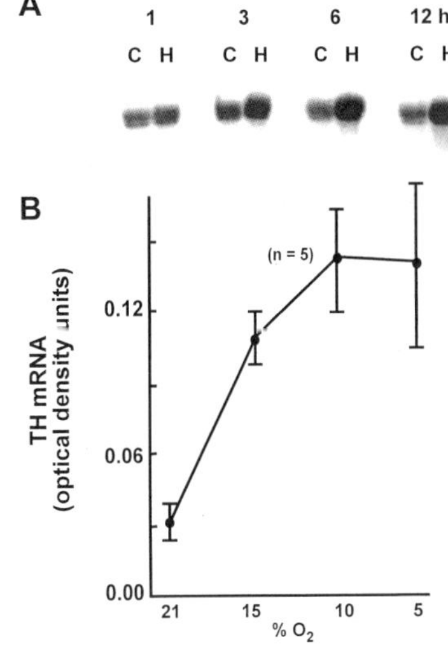

Figure 4. Effect of graded hypoxia on TH mRNA and TH enzyme levels in PC12 cells. **A.** Northern blot of TH mRNA from PC12 cells exposed for different duration to 5% O_2. **B.** Averaged data from 5 separate Northern blot experiments in which TH mRNA from PC12 cells was measured following exposure (6 h) to different levels of O_2. Quantitation performed by optical density reading of autoradiogram.

pression in PC12 cells is responsive to reductions in environmental O_2 within a moderate to severe range of hypoxia. In fact, these cells are exquisitely sensitive to reductions in O_2 tension and are therefore an excellent model system for investigations on the cellular and molecular basis of gene regulation by hypoxia.

The increase in TH mRNA in PC12 cells during hypoxia is due to increases in both the rate of gene transcription and stability of TH mRNA (Czyzyk-Krzeska et al, 1994a,b). We used PC12 cells to identify the *cis*-acting sequences on the TH gene that confers O_2 responsiveness and the *trans*-acting protein factors that interact with the sequences to regulate the rate of transcription. To identify the critical sequences that are responsible for regulating the rate of transcription during hypoxia, nested deletions of the 5' flanking region of the TH gene that were fused to the chloramphenicol transferase (CAT) reporter gene were transfected into PC12 cells prior to exposure to hypoxia. We found that the transcriptional response to hypoxia in PC12 cells is mediated by sequences that are located between -150 and -284, relative to the transcription start site (Czyzyk-Krzeska et al, 1994a; Norris & Millhorn, 1995) (Fig 5). TH promoter fragments shorter than -150 were unable to confer hypoxia responsiveness. The fragment of the TH gene confers O_2 responsiveness (-150 to -284) contains several *cis*-regulatory elements (AP1, AP2, HIF-1) that might be involved in regulation of the rate of transcription during hypoxia.

Gel mobility shift experiments were performed to determine if any of these elements are targets of hypoxia-induced protein regulatory factors. In these experiments, the fragment of the native TH gene that extends from -190 to -284 and contains the AP1, AP2 and HIF-1 sequences was used as a probe. The labeled probe was incubated with nuclear protein extracts from cells exposed to either 21 or 5% O_2 for 6 h. Results from a single gel shift experiment are shown in Figure 6. There was a constitutive level of binding activity with extracts from cells exposed to 21% O_2 (lane 2) that was markedly less than that measured with extracts from cells exposed to 5% O_2 (lane 3). Competition experiments using non-labeled oligonucleotide probes that contain sequences which corresponded to the TH regulatory motifs, AP1 and HIF-1, were performed to determine if these motifs are involved in the hypoxia-induced protein binding interaction with the TH gene. We found that competition probes (50X) that contained either the AP1 (lanes 4 and 5) or HIF-1 (lanes 6 and 7) sequence partially blocked binding of protein to the native TH gene fragment. These results show clearly that binding to the native TH fragment that contains the AP1 and HIF-1 elements is regulated by reduced O_2 tension. In another series of experi-

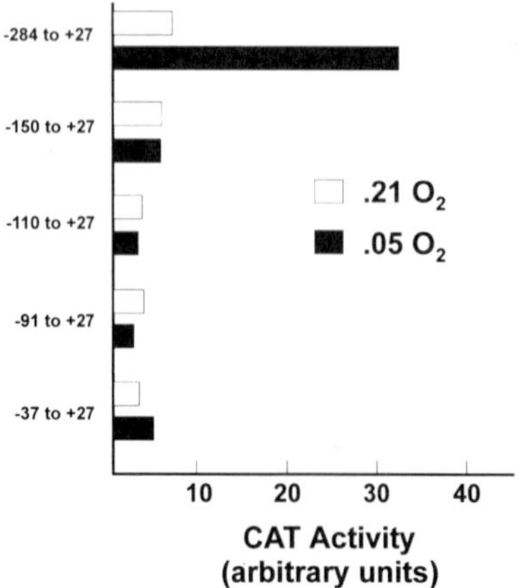

Figure 5. Effect of hypoxia on stimulation of a reporter gene (chloramphenicol acetyltransferase, CAT), that was cloned from fragments of 5' flanking region of TH gene. The sequence numbers indicating the fragment of the TH gene are relative to transcription start site. The -284 to +27 fragment of the TH gene was able to regulate transcription during hypoxia. TH promoter fragments less than -150 were unable to regulate transcription during hypoxia.

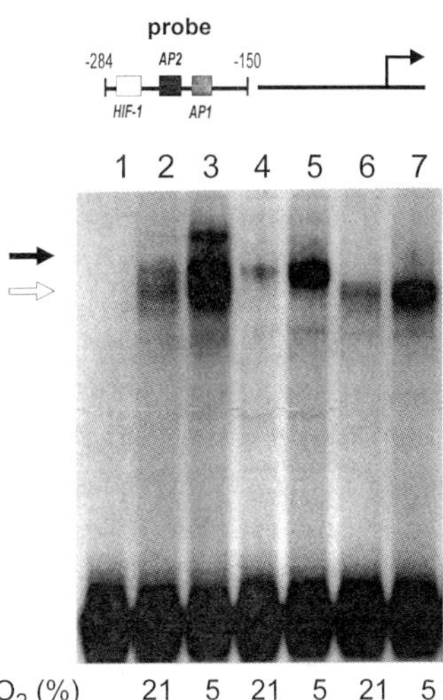

Figure 6. Effect of hypoxia on protein binding to the region of the 5' flanking region of the TH gene that confers O_2 responsiveness. Nuclear protein extracts (NPE) from PC12 cells exposed to either normoxia (21% O_2) or hypoxia (5% O_2) were used in the gel shift assay. The fragment of the TH DNA corresponding to -284 to -190 of the 5' flank was used as probe. Arrows denote protein-DNA binding complexes. Lane 1 = no protein, lane 2 = 21% O_2 (no competition), lane 3 = 5% O_2 (no competition), lane 4 = 21% O_2 (AP1 competition), lane 5 = 5% O_2 (AP1 competition), lane 6 = 21% O_2 (HIF-1 competition), and lane 7 = 5% O_2 (HIF-1 competition). (From Norris & Millhorn, 1995).

ments, double-stranded oligonucleotide probes that contained either the AP1 or HIF-1 sequence were used for gel shift experiments. We measured an increase in hypoxia-induced binding activity with the AP1, but not the HIF-1 probe (not shown). Binding to the AP1 oligoprobe was competed with unlabeled AP1 probe. Not only did binding to the AP1 sequence increase during hypoxia, but the binding activity was also persistent during prolonged hypoxia (24 h). These findings demonstrate that hypoxia-induced binding to the AP1 element is induced by reduced O_2 tension and persistent during chronic hypoxia conditions. Subsequent immunological experiments (super shift analysis and shift-western analysis) showed that c-Fos and JunB heterodimers are formed during hypoxia and bind to the AP1 site. We also performed site-specific mutation experiments which showed that the AP1 element is critical for activation of TH gene expression during hypoxia.

Hypoxia is often a chronic condition. We therefore performed experiments to determine if increased TH gene expression is sustained during chronic hypoxia. In these experiments individual dishes of PC12 cells were exposed to 10% O_2 for 3 to 14 days. Northern blot analysis showed that TH mRNA levels remained elevated during the entire 14 day period (Fig 7). A graphical representation of the Northern blot data is presented in the lower

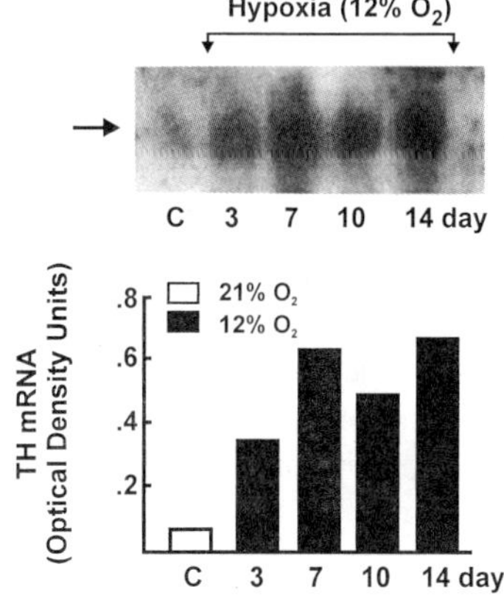

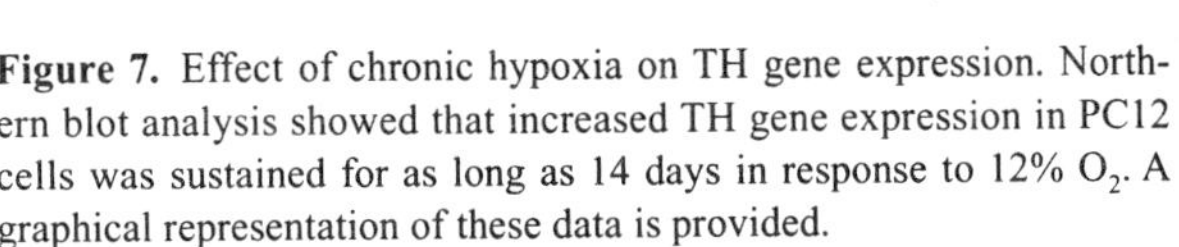

Figure 7. Effect of chronic hypoxia on TH gene expression. Northern blot analysis showed that increased TH gene expression in PC12 cells was sustained for as long as 14 days in response to 12% O_2. A graphical representation of these data is provided.

part of the figure. These findings certainly suggest that TH gene expression remains elevated during chronic hypoxia and that the gene regulatory mechanisms remain active during long-term exposure to hypoxia. To our knowledge this is the first study of long-term hypoxia on gene expression.

It has been shown previously that cAMP increases during hypoxia in carotid body type I cells (Wang et al, 1991) and that the TH gene is regulated by the cAMP-protein kinase A (PKA) signal transduction pathway in response to membrane depolarization in PC12 cells (Kilbourne et al, 1992). We have performed experiments to determine if this pathway is involved in regulation to TH gene expression in PC12 cells during hypoxia. Results from these experiments showed that PKA activity is actually decreased during hypoxia and that TH gene expression is regulated by hypoxia in a mutant PC12 cell line that is deficient in PKA. These findings indicate that the cAMP-PKA pathway is not required for regulation of TH gene expression during hypoxia in PC12 cells. The signal transduction pathway that is responsible for regulating TH gene expression during hypoxia remains unknown, but could involve membrane depolarization and Ca^{2+} mobilization.

3. MECHANISMS OF CELL RESPONSES TO OXYGEN CHANGES

The mechanisms by which O_2-sensitive cells respond to changes in O_2 tension remain uncertain. However, it has been reported that type I cells express a novel K channel that is reversibly and selectively inhibited by hypoxia (Lopez-Barneo et al, 1988; Delpiano & Hescheler, 1989; Lopez-Lopez et al, 1989; Ganfornina & Lopez-Barneo, 1991). We showed that the dopaminergic PC12 cells also express an O_2-sensitive K channel that displays ionic kinetics that are similar to those reported for type I cells and other O_2-sensitive tissue (Zhu et al, 1996). The O_2-sensitive K current in PC12 cells is inhibited in a graded fashion by exposure to progressively more severe hypoxia (Fig 2) and is blocked by tetraethylammonium (TEA). Hypoxia-induced inhibition of this current leads to membrane depolarization, an increase in intracellular free Ca^{2+}, and release of dopamine (not shown). It seems entirely possible that inhibition of the O_2-sensitive K channel, membrane depolarization and Ca^{2+} mobilization are important cellular mechanisms for sensing changes in O_2 tension and transduction of this signal into the appropriate cellular responses.

A primary response of the O_2-sensitive cells in the mammalian carotid body is activation of closely located sensory terminals by release of neurotransmitter. Both type I cells (Fidone et al, 1982; Obeso et al, 1992) and the O_2-sensitive PC12 cells (Zhu et al, 1995) release dopamine in response to reduced O_2 tension. Moreover, it has been shown that reduced O_2 leads to enhance the activity of the rate-limiting enzyme (TH) in dopamine synthesis (Gonzalez et al, 1979) and increased TH gene (Czyzyk-Krzeska et al, 1992) in the rat carotid body. We have used PC12 cells as a model system to identify the molecular genetic mechanisms responsible for regulation of TH gene expression during hypoxia (Czyzyk-Krzeska et al, 1994a,b; Norris & Millhorn, 1995). Results from these investigations revealed that the TH gene is regulated by specific interactions among *cis*-acting DNA sequences and protein regulatory factors. Results from experiments in which nested deletions of the 5' flanking region of the TH gene was cloned in front of a reporter gene revealed that a region of the TH promoter that extends from -150 to -284 is required for transcriptional activation by hypoxia. This region of the gene contains a number of cis-acting regulatory elements including an AP1, AP2, and HIF-1 sequence. Findings from gel shift experiments showed hypoxia-induced protein binding to this fragment of the TH gene. The HIF-1 element has been implicated in transcriptional regulation of the erythropoietin (EPO) gene during hypoxia (Semenza & Wang, 1993). Findings from gel shift assays in which short oligonucleotides that contained the AP1 site, but not the AP2 or HIF-1 sites, were used as probes, revealed that hypoxia caused increased binding to the AP1 sequence. It has been shown that the Fos/Jun family of proteins and other protein factors (*e.g.*, NFκB) are capable of binding to the AP1 site and regulating the rate of transcription of target genes (Stein et al, 1993). Our results indicate that interaction of proteins with the AP1 element on the TH gene play an important role in control of transcription during hypoxia. This is supported by our finding that site-specific mutation of the AP1 element abolished transcription of the TH-CAT construct is evidence that the hypoxia-induced binding to the AP1 element plays a role in regulation of transcription of the TH gene during hypoxia (Norris & Millhorn, 1995).

4. SUMMARY

We have shown that the PC12 cell line is an excellent model system for investigations of the molecular and cellular processes involved in O_2-chemosensitivity. We have identified an O_2-sensitive K channel in this cell line that mediates membrane depolarization, an increase in intracellular free Ca^{2+}, and dopamine release during hypoxia. We also presented evidence which shows that expression of the gene for tyrosine hydroxylase, the rate-limiting enzyme in dopamine biosynthesis, is stimulated by reduced O_2 tension in PC12 and type I carotid body cells. In addition, we have successfully identified the DNA sequences and trans-acting protein factors that regulate transcription of the TH gene during hypoxia. The mechanisms by which a reduction in O_2 tension is transduced into alter cell function including increased gene expression remain unknown. Unpublished results from our laboratory show that the increased TH gene expression during hypoxia does not require activation of the cAMP-PKA signal transduction pathway. We propose that the increase in intracellular free Ca^{2+} that occurs as a result of membrane depolarization might play an important role. Preliminary findings from our laboratory show that blockade of the voltage operated Ca^{2+} channel or chelation of intracellular Ca^{2+} prevent full activation of the TH gene during hypoxia.

5. ACKNOWLEDGMENTS

This work was supported by grants from the National Institutes of Health (HL-33831 and HD-28948).

6. REFERENCES

Czyzyk-Krzeska MF, Bayliss D, Lawson E & Millhorn DE (1992) Regulation of tyrosine hydroxylase gene expression in the rat carotid body by hypoxia. J Neurochem 58: 1538–1546

Czyzyk-Krzeska MF, Furnari B, Lawson E & Millhorn DE (1994a) Hypoxia increases rate of transcription and stability of tyrosine hydroxylase mRNA in pheochromocytoma (PC12) cells. J Biol Chem 269: 760–764

Czyzyk-Krzeska MF, Dominski Z, Kole R & Millhorn DE (1994b) Hypoxia stimulates binding of a cytoplasmic protein to a pyrimidine-rich sequence in the 3'-untranslated region of rat tyrosine hydroxylase mRNA. J Biol Chem 269: 9940–9945

Delpiano M & Hescheler J (1989) Evidence for a PO_2 sensitive K^+ channel in the type I cell of the rabbit carotid body. FEBS Lett 249: 195–198

Fidone SJ, Gonzalez C & Yoshizaki K (1982) Effects of low oxygen on the release of dopamine from the rabbit carotid body *in vitro*. J Physiol, London 333: 93–110

Ganfornina MD & Lopez-Barneo J (1991) Single K channels in membrane patches of arterial chemoreceptor cells are modulated by O_2 tension. Proc Natl Acad Sci USA 88: 2927–2930

Gonzalez C, Kwok Y, Gibb J & Fidone S (1979) Effects of hypoxia on tyrosine hydroxylase activity in rat carotid body. J Neurochem 33: 713–719

Kilbourne EJ, Nankova B, Lewis E, McMahon A, Osaka H, Sabban D & Sabban E (1992) Regulated expression of the tyrosine hydroxylase gene by membrane depolarization. Identification of the responsive element and possible second messenger systems. J Biol Chem 267: 7563–7569

Lopez-Barneo J, Lopez-Lopez J, Ureña J & Gonzalez C (1988) Chemotransduction in the carotid body: K^+ current modulated by PO_2 in type I chemoreceptor cells. Science 241: 580–582

Lopez-Lopez J, Gonzalez C, Ureña J & Lopez-Barneo J (1989) Low PO_2 selectively inhibits K^+ channel activity in chemoreceptor cells of the mammalian carotid body. J Gen Physiol 93: 1001–1015

Norris M & Millhorn DE (1995) Hypoxia induced protein binding to O_2-responsive sequences on the tyrosine hydroxylase gene. J Biol Chem 270: 23774–23779

Obeso A, Rocher A, Fidone S & Gonzalez C (1992) The role of dihydropyridine-sensitive Ca^{2+} channels in stimulus-evoked catecholamine release from chemoreceptor cells of the carotid body. Neuroscience 47: 463–472

Semenza GL & Wang G (1993) General involvement of hypoxia-inducible factor 1 in transcriptional response to hypoxia. Proc Natl Acad Sci USA 90: 4304–4308

Stein B, Baldwin AS, Ballard DW, Greene WC, Angel P & Herrlich P (1993) Cross-coupling of the NF-kappa B p65 and Fos/Jun transcription factors produces potentiated biological function. EMBO J 12: 3879–3891

Wang W, Chen G, Yoshizaki K, Dinger B & Fidone S (1991) The role of cyclic AMP in chemoreception in the rabbit carotid body. Brain Res 540: 96–104

Zhu W, Conforti L & Millhorn DE (1995) Excitation-secretion in PC12 cells during hypoxia. Soc Neurosci Abstr 21: 65a

Zhu W, Conforti L, Czyzyk-Krzeska MF & Millhorn DE (1996) Membrane depolarization in PC12 cells during hypoxia is regulated by an O_2-sensitive K^+ current. Am J Physiol: Cell Physiol (In press)

21

REGULATION OF TYROSINE HYDROXYLASE mRNA STABILITY BY OXYGEN IN PC12 CELLS

Maria F. Czyzyk-Krzeska, Waltke R. Paulding, Janusz Lipski, John E. Beresh, and Sandra L. Kroll

Department of Molecular and Cellular Physiology
University of Cincinnati Medical Center
Cincinnati, Ohio 45267–0576

1. INTRODUCTION

Mammals evolved to live in the environment that contains 21% of oxygen. In order to preserve optimal tension of oxygen (pO_2) in the blood, organisms developed specialized cells that are O_2-sensors and initiate adaptive and protective regulatory mechanisms during limited availability of oxygen in the environment (*i.e.* hypoxia). The best known of these O_2-sensitive cells are the carotid body type I glomus cells that immediately detect even relatively moderate reduction in pO_2 in the arterial blood and communicate this information via carotid sinus nerve to the central nervous system networks that regulate the respiratory and cardiovascular systems. A major neurotransmitter that is released during hypoxia from type I cells is catecholamine dopamine. In type I cells hypoxia stimulates the activity of tyrosine hydroxylase (TH), the rate limiting enzyme in dopamine synthesis (Gonzalez et al, 1977; Hanbauer et al, 1977), and induces dopamine synthesis and release (Fidone et al, 1982a,b; Fishman et al, 1985). Moreover, hypoxia causes a five-fold increase in TH mRNA in a mechanism that is intrinsic to the type I cells, *i.e.* independent from neural or hormonal inputs (Czyzyk-Krzeska et al, 1992). Further identification and characterization of the O_2-dependent mechanisms that regulate TH gene expression required analysis at the molecular level. This type of studies has been, however, hindered by paucity of tissue provided by carotid body (only approximately 10,000 oxygen sensitive cells per carotid body in the rat). Our laboratory has recently reported that a clonal cell line derived from adrenal medulla tumor -pheochromocytoma- (PC12 cells) demonstrates several characteristics very similar to the carotid body type I cells. During hypoxia PC12 cells depolarize and release dopamine (Zhu et al, 1996). In addition, hypoxia leads to augmentation of TH protein content and its enzymatic activity (Feinsilver et al, 1987), and induces TH gene expression (Czyzyk-Krzeska et al, 1994a). The sensitivity, magnitude and time course of these responses in PC12 cells are very similar to those measured in the carotid body O_2-sensitive type I cells. The hypoxia-induced increase in the TH mRNA is

Frontiers in Arterial Chemoreception, edited by Zapata *et al.*
Plenum Press, New York, 1996

mediated by a dual mechanism involving an increased rate of TH gene transcription and increased stability of TH mRNA (half life of TH mRNA increases from 10 h to 30 h) (Czyzyk-Krzeska et al, 1994a). During the first hours of hypoxia, the increase in the total TH mRNA results primarily from fast transcriptional induction and the contribution of increased mRNA stability is small. During sustained hypoxia, the transcriptional rate declines and posttranscriptional regulation contributes primarily to the overall increase in TH mRNA. Thus, an increase in TH mRNA stability is necessary to maintain TH mRNA at the elevated concentration during long-term hypoxia. In the present paper, we summarize our studies on the molecular mechanisms involved in regulation of TH mRNA stability during hypoxia.

2. IDENTIFICATION OF A NOVEL CIS-ELEMENT IN THE 3' UNTRANSLATED REGION OF TH mRNA THAT IS NECESSARY FOR OXYGEN-DEPENDENT REGULATION OF TH mRNA STABILITY

Increase in TH mRNA stability correlates with the enhanced binding of a cytoplasmic protein to a sequence in the 3′ untranslated region of TH mRNA (Czyzyk-Krzeska et al, 1994b). Figure 1A shows the pattern of binding of proteins extracted from PC12 cells exposed to 21% O_2 or 5% O_2 to the 3′UTR of TH mRNA, as assessed by RNA gel retardation assays. The formation of this complex is enhanced when proteins were extracted from cells exposed to 5% O_2 from 1 to 18 h (Fig 1A). This enhancement in the complex formation is maintained when cells are treated with inhibitors of transcription for up to three hours (the longest time measured), indicating that on-going transcription is not necessary, at least not for the initial induction in the binding (not shown). Analysis by RNase T1 revealed that the binding region was limited to the 27 base long (1552–1578), cytidine-rich fragment of TH mRNA that we refer to as the *hypoxia-inducible protein binding site* (HIPBS) (Czyzyk-Krzeska et al, 1994b). Figure 1B shows a schematic representation of TH mRNA, including the sequence and localization of the HIPBS.

We performed detailed mutational analysis of the protein binding site within HIPBS (Czyzyk-Krzeska & Beresh, 1996). The sequences of important mutants and the quantification of the averaged results of formation of RNA-protein complexes are shown in Figure 1C. As expected, substitution of purines within HIPBS by cytidines [$C_{(6,18,19)}$] and to lesser extent with uridines [$U_{(6,18,19)}$] increased the binding. Importantly, we have identified a mutation $\mathbf{A}_{\mathbf{(10,11,12)}}$ where the substitution of adenines for the CCU sequence completely abolished the binding. This mutated RNA does not compete for the binding of protein to the wild sequence. We further identified the optimal hypoxia-inducible protein binding site which is represented by the motif (U/C)(C/U)**<u>CC</u>**CU where the core binding site is indicated by the bold-typed and underlined cytidines (Czyzyk-Krzeska & Beresh, 1996). Substitutions of either one of the cytidines with purine or uridine abolished the protein binding. The HIPBS motif is highly conserved in TH mRNA from different species (Czyzyk-Krzeska & Beresh, 1996).

Because hypoxia simultaneously induces both an increase in the rate of TH gene transcription and an increase in TH mRNA stability, it is difficult to isolate the stimulant's effect on stability alone. We have developed a system, however, that focuses exclusively on the posttranscriptional regulation of TH gene expression during hypoxia. Our system uses stably transfected PC12 cell lines that, in addition to the endogenous TH gene, ex-

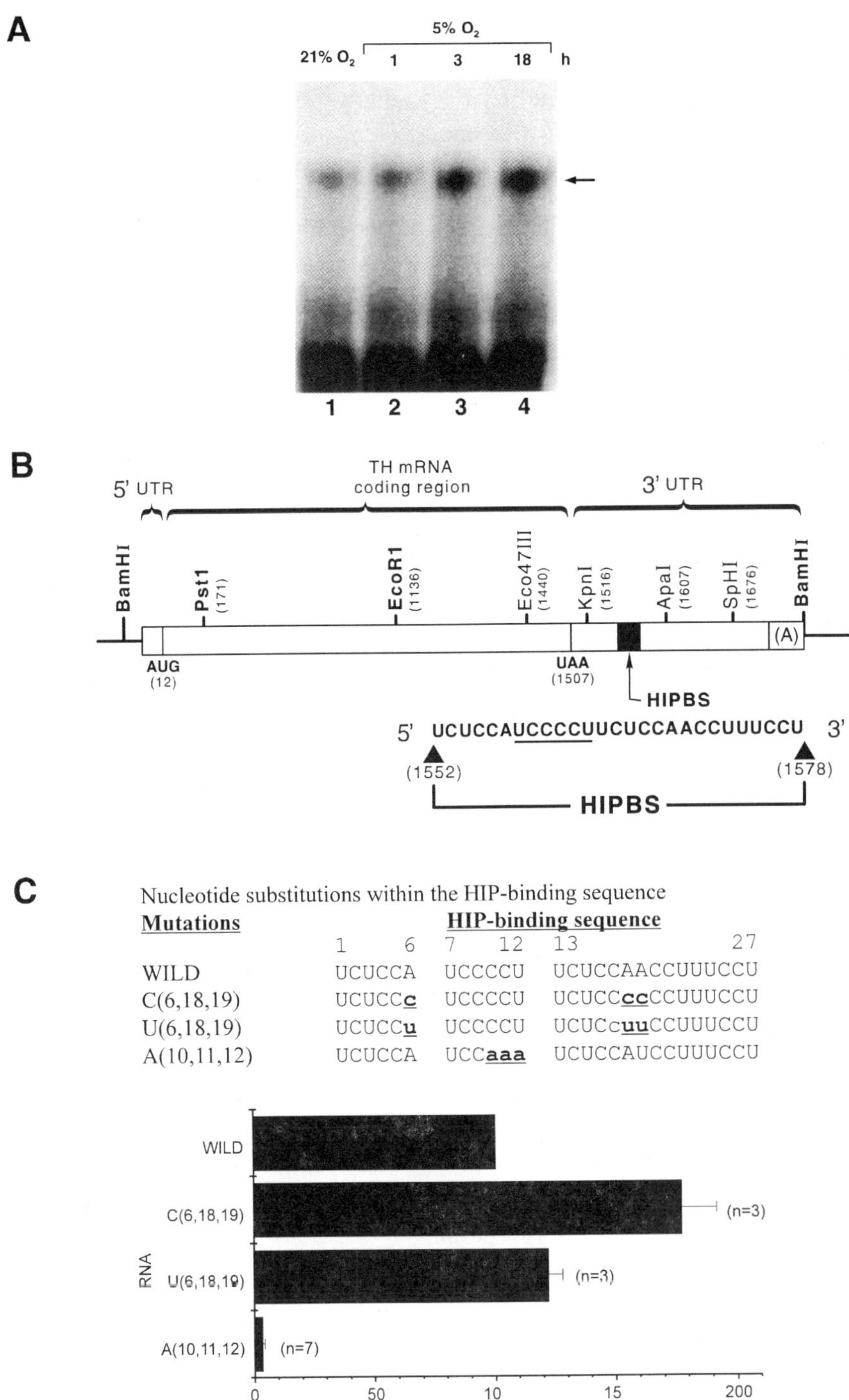

Figure 1. Identification of a novel *cis*-element in the 3′ untranslated region of TH mRNA. **A.** Gel retardation assay showing that protein binding to HIPBS is increased when protein extracts are obtained from PC12 cells exposed to hypoxia (1–18 h). **B.** Schematic representation of TH mRNA and position and sequence of HIPBS. **C.** Average results showing effects of mutations within HIPBS (Table) on the formation of HIPBS-protein complex.

press wild type (WT tTH mRNA) (UCC*CCUU*) or mutated within HIPBS ($MUT_{(10-13)}$ tTH mRNA) (UCC*AGAG*) TH mRNAs under control of a viral, hypoxia non-inducible cytomegalovirus (CMV) promoter in pcDNA3 eukaryotic expression vector. Both endogenous and transfected TH mRNAs are detected simultaneously using an RNase protection assay, with a probe that differentiates transfected mRNAs by an additional 30 bases located at the 5′ end of the 5′ untranslated region. Gel retardation assays in Figure 2A show that the $MUT_{(10-13)}$ transcript does not complex with PC12-cell cytoplasmic proteins. The degradation rates of transfected TH mRNAs were measured during normoxia (C) and hypoxia (H) 16 h after the inhibition of transcription with actinomycin D. Figure 2B shows the result of such experiment. The samples collected before actinomycin D was added are represented by C_0. It is clear that while hypoxia stabilizes the WT tTH mRNA (open arrow, lanes 1–3), similarly to the endogenous eTH mRNA (solid arrow; compare lanes 3 & 2 or 5 & 6); the $MUT_{(10-13)}$ tTH mRNA (lanes 4–6) is degraded after 16 h of transcriptional inhibition in both normoxic and hypoxic cells and is not stabilized by hypoxia during even shorter exposures to hypoxia.

Our results indicate that the interaction between the pyrimidine-rich HIPBS element and the hypoxia-inducible, poly(C) binding protein(s) is necessary for regulation of TH mRNA stability during hypoxia. The pyrimidine-rich sequences are primarily known to regulate splicing or translation (Morris et al, 1993), however, cytidine-rich elements were also shown to mediate the erythroid cell-specific stability of α_2-globin mRNA (Weiss & Liebhaber, 1994, 1995). This data is consistent with our hypothesis that cytidine-rich HIPBS and its binding protein regulate TH mRNA stability. The HIPBS-like elements are present in 3′ UTRs from other mRNAs that are likely to be regulated by hypoxia. We found HIPBS-like elements in the 3′ UTR of erythropoietin (EPO), inducible nitric oxide synthase (iNOS), tumor necrosis factor α (TNFα), myoglobin (MYO), tryptophan hydroxylase (TPH) and vascular endothelial growth factor (VEGF) mRNAs. In the case of EPO mRNA, binding of cytoplasmic protein to the HIPBS-like region was reported (Rondon et al, 1991). On the other hand, VEGF mRNA that is also stabilized during hypoxia is implicated to be regulated by a different mechanism although the HIPBS-like elements are also present in the 3′ UTR of VEGF mRNA (Levy et al, 1996). In other cases there is only indirect evidence for posttranscriptional regulation.

3. TRANS-ACTING ELEMENTS INVOLVED IN REGULATION OF TH mRNA STABILITY DURING HYPOXIA

HIPBS binding protein were analyzed on SDS-PAGE following UV-crosslinking of the RNA-protein complexes (Fig 3). The binding reactions were performed in the presence of poly(U) homopolymer that is used as a non specific competitor. A major 50 kD and a minor 80 kD bands were observed (arrows). Formation of both complexes was completely abolished when unlabeled 162 base TH transcript was added to the binding reaction, and neither band was formed when $MUT_{(10-13)}$ TH mRNA (see Fig 2A) was used in the binding reaction (not shown). Poly(C) RNA was a strong competitor of both complexes. Based on the above results, and on the fact that the protein core binding site is the UCCCCU motif, we concluded that the protein factors in both complexes show preferential affinity for the C-rich sequences and that the C-rich binding proteins are necessary for the formation of the complex with the TH mRNA. Most importantly, we found an enhancement of the 50 kD complex when proteins were extracted from hypoxic cells (Fig.

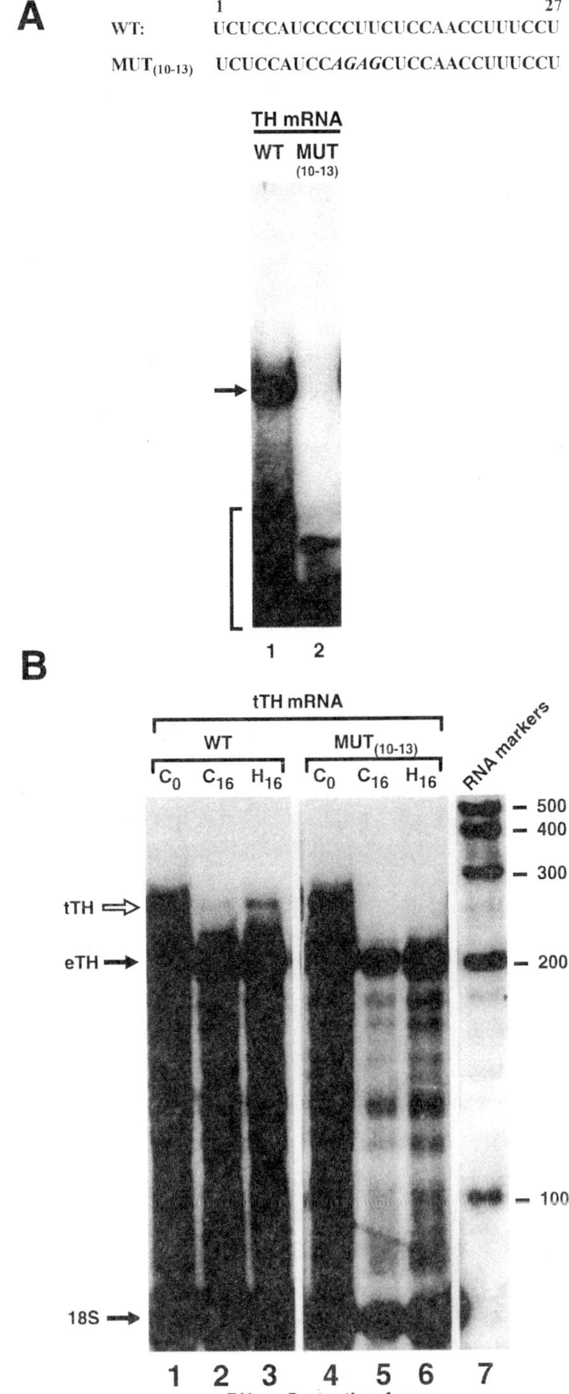

Figure 2. Mutations within HIPBS that abolish protein binding prevent regulation of TH mRNA stability during hypoxia. **A.** Gel retardation assay showing that mutation $MUT_{(10-13)}$ prevents formation of the RNA-protein complex. **B.** RNase protection assay showing regulation of mRNA stability for transfected wild type (WT, open arrow, lanes 1–3) or transfected mutated ($MUT_{(10-13)}$, lanes 4–6) TH mRNAs. Endogenous TH mRNA is indicated with a solid arrow. Cells expressing transfected TH mRNAs were treated with actinomycin D (5 μg/ml) and exposed to normoxia (C) or hypoxia (H) for 16 h.

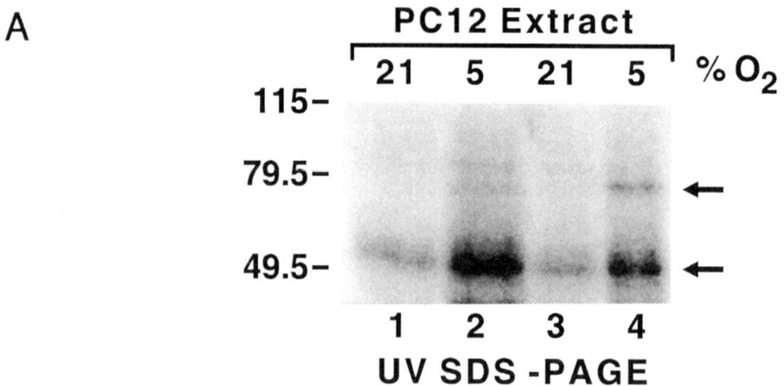

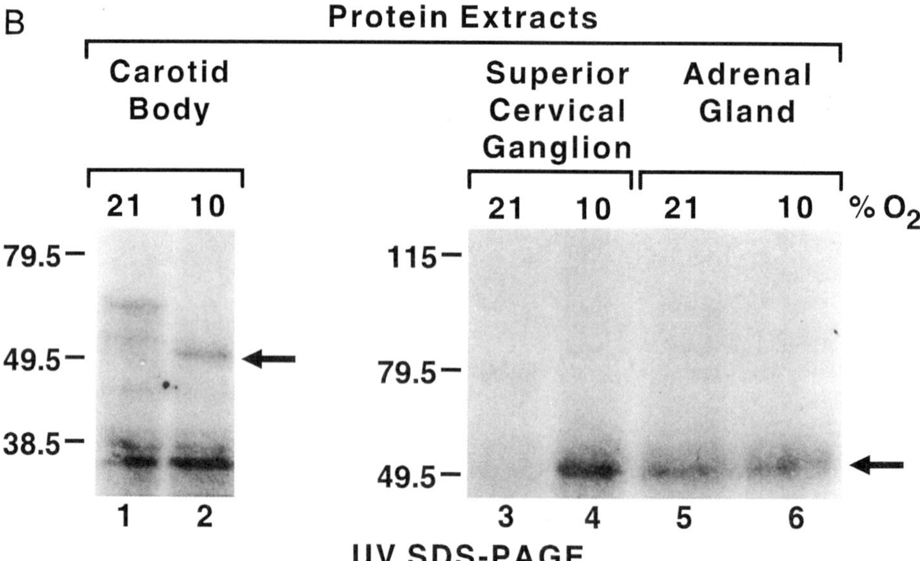

Figure 3. Identification of the HIPBS-protein complexes using UV-crosslinking. Two specific complexes -50 kD and 80 kD- are indicated with arrows. **A.** Formation of the 50 kD complex is induced when protein extracts are prepared from PC12 cells exposed to hypoxia (lanes 2 and 4) as compared to normoxia (lanes 1 & 3). **B.** Formation of the 50 kD complex is induced when protein extracts are prepared from carotid bodies (lanes 1 & 2) or superior cervical sympathetic ganglia (lanes 3 & 4) obtained from rats exposed to 10% hypoxia for 4 h. The formation of the 50 kD complex is not induced by hypoxia in adrenal gland.

3A, lanes 2 & 4) as compared to normoxic cells (Fig 3A, lanes 1 & 3). The formation of the 80 kD complex also increased.

Figure 3B shows the formation of UV-crosslinked complexes from crude protein extracts of either carotid bodies (Fig 3B, lanes 1 & 2), superior cervical ganglia (lanes 3 & 4) or adrenal glands (lanes 5 & 6). The carotid body is an extremely small structure (*ca.* 10,000 cells per carotid body), but 10 carotid bodies (from 5 rats) were sufficient to obtain approximately 80 μg of crude protein extract. The formation of the 50 kD complex was particularly enhanced when protein extracts were obtained from carotid bodies and superior cervical ganglia, but not adrenal glands, from rats exposed to 10% hypoxia (H) for 4 h.

We have previously reported that the HIPBS-protein complex was approximately 74 kD (Czyzyk-Krzeska et al, 1994b). Currently we see the 50 kD complex as the major one because we have used poly(U) RNA as a non-specific competitor. When UV-crosslinked complexes are formed without poly(U) RNA, a complex migrating at approximately 80 kD is dominant. After poly(U) is added, however, most of this complex disappears and the 50 kD complex becomes dominant. Since both 50 kD and 80 kD complexes are induced by hypoxia both can be involved in binding to TH mRNA. The currently known poly(C) binding proteins include the 66 and 64 kD nuclear proteins K and J (Matunis et al, 1992), the 43 kD cytoplasmic poly(C)-binding protein that binds to α_2 globin mRNA (α-PCBP) (Wang et al, 1995; Kiledjian et al, 1995), and the 48 kD LOX mRNA binding protein that binds to the multiple repeats of pyrimidine rich motifs C_4A/GC_3UCUUC_4AAG, and inhibits 15 lipoxygenase mRNA translation (Ostareck-Lederer et al, 1994). Based on our studies with the antibodies against the K protein (3C2 [22], gift from Dr G Dreyfuss' laboratory) we found that protein K was not involved in the formation of the TH mRNA-protein complex although it was present in the cytoplasmic extracts (data not shown). The 43 kD α-CP1 and α-CP2 proteins bind preferably to the CCUCCC sequences and are involved in regulation of the α_2 globin mRNA stability. These proteins show similarities with the TH mRNA binding protein that forms the 50 kD complex as far as molecular weight and affinity for the C-rich sequences. We have recently initiated purification of the HIP using poly(C) agarose affinity chromatography and found that we have enriched for two proteins of approximate molecular weight of 40 and 46 kD. We are presently continuing identification of these protein factors.

Regulation of gene expression at the posttranscriptional level may be particularly important during energy deprivation, such as hypoxia or ischemia, because it allows for increases in the steady-state levels or maintenance of mRNA that is already available in the cell. Very little is known about regulation of mRNA stability that physiologically occurs in the whole animal. Our data showing that binding of protein to HIPBS is increased when proteins are extracted from carotid bodies or superior cervical ganglia obtained from hypoxic animals indicate that TH mRNA may be regulated at the posttranscriptional level in these tissues during hypoxia. Thus, the induction of TH mRNA during hypoxia in type I cells of carotid body (Czyzyk-Krzeska et al, 1992) may involve posttranscriptional regulation. On the other hand, we previously reported that the TH mRNA is not increased in the superior cervical ganglion during short-term, mild hypoxia (Czyzyk-Krzeska et al, 1992). Thus, the present observation showing increased binding of protein to HIPBS during hypoxia indicates that if TH mRNA stability is increased in the sympathetic neurons during hypoxia, it may help to maintain the existing concentration of TH mRNA rather than to augment it.

4. ACKNOWLEDGMENTS

This work was supported by the NIH grant R29-HL51078 (MFC-K), American Heart Association Grant-in-Aid 94017440 (MFC-K) and NARSAD Young Investigator Award (MFC-K). MFC-K is a recipient of a Parker B Francis Fellowship. WRP and SLK are supported by the NIH Training Grant HL 07571.

5. REFERENCES

Czyzyk-Krzeska MF & Beresh JE (1996) Characterization of the hypoxia inducible protein binding site within the pyrimidine rich tract in the 3′ untranslated region of the tyrosine hydroxylase mRNA. J Biol Chem 271: 3293–3299

Czyzyk-Krzeska MF, Bayliss DA, Lawson EE & Millhorn DE (1992) Regulation of tyrosine hydroxylase gene expression in the rat carotid body by hypoxia. J Neurochem 58: 1538–1546

Czyzyk-Krzeska MF, Furnari BA, Lawson EE & Millhorn DE (1994a) Hypoxia increases rate of transcription and stability of tyrosine hydroxylase mRNA in pheochromocytoma (PC12) cells. J Biol Chem 269: 760–764

Czyzyk-Krzeska MF, Dominski Z, Kole R & Millhorn DE (1994b) Hypoxia stimulates binding of a cytoplasmic protein to a pyrimidine rich sequence in the 3′-untranslated region of rat tyrosine hydroxylase mRNA. J Biol Chem 269: 9940–9945

Feinsilver SH, Wong R & Rayabin DM (1987) Adaptation of neurotransmitter synthesis to chronic hypoxia in cell culture. Biochem Biophys Acta 928: 56–62

Fidone S, Gonzalez C & Yoshizaki K (1982a) Effects of hypoxia on catecholamine synthesis in rabbit carotid body *in vitro*. J Physiol, London 333: 81–91

Fidone S, Gonzalez C & Yoshizaki K (1982b) Effects of low oxygen on the release of dopamine from the rabbit carotid body *in vitro*. J Physiol, London 333: 93–110

Fishman MC, Greene WL & Platika D (1985) Oxygen chemoreception by carotid body cells in culture. Proc Natl Acad Sci USA 82: 1448–1450

Gonzalez C, Kwok Y, Gibb J & Fidone S (1977) Effects of hypoxia on tyrosine hydroxylase activity in rat carotid body. J Neurochem 33: 713–719

Hanbauer I, Lovenberg W & Costa E (1977) Induction of tyrosine 3-monooxigenase in carotid body of rats exposed to hypoxic conditions. Neuropharmacology 16: 277–282

Kiledjian M, Wang X & Liebhaber SA (1995) Identification of two KH domain proteins in the α-globin mRNP stability complex. EMBO J 14: 4357–4364

Levy AP, Levy NS, Goldberg MA (1996) Posttranscriptional regulation of vascular endothelial growth factor by hypoxia. J Biol Chem 271: 2746–2753

Matunis MJ, Michael WM & Dreyfuss G (1992) Characterization and primary structure of the poly(C)-heterogeneous nuclear ribonucleoprotein complex K protein. Mol Cell Biol 12: 164–171

Morris DR, Kakegawa T, Kaspar RL & White MW (1993) Polypyrimidine tracts and their binding proteins: regulatory sites for posttranscriptional modulation of gene expression. Biochemistry 32: 2931–2937

Ostareck-Lederer A, Ostareck DH, Standart N & Thiele BJ (1994) Translation of 15-lipoxygenase mRNA is inhibited by protein that binds to a repeated sequence in the 3′ untranslated region. EMBO J 13: 1476–1481

Rondon IJ, MacMillan LA, Beckman BS, Goldberg MA, Schneider T, Bunn HF & Malter JS (1991) Hypoxia upregulates the activity of a novel erythropoietin mRNA binding protein. J Biol Chem 266: 16594–16598

Wang X, Kiledjian M, Weiss IM & Liebhaber SA (1995) Detection and characterization of a 3′ untranslated region ribonucleoprotein complex associated with human α-globin mRNA stability. Mol Cell Biol 15: 1769–1777

Weiss IM & Liebhaber SA (1994) Erythroid cell-specific determinants of α-globin mRNA stability. Mol Cell Biol 14: 8123–8132

Weiss IM & Liebhaber SA (1995) Erythroid cell-specific mRNA stability elements in the α_2 globin 3′ untranslated region. Mol Cell Biol 15: 2457–2465

Zhu WH, Conforti L, Czyzyk-Krzeska MF & Millhorn DE (1996) Hypoxia modulates excitation and dopamine secretion in PC12 cells through an O_2-sensitive K^+ current. Am J Physiol: Cell Physiol (In press)

EFFECTS OF HYPOXIA ON THE INTERCELLULAR CHANNEL ACTIVITY OF CULTURED GLOMUS CELLS

Verónica Abudara[1,2] and C. Eyzaguirre[1]

[1] Department of Physiology
University of Utah School of Medicine
Salt Lake City, Utah
[2] Departamento de Fisiología
Facultad de Medicina
Universidad de la República
Montevideo, Uruguay.

1. SUMMARY

Dual voltage clamp experiments have shown that hypoxia induced by Na-dithionite or N_2 reduced junctional macroconductance (G_j) in about 70% of cultured and coupled glomus cell pairs while increasing it in the rest. To explore possible mechanisms for these effects, we studied the activity of gap junction channels under similar conditions. The calculated single channel conductances (g_j) fell into two categories. A low-conductance group, which was most frequently observed, had a mean g_j of 27.8 ± 0.29 pS (mean ± SEM; n = 968 events). The other group had higher conductances (47.6 ± 0.35 pS; n = 528). When PO_2 was reduced (hypoxia), the low conductances did not change significantly in any of the junctions. The high-conductance units appeared less frequently in some junctions whereas in others they remained unaltered. Thus, rapid channel flickering during hypoxia may not be the only mechanism determining G_j during coupling or uncoupling. It is possible that slow (seconds) opening and closing of the channels could play an important role in this phenomenon.

2. INTRODUCTION

Transmission of signals between two coupled cells is mediated by intercellular channels in gap junctions. Imaging with low-angle x-rays and electron microscopy show, embedded in the plasma membrane of each cell, six protein subunits (connexins, forming the connexon) surrounding an aqueous pore (Hille, 1992). Adjoining connexons from two ap-

Frontiers in Arterial Chemoreception, edited by Zapata *et al.*
Plenum Press, New York, 1996

posed cells form a dodecameric structure across the gap. These channels provide a non-selective pathway through which, ions and small molecules cross the junctions. The ease of passage can be regulated through different mechanisms leading to the opening or closing of the channels. As in many other systems, glomus cells of the carotid body are electrically coupled through gap junctions (McDonald, 1981; Monti-Bloch et al, 1993; Abudara & Eyzaguirre, 1994). In addition, large molecules such as Procion navy blue (intracellularly injected) can cross these junctions (Baron & Eyzaguirre, 1977).

The most accurate electrical parameter monitoring the strength of coupling and its variations, is the junctional conductance. Dual whole-cell voltage clamping has shown that hypoxia reduces G_j in most glomus cell pairs (about 70%) while developing tighter coupling in the others (Abudara & Eyzaguirre, unpublished). These results are in line with previous data obtained with dual current clamping in the whole organ (Monti-Bloch et al, 1993). The oxygen sensitivity of these intercellular junctions, raises important questions about the role of hypoxic modulation of coupling during chemoreception (Eyzaguirre & Abudara, 1995; also, this volume).

The mechanisms underlying the effects of hypoxia on junctional conductance, are unknown. Some results indicate that Ca^{+2} influx during PO_2 reduction may be responsible for this effect since high $[Ca^{2+}]_i$ disengages the glomus cells in a manner similar to hypoxia (Abudara & Eyzaguirre, 1996). However, hypoxia may modulate junctional conductance through various mechanisms: by altering the number of functional channels, the probability of opening, the open time and/or the elementary conductance of individual channels. It has been suggested that Ca^{+2} and H^+ bind to specific sites, and affect the gating kinetics of the channel, probably by conformational changes.

As a first step to investigate these mechanisms, we have started to characterize the behavior of intercellular channels under normoxia and hypoxia, using dual whole-cell voltage clamping.

3. METHODS

Carotid bodies were removed from the carotid bifurcations of anesthetized (Na-pentobarbital, 50 mg/kg) Wistar rats (40–60 g). The freed organs were suspended in 500 μl of growth medium in collagen-coated petri dishes and mechanically dissociated. After the cells settled on the bottom of the dish, 2 ml of serum-free growth medium was added to the dishes. This medium was a mixture of Dulbecco's Modified Eagle's Medium (DMEM) and Ham's Nutrient F-12, sodium bicarbonate 0.014 mM, insulin 80 U/l and 1% mixture penicillin/streptomycin/fungizone. pH was adjusted to 7.4 with HEPES-NaOH. The preparations were left in a humidified atmosphere of 5% CO_2, 95% air, at 37°C, for 1 to 7 days. During electrophysiological recordings, the cultures were superfused with Nutrient Mixture HAM F-12 supplemented with 1.18 g/l sodium bicarbonate, equilibrated with air or 100% O_2 , pH 7.4, at room temperature. Hypoxia was produced by brief exposure to 1–10 mM sodium dithionite ($Na_2S_2O_4$) or 100% N_2. PO_2 was continuously monitored in the bath with a small electrode.

Two adjacent glomus cells were simultaneously impaled with intracellular microelectrodes (3 M KCl, 10–20 MΩ) under phase-contrast optics at 450x magnification. Both electrodes were independently connected to the input stages of voltage-clamp amplifiers (WPI S-7050A Patch Clamp Systems). The resistance of the pipettes was corrected by a series resistance compensation circuit. The output of each amplifier was low-pass filtered at 100 Hz.

Both cells were voltage-clamped at identical holding potentials (V_H), resulting in zero transjunctional voltage (V_j). Command pulses applied to "driving" Cell 1 elicited a V_j across the junction. Currents recorded in the "passive" Cell 2 (ΔI_2) were produced only by the imposed V_j, being equal in magnitude but opposite in sign to I_j, the junctional current ($I_j = -\Delta I_2$). Thus, I_j was recorded as ΔI_2 during the V_j pulse (Fig 1). The junctional conductance G_j was calculated from the relationship $-\Delta I_2 / V_j$.

To study unitary conductances, a constant transjunctional voltage was imposed by holding each cell at a different potential. Thus, I_j flowed from the more positive cell to its more negative neighbor evoking an outward current (I_1) in this cell and an inward, junctional current in the other. Similarly, and considering that channels have open and closed states, the activity of intercellular channels (gating) are reflected by simultaneous step changes in both current traces (I_1 and I_2), which are equal in magnitude but opposite in polarity (mirror image).

Voltage and current recordings, were simultaneously stored on video tape for further analysis or connected on line to a MacIntosh Plus computer through a Mac Lab/4 interphase. Data were acquired by Scope v. 3.28 (sampling up to 1.23 kHz) and by Chart / 4 programs. The information was retrieved in digital form and stored in Statview 1.04 spread sheets for quantification.

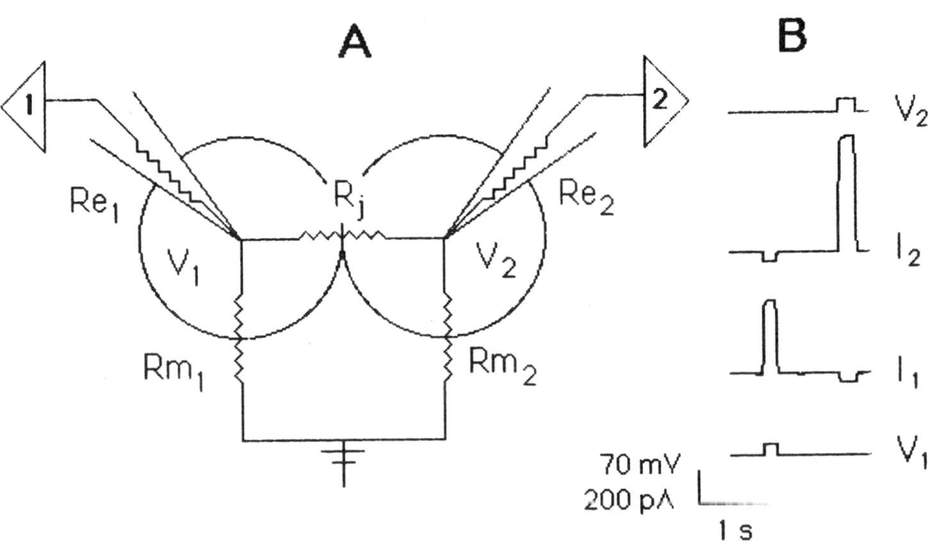

Figure 1. A. Equivalent circuit for a pair of coupled cells connected to two independent voltage-clamp amplifiers (1, 2). The non-junctional membrane (input) resistance of each cell is Rm_1 and Rm_2; R_j is the junctional resistance between the coupled cells. Re_1 and Re_2 represent the series resistances of the electrodes. The membrane potential of each cell (Vm_1 and Vm_2) is controlled by the voltage-clamp amplifiers 1 and 2. **B**. Measurement of macrojunctional conductance, G_j. Both cells were held at -20 mV while voltage steps of about 30 mV were alternately applied (V_1, V_2) to monitor G_j. Downward deflections in I_1 and I_2 represent junctional currents and upward deflections represent junctional plus non-junctional currents. Note the different duration of voltage steps in V_1 and V_2 for cells 1 and 2. In this pair, the value of $G_j = I_j / V_j$ was 1.74 nS.

4. RESULTS

4.1. Estimates of Single Junction Channel Conductance (G_j)

Unless otherwise stated, the channel data reported here were collected from naturally occurring low macrojunctional conductance pairs (< 2 nS). This was necessary to analyze a low-density channel population. The macroconductance G_j ranged from 0.19–1.93 nS, with a mean ± SEM of 0.77 ± 0.12 nS, in eight pairs. We selected recordings having low noise, no slow waves (see below) and symmetry of quantal changes of equal magnitude and opposite polarity in I_1 and I_2. To estimate the most likely single-channel conductance, two methods were used: 1) In some recordings from both cells, the amplitude of unitary events could be unambiguously seen. In these cases, current transitions from one level to another (without apparent partial steps) were measured by hand. The amplitude of the transitions was divided by V_j to obtain g_j. 2) Other recordings, showing a more dense channel population, were digitized by using the Statview Program. The amplitudes of all points from current records were measured from a baseline level, defined as the minimal value of current noise. At this reference level, which was arbitrarily set at zero pA, *n* intercellular channels remained open, and junctional noise increased when the channels switched from the closed to the open state. Therefore, the baseline, which was updated during each period of analysis, represented the more "closed" level of the selected period. The amplitude of the digitized points of the current records was then divided by V_j and the calculated conductances were plotted in frequency histograms. Such histograms showed a series of roughly Gaussian conductance peaks. Significant differences between the peaks reflected the conductance amplitude of single channels or g_j (Veenstra, 1990). The frequency histogram of unitary channel conductances g_j, calculated with both methods, showed two main peaks: a major one of conductances ≈ 20–35 pS, and a smaller one at about 40–55 pS. If we assume the presence of at least two independent normal distributions, we can define categories for both of them and calculate their mean conductances. The calculated mean values were 27.8 ± 0.29 pS), n = 968 events, for the first distribution and 47.6 ± 0.35 pS, n = 528 events for the second one. This is shown in Figure 2.

Figure 3 shows one recording of dual voltage-clamped cells where a steady driving voltage (150 mV) was applied across the junction (A). Junction channels falling within the two categories described above are shown in B by filled (small amplitude) and open (large amplitude) arrows. Note the opposite polarities of the flickering events in I_1 and I_2.

The mean open-time of junction channels was measured in 5 pairs. Its value was 109 ms (range 10–750 ms; n = 57) for the 20–35 pS conductance and 140 ms (range 17 ms-1.4 s; n = 52) for the 40–55 pS conductance. The time course of the transitions from the open to the closed states and vice versa was 10–20 ms. Nevertheless, as signals were low-pass

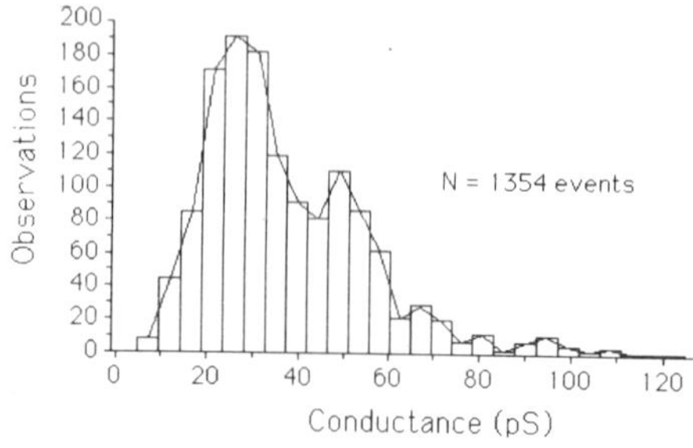

Figure 2. Frequency histogram of conductances determined from small steps in junction current I_j in 8 different pairs. Horizontal axis, single-channel conductance g_i, 30 bins; vertical axis, number of occurrences in each bin. Conductance changes of 20–35 pS appeared most frequently, followed by a smaller, peak at 40–55 pS. Bars represent the actual measurements. The superimposed line connects the peaks obtained from each bin.

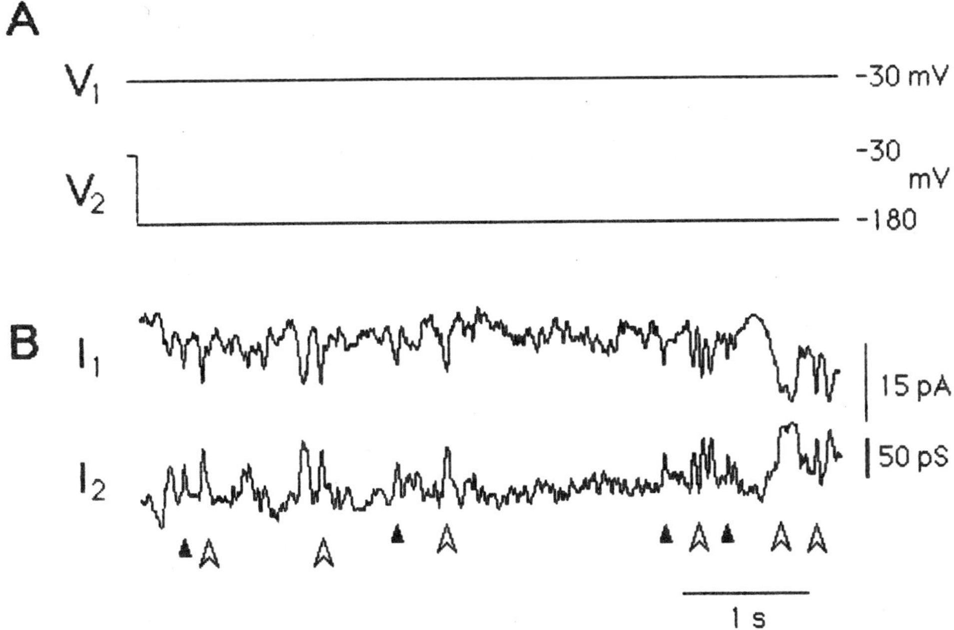

Figure 3. Gap junction channels between voltage-clamped glomus cells. **A**. A steady driving voltage of 150 mV was imposed through the junction by holding Cell 1 at -30 mV (V_1) and Cell 2 at -180 mV (V_2). **B**. Current recordings (I_1, I_2) show activity of intercellular channels. Channels with low (20–35 pS) and large (40–55 pS) conductances are shown by filled and open arrow heads respectively. Calibrations in B are for current (pA) and conductance (pS) of the channels.

filtered at 100 Hz to reduce noise, the possibility of an undetected higher frequency flickering cannot be ignored. Also, many of our recordings showed more than one open channel. In this situation, kinetic analysis of single intercellular events is difficult.

4.2. Effects of Hypoxia on Junction Channel Activity

At this writing we have analyzed only five pairs of coupled cells. During hypoxia, the peaks corresponding to the low-conductance channels were not changed in a statistically significant way in all pairs. In three instances (60%) the occurrence of high-conductance channels was significantly reduced (also, Eyzaguirre & Abudara, 1995). However, these high-conductance channels were not significantly affected in the other two pairs. Consequently, the effect of hypoxia on junction channel activity seems to be restricted to the high-conductance channels. What is interesting moreover is that hypoxic changes in G_j (macroconductance) were not always associated with changes in g_j (channel flickering). For instance, in one pair, G_j decreased from 4.87 nS to 2.77 nS (uncoupling) during superfusion with $Na_2S_2O_4$ 2 mM (PO_2 = 30 Torr). The unitary conductances were calculated and showed a bimodal distribution with peaks at 23.9 ± 0.17 pS and 40.8 ± 0.26 pS during normoxia. During hypoxia, in spite of the uncoupling, these peaks showed almost identical values (23.6 ± 0.16 pS, and 40.3 ± 0.16 pS).

5. DISCUSSION

Analyses of gap junction channel activity from a total of eight normoxic glomus cell pairs indicated that these events were grouped in two unitary conductance groups. The low-amplitude conductance group, most frequently observed, had a mean around 28 pS while the high-amplitude group had a mean of about 48 pS. Channels with single conductances of 50–60 pS have been reported in neonatal rats (Burt & Spray, 1988) and embryonic chick heart (Veenstra & De Haan, 1988). However, values of g_j ranging from 10 to 30 pS have been observed in fibroblasts (Jongsma & Rook, 1990), in transformed cells (Spray & Burt, 1990) and in cell lines derived from rat liver (Spray et al, 1991).

5.1. Is There More Than One Type of Junction Channel between Glomus Cells?

Several possibilities will be discussed immediately below:

A. We favor the idea that the two conductances (20–35 pS and 40–55 pS) represent activity of different junction channels, possibly formed by different proteins. Evidence favoring this hypothesis comes from the following observations: (a) Events of both amplitudes were recorded in all pairs although some transitions from one level of conductance to the other were observed. (b) When g_j was measured in two well coupled pairs ($G_j > 5$ nS), it showed a calculated mean conductance of 50.7 ± 0.1 pS, suggesting that large G_js result from many high-conductance channels at the junction. (c) Hypoxia preferentially affected the frequency of occurrence of high-conductance events whereas low-conductance channels were resistant to hypoxic exposure. Clearly, the possibility of having two types of junction channels, formed by different proteins, needs to be established by immunocytochemical studies.

B. The major peak at 20–35 pS represents the true unitary conductance and the larger one (40–55 pS) reflects simultaneous openings of two 20–35 pS channels. This possibility cannot be ruled out although the 40–55 pS peaks were too large to be solely explained by the random opening of two single low-conductance channels. Furthermore, in such case hypoxia should have depressed both peaks and this did not happen.

C. The smaller conductances of 20–35 pS are subconductance states of the true 40–55 pS single channel conductances. Multiple conductance states have been identified in a variety of ion channels (Auerbach & Sachs, 1984) probably representing different states of the channel proteins. Again, we refer to the effects of hypoxia. It is impossible to depress total channel conductance (presumably represented by the 40–55 pS peaks) without affecting the sub-conductances.

5.2. Possible Mechanism Responsible for Reduction in Conductance Peak during Hypoxia

In a junction with only one channel type, the macroconductance G_j is $= n \times P_o \times g_j$, where n represents the number of channels, P_o is the probability for a given channel to be in the open state and g_j the unitary conductance of the channel. When more than one channel type is present, identical terms are added to the equation (as many terms as types of channels). Thus, if n and g_j remained constant when hypoxia changed G_j, coupling or uncoupling could have been due to variations in the P_o of the channels. Hypoxia may have preferentially affected the frequency of occurrence of the high-conductance channels. If this is the case, it would not be unique. Delpiano & Hescheler (1989) and Ganfornina & López-Barneo (1991) have reported that hypoxia reduces the P_o of K^+ channels in the glomus cell membrane.

5.3. Role of Junction Channels in the Effects of Hypoxia on Macro Junctional Conductance

Hypoxia uncouples about 70% of the cell pairs but the rest undergo tighter coupling (Eyzaguirre & Abudara, this volume). These opposite effects may depend on the type of channel affected by hypoxia. One type of channel may always close under low PO_2 whereas others may open. On the other hand, a reduction in PO_2 may act on the same channel through different mechanisms. To decide between these possibilities, the channel kinetic properties should be studied during normoxia and low oxygenation. Recent data support the view that hypoxia affects junctional conductance through different intracellular mediators, *i.e.*, Ca^{2+} and H^+ ions, and cAMP. In glomus cells, an excess of Ca^{2+} ions decreases coupling in most cell pairs while cAMP increases it (Abudara & Eyzaguirre, 1996; also, unpublished). cAMP may act by phosphorylating the gap junction proteins as occurs in other systems (Saez et al, 1986). Therefore, the same intercellular channels may open or close depending on the relative amounts of available cytosolic factors.

An important point noted above, is that hypoxic uncoupling (or increased coupling) was not always followed by obvious changes in junction channel flickering, *i.e.*, the frequency of appearance of channel conductances did not change. It is possible that the junction channels of glomus cells open or close in two ways. One would be by rapid alternations in activity (flickering), and the other by slowly narrowing or enlarging the intercellular pore, like the shutter of a photographic camera. Detailed analyses of available data should shed light on this possibility. In fact, on numerous occasions we have obtained dual current recordings in which channel flickering was superimposed on slow waves (lasting seconds), as shown in Figure 3 of Eyzaguirre & Abudara (1995). Hypoxia did not equally affect flickering and the slow waves.

6. ACKNOWLEDGMENTS

Work supported by NIH grant NS 07938.

The presentation of this paper by VA received the Heymans-de Castro-Neil Award for young scientists.

7. REFERENCES

Abudara V & Eyzaguirre C (1994) Electrical coupling between cultured glomus cells of the rat carotid body: Observations with current and voltage clamping. Brain Res 664: 257–265

Abudara V & Eyzaguirre C (1996) Effects of calcium on the electric coupling of carotid body glomus cells. Brain Res (in press)

Auerbach A & Sachs F (1984) Patch clamp studies of single ionic channels. Annu Rev Biophys Bioeng 13: 269–302

Baron M & Eyzaguirre C (1977) Effects of temperature on some membrane characteristics of carotid body cells. Am J Physiol 233: C35-C46

Burt JM & Spray DC (1988) Single-channel events and gating behavior of the cardiac gap junction channel. Proc Natl Acad Sci USA 85: 3431–3434

Delpiano MA & Hescheler J (1989) Evidence for a PO_2-sensitive K^+ channel in the type-I cell of the rabbit carotid body. FEBS Lett 249: 195–198

Eyzaguirre C & Abudara V (1995) Possible role of coupling between glomus cells in carotid body chemoreception. Biol Signals 4: 263–270

Ganfornina MD & López-Barneo J (1991) Single K^+ channels in membrane patches of arterial chemoreceptor cells are modulated by O_2 tension. Proc Natl Acad Sci USA 88: 2927–2930

Hille B (1992) Ionic Channels of Excitable Membranes. Sunderland, MA: Sinauer

Jongsma H & Rook M (1990) Cardiac gap junctions: gating properties of single channels. In: Robards AW, Lucas WJ, Pitts JD, Jongsma HJ & Spray DC (eds) Parallels in Cell to Cell Junctions in Plants and Animals. Berlin: Springer. pp 87–99

Kessler JA, Spray DC, Saez JC & Bennett MVL (1985) Development and regulation of electrotonic coupling between cultured sympathetic neurons. In: Bennett MVL & Spray DC (eds) Gap Junctions. NY: Cold Spring Harbor Laboratory. pp 231–240

McDonald DM (1981) Peripheral chemoreceptors: structure-function relationships of the carotid body. In: Hornbein TF (ed) Regulation of Breathing, vol. 17, Lung Biology in Health and Disease. New York: Marcel Dekker. pp 105–319

Monti-Bloch L, Abudara V & Eyzaguirre C (1993) Electrical communication between glomus cells of the rat carotid body. Brain Res 622: 119–131

Saez JC, Spray DC, Nairen AC, Hertzberg E, Greengard P & Bennett MVL (1986) cAMP increases junctional conductance and stimulates phosphorylation of the 27-kDa principal gap junction polypeptide. Proc Natl Acad Sci USA 83: 2473–2477

Spray DC & Burt JM (1990) Structure-activity relations of the cardiac gap junction channel. Am J Physiol 258: C195-C205

Spray DC, Chanson M, Moreno AP, Dermietzel R & Meda P (1991) Distinctive gap junction channel types connect WB cells, a clonal cell line derived from rat liver. Am J Physiol 260: C513-C527

Veenstra RD (1990) Voltage-dependent gating of gap junction channels in an embryonic chick ventricular cell pairs. Am J Physiol 258: C662-C672

Veenstra RD & DeHaan RL (1988) Cardiac gap junction channel activity in embryonic chick ventricular cells. Am J Physiol 254: H170-H180

23

REFLECTIONS ON THE CAROTID NERVE SENSORY DISCHARGE AND COUPLING BETWEEN GLOMUS CELLS

C. Eyzaguirre[1] and Verónica Abudara[1,2]

[1] Department of Physiology
University of Utah School of Medicine
Salt Lake City, Utah
[2] Departamento de Fisiología
Facultad de Medicina
Universidad de la República
Montevideo, Uruguay

1. MORPHOLOGY AND ORIGIN OF THE SENSORY DISCHARGES

In most sensory receptors of vertebrates, the action potentials of myelinated fibers originate from the first node of Ranvier, closest to the nerve terminals (Loewenstein & Rathkamp, 1958). The spike origin is not established in receptors innervated by unmyelinated (C) fibers, but probably occurs in the fiber at some distance from the endings (Edwards & Ottoson, 1958; Ringham, 1971). The carotid body glomus cells are innervated by myelinated (A) and unmyelinated (C) fibers from the carotid nerve (Fidone & Sato, 1969), although it is not known where the action potentials originate in either type of fiber. These uncertainties are due to a large extent to the complex morphology of the carotid body innervation. A single carotid nerve fiber divides extensively to innervate up to 20 glomus cells (Eyzaguirre & Gallego, 1975; Kondo, 1976) forming what is, presumably, the sensory unit. Moreover, glomus cells may be innervated more than once by the same fiber, and some cells are innervated by more than one carotid nerve fiber (De Castro, 1940; 1951). Figure 1 is a composite drawing from De Castro's original microscope slides examined by Eyzaguirre & Gallego (1975). Axon 1 innervates glomeruli A and C. Cells marked by dots in glomerulus A are innervated by branches from axons 1 and 2. As shown below, this complex innervation pattern has to be considered when analyzing the origin of the sensory discharge.

2. GENERATOR ACTIVITY IN CAROTID NERVE TERMINALS

Intracellular recordings from single chemosensory nerve endings (within the carotid body) showed many small depolarizing potentials (s.d.p.s) of varying amplitudes

Frontiers in Arterial Chemoreception, edited by Zapata *et al.*
Plenum Press, New York, 1996

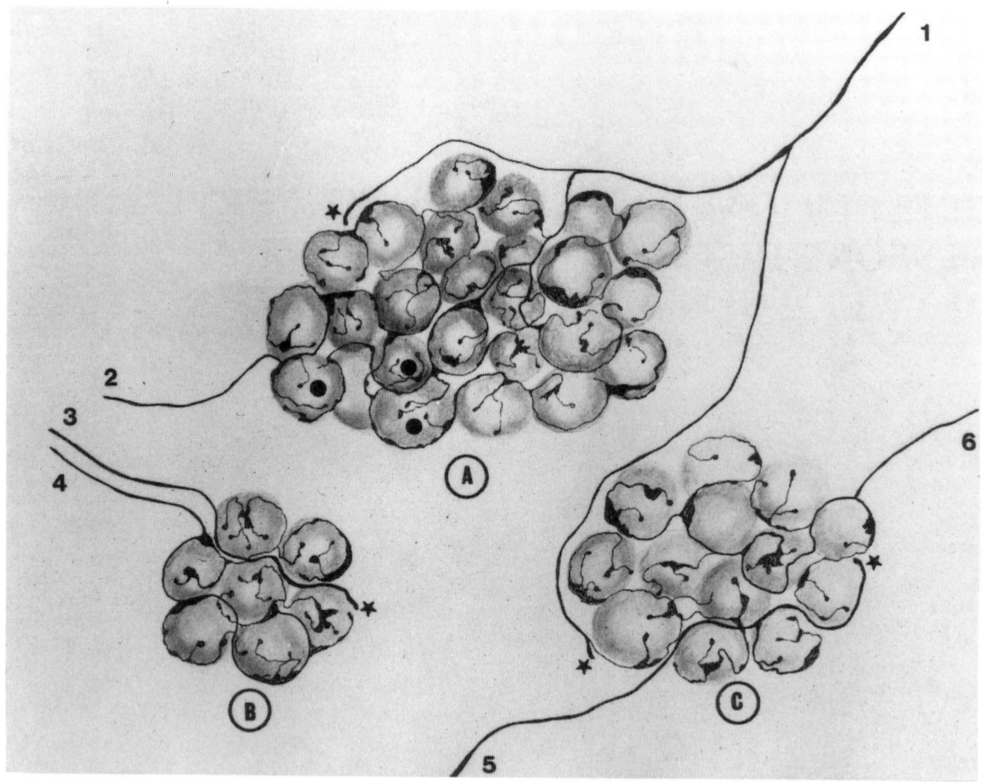

Figure 1. Drawing of carotid body innervation prepared from De Castro's original slides. Three glomeruli (A, B and C) are innervated by carotid nerve axons 1–6. Note branching of some fibers innervating more than one glomerulus. Some glomus cells (marked by dots) receive innervation from more than one fiber. Stars, nerve fibers leave the optical field. From Eyzaguirre & Gallego (1975).

(1–25 mV; mean around 5 mV). Their duration had a mean about 46 ms varying between 5 and 250 ms (Hayashida et al, 1980). The frequency of interval distribution approached that suggested for random events, and was similar to that of the discharge of single carotid nerve fibers (Biscoe & Taylor, 1963; Eyzaguirre & Koyano, 1965). It suggests that a single s.d.p. may trigger an action potential. Variations in the amplitude and rise time of different s.d.p.s suggested that they originated from different nerve terminals spreading electrotonically within the complex network of nerve fibers and endings. Another characteristic of s.d.p.s, important for our discussion, is that they are local and graded responses, insensitive to TTX. A summation of s.d.p.s was especially clear when the preparations were stimulated with ACh or cyanide. During stimulation, the s.d.p. frequency markedly increased, the local responses fused resulting in a large local depolarization accompanying an increased sensory discharge frequency. Consequently, s.d.p.s may be the unitary components of a receptor or generator potential driving the carotid nerve sensory discharge.

Figure 2A shows oscilloscope traces (1–7) from an intracellular recording of a single carotid nerve ending. The s.d.p.s occur in isolation (in 6), close together (in 1) or are fused (in 5). Attenuated spikes, probably from another nerve branch, are interspersed between the s.d.p.s (in 1- 4, 6 and 7). B, recorded from a different nerve terminal, shows

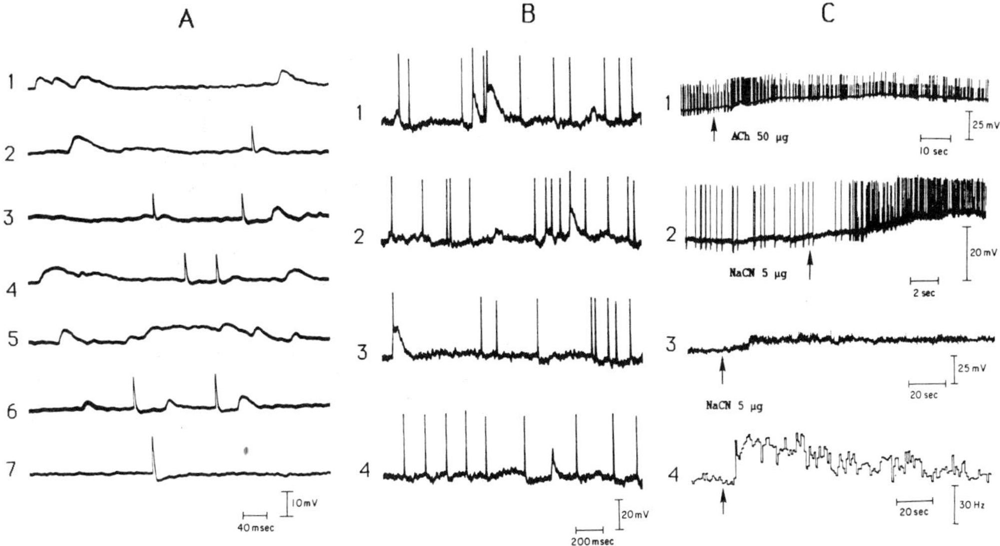

Figure 2. Intracellular recordings from single carotid nerve endings. **A**, small depolarizing potentials (s.d.p.s) and attenuated action potentials interspersed between them. **B**, local nerve ending depolarizations producing spikes. Numerous action potentials probably originated from another terminal. **C**, traces 1 and 2 show effects of ACh 50 μg and NaCN 5 μg on nerve terminal depolarization and sensory discharge frequency. Trace 3, similar effect elicited by NaCN 5 μg (very small spikes). Trace 4, frequency changes in s.d.p.s seen after filtering the spikes (from Hayashida et al, 1980).

multiple spikes probably elicited in another fiber. However, in a few instances the larger s.d.p.s produced action potentials (in 1–3). A smaller s.d.p. in 4 did not generate a spike. C, illustrates recordings from another terminal. This time, the carotid body was stimulated with ACh 50 μg (in 1) and with NaCN 5 μg (in 2). There is an increase in sensory discharge frequency riding on a slow nerve depolarization. In another recording (3), NaCN 5 μg depolarized the nerve terminal although the recorded spikes were very small. It was possible to record the frequency of the s.d.p.s, by adjusting the sensitivity of a window discriminator, as shown in 4. There was a sharp increase in s.d.p. frequency, which subsided after several sec. These experiments showed that when s.d.p.s occur in close succession they summate, fuse and contribute to the general depolarization of the nerve ending membrane (Hayashida et al, 1980).

We do not know how the s.d.p.s are generated since technical difficulties have prevented extensive studies on this subject. However, some suggestions can be advanced. S.d.p.s may be elicited by leakage of transmitters from the glomus cells. If leakage at rest is intermittent we can expect the near random pattern of occurrence already observed. Furthermore, if transmitters are released in "packets" of different sizes we could expect s.d.p.s of different amplitudes. During stimulation, release of transmitter packets may occur more frequently, resulting in more frequent s.d.p.s. as already shown. Also, s.d.p.s should summate when occurring frequently, producing a large nerve ending depolarization, since they are graded and slow local responses. Thus, s.d.p.s may be the postsynaptic expression of transmitter release from glomus cells.

3. GLOMUS CELL COUPLING AND TRANSMITTER RELEASE

McDonald (1981) first described the presence of gap junctions between glomus cells. This observation fitted well with that of Baron & Eyzaguirre (1977) who saw that injections of the membrane-impermeant dye, Procion navy blue, into one glomus cell spread to adjacent ones. This observation showed passage of substances between the cells, presumably through the gap junctions, and led to a series of studies on the electric coupling between glomus cells (Monti-Bloch & Eyzaguirre, 1990; Monti-Bloch et al, 1993; Abudara & Eyzaguirre, 1994; Eyzaguirre & Abudara, 1995). For this purpose, two adjacent glomus cells were simultaneously impaled with intracellular microelectrodes. One cell was stimulated with current pulses that elicited a voltage in this cell. When the adjacent cell was coupled to the stimulated one, the voltage was transferred to it with various degrees of attenuation. Thus, the coupling coefficient (K_C) was calculated as $K_C = E_2/V_1$, E_2, being the transferred voltage and V_1, the voltage elicited in the stimulated cell. K_C varied from zero (uncoupled cells) to one (maximal coupling). More recently, we have voltage-clamped both cells at the same holding potential (V_H) to establish the junctional macro conductance (G_J). Negative pulses applied to Cell 1 induce an inward current in this cell and an outward current when the pulse is positive. The pulses also elicited currents in coupled Cell 2, but of opposite polarities. Negative pulses induced current outflow and positive pulses current inflow. Thus, electric exchanges across the gap junctions allow to calculate G_J as I_2/V_j. I_2 is the current flowing in the coupled cell (inward or outward) and V_j, the transjunctional voltage. G_j varied from 0.05 to 34.4 nS with a mean around 1.5 nS. In other experiments, both cells have been voltage clamped at a different but steady V_H with a $\Delta V_H > 50$ mV. This imbalance has allowed to observe the activity of junction channels and calculate the junction channel conductances (g_j). (See Abudara & Eyzaguirre, this volume.)

Experiments done with current or voltage clamping yielded similar results. During hypoxia, hypercapnia, acidity or applications of putative neurotransmitters (cholinergic agents or dopamine), most glomus cell pairs (60–80%) became uncoupled to various degrees. The rest were unaffected or underwent tighter coupling. K_C (or G_J) was reduced during uncoupling but increased when coupling became tighter. Figure 3 shows the changes in G_J (voltage-clamp experiments) during hypoxia induced by Na-dithionite 1–10 mM, which reduced the mean PO_2 in the saline from about 130 to 10 Torr (range 1–18 Torr). Superfusions with 100% N_2 reduced PO_2 to about 80 Torr (range 42–105 Torr). Both stimuli uncoupled (decreased G_j) nearly 70% of the cells but there was increased coupling (increased G_j) in most of the others. The uncoupling and coupling induced by N_2 were more pronounced although the fall in PO_2 was less pronounced. We do not know the

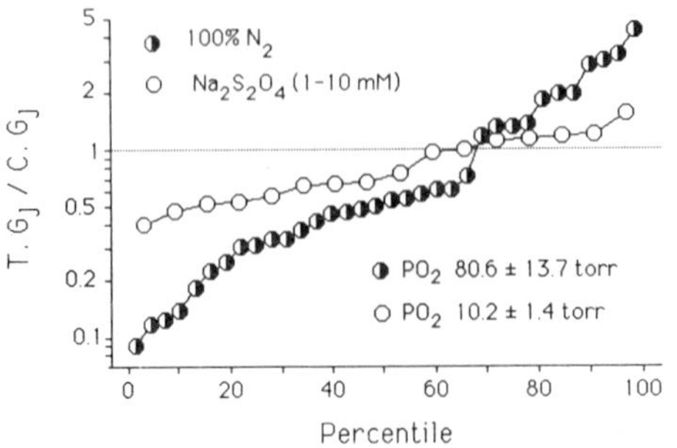

Figure 3. Cultures of glomus cell clusters. Percentile distribution of changes in junctional conductance (G_J) during hypoxia induced by $Na_2S_2O_4$ 1–10 mM boluses (open circles). The mean PO_2 in saline fell from about 130 to 10 Torr. Statistically different coupling and uncoupling effects were obtained with N_2-equilibrated solutions (half-filled circles) although the mean PO_2 fell only to about 80 Torr. Ordinate, ratio of conductance changes. C_{GJ} is control conductance and T_{GJ} the test conductance.

reason for these differences, unless there is an optimal hypoxic level to exert these effects. Deviations from this optimal level might weaken the engagement or disengagement of the cells. However, this possibility has yet to be tested at different PO_2 levels. Alternatively, Na-dithionite may have pharmacological effects opposing hypoxic coupling effects.

Concerning transmitter release, we would like to propose that it is related to intercellular coupling. Many exocrine and endocrine gland cells are coupled via intercellular gap junctions that allow exchange of materials (from ions to molecules). During stimulation most (but not all) cells disengage. It appears that secretion is enhanced by uncoupling, suggesting that secretory cells function best when isolated from their neighbors. For instance, secretagogues uncouple lacrimal cells (Neyton & Trautmann, 1986). More to the point, secretion of amylase by the exocrine pancreas increases when intercellular communications are blocked by alcohols (Meda et al, 1988). Carotid body glomus cells also are secretory elements, releasing their products (ACh, catecholamines -especially dopamine, and peptides) toward the blood vessels, their neighbors, and the nerve terminals. The endocrine effects of this release are probably minuscule. The effects of transmitters released toward other glomus cells may be important since these cells have autoreceptors that are affected by exogenous applications of these substances (for references see González et al, 1994). Our present focus is transmitter release toward the nerve terminals since it determines the frequency of the sensory discharge. Whatever the target of the released agents, secretion probably accompanies changes in intercellular coupling.

4. IS THE SENSORY DISCHARGE INFLUENCED BY GLOMUS CELL INTERACTIONS?

Gap junctions are cribriform, containing numerous aqueous pores connecting the cytoplasm of two or more adjacent cells. Each pore is surrounded by six proteins (connexins) on each side of the membranes, forming a total dodecameric structure, the connexon. Connexins allow the pore to stay open or, when they twist, shut it partially or totally. When the pores are open, coupling is tight and the junctional conductance is high. On the other hand, when the pores close (totally or partially) the cells are totally or partially uncoupled resulting in zero or very low junctional conductance. In practice, during incomplete uncoupling some pores are shut, others remain half open and the rest stay open. During total uncoupling, all pores are closed.

We have scant information about intercellular communications in the carotid body, except what was previously described. In other tissues, however, there is a wealth of knowledge ranging from the descriptive to basic molecular mechanisms operating at the connexin level. Consequently, in trying to find a physiological role for uncoupling we will adapt information available from other secretory cells, and will speculate regarding implications for the nerve discharge. We propose that coupling between glomus cells is related to transmitter release providing a chemical titration system that modulates the carotid nerve discharge. The schematic diagram in Figure 4 shows a parent fiber from the carotid nerve, branching to innervate three pairs of glomus cells. The upper pair is uncoupled (all connecting channels are closed) and there is maximal leakage of transmitters at rest. The middle pair is partly coupled because only a few channels (pores) are open, and leakage of transmitters is less pronounced. The lowest pair is tightly coupled because most intercellular channels are open and transmitter leaks have stopped or are minimal. Each of the three postsynaptic nerve endings is receiving chemical signals of different intensity that would affect the frequency and amplitude of the small depolarizing potentials (s.d.p.s). The s.d.p.

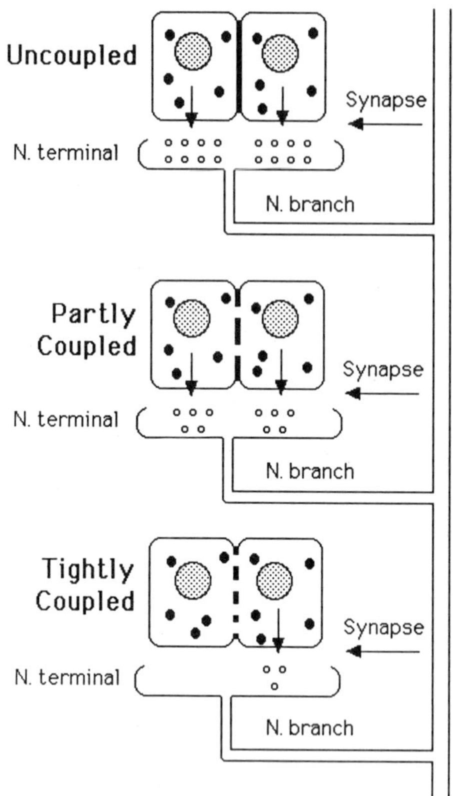

Figure 4. Model proposed to explain possible correlation between glomus cell uncoupling and transmitter release toward carotid nerve terminals. Three pairs of glomus cells show different degrees of coupling with resulting variations in transmitter release. Cell uncoupling leads to more release whereas tighter coupling stops release or this is reduced.

frequency and amplitude would be maximal in the ending apposed to the uncoupled cells, decreasing in amplitude and frequency as coupling gets tighter. The s.d.p.s may trigger action potentials in the upper two branches going to the parent fiber. Spikes may travel unimpeded in the parent fiber or, if they collide, only one will survive. Action potential collisions at this level may partly explain the aperiodic sensory discharge.

During stimulation, most glomus cells disengaged. That is, the coupling conditions shown in Figure 4 moved from the bottom to the top, resulting in increased transmitter release and more frequent and larger s.d.p.s. However, in a minority of cells coupling moved in the opposite direction, that is, it became tighter with reductions in transmitter release. This resulted in a decrease in the frequency and amplitude of the s.d.p.s. Why is it that coupling changes occur in opposite directions in different cell pairs? We do not have an answer, but a different preparation may provide a partial solution to this question. cAMP exerts coupling or uncoupling effects on vein endothelial cells depending on their physiological state. Active cells were uncoupled by cAMP whereas the same agent increased coupling in quiescent cells. This effect appeared related to $[Ca^{2+}]_i$ that was high during activity and low during quiescence (Spray et al, 1988). A similar mechanism may operate in glomus cells. However, if this comparison is appropriate "active" glomus cells would communicate better with each other than "inactive" ones. They would be more interested in exchanging materials across their gap junctions than in leaking transmitters toward the nerve endings. It may depend on the aerobic metabolism keeping oxygenation and pH higher than when such metabolism does not operate optimally. Such cells would be well oxygenated and tightly coupled saving their products rather than leaking them out. A hypoxic or acid challenge would close intercellular communications and transmitters will leak out. On the other hand, poorly oxygenated cells with low pH_i ("inactive") would be leaking transmitters toward the nerve terminals. Their intercellular communication is poor and the cells are partly uncoupled. A similar challenge would open their communications (to help each other) and save their products by reducing transmitter loss. Consequently, changes in coupling in opposite directions, and resulting differences in transmitter release, may help in preventing exhaustion of these products. If during stimulation all cells underwent uncoupling, there would be maximal transmitter release, a situation that would not allow repeated stimulations unless there is rapid restoration of the lost products. On the other hand, if stimulation induced tighter coupling in all glomus cells, there would be little or no transmitter release. We know that this is not so since stimulation by hypoxia, acidity or hypercapnia invariably increases transmitter release from glomus cells (for references see González et al, 1994). It is unknown whether cells that disengage or show tighter coupling during stimulation always do so, or if their roles change with time.

In all instances, whether there was an increase or decrease in glomus cell coupling during stimulation, the sensory discharge frequency must have increased, as has been extensively shown in other studies. Those observations agree with the proposed model since most glomus cells uncoupled during excitation, possibly leading to increased transmitter release. The minority of cells showing increased coupling may provide a restraining mechanism preventing excessive nerve firing, and/or saving transmitters for adequate responses during prolonged stimulation.

5. TESTING THE MODEL

It is extremely difficult to experimentally test the proposed model in a carotid body-nerve preparation because one must impale two adjacent glomus cells and the corresponding nerve endings. Impaling single nerve terminals and maintaining good penetrations for any length of time has been extremely laborious and infrequently successful (Hayashida et al, 1980). Experimental testing could be feasible, however, using an "artificial" preparation. Alcayaga & Eyzaguirre (1990) obtained functional contacts between nodose ganglion neurons co-cultured with glomus cell clusters. Stimulation of the glomus cells evoked neuron depolarization and increased frequency in spontaneous spike activity. In this preparation, processes from the soma (neurites) innervated the glomus cells. Thus, depolarizations occurring in the neurites were detected in the soma because of electrotonic spread. It is much easier to impale a large soma (20–60 μm) rather than very small nerve terminals.

In other studies, we have frequently impaled cultured and adjacent glomus cells to study intercellular coupling (Abudara & Eyzaguirre, 1994; Eyzaguirre & Abudara, 1995; also Fig 3). Consequently, one could co-culture glomus cells (in monolayers) with dispersed sensory neurons. It may be better to use neurons from the petrosal rather than the nodose ganglion for two reasons: 1) There are many more arterial chemosensory afferents in the former; and 2) Cultured petrosal neurons may keep their affinity (tropism) toward their original targets, the glomus cells in this case, as occurs in the intact animal (Dinger et al, 1985; Zapata et al, 1969; 1976). Thus, a petrosal neuron-glomus cell preparation may yield more frequent, and functionally active synaptic contacts than the nodose neuron-glomus cell preparation.

It should be feasible to impale the neurons and two adjacent glomus cells, once functional contacts between these elements have been established. Thus, one could establish direct correlations between neuronal activity and connections between glomus cells. There may be problems however. Alcayaga & Eyzaguirre (1990) did not record s.d.p.s from nodose neurons although this failure may have been due to the length (about 100 μm) of the very thin neurites emerging from the somata. Seeding petrosal neurons over monolayers of glomus cells may produce functional contacts through shorter neurites. This arrangement should help the electrotonic spread of very small potentials occurring at the points of contact with the glomus cells. When s.d.p.s are recorded from neuron somata one could do extensive pharmacological tests to establish the nature of the transmitters eliciting them. An experimental model along these lines has already been developed (see Zhong & Nurse, 1996).

6. ACKNOWLEDGMENTS

Work supported by NIH grant NS 07938

7. REFERENCES

Abudara V & Eyzaguirre C (1994) Electrical coupling between cultured glomus cells of the rat carotid body: observations with current and voltage clamping. Brain Res 664: 257–265

Alcayaga J & Eyzaguirre C (1990) Electrophysiological evidence for the reconstitution of chemosensory units in co-cultures of carotid body and nodose ganglion neurons. Brain Res 534: 324–328

Baron M & Eyzaguirre C (1977) Effects of temperature on some membrane characteristics of carotid body cells. Am J Physiol 233: C35-C46

Biscoe TJ & Taylor A (1963) The discharge pattern recorded in chemoreceptor afferent fibres from the cat carotid body with normal circulation and during perfusion. J Physiol, London 168: 332–344

De Castro F (1940) Nuevas observaciones sobre la inervación de la región carotídea. Los quimio- y preso-receptores. Trab Lab Invest Biol Univ Madrid 32: 297–385

De Castro F (1951) Sur la structure de la synapse dans les chemocepteurs: leur mécanisme d'excitation et rôle dans la circulation sanguine locale. Acta Physiol Scand 22: 14–43

Dinger B, Stensaas LJ & Fidone S (1985) Cat carotid bodies reinnervated by normal or foreign nerves. Brain Res 344: 21–32

Edwards C & Ottoson D (1958) The site of impulse initiation in a nerve cell of a crustacean stretch receptor. J Physiol, London 143: 138–148

Eyzaguirre C & Abudara V (1995) Possible role of coupling between glomus cells in carotid body chemoreception. Biol Signals 4: 263–270

Eyzaguirre C & Gallego A (1975) An examination of De Castro's original slides. In: Purves MJ (ed) The Peripheral Arterial Chemoreceptors. London: Cambridge Univ Press. pp 1–23

Eyzaguirre C & Koyano H (1965) Effects of hypoxia, hypercapnia, and pH on the chemoreceptor activity of the carotid body *in vitro*. J Physiol, London 178: 385–409

Fidone SJ & Sato A (1969) A study of chemoreceptor and baroreceptor A and C-fibres in the cat carotid nerve. J Physiol, London 205: 527–548

González C, Almaraz L, Obeso A & Rigual R (1994) Carotid body chemoreceptors: From natural stimuli to sensory discharges. Physiol Rev 74: 829–898

Hayashida Y, Koyano H & Eyzaguirre C (1980) An intracellular study of chemosensory fibers and endings. J Neurophysiol 44: 1077–1088

Kondo H (1976) Innervation of the carotid body of the adult rat. Cell Tiss Res 173: 1–15

Loewenstein WR & Rathkamp R (1958) The sites for mechano-electric conversion in a pacinian corpuscle. J Gen Physiol 41: 1245–1265

McDonald DM (1981) Peripheral chemoreceptors: Structure-function relationships of the carotid body. In: Hornbein TF & Lenfant C (eds) Lung Biology in Health and Disease, vol 17: Regulation of Breathing. New York: Dekker. pp 105–320

Meda P, Bruzzone R, Chanson M & Bosco D (1988) Junctional coupling and secretion of pancreatic acinar cells. In: Hertzberg GL & Johnson RG (eds) Gap Junctions. Modern Cell Biology, vol 7. New York: Liss. pp 353–364

Monti-Bloch L & Eyzaguirre C (1990) Effects of different stimuli and transmitters on glomus cell membranes and intercellular communications. In: Eyzaguirre C, Fidone SJ, Fitzgerald RS, Lahiri S & McDonald DM (eds) Arterial Chemoreception. New York: Springer. pp 157–167

Monti-Bloch L, Abudara V & Eyzaguirre C (1993) Electrical communication between glomus cells of the rat carotid body. Brain Res 622: 119–131

Neyton J & Trautmann A (1986) Acetylcholine modulation of the conductance of intercellular junctions between rat lacrimal cells. J Physiol, London 377: 283–295

Ringham GL (1971) Origin of nerve impulse in slowly adapting stretch receptor of crayfish. J Neurophysiol 34: 773–784

Spray DC, Sáez JC, Burt JM, Watanabe T, Reid LM, Hertzberg EL & Bennett MVL (1988) Gap junctional conductance: multiple sites of regulation. In: Hertzberg EL & Johnson RG (eds) Gap Junctions. Modern Cell Biology, vol 7. New York: Liss. pp 227–244

Zapata P, Hess A & Eyzaguirre C (1969) Reinnervation of carotid body and sinus with superior laryngeal nerve fibers. J Neurophysiol 32: 215–228

Zapata P, Stensaas LJ & Eyzaguirre C (1976) Axon regeneration following a lesion of the carotid nerve: Electrophysiological and ultrastructural observations. Brain Res 113: 235–253

Zhong H & Nurse C (1996) Co-cultures of rat petrosal neurons and carotid body type 1 cells: A model for studying chemosensory mechanisms. Adv Exp Med Biol 410: 189–193

24

GENERATION OF INTERSPIKE INTERVALS OF RAT CAROTID BODY CHEMORECEPTORS

David F. Donnelly

Department of Pediatrics
Section of Respiratory Medicine
Yale University School of Medicine
New Haven, Connecticut 06520

1. INTRODUCTION

Hypoxia is well established to stimulate carotid body chemoreceptors leading to an increase in sinus nerve activity, but the mechanism by which the nerve activity increases is unresolved. It is generally assumed that spike initiation is solely dependent on presynaptic transmitter secretion, but, synaptic blockade with low calcium solutions causes little change in baseline nerve activity (although it does eliminate the hypoxia response) (Donnelly & Kholwadwala, 1992). This suggests that the nerve endings can initiate action potentials independent of glomus cell secretion. However, it is difficult to study this directly because of the small size of the nerve terminals and uncertainty regarding the site of action potential generation. The present study was undertaken to better understand the process of spike initiation by examination of the interspike interval pattern from rat chemoreceptors. The results show that spike generation during normoxia and during hypoxia stimulation is a Poisson-type random process, and this generator characteristic is highly sensitive to the Na^+ channel agonist, veratridine.

2. METHODS

Carotid bodies were harvested from anesthetized rats of 20–30 days of age. The carotid body was dissected free along with a length of the cut sinus nerve and cleaned by a 30 min exposure to collagenase/trypsin, as previously described (Kholwadwala & Donnelly, 1992). The organ was placed in a perfusion chamber mounted on an inverted microscope and superfused with Ringer's saline (in mM: 125 NaCl, 3.1 KCl, 1.25 NaH_2PO_4, 2.4 $CaCl_2$, 1.3 $MgSO_4$, 26 $NaHCO_3$, 10 glucose). Single-fiber nerve activity was recorded with a suction electrode, discriminated (BAK DIS-1), and the interspike-intervals were timed to 1 msec accuracy. Interval trains of 1000–2000 successive spikes were recorded

Frontiers in Arterial Chemoreception, edited by Zapata *et al.*
Plenum Press, New York, 1996

during steady-state stimulation with normoxia solution ($PO_2 \approx 150$ Torr), and with moderately hypoxic solution ($PO_2 \approx 70$ Torr). From the interval train, a series of 500 consecutive intervals was selected for further analysis based on a constant mean frequency of discharge.

In some experiments, the carotid body was exposed to a dilute solution of veratridine (0.5–1 μM) for 5 min. Veratridine is a Na^+ channel agonist which binds to open Na^+ channels and causes a prolongation of the open state (Sunami et al, 1993). After the treatment period, the drug was washed out with normoxic saline for a period of 30–60 min. Samples of the afferent spike train were periodically timed during the washout period.

Spike trains were analyzed at two levels. In the first, the interspike interval histogram was calculated and compared against that expected from a Poisson-type random process. Expected-to-observed values were compared using a X^2 statistic. In the second level of analysis, the ordering of the intervals was considered. This was primarily accomplished by computing expectation density (Poggio & Viernstein, 1966). This parameter, akin to a serial correlation coefficient in the time domain, is computed by placing a time ruler on the first spike of the series and marking the occurrence times of spikes 5 sec into the future. The ruler is then moved to the second spike and the occurrence times marked, and so on.

3. RESULTS

For chemoreceptor spike trains recorded during normoxia ($PO_2 \sim 150$ Torr), the interspike interval histogram was not different from Poisson for 10/15 trains (Fig 1). In the 5 trains in which the trains were different, this difference was slight and was always confined to a decrease in the number of short intervals. If the shortest 1/3 of the bins were excluded from the analysis then no histogram for chemoreceptors recorded during normoxia was different than Poisson. During stimulation with moderate hypoxia ($PO_2 \sim 70$ Torr) about half (7/15) of the series were not different than Poisson. In all cases where the histogram was different from expected, the deviation was confined to short intervals: during hypoxia there was an increased number of short intervals (Fig 2).

During normoxia and during hypoxia, there was no evidence of serial ordering. The expectation density for all interval trains was constant and unchanging (Figs 1, 2). This was confirmed by taking the original train, shuffling the intervals and calculating the expectation density on the shuffled series. This shuffling and recomputation was done multiple times, resulting in a population of expectation density values based on multiple shuffling. The mean ± SD for this population are shown by dotted lines (Figs 1, 2). At this point, the chemoreceptor interval generation pattern could be fully characterized by a single parameter - a constant probability of a spike in any time period, Δt.

This characterization was greatly altered by a brief exposure to the Na^+ channel agonist, veratridine. Veratridine was applied for 5 min at 0.5–1 μM and then washed out for 30–60 min. The discharge rate was unstable during veratridine exposure, which precluded analysis, but was stable over short times in the washout period. Veratridine exposure imposed an ordering on the spike generation process such that the occurrence of a spike greatly increased the probability or expectation of more spikes (Fig 3). This was more than just an increase in the number of short duration intervals since the original series was significantly different from the interval series placed in shuffled order (Fig 3).

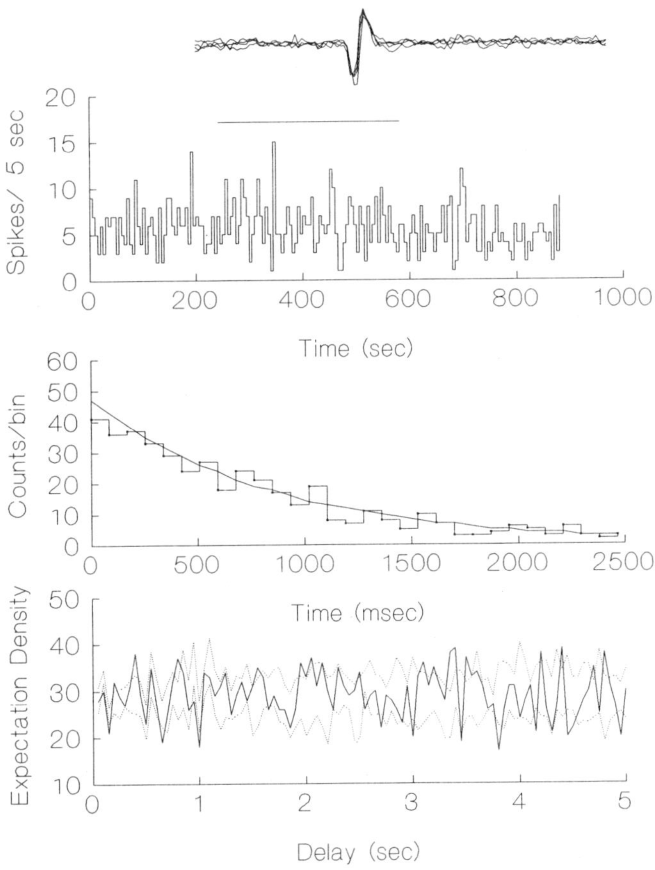

Figure 1. Analysis of single-fiber chemoreceptor interspike intervals during normoxia. Top, frequency *vs* time (5 sec/bin). Bar indicates analysis period of 500 consecutive spikes. Middle, interspike interval histogram. Smooth line is the predicted values from a Poisson generator of the same mean frequency. The histogram was not significantly different from that predicted by a Poisson generator. Lower, expectation density. Solid line is the original spike series. Dotted line is mean ± SD of population of values arising from multiple shuffling of the original series.

4. DISCUSSION

These results demonstrate that rat chemoreceptor discharge, *in vitro*, may be well characterized by a single parameter - a constant probability that a spike will be generated in time period, Δt. This characterization is the same as for radioactive decay and gives rise to an exponential interspike interval distribution and to a constant expectation density. Since the characterization is the same during normoxia and during hypoxia, it suggests that the process of spike generation is the same in both conditions.

It may be particularly important that the spike generation process is very sensitive to the Na^+ channel agonist, veratridine. This drug binds to open Na^+ channels and increases the duration of the open state (Sunami et al, 1993). Typically the drug is used at concentrations of 50–100 μM in order to study Na-dependent secretion from synaptosomes or, in some cases, catecholamine release from glomus cells (Rocher et al, 1994). The concentra-

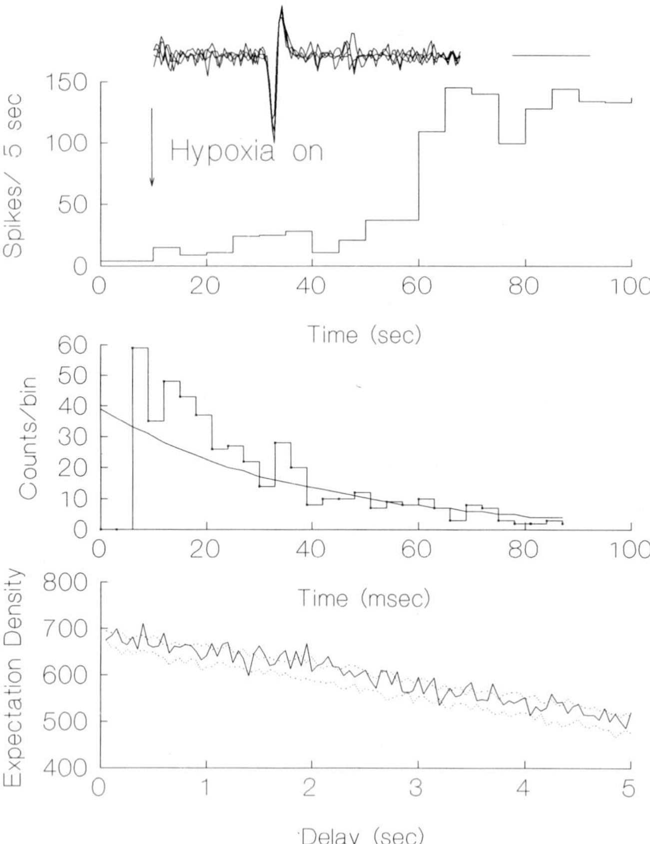

Figure 2. Analysis of single-fiber chemoreceptor interspike intervals during hypoxia. Legend as in Figure 1. In this case, the interspike interval distribution was significantly different from exponential, but the difference was small and was due to a greater-than-predicted number of short intervals. Downward slope of expectation density is due to short duration of the spike train.

tion used in the present study was only 1–2% of the typical dosage and data were collected up to 1 hour into the washout period - at a time when the effective concentration was undoubtedly much less. Still, at these low concentrations the spike generation process was radically altered such that the spikes became interdependent. Since rat glomus cells have little or no fast Na^+ channels (Fieber & McCleskey, 1993), it is likely that the veratridine effect is solely on the nerve endings. This suggests that spike generation is dictated by the state of the Na^+ channels in the nerve endings.

A model consistent with these observations is as follows: the action potential generation region has a small number of channels, but the current through individual channels may significantly change the terminal voltage. We may speculate that the nerve terminals have 100 Na^+ channels, each with a probability, P, of being open (*e.g.*, 0.05). Threshold is reached if 5 or more channels are simultaneously open. The theoretical nerve spiking frequency is the sum of the binomial probabilities of having 5, 6, 7...100 simultaneously open Na^+ channels. An increase in nerve activity during hypoxia may be caused by an increase in open probability (*e.g.*, P goes from 0.05 to 0.06) or by a decrease in threshold requirements (*e.g.*, 5 to 4 channels).

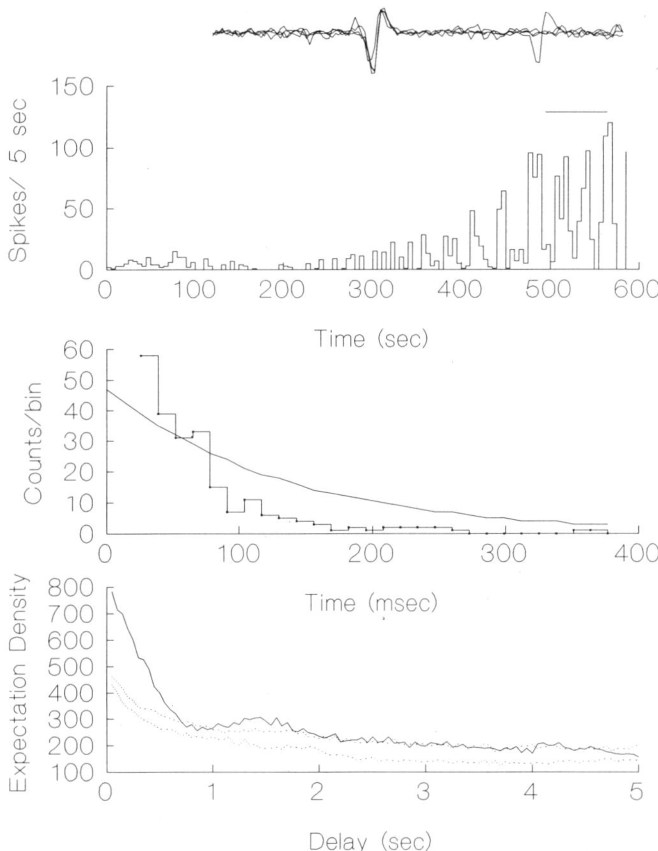

Figure 3. Analysis of chemoreceptor spike train recorded during the washout period from veratridine. Veratridine (0.5 μM) was applied for 5 min and the washout period was started at time 0 on the above scale. Bar on upper panel indicates the analysis period. Note change in expectation density compared to Figures 1, 2.

This model is consistent with a number of experimental observations: 1) the exponential interspike interval histogram; 2) constant expectation density; 3) veratridine sensitivity; and 4) lack of effect of calcium-free solution on normoxic spike generation. Although undoubtedly oversimplified this model suggests that glomus cell excitatory transmitter(s) may target nerve Na^+ channel as a means of modulating nerve activity, perhaps through modulation of "window" currents (amount of steady-state Na-channel activation). The model also makes testable predictions regarding the consequences of perturbations of Na^+ gradient or Na^+ channel number - both of which can be readily addressed experimentally. These predictions are currently being done in our laboratory.

5. REFERENCES

Donnelly DF & Kholwadwala D (1992) Hypoxia decreases intracellular calcium in adult rat carotid body glomus cells. J Neurophysiol 67: 1543–1551

Fieber LA & McCleskey EW (1993) L-type calcium channels in type I cells of the rat carotid body. J Neurophysiol 70: 1378–1384

Kholwadwala D & Donnelly DF (1992) Maturation of carotid chemoreceptor sensitivity to hypoxia: *in vitro* studies in the newborn rat. J Physiol, London 453: 461–473

Poggio GF & Viernstein LJ (1966) Time series analysis of impulse sequences of thalamic somatic sensory neurons. J Neurophysiol 27: 517–545

Rocher A, Obeso A, Herreros B & González C (1994) Assessment of Na^+ channel involvement in the release of catecholamines from chemoreceptor cells of the carotid body. Adv Exp Med Biol 360: 201–204

Sunami A, Sasano T, Matsunaga A, Fan Z, Sawanobori T & Hiraoka M (1993) Properties of veratridine-modified single Na^+ channels in Guinea pig ventricular myocytes. Am J Physiol 264: H454-H463

25

THE COUPLING BETWEEN INTRACELLULAR pH, ION TRANSPORT, AND CHEMOSENSORY DISCHARGE

R. Iturriaga,[1,2] A. Mokashi,[2] and S. Lahiri[2]

[1] Laboratory of Neurobiology
Catholic University of Chile
Santiago, Chile
[2] Department of Physiology
University of Pennsylvania School of Medicine
Philadelphia, Pennsylvania 19104–6085

1. INTRODUCTION

The current model of chemoreception in the carotid body (CB) recognizes the glomus cell as the site of transduction of O_2, CO_2 and $[H^+]$ stimuli. In response to hypoxia or acid hypercapnia, glomus cells are expected to release a neurotransmitter which in turn should increase the firing rate of chemosensory discharges. Consequently, the chemosensory discharges recorded from the carotid sinus nerve could be used to monitor the cellular responses of the chemoreceptor cells.

Recently, Buckler et al (1991) and Wilding et al (1992) reported that isolated glomus cells in saline solution buffered with HEPES showed a prolonged acidosis in response to an acid load when the cells were bathed with 5-(N-ethyl-N-isopropyl)-amiloride (EIPA), 5-(N,N-hexamethylene)-amiloride (HMA) or with a solution without Na^+. This acidification was attributed to the selective inhibition of the Na^+-H^+ exchanger that works as an acid extruder in glomus cells. In a solution containing CO_2-HCO_3^-, the effects of EIPA and zero Na^+ on the pH_i of the glomus cells were less marked because other mechanisms for pH_i regulation were operative. Accordingly, an acid hypercapnic stimulus applied during the blocking of the Na^+-H^+ exchanger with amiloride -a Na^+ channel inhibitor that also inhibits the Na^+-H^+ exchanger- (Benos, 1982), or EIPA would produce a prolonged acidification of the glomus cells and, consequently, an increased frequency of chemosensory discharge.

To test the above hypothesis we studied the effects of amiloride and EIPA on the chemosensory response to hypercapnia. We also studied the effects of these agents on the responses to hypoxia, cyanide and nicotine, because these responses are not initiated by acidification of glomus cells (Mokashi et al, 1995). Since these drugs may impair other

Frontiers in Arterial Chemoreception, edited by Zapata *et al.*
Plenum Press, New York, 1996

Na^+ transport system in the CB cells we also tested the effects of 2–4 dimethyl benzamil, an amiloride analog that is a selective inhibitor of the Na^+-Ca^{2+} exchanger, but not of the Na^+-H^+ exchanger (Kleyman & Cragoe, 1988).

2. METHODS

Carotid bodies obtained from pentobarbitone anesthetized cats were perfused and superfused *in vitro* as described previously (Iturriaga et al, 1991). The carotid bifurcation including the CB was perfused *in vitro* with a Tyrode's solution equilibrated at PO_2 of 120 Torr, PCO_2 of 35 Torr at pH 7.40, and superfused with the same Tyrode equilibrated at $PO_2 < 20$ Torr. The composition of the Tyrode was (in mM) Na^+ 154; K^+ 4.7; Ca^{2+} 2.2; Mg^{2+} 1.1; glutamate 21; HCO_3^- 21.4 mM, Cl^- 123.3, D-Glucose 5.5 mM, and HEPES 5 mM. The fluid temperature was regulated at 37.0 ± 0.5°C.

The chemosensory discharges were recorded from the whole carotid sinus nerve placed on a pair of platinum electrodes and lifted into paraffin oil. The signals were preamplified, amplified, filtered and fed to an electronic amplitude discriminator. The resulting standardized pulses were counted by a frequency meter. The signals were stored in a digital-analog VCR recording system for later analyses. The responses to hypoxia (PO_2 of 30–50 Torr) and acid hypercapnia (PCO_2 of 60–85 Torr at pH 7.20) were tested. NaCN (2 nmol) and nicotine (2 nmol) were injected as boluses of 0.2 ml into the perfusate.

3. RESULTS

Figure 1 shows the effects of amiloride hydrochloride (1 mM) on the chemosensory responses to acid hypercapnia and hypoxia. Perfusion with Tyrode containing amiloride reversibly reduced the chemosensory responses to hypercapnia, while the response to hypoxia was less altered. In control conditions in 5 CBs, hypoxia and acid hypercapnia increased chemosensory discharges from 37.5 ± 12.3 impulses/s to 378.3 ± 21.4 and 250.5 ± 44.5 impulses/s, respectively. During perfusion with Tyrode containing amiloride, hypoxia and acid hypercapnia increased chemosensory discharges to 313.1 ± 57.8 impulses/s and 130.1 ± 26.3 impulses/s ($p < 0.05$), respectively. The increase in chemosensory activity induced by hypoxia and hypercapnia was reduced by amiloride by 17.2% and 48.1%, respectively.

The chemosensory responses evoked by 2 nmol nicotine in 5 CBs decreased by 82% during perfusion with Tyrode containing amiloride. Since amiloride is a blocker of Na^+ channels (Benos, 1982; Kleyman & Cragoe, 1988), we also used EIPA, a more selective inhibitor of the Na^+-H^+ exchanger (Kleyman & Cragoe, 1988). Figure 2 shows the effects of EIPA (20 μM) on the chemosensory responses to acid hypercapnia (Fig 2A) and to hypoxia (Fig 2B). The overall responses to hypercapnia and hypoxia were almost abolished in all of the 6 CBs studied during perfusion with Tyrode containing EIPA (20 μM). The effect of EIPA at low concentration (20 μM) for 10–15 min was reversible as is it shown in Figure 2.

EIPA also blocked the chemosensory responses to 2 nmol NaCN and to 2 nmol nicotine injected into the perfusate as shown in Figure 3. The effect of EIPA was reversible.

Perfusion of Tyrode containing 2–4 dimethyl benzamil (10 μM) reversibly reduced the responses to hypoxia and to hypercapnia (Fig 4).

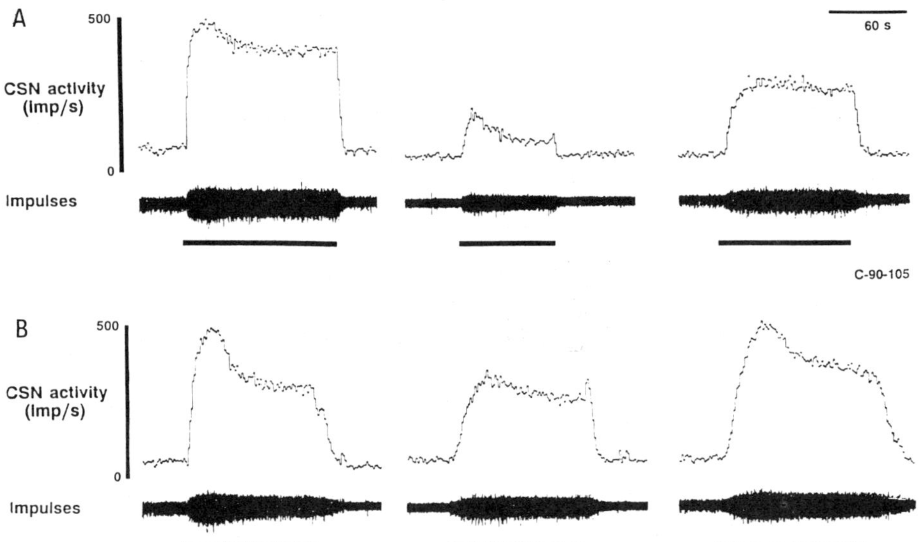

Figure 1. Effects of amiloride (1 mM) on carotid chemosensory responses to acid hypercapnia (A, PCO_2 80 Torr at pH 7.00) and to hypoxia (B, PO_2 40 Torr at pH 7.40). Bars indicate duration of hypercapnia and hypoxia. First panel, control response; Second panel, amiloride; Third panel, recovery after 20 min.

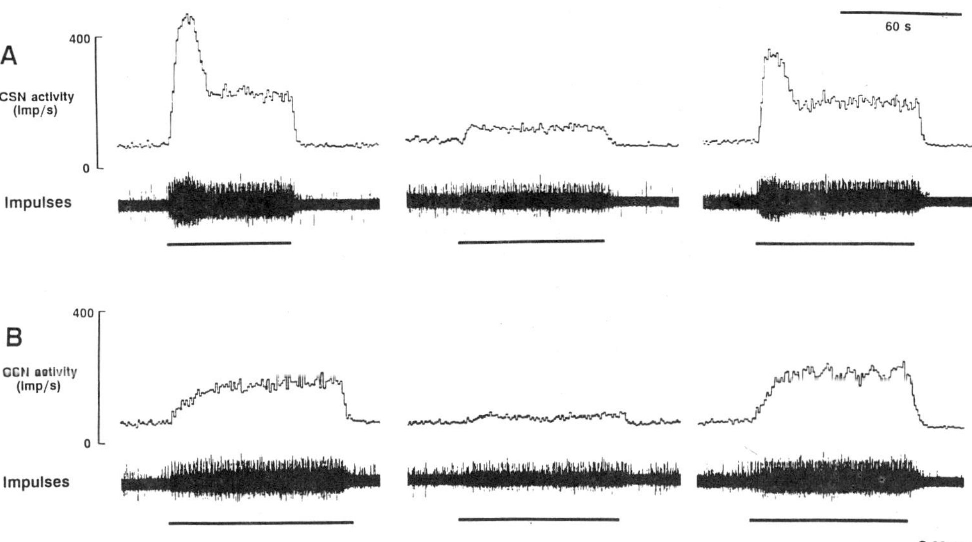

Figure 2. Effects of EIPA (20 μM) on carotid chemosensory responses to acid hypercapnia (A, PCO_2 80 Torr and pH 7.00) and to hypoxia (B, PO_2 50 Torr at pH 7.40). Bars indicate duration of hypercapnia and hypoxia. First panel, control response; Second panel, EIPA; Third panel, recovery after 20 min.

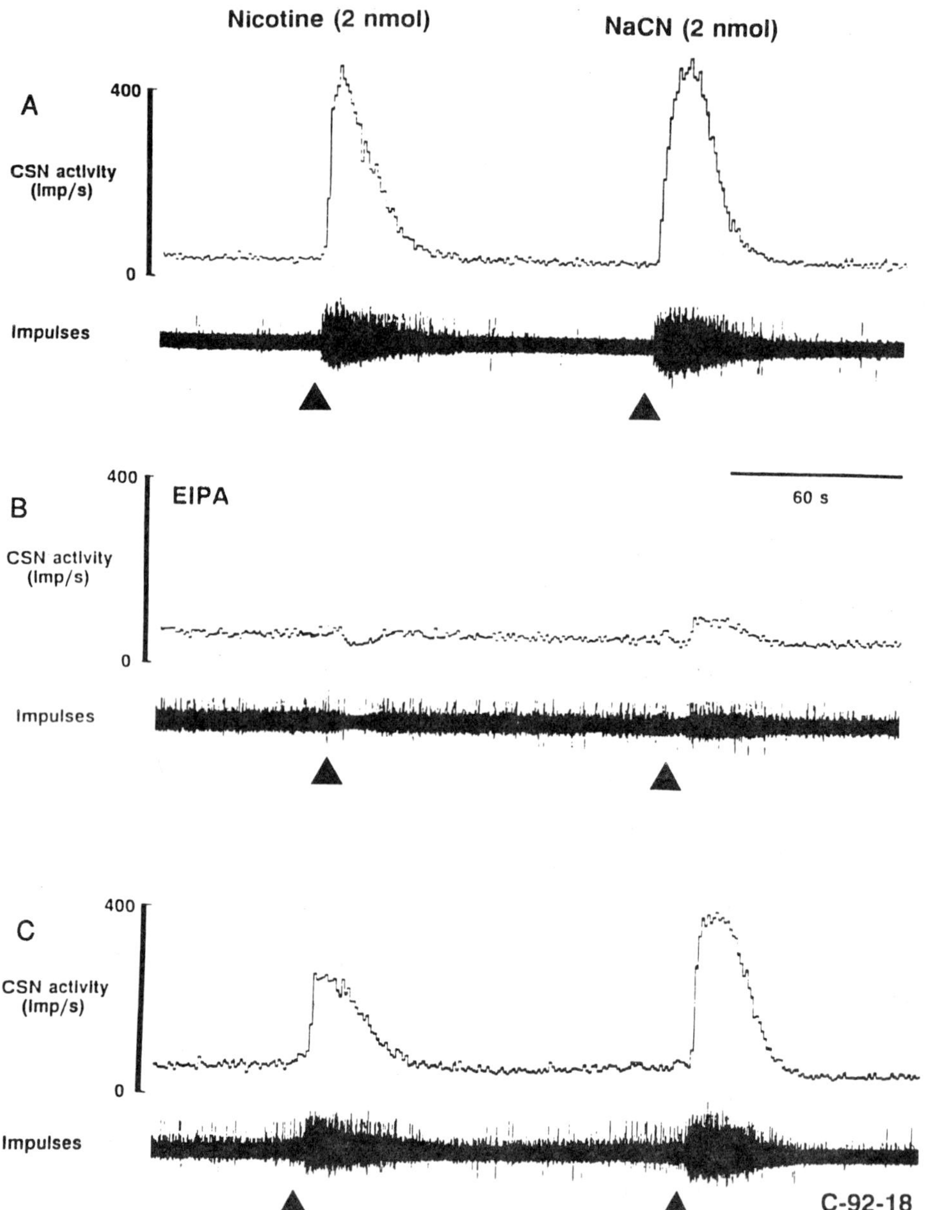

Figure 3. Effects of EIPA (20 μM) on carotid chemosensory responses to nicotine and NaCN. Arrows indicate nicotine and NaCN injections. A, control; B, EIPA; C, recovery after 20 min.

4. DISCUSSION

Buckler et al (1991) and Wilding et al (1992) found that EIPA and HMA produced a prolonged acidosis in isolated glomus cells in response to an acid load. Since the chemosensory discharges are the result of the integration of the secretory response of glomus cells, we expected that EIPA could produce a prolonged acidification of glomus cells in

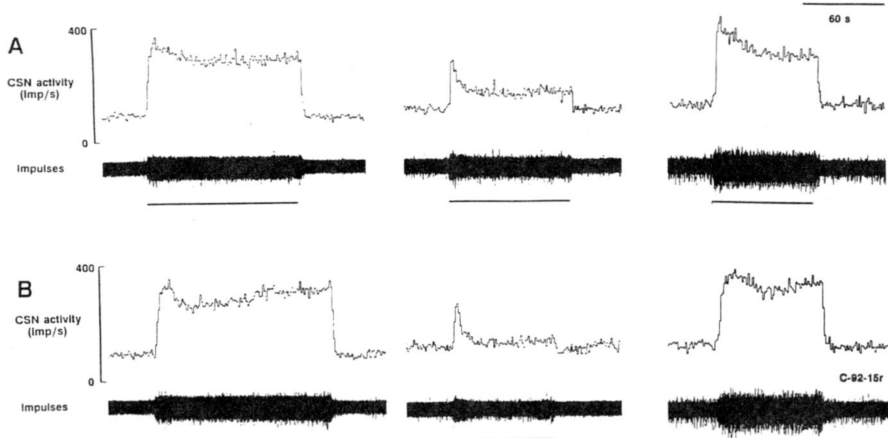

Figure 4. Effects of 2–4 dimethyl benzamil (20 μM) on chemosensory responses to acid hypercapnia (A, PCO_2 80 Torr at pH 7.0) and to hypoxia (B, PO_2 50 Torr, pH 7.40). Bars indicate duration of hypercapnia and hypoxia. First panel, control. Second panel, 2–4 dimethyl benzamil. Third panel, recovery after 20 min.

response to acid hypercapnia. This acidification could be followed by an increased frequency of chemosensory discharges. Contrarily to this expectation, our results showed that amiloride and EIPA reversibly reduced or almost abolished the cat carotid chemosensory responses to hypercapnia as well as hypoxia, cyanide and nicotine. These nonspecific actions suggest that the effects of these drugs were not due to specific blockade of Na^+-H^+ exchanger in glomus cells.

A general question raised from our results concerns the specificity of the effect of EIPA on the neurotransmitter release in glomus cells. If CB efflux of dopamine is an indicator of the activation of glomus cells (González et al, 1994) we would anticipate that EIPA, which produced a prolonged acidification of isolated glomus cells, should also enhance the efflux of dopamine from the CB. However, Rocher et al (1991) reported that EIPA (40 μM) did not modify the dopamine efflux from rabbit CB superfused with CO_2-HCO_3^- buffered medium, but decreased the dopamine efflux (by 60%) elicited by propionate or acid hypercapnia (20% CO_2 at pH 6.6) when the CBs were superfused with CO_2-HCO_3^- free medium. Thus, we expected that the chemosensory response to acid hypercapnia were not modified by EIPA. Contrarily to this expectation, our results showed that EIPA reduced all the chemosensory responses in CO_2-HCO_3^- buffered medium.

Rocher et al (1991) proposed that a rise in glomus cells $[H^+]$ elicited by acid hypercapnia is followed by an activation of the Na^+-H^+ exchanger and a subsequent rise in $[Na^+]_i$, which in turn reverses the Na^+-Ca^{2+} exchanger function, accumulating Ca^{2+}, and finally leading to dopamine release. Recently, Buckler and Vaughan-Jones (1993) reported that acid hypercapnia raised $[Ca^{2+}]_i$ in isolated glomus cells from neonatal rats. This increase was almost abolished by Ca^{2+} free medium and was reduced by the Ca^{2+} blocker D600, indicating the probable involvement of Ca^{2+} influx from the extracellular space.

Our results showing that 2–4 dimethyl benzamil reduced all the chemosensory responses do not further contribute to clarify the role of extracellular Ca^{2+} in chemoreception. A plausible explanation for the effects of EIPA and 2–4 dimethyl benzamil is that Na^+-H^+ and Ca^{2+}-Na^+ exchangers are widely distributed in the CB cells (*i.e.*, sensory nerve terminals, type I and II cells) as in other tissues (Madshus, 1988; Roos & Boron, 1981). If this is the case, the blockers used here could impair not only mechanisms involved in the pH_i regulation of glomus cells, but also could impair the generation of the chemosensory discharges by blocking ion transport in sensory nerve terminals. Amiloride and its analogues may accumulate within the cells and alter other cellular processes because these molecules are permeable weak bases that easily cross the cell membrane (Kleyman and Cragoe, 1988). Indeed, its is well known that amiloride and its analogues inhibit enzymes and proteins such as protein kinases, adenylate cyclases, monoamine oxidases, alpha and beta adrenergic receptors and nicotinic receptors (See Kleyman & Cragoe, 1988).

In summary our results show that amiloride and EIPA suppress all the chemosensory responses *in vitro*, and therefore do not allow the conclusion that the chemoreceptor cell acidification induced by the inhibition of the Na^+-H^+ exchanger mechanism is followed by an augmented chemosensory discharge.

5. ACKNOWLEDGMENTS

Work supported in part by grants HL-50180–02, USA, to SL, and FONDECYT 1950997, Chile, to RI.

6. REFERENCES

Benos DJ (1982) Amiloride: a molecular probe of sodium transport in tissue and cells. Am J Physiol 242: C131-C145

Buckler KJ & Vaughan-Jones RD (1993) Effects of acidic stimuli on intracellular calcium in isolated type I cells of the neonatal rat carotid body. Pflügers Arch 425: 22–27

Buckler KJ, Vaughan-Jones RD, Peers C & Nye PCG (1991) Intracellular pH and its regulation in the isolated type I carotid body cells of the neonatal rat. J Physiol, London 436: 107–129

González C, Almaraz L, Obeso A & Rigual R (1994) Carotid body chemoreceptors: From natural stimuli to sensory discharges. Physiol Rev 74: 829–898

Iturriaga R, Rumsey WL, Mokashi A, Spergel D, Wilson, DF & Lahiri, S (1991) *In vitro* perfused-superfused cat carotid body for physiological and pharmacological studies. J Appl Physiol 70: 1393–1400

Kleyman TR & Cragoe EJ (1988) Amiloride and its analogs as tools in the study of ion transport. J Membr Biol 105: 1–21

Madshus IH (1988) Regulation of intracellular pH in eukaryotic cells. Biochem J 250: 1–8

Mokashi A, Ray D, Botre F, Katayama F, Osanai S & Lahiri S (1995) Effect of hypoxia in intracellular pH of glomus cells cultured from cat and rat carotid bodies. J Appl Physiol 78: 1875–1881

Rocher A, Obeso A, González C & Herreros B (1991) Ionic mechanisms for the transduction of acidic stimuli in the rabbit carotid body glomus cells. J Physiol, London 433: 533–548

Roos A & Boron WF (1981) Intracellular pH. Physiol Rev 61: 296–434

Wilding TJ, Cheng B & Roos A (1992) pH regulation in adult rat carotid body glomus cells: Importance of extracellular pH, sodium and potassium. J Gen Physiol 100: 593–608

26

DEPOLARIZATION IS A CRITICAL EVENT IN HYPOXIA-INDUCED GLOMUS CELL SECRETION

Nirit Weiss and David F. Donnelly

Section of Respiratory Medicine
Yale University School of Medicine
New Haven, Connecticut 06510

1. INTRODUCTION

Hypoxia chemotransduction within the carotid body is generally believed to be mediated by the glomus cells. Neurotransmitters (primarily dopamine) are stored within glomus cells in dense-cored vesicles, and catecholamine secretion is enhanced by hypoxia. Glomus cells are apposed to afferent terminals of the sinus nerve, and hypoxia-induced release of catecholamines leads to increased sinus nerve spiking activity. Two theories have evolved in an attempt to elucidate the cellular mechanisms involved in hypoxia-induced glomus cell secretion. In one model, hypoxia inhibits an oxygen-sensitive K^+ channel, leading to depolarization, activation of voltage-dependent Ca^{2+} currents, and enhanced secretion of catecholamine due to increased intracellular calcium (Gonzalez et al, 1994). In support of this model, several investigators have observed an inhibition of glomus cell K^+ current by hypoxia during patch-clamp recording of isolated glomus cells, and this inhibition appears to be correlated with an increase in $[Ca^{2+}]_i$ and enhanced secretion (Montoro et al, 1996). In contrast, others have observed an increase in $[Ca^{2+}]_i$ during hypoxia in the absence of extracellular calcium, implicating a second model, in which hypoxia causes release of calcium from intracellular stores, leading to enhanced secretion (Biscoe et al, 1989a; Biscoe & Duchen, 1990). In this second model, depolarization and calcium influx are not important events in the stimulus cascade. This is supported further by observations that membrane potential may actually hyperpolarize, rather than depolarize, during stimulation (Biscoe & Purves, 1989b).

In the present experiments we attempted to resolve this issue by measuring secretion (or vesicular fusion events) from individual glomus cells in an intact carotid body during hypoxia stimulation and during depolarization. Fusion of the dense-cored vesicles with the cell membrane causes a slight increase in cell size and capacitance. Detection of secretory activity was therefore accomplished by high-resolution calculation of membrane capacitance during patch-clamp recordings. We focused primarily on addressing two questions:

Frontiers in Arterial Chemoreception, edited by Zapata *et al.*
Plenum Press, New York, 1996

1) Does glomus cell membrane potential change during hypoxia? 2) Is depolarization necessary or sufficient to account for the enhanced secretion observed during hypoxia?

2. METHODS

The region of the carotid bifurcation was removed from anesthetized, decapitated rats. The carotid body and a portion of the cut sinus nerve were carefully dissected free and the connective tissue was removed by exposure to a dilute solution of collagenase/trypsin for 30 min. The tissue was placed in a perfusion chamber mounted on an inverted microscope and superfused with Ringer's saline (in mM: 125 NaCl, 3 KCl, 24 $NaHCO_3$, 1.25 NaH_2PO_4, 1.2 $CaCl_2$, 1.2 $MgSO_4$, and 10 glucose) bubbled with 20% O_2, 5% CO_2, balance N_2. The PO_2 next to the carotid body was measured with a platinum wire electrode insulated in a glass pipette, and covered with a butylacetate membrane. Whole-cell patch clamp recording of surface cells was undertaken as previously described (Donnelly, 1995). Most experiments were performed with perforated-patch access using amphotericin B as the pore-forming agent at a final concentration of 250 μg/ml (Rae, 1991). Pipette solution was based on K-gluconate (140 mM K-gluconate, 10 mM HEPES, 0.5 mM Ca^{2+}, pH 7.2).

Cells were initially characterized in the voltage-clamp mode, by developing an I/V profile over the voltage range of -60 to +60 mV. Glomus cells were identified based on the I/V profile of voltage-dependent currents: little inward current and pronounced outward current above -20 mV. The compensation circuit was switched off and the current response to a step hyperpolarization of 20 mV was recorded. The waveform of the current relaxation was fit to a 3rd order exponential equation and the values were used to calculate access resistance, membrane capacitance and membrane resistance. For the first part of the study, the recording mode was switched to current-clamp. Every 10 s a hyperpolarizing current of 10 pA was applied for calculation of input resistance. For the second part of the study, high resolution measurement of membrane capacitance was made by calculating the electrode/cell impedance at two frequencies and solving for the equivalent circuit (Donnelly, 1994).

3. RESULTS

3.1. Voltage Response of Glomus Cells

Under current-clamp conditions, the input resistance and membrane potential of glomus cells were measured before and during hypoxia. Average resting potential, recorded using the perforated-patch technique, was -33.6 ± 3.4 mV (mean ± SEM), and input resistance was 845.2 ± 64.6 MΩ (n= 22). After switching to a hypoxia solution superfusate (PO_2 = 0 Torr, glucose oxidase as oxygen scavenger, 1 min duration), the membrane potential rapidly depolarized in 19 of 22 cells. The average magnitude of depolarization was 10.7 ± 1.7 mV (Fig 1). In 3 of 22 cells, hypoxia caused no change in membrane potential.

3.2. Control of Glomus Cell Secretion

The initial part of this experiment addressed whether depolarization alone is sufficient to evoke secretion. At a holding potential of -60 mV, membrane capacitance was sta-

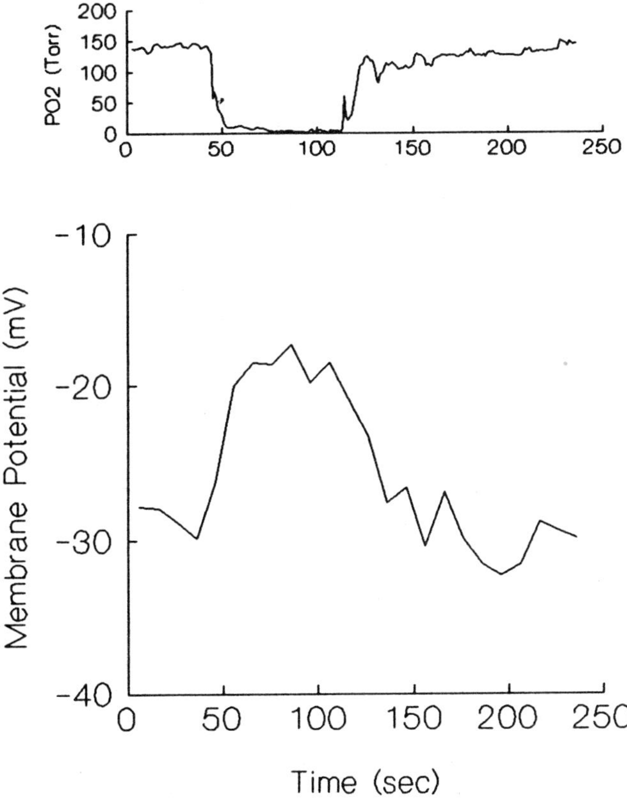

Figure 1. Glomus cells depolarize during hypoxic stimulus.

ble, but following depolarization to 0 mV there was a rapid increase in membrane capacitance. In 12/15 cells, capacitance increased at an initial rate of 325 ± 63 fF/sec, corresponding to an approximate vesicular fusion rate of 1,000 vesicles/sec (based on the average surface area of dense-cored vesicles measured in EM studies) (McDonald & Mitchell, 1975). During sustained depolarization for approximately 60 sec, membrane capacitance increased and plateaued (Fig 2). On average, the total change in capacitance was 1,000 ± 200 fF, corresponding to approximately 3,000 fusion events. After repolarization, capacitance returned to initial values at an average rate of 274 ± 52 fF/sec.

Having determined that depolarization alone can evoke secretion, we asked whether hypoxia alone, at a fixed membrane potential, can evoke secretion. At a holding potential of -60 mV, hypoxia alone (1 min duration) caused no significant change in cell capacitance (0 ± 1 fF, n= 6), but depolarization during the hypoxia trial caused a rapid increase in capacitance in all cells (Fig 3A and 3B).

In contrast to results obtained with perforated-patch recording, depolarization of cells recorded using conventional whole-cell recording caused no change in membrane capacitance (0 ± 1 fF, n= 20). For these experiments, the pipette fluid contained 1 mM EGTA, with no added calcium. Since EGTA may buffer the change in intracellular calcium by calcium influx, we tried to directly stimulate secretion by adding calcium to the pipette fluid. However, increasing pipette calcium to 2–10 μM was not associated with an increase in membrane capacitance following establishment of the whole-cell condition.

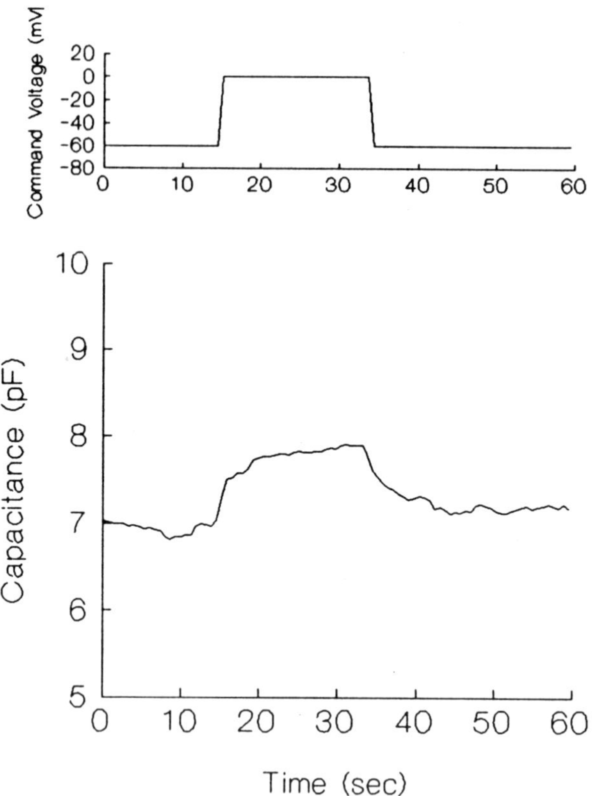

Figure 2. Capacitance increase during depolarization stimulus.

4. DISCUSSION

We have shown that glomus cells depolarize in response to hypoxia, and that hypoxia in the absence of a depolarization does not induce secretion. Depolarization closely follows the onset of hypoxia in our cells, and thus the timing of the depolarization is appropriate for mediating the physiologic increase in secretion. Our results are consistent with the first model of chemotransduction presented in the introduction, in which glomus cell depolarization is a critical event in initiating secretion.

There has been considerable uncertainty regarding the direction and magnitude of the change in glomus cell membrane potential with hypoxia. Some investigators using patch-clamp techniques reported a hyperpolarization during stimulation (Biscoe & Purves, 1989b), while others reported a depolarization using the same type of stimulation (Donnelly, 1993; Peers, 1990). Sharp electrode impalement studies of isolated rat glomus cells showed a hyperpolarization in the majority of isolated cells during hypoxia. These same investigators found that glomus cells which were part of cell clusters (rather than isolated cells) depolarized during hypoxia (Pang & Eyzaguirre, 1992). This implies that cell/cell interactions are critical in establishing the direction of the membrane potential change. A resolution to this issue is beyond the scope of the present study, but our study offers a unique perspective on the issue. Our patch-clamp recordings were obtained in individual

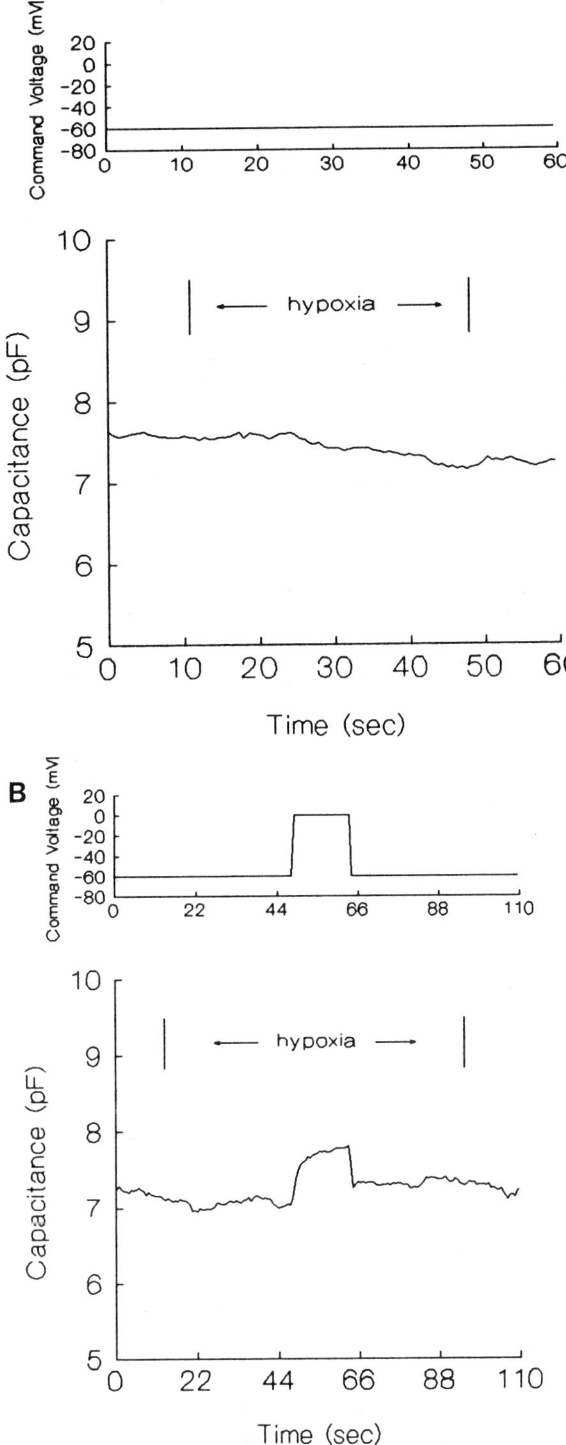

Figure 3. A. No change in capacitance during hypoxic stimulus at constant command potential. **B**. Same cell as in 3A. Depolarization during hypoxia evokes expected change in capacitance.

cells of an intact carotid body, thus preserving the morphology and cell/cell interactions which would have been lost in a dissociated preparation.

The role of intracellular calcium in glomus cell secretion is also uncertain. Many investigators record an increase in intracellular calcium with hypoxia (Biscoe et al, 1989a; Buckler & Vaughan-Jones, 1994), but, in other laboratories, hypoxia often fails to increase calcium (Chou et al, 1995; Roumy, 1994) or decreases calcium (Donnelly & Kholwadwala, 1992). Furthermore, the source of the calcium increase (when present) is uncertain, either from extracellular fluid (Buckler & Vaughan-Jones, 1994) or from intracellular stores (Biscoe et al, 1989a). Although we have no direct information on the calcium dynamics of our glomus cells, we found that membrane depolarization was a necessary step in the secretory response to hypoxia. This suggests that membrane potential, and hence, voltage-dependent activation of calcium currents, is an essential element in the control of secretion.

Although calcium is likely to be the most critical secretagogue in glomus cells, other intracellular factors may also be critical. In our studies, secretion could not easily be evoked using conventional whole-cell recording. A major complication (or advantage) of the conventional whole-cell technique is that intracellular dialysis of cytoplasmic factors may take place. Because secretion was reduced or blocked in this recording mode, it suggests that critical intracellular factors are reduced or lost in this mode. As mentioned, the most likely secretagogue is calcium, which would be buffered by the EGTA present in the pipette, but we were unable to overcome the inhibitory effect using high levels of pipette calcium. Alternatively, cyclic nucleotides and G-proteins have been implicated as playing a critical role in control of secretion from non-excitable cells, for instance, from mast cells (Neher, 1988) and melanotrophs (Okano et al, 1993). Although its too early to speculate on the importance of these other factors in control of glomus cell secretion, the difficulty in evoking secretion in the conventional whole-cell mode implies that diffusible factors, other than calcium, may be of considerable importance.

5. REFERENCES

Biscoe TJ, Duchen MR, Eisner DA, O'Neill SC & Valdeolmillos M (1989a) Measurements of intracellular calcium in dissociated type I cells of the rabbit carotid body. J Physiol, London 416: 421–434

Biscoe TJ & Purves MJ (1989b) Electrophysiological responses of disassociated type I cells of the rabbit carotid body to cyanide. J Physiol, London 413: 447–468

Biscoe TJ & Duchen MR (1990) Responses of type I cells dissociated from the rabbit carotid body to hypoxia. J Physiol, London 428: 39–59

Buckler KJ & Vaughan-Jones RD (1994) Effects of hypoxia on membrane potential and intracellular calcium in rat neonatal carotid body type I cells. J Physiol, London 476: 423–428

Chou CL, Shamri JSK, Ishizawa Y & Shirahata M (1995) Hypoxia depolarizes cultured cat glomus cells but does not increase intracellular calcium. Soc Neurosci Abstr 21:1883

Donnelly DF & Kholwadwala D (1992) Hypoxia decreases intracellular calcium in adult rat carotid body glomus cells. J Neurophysiol 67: 1543–1551

Donnelly DF (1993) Response to cyanide of two types of glomus cells in mature rat carotid body. Brain Res 630:157–168

Donnelly DF (1994) A novel method for rapid measurement of membrane resistance, capacitance, and access resistance. Biophys J 66: 873–877

Donnelly DF (1995) Modulation of glomus cell membrane currents of intact rat carotid body. J Physiol, London 489: 677–688

Gonzalez G, Almaraz L, Obeso A & Rigual R (1994) Carotid body chemoreceptors: from natural stimuli to sensory discharges. Physiol Rev 74: 829–898

McDonald DM & Mitchell RA (1975) The innervation of glomus cells, ganglion cells and blood vessels in the rat carotid body: a quantitative ultrastructural analysis. J Neurocytol 4: 177–230.

Montoro RJ, Ureña J, Fernandez-Chacon R, Alvarez De Toledo G & Lopez-Barneo J (1996) Oxygen sensing by ion channels and chemotransduction in single glomus cells. J Gen Physiol 107: 133–143

Neher E (1988) The influence of intracellular calcium concentration on degranulation of dialyzed mast cells from rat peritoneum. J Physiol, London 395: 193–214

Okano K, Monck JR & Fernandez JM (1993) GTPgammaS stimulates exocytosis in patch-clamped rat melanotrophs. Neuron 11: 165–172

Pang L & Eyzaguirre C (1992) Different effects of hypoxia on the membrane potential and input resistance of isolated and clustered carotid body glomus cells. Brain Res 575: 167–173

Peers C (1990) Hypoxic suppression of K^+ currents in type I carotid body cells: selective effect on the Ca^{2+}-activated K^+ currents. Neurosci Lett 119: 253–256

Rae J (1991) Low access resistance perforated patch recording using Amphotericin B. J Neurosci Meth 37: 15–26

Roumy M (1994) Cytosolic calcium in isolated type I cells of the adult rabbit carotid body: effects of hypoxia, cyanide, and changes in intracellular pH. Adv Exp Med Biol 360: 175–178

CO-CULTURES OF RAT PETROSAL NEURONS AND CAROTID BODY TYPE 1 CELLS

A Model for Studying Chemosensory Mechanisms

Huijun Zhong and Colin Nurse

Department of Biology
McMaster University
Hamilton, Ontario, Canada, L8S 4K1

1. INTRODUCTION

In mammals reflex hyperventilation following acute hypoxia is mediated via impulses in the carotid sinus nerve (CSN) which supplies afferent innervation to O_2- sensitive type 1 cells of the carotid body (Eyzaguirre & Zapata, 1984; Gonzalez et al, 1994). Type 1 cells contain multiple neurotransmitters, several of which are potential candidates for initiating or modulating CSN discharge during chemosensory signaling. The underlying synaptic events are poorly understood, and even controversial, in part because it is difficult to obtain reliable recordings from the afferent nerve endings *in situ* (see Eyzaguirre et al, 1983), and the transmitter sensitivity of these endings or of their parent cell bodies are unknown. Here we describe a preparation based on co-culture of rat type 1 cells and their afferent (petrosal) neurons which, combined with electrophysiological perforated-patch recording from identified neurons, provide an attractive approach for studying these mechanisms. Previous attempts using co-cultures of rat type 1 cells and nodose (sensory) neurons were hampered by the paucity of successful contacts, probably due to the low frequency of 'appropriate' chemosensory neurons present (Alcayaga & Eyzaguirre, 1990).

2. METHODS

The procedures for preparing separate cultures and co-cultures of dissociated carotid body (CB) type 1 cells and petrosal neurons from 6–12 day-old rat pups have been described elsewhere (Stea & Nurse, 1991; 1992). Nystatin perforated-patch recordings were obtained from the cell bodies of petrosal neurons grown for 4–7 days with or without type 1 cells, as previously described (Stea & Nurse, 1991; 1992). Typically, the extracellular fluid had the following composition (mM): NaCl 135; KCl 5; $CaCl_2$ 2; $MgCl_2$ 1; glucose

Frontiers in Arterial Chemoreception, edited by Zapata *et al.*
Plenum Press, New York, 1996

10; Hepes, 10 at pH 7.4; in a few experiments 24 mM $NaHCO_3$ was present (substituted for NaCl) and the pH was maintained by bubbling 5% CO_2. The pipette solution contained (mM): KCl 35; K gluconate 105; $CaCl_2$ 1; NaCl 10; Hepes 10, and nystatin 300 μg/ml, at pH 7.2. To facilitate recording of synaptic events in co-culture, neurons juxtaposed (within a few microns) to glomus cell clusters were selected, and the temperature of the bath was raised to 35°C. In experiments designed to test the sensitivity of petrosal neurons to putative neurotransmitters, the latter were applied by bath perfusion or by pressure ejection from a nearby 'puffer' pipette. In a few cases, the chemosensory identity of the recorded petrosal neuron was confirmed after fixation and immuno-staining for tyrosine hydroxylase (TH), probably the best available marker for CB chemoafferents in the rat (see Katz et al, 1993). Also in co-cultures, the relation between the processes of petrosal neurons and type 1 cell clusters could be revealed by double-label immunofluorescence, using antibodies against neurofilament (Texas red label) and TH (fluorescein label) respectively (see Fig 1). Immunofluorescent procedures are described in detail elsewhere (Jackson & Nurse, 1995).

3. RESULTS

In co-cultures (*e.g.*, Fig 1), recordings of membrane potential from petrosal neurons by the nystatin whole-cell technique revealed the frequent occurrence of spontaneous activity. Such activity was rare or absent in dissociated cell cultures of petrosal ganglia alone (see also, Stea & Nurse, 1992). Evidence for the presence of 'functional' synaptic contacts between type 1 cells and petrosal terminals was revealed by the occurrence of spontaneous spikes and subthreshold potentials, similar to spontaneous excitatory post-synaptic potentials or e.p.s.p.'s seen at conventional chemical synapses (Fig 2A). These sub-

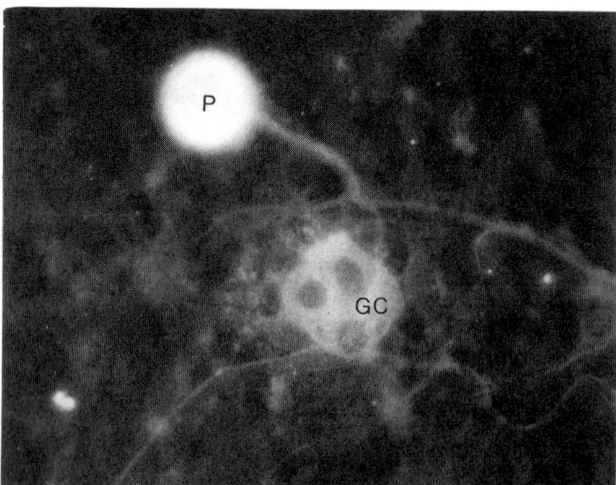

Figure 1. Fluorescence micrograph from an immunostained co-culture of rat petrosal neurons and type 1 cells. The cell body of the petrosal neuron (P) and its processes were stained with a mouse monoclonal antibody against neurofilament (NF 68 kDa) protein, and visualized with a Texas red -conjugated secondary antibody. The small cluster of three type 1 or glomus cells (GC) were stained with a rabbit antibody against tyrosine hydroxylase (TH), and visualized with a fluorescein- conjugated secondary antibody (for procedures, see Jackson & Nurse, 1995). The 3 nuclei of the type 1 cells are unstained and appear dark; note neuronal processes crossing over the type 1 cell cluster. Background cells (*e.g.*, fibroblasts and sustentacular cells) are unstained.

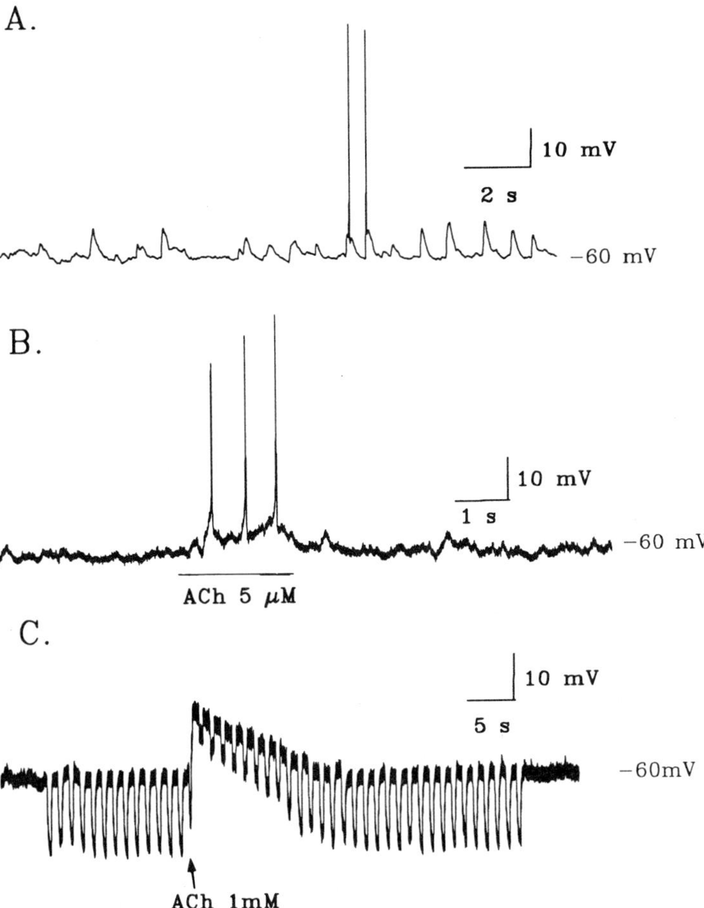

Figure 2. Membrane potential recordings from cultured petrosal neurons using the perforated-patch whole cell technique. In A and B, the neurons were juxtaposed (within a few microns) to type 1 cell clusters (*e.g.*, Fig 1B in Stea & Nurse, 1992). **A**. Spontaneous action potentials and subthreshold potentials, similar to excitatory post synaptic potentials or e.p.s.p.'s, were recorded in the neuronal cell body. **B**. Bath perfusion of ACh, during the period indicated by the lower horizontal bar, resulted in a small depolarization and spike activity in the neuron and the effect was reversible. **C**. In this culture of petrosal neurons alone, a 'puff' of ACh was applied to a petrosal cell body by pressure ejection from a nearby pipette, at the time indicated by the vertical arrow. Note ACh caused membrane depolarization associated with a conductance increase; constant hyperpolarizing current pulses were applied during the downward deflections. In all cases the resting membrane potential was ~ -60 mV.

threshold potentials were often present in recordings from petrosal cell bodies that were juxtaposed within a few microns to type 1 cell clusters (see Fig 1B in Stea & Nurse, 1992), suggesting the electrode was within a favorable electrotonic distance from the synaptic contact(s). As will be described in more detail elsewhere, application of hypoxic stimuli to similar co-cultures led in several cases to an excitatory response in juxtaposed' petrosal neurons, suggesting these cultures can also transduce and relay chemosensory information.

The neurotransmitter mechanisms that gave rise to the post-synaptic potentials and spike activity seen in Figure 2A are currently under investigation. Several excitatory neurotransmitters, localized to type 1 cells, have been implicated in carotid body function though there is some controversy over the one(s) that actually mediate hypoxic signaling (see Eyzaguirre & Zapata, 1984; Gonzalez et al, 1994). Since acetylcholine (ACh) has for some time been a leading candidate (Eyzaguirre & Zapata, 1984; Fitzgerald et al, 1995; see also this issue), we tested whether petrosal neurons are sensitive to ACh. As illustrated in Figure 2B, bath application of 5 μM ACh in co-cultures resulted in excitation of several petrosal neurons, with occasional spike activity. However, since nicotinic ACh receptors are also present on rat type 1 cells (Wyatt & Peers, 1993; our unpublished observations) it is possible that some of the activity seen in Figure 2B is mediated indirectly, via the secondary action of other transmitters. To test whether petrosal neurons were directly sensitive to ACh, the transmitter was applied focally to isolated cell bodies by pressure ejection from a 'puffer' pipette, in both petrosal (alone) cultures and co-cultures. As shown in Figure 2C, > 60% of petrosal neurons were sensitive to puffer-applied ACh, and in all cases the effect was excitatory and associated with a conductance increase. In several cases (not shown) the ACh-induced depolarization was substantially reduced by the ganglionic blocker hexamethonium (50 μM). In a few cases an ACh-sensitive petrosal neuron, identified electrophysiologically, was subsequently found to be positive for TH-immunoreactivity, a well-characterized marker for rat CB chemoafferents (Katz et al, 1993).

In preliminary studies the sensitivity of petrosal neurons to other potential transmitters present in type 1 cells was also tested. Whereas both 5-HT and substance P were found to be excitatory when applied to at least a subpopulation of petrosal neurons, results with dopamine were less consistent and may depend on the dose used.

4. DISCUSSION

In this communication we describe a preparation, consisting of co-culture of rat petrosal neurons and carotid body (CB) type 1 cells, which is potentially attractive for studying chemosensory mechanisms. The available evidence suggests that *de novo* functional synapses develop in these cultures between some neurons and type 1 cell clusters. Since the petrosal neurons that are carried into culture include subpopulations that subserve other sensory modalities, perhaps it is not surprising that some neurons may fail to form functional contacts. In particular, we found there was an increase in spontaneous electrical activity in co-cultured neurons, including the presence of both spike discharges and spontaneous potentials that resemble post-synaptic potentials. Most importantly, excitatory responses to normal CB chemostimuli, such as hypoxia and acidity, have been observed in petrosal neurons in co-culture (in preparation). The ability to record synaptic events in petrosal cell bodies, fortuitously located close to type 1 cell clusters, obviates some of the problems usually encountered during attempts to record from the nerve terminals *in situ* (see Eyzaguirre et al, 1983). Finally, since it is now possible to study the effects of CB neurotransmitters on both type 1 cells and *identified* chemoafferent neurons, these co-cultures should prove useful for understanding synaptic mechanisms during chemosensory signaling in the carotid body.

5. ACKNOWLEDGMENTS

We acknowledge the expert technical assistance of Cathy Vollmer, who refined the techniques for obtaining successful co-cultures. This work was supported by a grant from the Medical Research Council of Canada.

6. REFERENCES

Alcayaga J & Eyzaguirre C (1990) Electrophysiological evidence for the reconstitution of chemosensory units in co-cultures of carotid body and nodose ganglion neurons. Brain Res 534: 324–328

Eyzaguirre C, Monti-Bloch L, Hayashida Y & Baron M (1983) Biophysics of the carotid body receptor complex. In: Acker H & O'Regan RG (eds) Physiology of the Peripheral Arterial Chemoreceptors. Amsterdam: Elsevier. pp 59–87

Eyzaguirre C & Zapata P (1984) Perspectives in carotid body research. J Appl Physiol 57: 931–957

Fitzgerald RS, Shirahata M, Ide T & Lydic R (1995) The cholinergic hypothesis revisited- An unfinished story. Biol Signals 4: 298–303

Gonzalez C, Almaraz L, Obeso A & Rigual R (1994) Carotid body chemoreceptors: From natural stimuli to sensory discharges. Physiol Rev 74: 829–898

Jackson A & Nurse C (1995) Plasticity in cultured carotid body chemoreceptors: Environmental modulation of GAP-43 and neurofilament. J Neurobiol 26: 485–496

Katz DM, Finley JCW & Polak J (1993) Dopaminergic and peptidergic sensory innervation of the rat carotid body: Organization and development. Adv Exp Med Biol 337: 43–49

Stea A & Nurse CA (1991) Whole-cell and perforated-patch recordings from O_2-sensitive rat carotid body cells grown in short and long-term cultures. Pflügers Arch 418: 93–101

Stea A & Nurse CA (1992) Whole-cell currents in two subpopulations of cultured rat petrosal neurons with different tetrodotoxin sensitivities. Neuroscience 47: 727–736

Wyatt CN & Peers C (1993) Nicotinic acetylcholine receptors in isolated type 1 cells of the neonatal rat carotid body. Neuroscience 54: 275–281

28

RESPONSES OF CAT PETROSAL GANGLION NEURONS ARE MODIFIED BY THE PRESENCE OF CAROTID BODY CELLS IN TISSUE CULTURES

J. Alcayaga and J. Arroyo

Laboratorio de Neurobiología
Departamento de Biología, Facultad de Ciencias
Universidad de Chile
Santiago, Chile

1. CAROTID BODY SENSORY INNERVATION

The carotid body glomus (type I, receptor) cells are the sensory elements of the arterial chemoreceptor system. They are innervated by petrosal ganglion neurons that convey chemosensory information to the central nervous system. It is accepted that the transduction of the chemosensory stimuli in the glomus cells produces the exocytotic release of several transmitters and/or modulators that, acting on the neuronal terminal, drive the sensory activity (for review see González et al, 1994). However, there is limited information on the membrane potential changes induced in the petrosal ganglion neurons by effect of carotid chemosensory stimulation. Intracellular recordings from the nerve terminals within the carotid body showed the existence of slow, graded potentials that could generate spikes when they reach threshold (Hayashida et al, 1980), resembling synaptic or receptor potentials. Recently, acid-induced depolarizing responses, generating trains of action potentials when threshold was reached, were recorded from vagal sensory neurons co-cultured with carotid body cells (Alcayaga & Eyzaguirre, 1990). There is though, a degree of specificity in the formation of synapses between neurons and their target tissues, so we investigated the properties and responses of petrosal ganglion neurons of adult cats, both alone and in presence of carotid body tissue.

2. CULTURE AND RECORDING METHODS

2.1. Tissue Culture Preparation

The petrosal ganglia and carotid bodies were excised from adult cats of either sex (2250–3950 g), under pentobarbitone anaesthesia (40 mg/kg, ip). The neck was opened

Frontiers in Arterial Chemoreception, edited by Zapata *et al.*
Plenum Press, New York, 1996

and the carotid bifurcation reached. The glossopharyngeal nerve was localized and followed into the cranium, the ganglion reached, removed, and placed in ice-chilled, Ca^{2+}- and Mg^{2+}-free, Hanks' solution (mHBSS). The carotid bifurcation was vascularly isolated, excised and placed in mHBSS. The whole procedure was repeated contralaterally. The tissues were rinsed twice in mHBSS, the carotid bodies isolated from the bifurcation and the ganglia desheathed. Homologous tissues were pooled together, minced into 12 to 20 pieces, and enzymatically dissociated in mHBSS supplemented with 0.1% collagenase, 0.05% trypsin and 150 U/ml DNAse. Dissociation, carried out under agitation at 37°C for 30–75 min, was ended adding an excess of protein and soybean trypsin inhibitor, to final concentrations of 10% and 0.01%, respectively. After 10 min of additional incubation, the cell suspensions were centrifuged for 10 min at 1800 rpm, and the pellets suspended in medium 199 supplemented with 10% horse serum, 10% fetal bovine serum, 20 mM HEPES and nerve growth factor (15 ng/ml). The cell were then seeded into 35 mm Petri dishes previously covered with poly-L-lysine (0.1 mg/ml). Aliquots of petrosal ganglion neurons and carotid body tissue suspensions were mixed to obtain co-cultures. The cultures were maintained at 37°C in water-saturated 5% CO_2 in air atmosphere. The culture medium was changed every other day after a 3-day initial lag, during which the cells were undisturbed.

2.2. Recording Procedure

The cultures were placed in the stage of an inverted microscope, and superfused at room temperature (20–22°C) with 95% O_2-, 5% CO_2-equilibrated Earl's solution (EBSS). Petrosal ganglion neurons were impaled with 15–70 MΩ glass microelectrodes filled with 3 M KCl. Acid stimulus (EBSS + 10 mM PIPES buffer; pH 6.5) was delivered by amplitude and duration controlled pressure pulses applied to 10 μm tip glass pipettes located at 50–100 μm from the recorded neuron. The membrane potential, the current pulses and the pressure pulses, recorded through a pressure transducer, were stored on FM magnetic tape recorder (frequency response DC to 2500 Hz). The data were digitized off-line through a 12 bits, 100 kHz, digital to analog converter.

3. ELECTRICAL PROPERTIES OF CULTURED PETROSAL GANGLION NEURONS

The impalement of the cultured petrosal ganglion neurons permitted stable recordings, with resting membrane potentials ranging between -75 and -40 mV. Action potentials, evoked by brief (< 5 ms duration) depolarizing pulses, had amplitudes of 60 to 100 mV, with overshoots of 10 to 50 mV (Fig 1). No differences were found between the values recorded from neurons in petrosal ganglia cultures or ganglia-carotid bodies co-cultures (Table I). Our values agree with those previously recorded from cat petrosal ganglion neurons *in vitro* (Belmonte & Gallego, 1983; Gallego, 1983; Gallego et al, 1987; Morales et al, 1987). Most evoked action potentials presented a "hump" in the repolarizing phase (Fig 1), a characteristic of a vast population of the petrosal neurons (Belmonte & Gallego, 1983; Morales et al, 1987), but also present in other visceral (Gallego & Eyzaguirre, 1978; Jaffe & Sampson, 1976; Stansfeld & Wallis, 1985) and somatic sensory neurons (Matsuda et al, 1976; Ransom & Holz, 1977; Yoshida et al, 1978).

The action potential duration ranged from 1 to 7 ms (Table 1), similar to those previously reported for petrosal ganglion neurons (Belmonte & Gallego, 1983; Gallego, 1983;

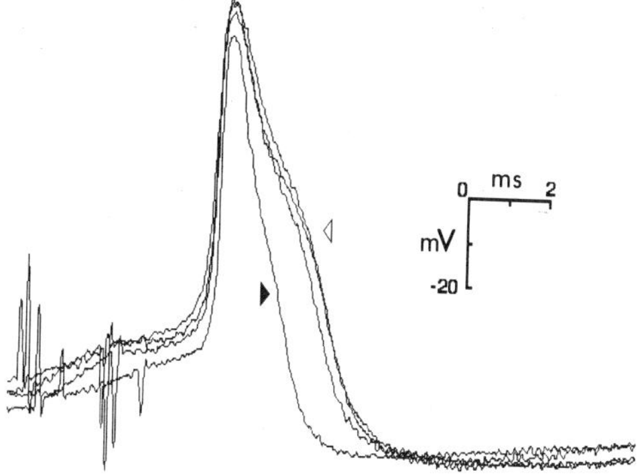

Figure 1. Action potentials of 4 petrosal ganglion neurons from a 6-day culture evoked by brief depolarizing pulses. Most responses presented a clear "hump" in the repolarizing phase (open arrowhead), while few presented a smaller hump (filled arrowhead).

Morales et al, 1987). However, the mean duration of the action potential in our preparation (Table 1) was slightly longer than that previously reported (Belmonte & Gallego, 1983; Morales et al, 1987). It must be considered that our recordings were performed at 20–22°C, about 15.5°C lower than previously reported data and that the action potential duration of cultured petrosal ganglion neurons should be reduced at higher temperatures. The after-hyperpolarizations, which followed the spikes lasted from 10 ms to about 100 ms, thus being in the lower part of the range previously reported for petrosal ganglion neurons (Belmonte & Gallego, 1983; Morales et al, 1987) and never reaching the duration showed by the fastest conducting petrosal ganglion neurons that project through the carotid nerve (Belmonte & Gallego, 1983) or by the H-neurons projecting through the pharyngeal branch of the glossopharyngeal nerve (Morales et al., 1987). However, the after-hyperpolarization is the neuronal property that most slowly recovers after peripheral axotomy (Gallego et al, 1987), and its recovery probably depends on peripheral target reinnervation (Belmonte et al, 1988). Thus, the axotomy produced during neuronal isolation and/or the lack of target reinnervation in the culture conditions could account for the observed differences. Moreover, our recordings, in contrast with previous ones, were performed using HCO_3^--CO_2 buffered media, lacking HEPES buffer. Good-buffers are known to alter the buffer capabilities of the intracellular medium (Walsh, 1990), probably altering intracellular pH and modifying neuronal passive and active properties with respect to HCO_3^--CO_2 buffered media (Church, 1992). Despite the mentioned differences, our data indicates that adult cat petrosal ganglion neurons in culture maintain electrophysiological characteristics similar to those described for acutely isolated petrosal ganglion neurons. The observed differences can be attributed to the recording methods and the axotomy during cellular isolation.

When the cells were depolarized by long-lasting pulses (> 500 ms) the neurons responded by firing a single, two or multiple action potentials, comprising 40%, 20% and 40% of the neuronal population in culture, respectively. The neurons that fired one and two action potentials maintained their response even if the membrane potential was reduced to zero. Multiple-spiking neurons increased the number and frequency of the spikes with the strength of depolarization. In the co-cultures, the number of neurons that fired a single action potential was reduced to 15%, while the multiple-spiking neurons comprised 70% of the recorded population. The increased number of spiking neurons in presence of carotid body tissue may be due either to the selection of a certain subpopulation of petrosal ganglion neurons or to a modification of the expression of membrane channels. The latter seems unlikely because the major electrical properties of the neurons were undistinguishable between the petrosal cultures and the co-cultures (Table 1).

Table 1. Electrical parameters of petrosal ganglion (PG) neurons cultured alone and in co-culture with carotid body (CB) tissue

Culture	Membrane potential (mV)	Spike amplitude (mV)	Spike duration (ms)	AHP amplitude (mV)	AHP duration (ms)
PG	56.7±7.4 (n=49)	83.2±9.9 (n=49)	2.7±1.2 (n=33)	14.1±2.8 (n=45)	31.7±16.2 (n=46)
PG + CB	53.9±6.5 (n=40)	85.9±8.1 (n=40)	3.0±1.2 (n=24)	15.1±3.4 (n=37)	30.6±11.0 (n=37)
Total	55.4±7.1 (n=89)	84.4±9.2 (n=89)	2.8±1.2 (n=57)	14.5±3.1 (n=82)	31.2±14.0 (n=83)

4. PETROSAL GANGLION RESPONSES TO LOCAL ACIDIFICATION

4.1. Petrosal Ganglion Cultures

Local acidification of the media surrounding the neurons had no effect on electrically evoked action potentials in 19.2% (5/26) of the recorded neurons, blocking the response in the remaining neurons (21/26). Blockade of the evoked action potentials was accompanied by a small (< 5 mV) depolarization (20/21) or hyperpolarization (1/21) that lasted during the whole stimulation period. The blocking effect of acidification could be overcome by increasing the magnitude of the depolarizing pulses. A similar blocking effect was evoked by extracellular acidification in cultured nodose ganglion neurons (Alcayaga & Eyzaguirre, 1990). Increased extracellular $[H^+]$ could block evoked action potentials by acting on Na- and K-conductances (Hille, 1968), depolarizing the neurons and increasing the action potential threshold (Gruol et al, 1980). The effect of extracellular acidification on petrosal ganglion neuron responses appears as the result of the direct effects of increased $[H^+]_e$ on the neuronal membrane and its ion fluxes. Thus, petrosal ganglion neurons, located downstream the chemosensory transduction process, are devoid of a specific acid-induced response as well as a specific hypoxic response (Stea & Nurse, 1992).

4.2. Petrosal Ganglion-Carotid Body Co-Cultures

In general, acidification produced similar effects to those already described for petrosal neurons cultured alone. The population of cells unaffected by acid was similar (4/20; 20%), but the number of neurons blocked by acid was reduced to 70% (14/20). Blockade of evoked action potentials was accompanied by depolarization (8/14; 57%), hyperpolarization (2/14; 14%) or no membrane potential changes (4/14; 29%). The remaining neurons (2/20; 10%) responded to a single, brief, acid pulse (≤500 ms) with a depolarization that triggered a train of action potentials once the threshold was attained (Fig 2), repolarizing to their previous resting membrane potential within 1–2 s (Fig 3a).

The magnitude of the depolarization and the number of action potentials in the train increased with increasing stimulus duration (Fig 2), suggesting a relation between the magnitude of the response and the amount of H^+ delivered to the neuron environs. This acid-induced response was recorded only from petrosal ganglion neurons co-cultured with glomus tissue. A similar acid-induced response was recorded from a population of nodose ganglion neurons in the presence of carotid body cells (Alcayaga & Eyzaguirre, 1990).

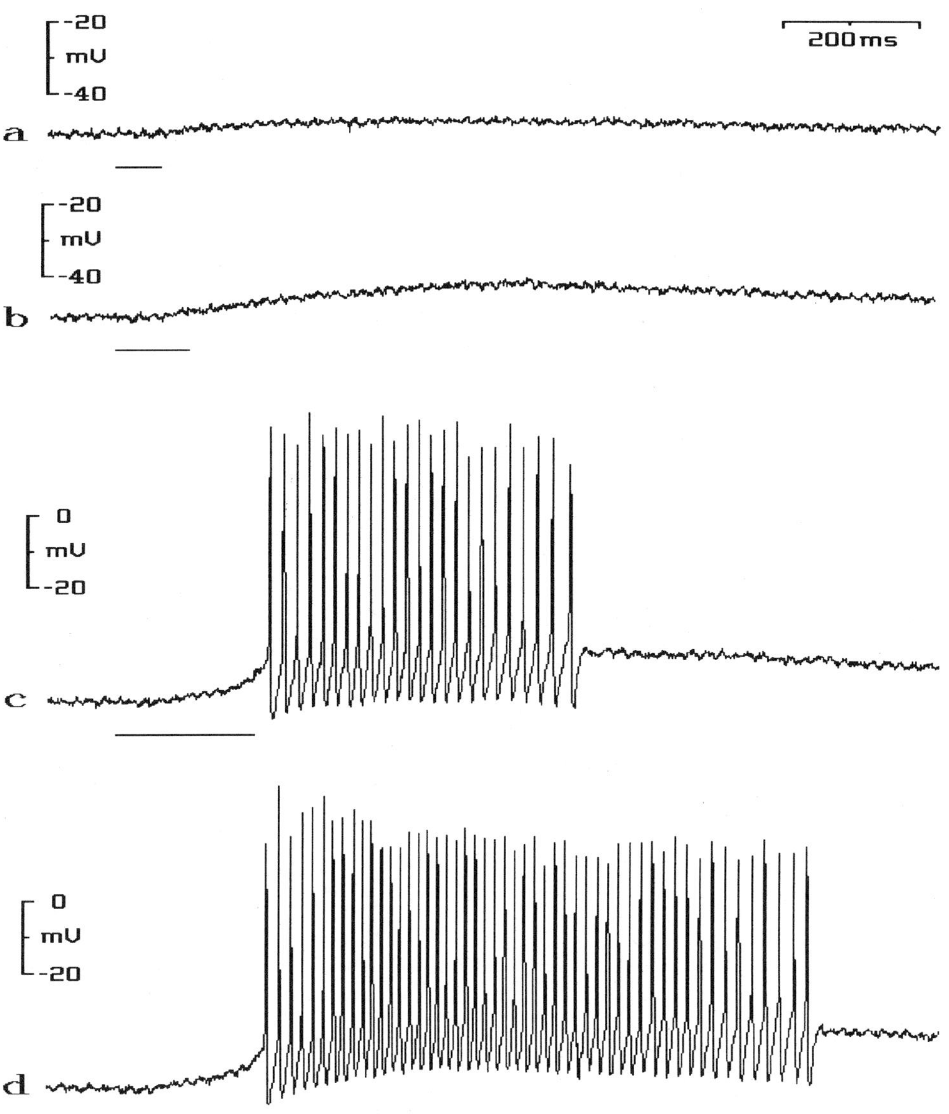

Figure 2. Acid-induced responses of a petrosal ganglion neuron co-cultured with carotid body tissue for 6 days. Magnitude of depolarization and number of action potentials fired increased with stimulus duration: **a**, 50 ms; **b**, 100 ms; **c**, 200 ms; **d**, 400 ms.

Our data indicate that the carotid body tissue is necessary for the development of this response, suggesting that functional restoration of synapses and/or trophic relations between glomus cells and sensory neurons are necessary to reestablish chemosensory-related activity in petrosal ganglion neurons.

When the acid stimulus was repeated, the responses to following stimuli consisted of depolarizations that never reached the threshold level to evoke an action potential (Fig. 3b). Similarly, during continuous local acidification the neurons remained depolarized after an initial burst of action potentials. These data indicate that acid-induced responses present adapta-

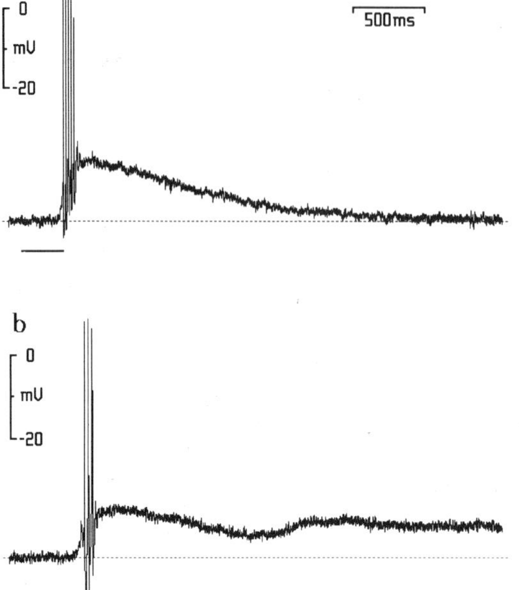

Figure 3. Acid-induced responses of petrosal ganglion neurons co-cultured with carotid body tissue. **a.** Response to a single supra-threshold stimulus, returning to basal level within 2 s. **b.** Sustained depolarization in response to repetitive stimulation, without reaching threshold after first stimulus. Dotted line, basal membrane potential.

tion during repetitive or continuous stimulation. Conversely, carotid sinus nerve activity presents little or no adaptation when continuously stimulated with acid (Eyzaguirre & Koyano, 1965). This difference can be partly explained by non-specific effects of H^+ on neuronal responses, counteracting the functional relations reestablished between glomus cells and sensory neurons. On the other hand, the exact extent of functional recovery of the glomus cell-petrosal ganglion relation has yet to be established.

5. CONCLUSIONS

Petrosal ganglion neurons in culture retain most of their electrophysiological characteristics, except for a reduction in after-hyperpolarization duration, that could be explained in terms of axotomy effects and lack of functional restoration with target tissue. The presence of carotid body tissue has no effect on these electrophysiological parameters, but a distinct acid-induced response developed in a population of petrosal ganglion neurons under these culture conditions. This acid-induced response was proportional to the amount of H^+ delivered in the neuron vicinity and presented adaptation to continuous or repetitive stimulation.

The petrosal ganglion-carotid body tissue co-cultures appear to restore some properties of the chemosensory afferent pathway and could be used to explore functional and trophic relations between their cellular components.

6. ACKNOWLEDGMENTS

This work was supported by the *Fondo Nacional de Investigación Científica y Tecnológica* (FONDECYT, grant 1133/92).

J. Alcayaga received the Data Foundation Award at the end of the XIIIth International Symposium on Arterial Chemoreceptors, Santiago, Chile, March 1996.

7. REFERENCES

Alcayaga J & Eyzaguirre C (1990) Electrophysiological evidence for the reconstitution of chemosensory units in co-cultures of carotid body and nodose ganglion neurons. Brain Res 534: 324–328

Belmonte C & Gallego R (1983) Membrane properties of cat sensory neurones with chemoreceptor and baroreceptor endings. J Physiol, London 342: 603–614

Belmonte C, Gallego R & Morales A (1988) Membrane properties of primary sensory neurones of the cat after peripheral reinnervation. J Physiol, London 405: 219–232

Church J (1992) A change from HCO_3^--CO_2 to HEPES-buffered medium modifies membrane properties of rat CA1 pyramidal neurones *in vitro*. J Physiol, London 455: 51–71

Eyzaguirre C & Koyano H (1965) Effects of hypoxia, hypercapnia, and pH on the chemoreceptor activity of the carotid body *in vitro*. J Physiol, London 178: 385–409

Jaffe RA & Sampson SR (1976) Analysis of passive and active electrophysiological properties of neurons in mammalian nodose ganglia maintained *in vitro*. J Neurophysiol 39: 802–815

Gallego R (1983) The ionic basis of action potentials in petrosal ganglion cells of the cat. J Physiol, London 342: 591–602

Gallego R & Eyzaguirre C (1978) Membrane and action potential characteristics of A and C nodose ganglion cells studied in whole ganglia and in tissue slices. J Neurophysiol 41: 1217–1232

Gallego R, Ivorra I & Morales A (1987) Effects of central or peripheral axotomy on membrane properties of sensory neurones in the petrosal ganglion of the cat. J Physiol, London 391: 39–56

González C, Almaraz L, Obeso A & Rigual R (1994) Carotid body chemoreceptors: from natural stimuli to sensory discharges. Physiol Rev 74: 829–898

Gruol DL, Barker JL, Huang L-YM, MacDonald JF & Smith TG Jr (1980) Hydrogen ions have multiple effects on the excitability of cultured mammalian neurons. Brain Res 183: 247–252

Hayashida Y, Koyano H & Eyzaguirre C (1980) An intracellular study of chemosensory fibers and endings. J Neurophysiol 44: 1077–1088

Hille B (1968) Changes and potentials at the nerve surface: divalent ions and pH. J Gen Physiol 51: 221–236

Matsuda Y, Yoshida S & Yonezawa T (1976) A Ca-dependent regenerative response in rodent dorsal root ganglion cells cultures *in vitro*. Brain Res 115: 334–338

Morales A, Ivorra I & Gallego R (1987) Membrane properties of glossopharyngeal sensory neurons in the petrosal ganglion of the cat. Brain Res 401: 340–346

Ransom BR & Holz RW (1977) Ionic determinants of excitability in cultured mouse dorsal root ganglion and spinal cord cells. Brain Res 136: 445–453

Stea A & Nurse CA (1992) Whole-cell currents in two subpopulations of cultured rat petrosal neurons with different tetrodotoxin sensitivities. Neuroscience 47: 727–736

Stansfeld CE & Wallis DI (1985) Properties of visceral primary afferent neurons in the nodose ganglion of the rabbit. J Neurophysiol 54: 245–260

Walsh PJ (1990) Fish hepatocytes accumulate HEPES: a potential source of error in studies of intracellular pH regulation. J Exp Biol 148: 495–499

Yoshida S, Matsuda Y & Samejima A (1978) Tetrodotoxin-resistant sodium and calcium components of action potentials in dorsal root ganglion cells of the adult mouse. J Neurophysiol 41: 1096–1106

MODIFICATIONS OF CAROTID BODY CO_2 CHEMOSENSITIVITY *IN VITRO*

P. Kumar, R. C. Landauer, and D. R. Pepper

Department of Physiology, The Medical School
University of Birmingham
Birmingham B15 2TT, United Kingdom

1. INTRODUCTION

The peripheral chemoreceptor functions as a transducer of a number of blood-borne stimuli, signalling via changes in action potential frequency in the carotid sinus branch of the glossopharyngeal nerve. Of these stimuli the response to blood gas tensions (PO_2 and PCO_2) and pH has received the most research attention, as transduction of these stimuli is believed to be the primary purpose of this receptor system, giving it a pivotal role in the maintenance of cardio-respiratory homeostasis.

It is evident that all afferent chemoreceptor fibres have the ability to convey information irrespective of the nature of the stimulus, *i.e.*, separate fibres for the transmission of PCO_2 or PO_2-derived information do not appear to exist. Clearly the two stimuli have to converge at some point in the chemotransduction process downstream of the generation of an afferent action potential. Such convergence would allow for stimulus interaction and indeed CO_2 and hypoxia do interact at the level of action potential discharge in an interdependent manner (Lahiri & Delaney, 1975). Thus, the slope of the linear PCO_2 stimulus-response curve is increased and its intercept with the PCO_2-axis decreased as PO_2 is decreased or, put another way, increasing PCO_2 shifts the exponential PO_2 stimulus response curve rightwards and upwards. The interaction between PCO_2 and hypoxia is therefore greater than additive, *i.e.*, multiplicative. The effect is best described as a "fan" of CO_2 response curves and is very similar to the fan observed when the ventilatory response to PCO_2 is measured at different levels of PO_2 (Nielson & Smith, 1952). Indeed, more recent data appears to ascribe all of the observed CO_2-O_2 ventilatory interaction to that occurring at the peripheral chemoreceptor with no further multiplication centrally (Clement et al, 1995).

The existence of a postnatal increase in the magnitude of the initial phase of the reflex ventilatory response to an acute hypoxic challenge (resetting) is well established for a number of species, including man, and recordings of afferent discharge, *in vivo*, have revealed that this maturation occurs at the carotid and aortic chemoreceptors (see Hanson & Kumar, 1994). More recently, it was demonstrated that this postnatal increase in the chemoreceptor discharge

Frontiers in Arterial Chemoreception, edited by Zapata *et al.*
Plenum Press, New York, 1996

frequency was maintained in the *in vitro* rat carotid body preparation (Kholwadwala & Donnelly, 1992), thus indicating resetting to be a process intrinsic to the chemoreceptor tissue and not due, for example, to changes in the concentration of circulating factors or in the efferent neural supply to the organ. Subsequently, we have shown that the greater than additive effect of hypoxia and hypercapnia upon single fibre chemoreceptor discharge described *in vivo* is also retained in the adult rat carotid body preparation *in vitro* but, more interestingly, is not present in neonatal tissue, where only an additive interaction between the two stimuli occurs (Pepper et al, 1995). Thus, in the neonate, increasing hypoxia, whilst increasing discharge, is without effect upon CO_2 sensitivity, giving rise to a set of essentially parallel CO_2 response curves and not the classical "fan" as observed in the adult. Further, the development of resetting, as measured by the ventilatory response to hypoxia, can be "blunted" by chronic hypoxaemia from birth (Eden & Hanson, 1987), suggesting the maturation to be an O_2-dependent process and, accordingly, the development of multiplicative interaction at the level of carotid chemoreceptor discharge can likewise also be prevented by chronic hypoxaemia from birth (Landauer et al, 1995). We have therefore suggested that a postnatal development of this multiplicative interaction rather than a development to hypoxia *per se*, might underlie the development of hypoxic chemosensitivity observed in the newborn.

In an attempt to understand the mechanisms which might determine resetting, we have begun to examine factors which might affect CO_2 chemosensitivity in the adult rat carotid body, *in vitro*. In this paper we will present data from three such factors.

1.1. Temperature

As well as their much documented responses to blood gas tensions and pH, chemoreceptors also exhibit a thermal sensitivity (Bernthal & Weeks, 1939; McQueen & Eyzaguirre, 1974; Gallego et al, 1979; Alcayaga et al, 1993) with elevations and reductions in both local and systemic temperature being well correlated with increases and decreases, respectively, in chemoreceptor discharge. Whether this effect is of reflex consequence in its own right or acts as a modifier of the chemotransduction process is not known. However, whilst the effect of changes in PO_2, PCO_2 and pH upon the thermal response of chemoreceptors has been described previously, the effect of temperature changes upon the sensitivity of the chemoreceptors to CO_2 had not been previously reported.

1.2. Extracellular Potassium Ion Concentration ($[K^+]_o$)

Jarisch et al (1952) proposed that elevations in $[K^+]_o$ could increase peripheral chemoreceptor discharge by a direct, depolarising effect at the post-synaptic afferent terminals of the carotid sinus nerve. More recently, results from *in vivo* studies have shown that the sensitivity of the chemoreceptor to hypoxia but not to hypercapnia or pH, is increased by elevations in $[K^+]_o$ and the role of elevations in $[K^+]_o$ in the (part) mediation of exercise hyperpnoea has been re-examined (see Linton & Band, 1990; Paterson, 1992, for reviews). The hypothesis that $[K^+]_o$ could perhaps be an "anaerobic work substance" had never been tested in an *in vitro* preparation where additional, indirect neural and humoural factors could be eliminated.

1.3. Adenosine

Adenosine is released ubiquitously during hypoxia (Moss et al, 1987), plays a neuromodulatory role in many physiological systems and may even act as a neurotransmitter in parts of the CNS. Its link with cellular metabolism makes it an attractive candidate for study in the carotid body and previous reports have described a stimulatory action of adenosine upon chemoreceptor afferent discharge (McQueen & Ribeiro, 1981) that is independent of effects upon blood flow (Runold et al, 1990). If adenosine is indeed acting like hypoxia then it could cause a dose-dependent increase in CO_2 sensitivity at the carotid body, a possibility which has not been previously investigated.

2. METHODS

Adult male Wistar rats were anaesthetized (1.5–2.5% halothane in 100% O_2) and carotid bodies were prepared for *in vitro* recording as described previously (Pepper et al, 1995). In all control situations, carotid bodies were superfused at 3 ml/min with warmed (37°C), gassed (95% O_2 / 5% CO^2), bicarbonate-buffered saline solution (125 mM NaCl, 3 mM KCl, 1.25 mM NaH_2PO_4, 5 mM Na_2SO_4, 1.3 mM $MgSO_4$, 24 mM $NaHCO_3$, 2.4 mM $CaCl_2$, 10 mM glucose - pH 7.38). Extracellular recordings of afferent single-fibre activity were made from the cut end of the carotid sinus nerve using glass suction electrodes. The PO_2 and temperature of the superfusate were continually monitored in the superfusion line immediately before the bath by a membrane oxygen electrode (N° 733, Diamond General, Ann Arbor, MI, USA) and meter (O_2/ CO_2 Analyser, Cameron Instrument Company, Port Aransas, Texas, USA) and thermocouple (871A, Tegam Inc, Madison, Ohio, USA). The oxygen electrode was calibrated against, and PCO_2 was determined from, superfusate samples collected just distal to the carotid body and measured on a blood gas analyser (NovaStat 3, Nova Biochemical, Waltham, MA, USA). Afferent spike activity and superfusate PO_2 were monitored on an oscilloscope and thermal pen recorder and stored during each experiment on a VHS video recorder via a DC modified PCM digital unit (Sony 501ES). Action potentials were digitised on line at 20 kHz and converted to TTL pulses via a window discriminator (Neurolog NL200). Superfusate PO_2 was altered by bubbling the superfusate reservoir with differing mixtures of N_2, O_2 and CO_2 to produce slow ramp (*ca.* 100 mm Hg PO_2/min) decreases in PO_2 which were sampled throughout at 10 kHz by a computer (Macintosh IIci with National Instruments NB - MIO-16 DA and NB-MIO-8G DMA cards) running customised LabVIEW 2 (National Instruments Co, Austin, Texas, USA) software. TTL pulses were counted and binned into 10 s periods and correlated against the mean PO_2 during the 10 s period and steady state PCO_2. A single exponential with offset was fitted to the response to decreases in PO_2 using an iterative routine (ProFit, Cherwell Scientific, Oxford, UK), described by the following equation:

$$y = A \cdot e^{-(x-x_0)/t_0} + \text{const}$$

where *y* is chemoreceptor discharge frequency and *x* the PO_2; *A*, the discharge at an arbitrarily selected PO_2 equivalent to x_0; t_0, the rate constant, and *const*, the horizontal offset. Responses to increases in PCO_2 were fitted by linear regression. The protocols used for each of the three factors are explained in the appropriate result section.

Data are expressed as means ± SEM's and tested for significant differences with ANOVA (single factor unless stated otherwise), *t*-test or regression analysis as indicated, using Statview II (Abacus Concepts, Berkeley, CA, USA) software.

3. RESULTS

3.1. Temperature

Carotid bodies (n= 6) were superfused with HCO_3^--buffered saline, initially held at a constant control temperature of 37°C and then held at 35°C and 39°C in a randomly selected order. At each temperature the preparations were equilibrated at 3 levels of steady-state PCO_2 (38.5 ± 0.8, 57.6 ± 3.8, and 79.2 ± 5.7 mm Hg) in hyperoxia (PO_2 > 400 mm Hg) and chemoreceptor discharge frequency recorded. Steady state discharge was correlated with PCO_2 at each temperature and with temperature at each PCO_2. The gradients of these plots were taken as measures of the CO_2 (SCO_2, Hz/mm Hg) and thermal (S_T, Hz/°C) sensitivities, respectively. Arrhenius plots were constructed (McQueen & Eyzaguirre, 1974) and apparent activation energy (μ, kJ/mol) calculated on the assumption that the velocity of the reaction(s) was proportional to the discharge frequency. Significance was established by linear regression analysis.

At each temperature, chemoreceptor discharge increased linearly with PCO_2. Increasing temperature significantly increased SCO_2 (Fig 1A) across the temperature range studied ($SCO_2 = 0.006 \pm 0.003 \cdot °C - 0.213$; $p < 0.05$). Likewise, a significant and similar increase in S_T was observed with increasing PCO_2 ($S_T = 0.006 \pm 0.002 \cdot$ mm Hg $PCO_2 - 0.200$; $p < 0.01$). Apparent activation energies were unaffected by CO_2 ($\mu = 4.384 \pm 2.502 \cdot$ mm Hg $PCO_2 - 91.543$; $p > 0.10$).

3.2. Extracellular Potassium Ion Concentration

$[K^+]_o$ was raised in steady state steps from a control level of 3.0 to 5.3, 9.5 and 16.8 mM and chemoreceptor responses to hypoxia and hypercapnia examined. Increasing $[K^+]_o$ significantly increased baseline chemoreceptor discharge in hyperoxia (PO_2 > 400 mm Hg) in a non-linear fashion ($p < 0.001$, ANOVA, n= 10) when all levels of $[K^+]_o$ were included in the analysis but discharge was not increased significantly between 3.0 and 5.3 mM $[K^+]_o$ ($p > 0.40$, paired *t*-test). The elevation in discharge at the highest level of $[K^+]_o$ was relatively modest (*ca.* 20% maximum discharge) when compared to that obtained in severe hypoxia (*ca.* 100% maximum discharge). Chemoreceptor sensitivity to $[K^+]_o$ increased non-linearly as $[K^+]_o$ was increased but this effect was not dependent upon the PO_2 ($p > 0.90$, two factor ANOVA).

Increasing PCO_2 in hyperoxia increased chemoreceptor discharge linearly at all levels of $[K^+]_o$ (Fig 1B). Whilst discharge at any level of PCO_2 was elevated by increased levels of $[K^+]_o$, raising $[K^+]_o$ did not increase SCO_2 ($SCO_2 = 0.009) \cdot [K^+]_o + 0.24$; $p > 0.20$, regression analysis, n= 6). Similarly, increasing PCO_2 did not increase chemosensitivity to $[K^+]_o$. The lack of effect of $[K^+]_o$ upon CO_2 chemosensitivity was also observed as PO_2 was decreased to hypoxic levels ($p > 0.10$, two factor ANOVA, n=5).

3.3. Adenosine

Steady state discharge was recorded as adenosine was superfused at increasing concentrations, between 1 and 100 μM, whilst the PO_2 was maintained > 400 mm Hg and the PCO_2 held firstly at 34 mm Hg and then at 69 mm Hg. CO_2 sensitivities were derived at each level of adenosine. In a second protocol, CO_2 sensitivity was calculated again but this time at different levels of PO_2, from analysis of the chemoresponse to ramp decreases in superfusate PO_2, at steady PCO_2's of 34 mm Hg and 69 mm Hg, both before and during

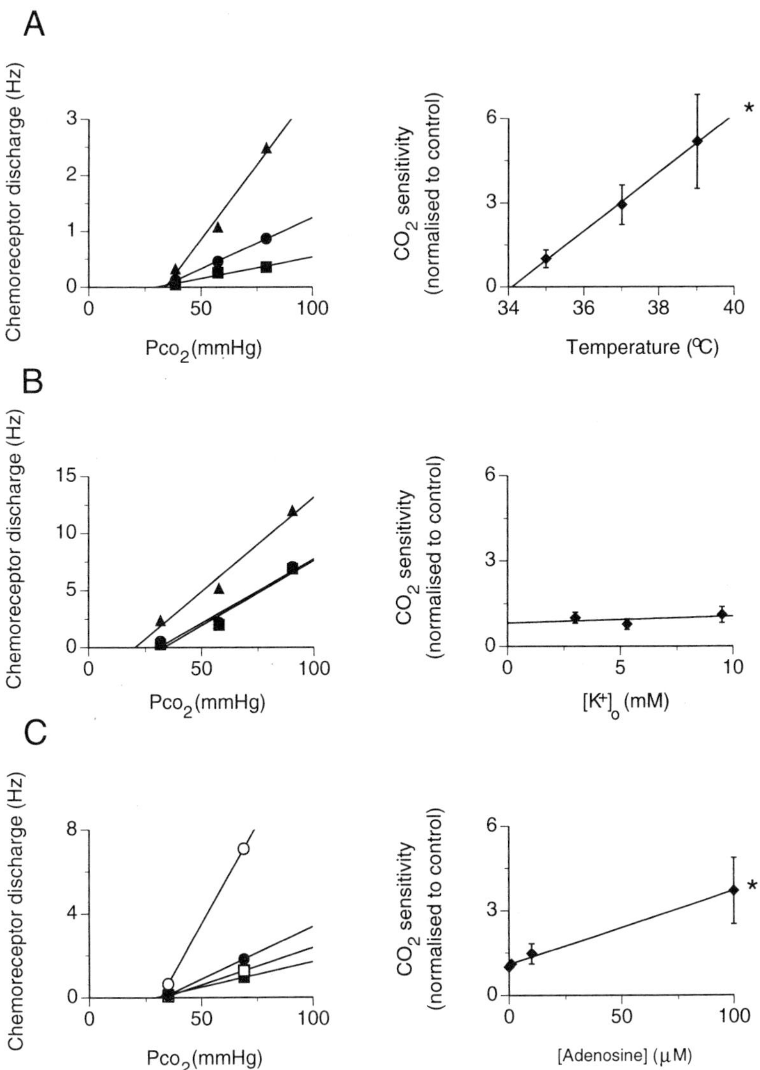

Figure 1. CO_2 sensitivity is increased by increasing temperature (**A**) and exogenous adenosine (**C**) but is unaffected by $[K^+]_o$ (**B**). **A**. Left, Steady-state single fibre chemoreceptor discharge recorded in hyperoxia ($PO_2 > 400$ mm Hg). Superfusate PCO_2 was increased from 39 to 58 and then to 79 mm Hg whilst the temperature was held at 37°C (filled circles), 35°C (filled squares) or 39°C (filled triangles). Right, Mean ± SEM (n= 6) CO_2 sensitivity (SCO_2, Hz/mm Hg) at each temperature significantly increased with increasing temperature ($p < 0.05$, regression analysis). Data was normalised to the SCO_2 at 35°C. **B**. Left, Steady-state PCO_2 stimulus response from a 3-fibre chemoreceptor preparation recorded in hyperoxia. Superfusate PCO_2 was increased from 32 to 58 and then to 90 mm Hg at each $[K^+]_o$ level; 3 mM (filled squares), 5.3 mM (filled circles) and 9.5 mM (filled triangles). Right, mean ± SEM (n = 6) SCO_2 was derived as the slope of the PCO_2 response curves at each level of $[K^+]_o$. Linear regression analysis revealed that SCO_2 was unaffected by $[K^+]_o$ ($p > 0.60$). Data was normalised to the SCO_2 at 3.0 mM $[K^+]_o$. **C**. Left, Steady-state single fibre chemoreceptor discharge recorded in hyperoxia. Superfusate PCO_2 was stepped from 34 to 69 mm Hg at each concentration of adenosine; control (0 μM) (filled squares), 1 μM (open squares), 10 μM (filled circles) and 100 μM (open circles). Right, mean ± SEM (n = 5) SCO_2 was derived as the slope of the PCO_2 response curves at each concentration of adenosine and was found to increase significantly ($p < 0.03$, ANOVA) with increasing [adenosine]. Data was normalised to the control SCO_2.

superfusate application of the adenosine receptor antagonist, aminophylline at a concentration of 100 μM.

Adenosine increased chemoreceptor discharge at both levels of PCO_2 and increased CO_2 chemosensitivity in hyperoxia (Fig 1C) from a control level of 0.04 ± 0.01 Hz·mm Hg^{-1} PCO_2 to 1.10 ± 0.09, 1.47 ± 0.36 and 3.70 ± 1.18 of control at 1, 10 and 100 μM, respectively ($p < 0.03$, ANOVA, n= 5). This effect was reversible, with a post-control CO_2 sensitivity of 0.97 ± 0.50 of the initial control ($p > 0.90$, ANOVA).

In the second protocol (n= 9), aminophylline decreased chemoreceptor discharge in hyperoxia from 0.74 ± 0.19 to 0.30 ± 0.12 ($p < 0.05$, paired *t*-test) and from 8.20 ± 2.27 to 3.72 ± 0.60% maximum discharge ($p < 0.02$, paired *t*-test) at 34 mm Hg and 69 mm Hg PCO_2, respectively. Chemoreceptor discharge (at 34 and 69 mm Hg PCO_2) was significantly ($p < 0.05$, ANOVA in all cases) elevated by decreases in PO_2 both before and during aminophylline. During control runs and in the presence of aminophylline, CO_2 sensitivity increased exponentially and significantly as PO_2 was reduced $p < 0.01$, ANOVA). Paired *t*-tests between the two groups of data at levels of PO_2 (400–100 mm Hg) revealed that the CO_2 sensitivity during aminophylline superfusion was lower than control ($p < 0.05$) except when the preparation approached the severest level of hypoxia (100 mm Hg; $p > 0.05$), where discharge was increasing sharply towards its maximum.

4. DISCUSSION

We have utilised an *in vitro* carotid body preparation to investigate factors which could affect CO_2 chemosensitivity. The use of such a preparation has advantages over the *in vivo* approach as the effect upon the carotid body can be investigated in the absence of systemic effects. The disadvantage of such an approach lies in a poor knowledge of the actual tissue level of a gas stimulus, which will of course depend upon the surface level of the stimulus, its solubility, the metabolic rate of the tissue and the depth from the surface. Whilst a significant gradient exists between the surface PO_2 and that at the core of a metabolising, *in vitro* carotid body, due to its greater solubility the maximum, steady-state PCO_2 gradient through a similar sized sphere of cells is considerably less than that of PO_2 and can be calculated to be < 4 mm Hg. The data regarding CO_2 sensitivity in hyperoxia should therefore be directly applicable to the *in vivo* situation.

Our results from the temperature experiments confirm previous findings (Gallego et al, 1979) of a relatively high apparent activation energy for the reactions underlying CO_2 transduction which is unaffected by hypercapnic acidosis. In addition, we have shown that increasing temperature increases CO_2 sensitivity and increasing PCO_2 increases thermal sensitivity. These findings may have physiological importance during exercise in the adult and in the developing O_2 and CO_2 sensitivities seen during the post-natal period, although other consequences of temperature changes *in vivo* may attenuate the effect observed *in vitro* (Zapata et al, 1994). Additionally, these findings should encourage caution when interpreting data obtained from *in vitro* studies performed at room temperature.

We have also demonstrated that an elevation of $[K^+]_o$ can increase chemoreceptor discharge in the *in vitro* carotid body in a PO_2- and PCO_2-independent manner, suggesting that the PO_2-dependent effects of $[K^+]_o$, previously reported by some authors *in vivo*, may be due to other, indirect effects of $[K^+]_o$ or hypoxia. We have also confirmed that increases in $[K^+]_o$ do not affect CO_2 chemosensitivity. Additionally, the finding that the significant depolarisation that would be induced by 16.8 mM $[K^+]_o$ did not cause as great an increase in chemoreceptor discharge as that induced by hypoxia, might suggest that hypoxia has additional pre-synaptic effects apart from depolarisation of the type I cell, although, of course, a post-synaptic effect in this preparation cannot be ruled out. Since its inception the so-called "acid hypothesis" remains one of the few which attempts to account for CO_2-O_2 interaction at the carotid body (see Hanson et al, 1981). Whilst some of its initial premises have not been proven, the broad proposals of the acid hypothesis remain intact to date. Thus, metabolic and respiratory acidosis both cause decreases in type I cell intracellular pH and subsequent elevations in intracellular $[Ca^{2+}]$ as a necessary prerequisite to transmitter release (Buckler & Vaughan-Jones, 1994a). The details of how this elevation in $[Ca^{2+}]$ is achieved differs between groups but in one proposal a decrease in pH causes inhibition of a Ca^{2+}-dependent component of the total K^+ -current, cell depolarisation and Ca^{2+} entry through L-type Ca^{2+}-channels. Interestingly, hypoxia has also been shown to be capable of inhibiting the same component of the K^+ -current (Buckler & Vaughan-Jones, 1994b; Peers, 1990) to cause depolarisation. Thus, a point of convergence between CO_2 and hypoxia may occur at the level of type I cell depolarisation. However, in the experiments reported here, the lack of effect of $[K^+]_o$ upon CO_2 sensitivity may place the site of hypoxia-CO_2 interaction more "upstream" of type I cell depolarisation.

In our third series of experiments we have shown that exogenous adenosine can act like hypoxia to increase peripheral chemoreceptor CO_2 sensitivity, which together with the aminophylline data could be taken to suggest that endogenous adenosine may be involved in the genesis of a multiplicative interaction between hypoxia and CO_2. The source of the endogenous adenosine was not established by these experiments but as a breakdown product of ATP, a link with hypoxia is apparent.

Taken together our data demonstrate that CO_2 sensitivity can be modified by external factors as well as by hypoxia. It remains to be established if any of these are involved in the postnatal maturation of chemosensitivity.

5. ACKNOWLEDGMENTS

This work was supported by the Wellcome Trust and the MRC. PK is a Lister Institute Research Fellow.

6. REFERENCES

Alcayaga J, Sanhueza Y & Zapata P (1993) Thermal dependence of chemosensory activity in the carotid body superfused *in vitro*. Brain Res 600: 103–111

Bernthal T & Weeks WF (1939) Respiratory and vasomotor effects of variations in carotid body temperature. Am J Physiol 127: 94–105

Buckler KJ & Vaughan-Jones RD (1994a) Effects of hypercapnia on membrane potential and intracellular calcium in rat carotid body type I cells. J Physiol, London 478: 157–171

Buckler KJ & Vaughan-Jones RD (1994b) Effects of hypoxia on membrane potential and intracellular calcium in rat neonatal carotid body type I cells. J Physiol, London 476: 423–428

Clement ID, Pandit JJ, Bascom DA, Dorrington KL, O'Connor DF & Robbins PA (1995) An assessment of central-peripheral ventilatory chemoreflex interaction using acid and bicarbonate infusions in humans. J Physiol, London 485: 561–570

Eden GJ & Hanson MA (1987) Effects of chronic hypoxia from birth on the ventilatory responses to acute hypoxia in the newborn rat. J Physiol, London 392: 11–19

Gallego R, Eyzaguirre C & Monti-Bloch L (1979) Thermal and osmotic responses of arterial receptors. J Neurophysiol 42: 665–680

Hanson MA & Kumar P (1994) Chemoreceptor function in the foetus and neonate. Adv Exp Med Biol 360: 99–108

Hanson MA, Nye PCG & Torrance RW (1981) The exodus of an extracellular bicarbonate theory of chemoreception and the genesis of an intracellular one. In: Belmonte C, Pallot D, Acker H & Fidone S (eds) Arterial Chemoreceptors. Leicester: Leicester Univ Press. pp 403–416

Jarisch A, Landgren S, Neil E & Zotterman Y (1952) Impulse activity in the carotid sinus nerve following intra-carotid injection of potassium chloride, veratrine, sodium citrate, adenosinetriphosphate and alpha dinitrophenol. Acta Physiol Scand 25: 195–211

Kholwadwala D & Donnelly DF (1992) Maturation of carotid chemoreceptor sensitivity to hypoxia: *in vitro* studies in the newborn rat. J Physiol, London 453: 461–473

Lahiri S & Delaney RG (1975) Stimulus interaction in the responses of carotid body chemoreceptor single afferent fibres. Respir Physiol 24: 249–266

Landauer RC, Pepper DR & Kumar P (1995) Effect of chronic hypoxaemia from birth upon chemosensitivity in the adult rat carotid body *in vitro*. J Physiol, London 485: 543–550

Linton RAF & Band DM (1990) Potassium and breathing. News Physiol Sci 5: 104–107

McQueen DS & Eyzaguirre C (1974) Effects of temperature on carotid chemoreceptor and baroreceptor activity. J Neurophysiol 37: 1287–1296

McQueen DS & Ribeiro JA (1981) Effect of adenosine on carotid chemoreceptor activity in the cat. Br J Pharmacol 74: 129–136

Moss IR, Runold M, Dahlin I, Fredholm BB, Nyberg F & Lagercrantz H (1987) Respiratory and neuroendocrine responses of piglets to hypoxia during postnatal development. Acta Physiol Scand 131: 533–541

Neilson M & Smith H (1952) Studies on the regulation of respiration in acute hypoxia. Acta Physiol Scand 24: 293–313

Paterson DJ (1992) Potassium and ventilation in exercise. J Appl Physiol 72: 811–820

Peers C (1990) Hypoxic suppression of K^+-channels in type I carotid body cells: Selective effect on the Ca^{2+}-activated K^+-current. Neurosci Lett 119: 253–256

Pepper DR, Landauer RC & Kumar P (1995) Postnatal development of CO_2-O_2 interaction in the rat carotid body *in vitro*. J Physiol, London 485: 531–541

Runold M, Cherniack NS & Prabhakar NR (1990) Effect of adenosine on isolated and superfused cat carotid-body activity. Neurosci Lett 113: 111–114

Zapata P, Larraín C, Iturriaga R & Alcayaga J (1994) The carotid bodies as thermosensors: Experiments *in vitro* and *in situ*, and importance for ventilatory regulation. Adv Exp Med Biol 360: 253–255

30

INTRACELLULAR ACIDOSIS POTENTIATES CAROTID CHEMORECEPTOR RESPONSES TO HYPOXIA IN THE ABSENCE OF CO_2-HCO_3^-

R. Iturriaga

Laboratory of Neurobiology
Catholic University of Chile
Santiago, Chile

1. EFFECTS OF CO_2-HCO_3^- ON CHEMOSENSORY RESPONSE TO HYPOXIA

Experiments *in vitro* showed that the frequency of carotid chemosensory discharges (f_x) increases in response to appropriate physiological and pharmacological stimuli in the nominal absence of CO_2-HCO_3^- (Eyzaguirre & Lewin 1961; Iturriaga & Lahiri, 1991). In studies with isolated glomus cells bathed with media without CO_2-HCO_3^-, hypoxia diminished the membrane K^+ conductance (López et al, 1989; Peers & Green 1991) and increased intracellular free [Ca^{2+}] (Biscoe & Duchen, 1988). Thus, the presence of CO_2-HCO_{3-} in the *in vitro* medium is not required for the generation of the hypoxic chemosensory response. Nevertheless, the presence of CO_2-HCO_3^- in the *in vitro* medium sped up the onset and the rate of rise of the cat chemosensory responses to hypoxia, flow interruption and NaCN, as compared with the responses obtained when the CBs were perfused with medium buffered at the same pH 7.40 (Iturriaga & Lahiri, 1991; Shirahata & Fitzgerald, 1993).

It is well known that f_x shows a strong non-linear interaction between hypoxic and CO_2-H^+ stimuli (Lahiri & DeLaney, 1975). A possible explanation for this interaction was advanced by Torrance and colleagues (see Hanson et al, 1981), who proposed that a common mechanism of intracellular acidosis would mediate the transduction of both O_2 and CO_2-H^+ stimuli in the carotid body (CB). Recent studies have found that high PCO_2 and [H^+] consistently reduced the intracellular pH (pH_i) in isolated glomus cells (Buckler et al, 1991; He et al, 1991; Mokashi et al, 1995; Sato, 1994; Wilding et al, 1992) and in the whole CB (Iturriaga et al, 1992). However, the same studies found that hypoxia did not consistently reduce the pH_i in isolated glomus cells (He et al, 1991; Mokashi et al, 1995;

Wilding et al, 1992) nor in the whole CB (Iturriaga et al, 1992). Thus, transduction of O_2 is not triggered by intracellular acidosis, but these results are not against the idea that the rate of rise of the chemosensory response to hypoxia may depend on the CO_2-HCO_3^--dependent mechanisms which regulate the pH_i in the chemoreceptor cells.

The effects of CO_2-HCO_3^- on hypoxic chemoreception seem to be mediated by a reduction in the glomus cell pH_i due to intracellular CO_2 hydration catalyzed by the enzyme carbonic anhydrase (Black et al, 1971; Hanson et al, 1981; Iturriaga et al, 1993). In fact, permeable inhibitors of carbonic anhydrase that produced in isolated glomus cells alkalinization and slowed the pH_i fall induced by high PCO_2 (Buckler et al, 1991) also delayed the cat chemosensory responses to hypercapnia and hypoxia *in situ* (Black et al, 1971) and *in vitro* (Iturriaga et al, 1993). These observations suggest that the catalyzed production of H^+ in the presence of CO_2-HCO_3^- maintains a relative acid pH_i (6.9 to 7.2) inside the glomus cell (Buckler et al, 1991; He et al, 1991; Mokashi et al, 1995; Wilding et al, 1992). However, a rise in intracellular PCO_2 may reduce the glomus cell pH_i not only because of CO_2 hydration, but also because HCO_3^- extrusion through the Cl^--HCO_3^- exchangers and anion channels present in glomus cells (Buckler et al, 1991). In fact, blockade of the Cl^--HCO_3^- exchanger by eliminating external Cl^- made rat glomus cells alkaline in the presence of CO_2-HCO_3^- (Buckler et al, 1991) and slowed the cat chemosensory response to hypoxia (Lahiri & Iturriaga, 1993).

2. IS CO_2-HCO_3^- ESSENTIAL FOR HYPOXIC CHEMORECEPTION?

Shirahata and Fitzgerald (1993) proposed that CO_2-HCO_3^- is essential for O_2 chemoreception because they did not observe any effect of sodium butyrate (5–20 mM) on basal f_x or any significant response to hypoxia in the nominal absence of CO_2-HCO_3^- from the perfusate of their *in situ* cat CB preparation. However, several reports have shown that hypoxia does stimulate carotid chemoreceptor discharge *in vitro* in the nominal absence of CO_2-HCO_3^- (see González et al, 1994, for review).

A major difference between experiments performed in the *in vitro* perfused-superfused and superfused cat CB preparations and the experiments performed in the perfused *in situ* preparation is the duration of the hypoxic stimulation. In the *in vitro* experiments, the hypoxic challenges -made with the same saline solutions- were maintained for 5 or more min. On the contrary, in the perfused *in situ* experiments, the CBs perfused with its own arterial blood were stimulated with saline solutions for just 90 s (Shirahata & Fitzgerald, 1993). Thus, a brief hypoxic stimulus without CO_2-HCO_3^- could not produce a significant chemosensory response giving the impression that CO_2-HCO_3^- is essential for hypoxic chemoreception.

Certainly, CO_2-HCO_3^- plays an important function speeding up the chemosensory response to hypoxia. Without CO_2-HCO_3^- the rate of rise of responses to hypoxia is greatly attenuated (Iturriaga & Lahiri, 1991) due to an alkaline pH_i, as reported in isolated glomus cells (Buckler et al 1991; He et al, 1991; Mokashi et al, 1995; Wilding et al, 1992). This alkaline pH_i caused by the absence of CO_2-HCO_3^- has been attributed to the blockade of the glomus cell Cl^--HCO_3^- exchanger which is an acid loader (Buckler et el, 1991). Thus, the available data suggest that the rate of rise of the chemosensory response to hypoxia may depend on the glomus cell pH_i setting, but not on the presence of exogenous CO_2-HCO_3^- itself.

3. TESTING THE EFFECTS OF AN INTRACELLULAR ACIDOSIS ON THE CHEMOSENSORY RESPONSES TO HYPOXIA IN THE ABSENCE OF CO_2-HCO_3^-

If CO_2-HCO_3^- is not essential for carotid hypoxic chemoreception, but the response depends on a relative acid pH_i in the glomus cells, we would expect that a permeable weak acid such as acetic acid, which produced predictable acidosis in isolated glomus cells and in the whole CB (Iturriaga et al, 1992; Sato, 1994), should raise the basal f_x and enhance the chemosensory response to hypoxia in the absence of CO_2-HCO_3^- at constant pH 7.40.

To test the above hypothesis, I used an *in vitro* preparation of the cat CB. Briefly, carotid bifurcations including the CBs were excised from sodium pentobarbitone anesthetized cats and perfused-superfused *in vitro* as previously described (Iturriaga & Lahiri, 1991). The CBs were perfused with a modified Tyrode's solution (36.5 ± 0.5°C) without CO_2-HCO_3^-, buffered with HEPES (5 mM) at pH 7.40, equilibrated at PO_2 of 120 Torr and simultaneously superfused with the same Tyrode equilibrated at $PO_2 < 20$ Torr. The f_x was recorded from the whole carotid sinus nerve. The CBs were perfused and superfused first with Tyrode without acetate for about 45 min, and then with Tyrode containing 30 mM sodium acetate (replacing the same amount of sodium glutamate).

The effect of acetate on the chemosensory response to hypoxia is shown in Figure 1. In the absence of acetate, hypoxia slowly increased f_x to a steady level in about 6 min (Fig. 1A). When the CB was perfused and superfused with Tyrode containing 30 mM sodium acetate (pH 7.40), the basal f_x increased and the response to the same hypoxic stimulus was strikingly faster (Fig. 1B). During perfusion with acetate, the half-time of the hypoxic response in 5 CBs was reduced in 156.2 ± 57 s ($p < 0.05$) and the maxf_x increased by a 78.6% (range: 12 to 125%).

In the absence of acetate, the interruption of the perfusate flow increased f_x after a delay of about 20 s (Fig 2A). The presence of acetate markedly sped up the onset and the rate of rise of the chemosensory response to perfusate stop flow (Fig 2B). The half-time required to reach the maximum f_x during perfusion with acetate decreased in 29.6 ± 5.3 s ($p < 0.05$; $n = 5$). The maxf_x attained during flow interruptions increased by 27.3% (range: 9.7 to 65%).

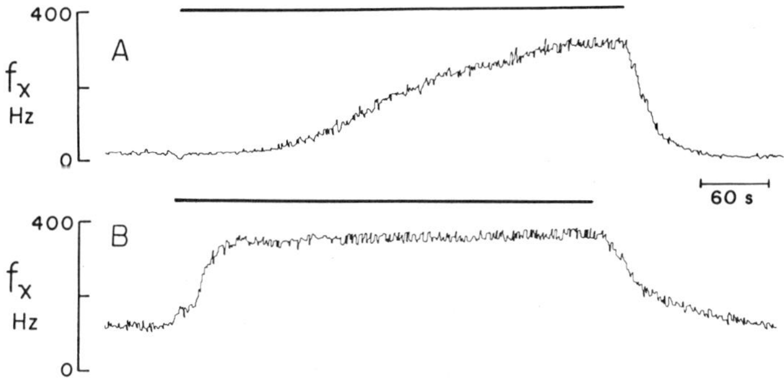

Figure 1. Effects of acetate on the chemosensory response to hypoxia (PO_2 from 125 Torr to 25 Torr) during perfusion with Tyrode free of CO_2-HCO_3^- at pH 7.40. **A**, Tyrode without acetate. **B**, Tyrode with 30 mM sodium acetate. Bars indicate duration of hypoxic perfusion.

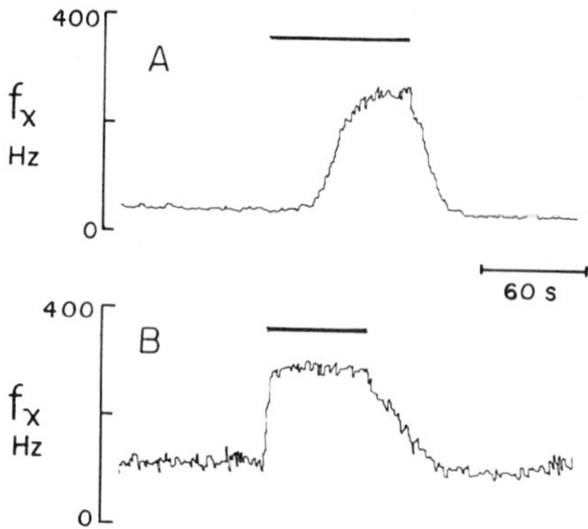

Figure 2. Effects of acetate on the chemosensory response to flow interruption during perfusion with Tyrode (PO_2 = 125 Torr) free of CO_2-HCO_3^- at pH 7.40. **A**, Tyrode without acetate. **B**, Tyrode with 30 mM sodium acetate. Bars indicate duration of flow interruption.

Figure 3 shows the effect of acetate on the chemosensory responses to several doses of NaCN (0.01–10 μg). In the absence of acetate, only the larger dose of NaCN (10 μg) increased f_x (Fig 3A). In the presence of acetate, the chemosensory response to the larger doses of NaCN was augmented (Fig 3B).

4. ACETATE MIMICS THE EFFECTS OF CO_2-HCO_3^- ON HYPOXIC CHEMORECEPTION

Present results show that the presence of acetate (30 mM) in the perfusate-superfusate medium -without CO_2-HCO_3^- and buffered with HEPES at pH 7.40- markedly increased basal f_x and the rate of rise of the chemosensory responses to hypoxia and stop flow. Acetate also increased the amplitude of the response to NaCN and to a less extent the responses to stop flow and hypoxia. Clearly, acetate mimics the enhancing effects of CO_2-HCO_3^- on the chemosensory responses to hypoxia, stop flow and NaCN (Iturriaga & Lahiri, 1993). Acetic acid, like CO_2, rapidly diffused into the cells and reduced the pH_i in isolated glomus cells and in the whole cat CB (Iturriaga et al, 1992; Sato, 1994).

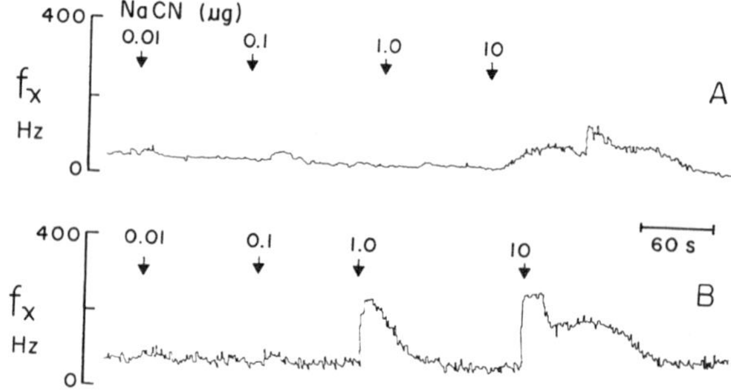

Figure 3. Effects of acetate on carotid chemosensory response to NaCN during perfusion with Tyrode (PO_2 = 125 Torr) free of CO_2-HCO_3^- at pH 7.40. **A**, Tyrode without acetate. **B**, Tyrode containing 30 mM sodium acetate. Arrows indicate NaCN injections.

5. PHYSIOLOGICAL ROLE OF CO_2-HCO_3^- ON CAROTID CHEMORECEPTION

The above results extend the observations of Shirahata & Fitzgerald (1993), who reported that hypoxic perfused medium without CO_2-HCO_3^- but containing sodium butyrate (5–20 mM) increased the cat f_x as much as during hypoxic perfusion with CO_2-HCO_3^-. Present results show that perfusion with Tyrode containing acetate not only potentiated the response to hypoxia, stop flow and NaCN but also increased basal f_x suggesting that weak acids raise basal f_x and speed up the hypoxic response by a common mechanism of lowering the CB pH_i. Thus, CO_2-HCO_3^- seems not to be so critical for O_2 chemoreception. Perhaps it is more critical a relative elevated $[H^+]_i$ within the glomus cells. However, CO_2-HCO_3^--H^+ is the major buffer system in the whole animal. Clearly, *in situ* CO_2-HCO_3^- plays a prominent physiological function by speeding up the hypoxic chemoreception in the CB. Moreover, in the presence of CO_2-HCO_3^-, carbonic anhydrase performs a facilitatory role in the physiological chemosensory responses to CO_2 and O_2 (Hanson et al, 1981, Iturriaga et al, 1993).

6. POSSIBLE MECHANISMS FOR THE POTENTIATION OF CHEMOSENSORY RESPONSES TO HYPOXIA INDUCED BY INTRACELLULAR ACIDIFICATION IN THE ABSENCE OF CO_2-HCO_3^-

According to the membrane model of chemoreception, O_2 transduction is initiated by a depolarization of glomus cells due to the closing of PO_2-dependent K^+ channels and the subsequent opening of voltage-gated Ca^{2+} channels leading to a rise in $[Ca^{2+}]_i$ (See González et al, 1994, for review). Intracellular acidosis may converge on the O_2 sensing pathway; indeed glomus cell acidosis produced by acetate, propionate or CO_2 at constant external pH of 7.40 reduced the PO_2-dependent K^+ current (Peers & Green, 1991; Stea et al, 1991), depolarized the glomus cells and augmented $[Ca^{2+}]_i$ (Buckler & Vaughan-Jones, 1993; Sato, 1994). Thus, it is likely that intracellular acidosis would enhance the rate of rise of $[Ca^{2+}]_i$ induced by hypoxia. A $[Ca^{2+}]_i$ potentiation is expected to enhance the release of an excitatory transmitter from the glomus cells and then enhance the chemosensory discharges. Accordingly, weak acid such as acetate or CO_2 would enhance the release of the excitatory transmitter from the glomus cells during hypoxia.

Present results also show that acetate sped up the rate of rise of the response to flow interruption. In this *in vitro* CB preparation, during stop flow f_x increased as PO_2 declined to 0 Torr due to O_2 consumption by the CB cells. Thus, we can not preclude the possibility that acetate could increase the rate of O_2 disappearance from the CB by augmenting the O_2 consumption of the CB cell.

7. CONCLUSIONS

In summary, present results show that O_2 chemoreception occurs in the nominal absence of CO_2-HCO_3^- in the extracellular medium but the presence of acetate in the perfused and superfused medium potentiated the CB chemosensory response to hypoxia, flow interruption and NaCN at pH of 7.40. These results strongly suggest that intracellular acidosis contributes to potentiate the hypoxic response.

8. ACKNOWLEDGMENTS

Work supported by grant FONDECYT 195–0997, Chile.

Thanks are due to Mrs Carolina Larraín for her valuable help during the experiments, as well as in the preparation of the illustrations.

9. REFERENCES

Biscoe TJ & Duchen MR (1988) Electrophysiological responses of dissociated type I cells of the rabbit carotid body to cyanide. J Physiol, London 405: 210–232

Black AMS, McCloskey DI & Torrance RW (1971) The response of carotid body chemoreceptors in the cat to sudden changes of hypercapnic and hypoxic stimuli. Respir Physiol 13: 36–49

Buckler KJ & Vaughan-Jones RD (1993) Effects of acidic stimuli on intracellular calcium in isolated type I cells of the neonatal rat carotid body. Pflügers Arch 425: 22–27

Buckler KJ, Vaughan-Jones RD, Peers C & Nye PCG (1991) Intracellular pH and its regulation in the isolated type I carotid body cells of the neonatal rat. J Physiol, London 436: 107–129

Eyzaguirre C & Lewin J (1961) Effects of different oxygen tension of the carotid body *in vitro*. J Physiol, London 159: 238–250

González C, Almaraz L, Obeso A & Rigual R (1994) Carotid body chemoreceptors: From natural stimuli to sensory discharges. Physiol Rev 74: 829–898

Hanson MA, Nye PCG & Torrance RW (1981) The exodus of an extracellular bicarbonate theory of chemoreception and the genesis of an intercellular one. In: Belmonte C, Pallot C, Acker H & Fidone S (eds) Arterial Chemoreceptors. Leicester: Leicester University Press. pp 403–416

He S-F, Wei J-Y & Eyzaguirre C (1991) Effects of relative hypoxia and hypercapnia on intracellular pH and membrane potential of cultured carotid body glomus cells. Brain Res 556: 333–338

Iturriaga R & Lahiri S (1991) Carotid body chemoreception in the absence and presence of CO_2-HCO_3^-. Brain Res 568: 253–260

Iturriaga R, Rumsey WL, Lahiri S, Spergel D & Wilson DF (1992) Intracellular pH and O_2 chemoreception in the cat carotid body *in vitro*. J Appl Physiol 72: 2259–2266

Iturriaga R, Mokashi A & Lahiri S (1993) Dynamics of the carotid body responses *in vitro* in the presence of CO_2-HCO_3^-: Role of carbonic anhydrase. J Appl Physiol 75: 1587–1594

Lahiri S & DeLaney RG (1975) Stimulus interaction in the responses of carotid body chemoreceptors single fibers. Respir Physiol 24: 249–266

Lahiri S & Iturriaga R (1993) Role of ion exchangers in the carotid body chemotransduction. Adv Exp Med Biol 337: 177–182

López-López J, González C, Ureña J & López-Barneo J (1989) Low PO_2 selectively inhibits K channel activity in chemoreceptor cells of the mammalian carotid body. J Gen Physiol 93: 1001–1015

Mokashi A, Ray D, Botre F, Katayama M, Osani S & Lahiri S (1995) Effect of hypoxia on intracellular pH of the glomus cell cultured from cat and rat carotid bodies. J Appl Physiol 78: 1875–1881

Peers C & Green FK (1991) Inhibition of Ca^{2+}-activated K^+ current by intracellular acidosis in isolated type I cells of the neonatal rat carotid body. J Physiol, London 437: 589–602

Sato M (1994) Effects of CO_2, acetate and lowering extracellular pH on Ca^{2+} and pH on cultured glomus cells of the newborn rabbit carotid body. Neurosci Lett 173: 159–162

Shirahata M & Fitzgerald RS (1993) Role of carbon dioxide for hypoxic chemotransduction of the cat carotid body. Adv Exp Biol Med 337: 213–219

Stea A, Alexander SA & Nurse CA (1991) Effect of pH_i and pH_e on membrane currents recorded with perforated-patch method from cultured chemoreceptors of the rat carotid body. Brain Res 567: 83–90

Wilding TJ, Cheng B & Roos A (1992) pH regulation in adult rat carotid body glomus cells. Importance of extracellular pH, sodium and potassium. J Gen Physiol 100: 593–608

31

CENTRAL pH CHEMOSENSITIVITY IN THE NEWBORN OPOSSUM *MONODELPHIS DOMESTICA*

Jaime Eugenín[1,2]

[1] Facultad de Ciencias Médicas
Universidad de Santiago de Chile
Santiago 2, Chile
[2] Abteilung Pharmakologie
Biozentrum der Universität Basel
Basel, CH 4056, Switzerland

1. INTRODUCTION

Central and peripheral chemoreceptors provide tonic drive to the neuronal network that generates respiratory rhythm. The peripheral chemoreceptor organs (carotid and aortic bodies) are well defined, whereas the identity of the structures in charge of mammalian central chemoreception are still uncertain (Coates et al, 1993).

A recent strategy to study central chemoreception and its effects on respiration has been the development of *in vitro* preparations. In these *in vitro* preparations fictive respiration can be recorded from C3-C5 ventral roots of isolated mammalian CNS (Suzue, 1984). Among these *in vitro* preparations, only the isolated CNS of the newborn opossum *Monodelphis domestica* presents respiratory frequency over 40 per min at room temperature, which is closer to the respiratory rate observed in intact pups. This marsupial preparation shows remarkable properties of survival, growth and development (Nicholls et al, 1990; Stewart et al, 1991; Woodward et al, 1993; Zou et al, 1991), in special when compared to a similar preparation from neonatal rat for which only hours of survival have been reported (Suzue, 1984).

Fictive respiration in newborn opossum *in vitro* increases after acidification of the superfusion medium (Zou, 1994). Superfusion of the brain stem, but not the spinal cord, with low pH solutions increased both amplitude and frequency of fictive respiration, while high pH solutions had the opposite effect (Eugenín, 1994). Here, a preliminary study about the localization of pH-sensitive areas on the surface of the isolated CNS in seven newborn opossums is reported.

Frontiers in Arterial Chemoreception, edited by Zapata *et al.*
Plenum Press, New York, 1996

2. METHODS

Newborn *Monodelphis domestica* (4–14 days old) were anaesthetized with methoxyflurane (Metofane, Pitman-Moore). The CNS was removed and transferred to a recording chamber 0.5 ml in volume. The brain stem was superfused separately from the spinal cord using a thin film partition sealed with vaseline at the level of C1-C2. Both parts were superfused at continuous flows of 0.6 to 0.8 ml·min^{-1} with BME (Basal Medium Eagle's, Gibco) supplemented with D-glucose to a final concentration of 30 mM and equilibrated with O_2:CO_2 (95%:5%, pH 7.37–7.40) at room temperature (22–25°C).

Spontaneous activity from C3-C5 ventral roots was recorded by means of glass suction microelectrodes. Single respiratory-related units from the lower brain stem were recorded extracellularly by means of a 2–4 MΩ glass microelectrode filled with 1 M NaCl and driven by a micromanipulator. Electrical signals were amplified by low-noise differential amplifiers and bandpass filtered at 3–3000 Hz. The multiunitary activity and its integration obtained by full-wave rectification (time constant, 50–100 ms) were displayed on an oscilloscope and a chart recorder. The raw signal was stored on a videotape at a sampling frequency of DC-9 kHz or DC-18 kHz.

Topical application of BME at pH 6.5 (supplemented with 5 mM HEPES and titrated with HCl) or BME at pH 7.4 was done through a glass pipette of 100 μm of outer diameter. Inside the pipette a triple barrel electrode was placed. One barrel contained BME control (pH 7.4) and another a test solution. The third barrel was used for internal drain, to renew medium inside the pipette and to avoid leakage specially when the glass pipette was advanced towards the nervous tissue. Once the tip touched the surface of the CNS, a gentle suction was generated inside the pipette to produce a seal between the glass and the tissue. Test medium was released from one barrel to the pipette interior and the internal drain was stopped. Leaking and diffusion of test medium into nearby tissue was minimized by increasing the rate of flow to 1.2–1.5 ml·min^{-1} in each chamber and by adding an external drain for suction of medium through a glass pipette placed about 200 μm from the tip of the stimulating pipette.

Ventral root activity was regular and stable for at least 3–5 min before each topical application of test solutions.

3. RESULTS

Basal fictive respiration recorded from C3-C5 ventral roots of newborn opossums consisted of a regular, short duration (about 300 ms), and high frequency rhythm (44 ± 6 min^{-1}, mean ± SEM; n= 10) of bursts of action potentials (Fig 1).

Ventral and dorsal surfaces of the isolated CNS of seven newborn opossums were explored systematically by touching the nervous tissue with the tip of a glass micropipette containing BME, pH 6.5. Only topical application of acid confined to the ventral medulla increased respiratory activity. Respiratory frequency increased by 25 to 100% and the amplitude of integrated activity by 20 to 200% (Fig 2).

The most sensitive area, that is, that area on which stimuli produced more often and bigger responses, corresponded to a zone located medial to the hypoglossal roots.

4. DISCUSSION

The results show that the ventral medulla of newborn opossum has chemosensory areas able to drive the respiratory rhythm. Chemosensory areas were found to be distrib-

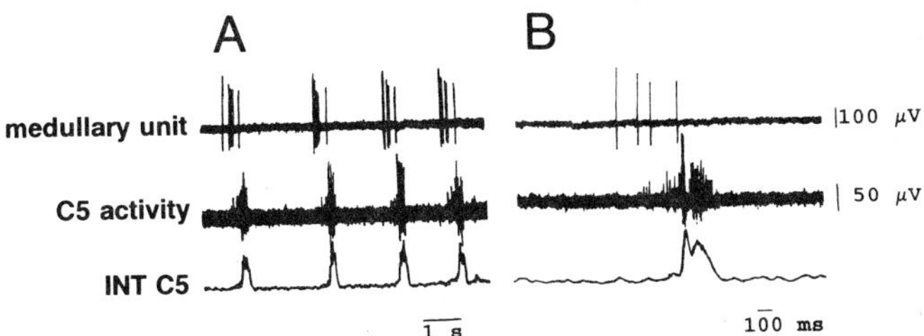

Figure 1. Fictive respiration recorded from C5 ventral roots in the isolated CNS preparation of 9 day old opossum (C5). Integration of C5 activity using a full-wave rectifier (INT C5). Upper trace, an extracellular recording of an pre-inspiratory medullary unit. In B, a fast sweep of respiratory activity is shown.

uted on the ventral medulla following a similar topography to those described in other mammals (Bruce & Cherniack, 1987; Loeschcke, 1982; Mitchell et al, 1963; Monteau et al, 1990); they extended from zones analogous to the classical area of Mitchell (rostral) to the classical area of Loeschcke (caudal).

To what extent test solutions could diffuse into nearby tissue and thus, to affect structures located far away from the site of application could not be determined. However,

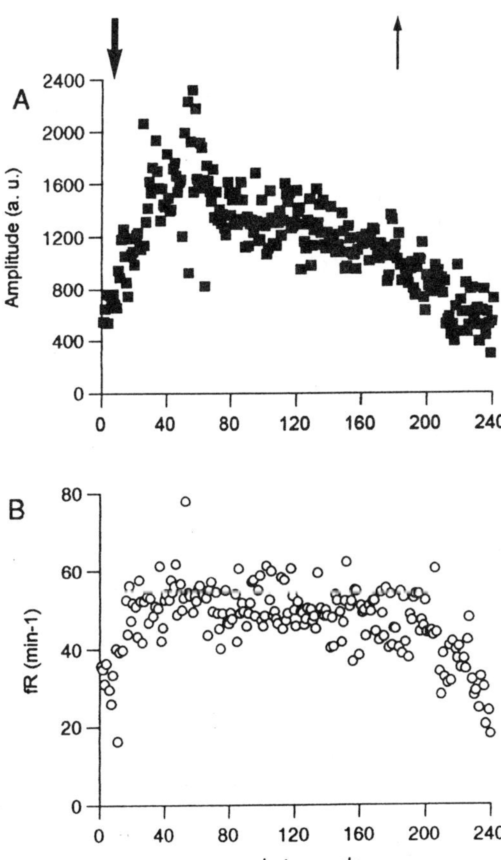

Figure 2. Local application of BME, pH 6.5 to ventral medulla in a 5 day old opossum. **A**, amplitude of the integrated activity from C5 ventral root (time constant, 100 ms) expressed in arbitrary units. **B**, instantaneous respiratory frequency. Each point represents a cycle. Big and thin arrows indicate beginning and ending of topical application of BME, pH 6.5, respectively.

the fact that stimulation of very precise spots of the surface of ventral medulla was required to elicit a respiratory response makes unlikely such possibility. For example, stimuli applied on dorsal medulla, pons or cervical spinal cord were unsuccessful to evoke any respiratory responses.

Since fictive respiration of isolated CNS of newborn opossum maintains most of its *in situ* properties, this *in vitro* preparation could prove to be useful for detailed anatomical and electrophysiological study of the structures responsible for central chemoreception.

5. ACKNOWLEDGMENTS

I am particularly grateful to Dr JG Nicholls for his support, encouragement and advice to perform this work. Thanks are also due to Eric Hardman, Marlies Thalmer and Urs Berglas for maintaining the colony of *Monodelphis*. I thank to Dr WB Adams for his help with the electronics and Paul Bättig for photography. This work was supported by the Swiss Nationalfonds Grant (# 313626292) to JG Nicholls.

The author of this paper received the Data Foundation Award at the end of the XIIIth International Symposium on Arterial Chemoreceptors, Santiago, Chile, March 1996.

6. REFERENCES

Bruce EN & Cherniack NS (1987) Central chemoreceptors. J Appl Physiol 62: 389–402

Coates EL, Li A & Nattie EE (1993) Widespread sites of brain stem ventilatory chemoreceptors. J Appl Physiol 75: 5–14

Eugenín J (1994) pH sensitivity and cholinergic modulation of fictive respiration of the newborn opossum (*Monodelphis domestica*) *in vitro*. Soc Neurosci Abstr 20: 544

Loeschcke HH (1982) Central chemosensitivity and the reaction theory. J Physiol, London 332: 1–24

Mitchell RA, Loeschcke HH, Massion WH & Severinghaus JW (1963) Respiratory responses mediated through superficial chemosensitive areas on the medulla. J Appl Physiol 18: 523–533

Monteau R, Morin D & Hilaire G (1990) Acetylcholine and central chemosensitivity: *in vitro* study in the newborn rat. Respir Physiol 81: 241–254

Nicholls JG, Stewart RR, Erulkar SD & Saunders NR (1990) Reflexes, fictive respiration and cell division in the brain and spinal cord of the newborn opossum, *Monodelphis domestica*, isolated and maintained *in vitro*. J Exp Biol 152: 1–15

Stewart RR, Zou DJ, Treherne JM, Mollgard K, Saunders NR & Nicholls JG (1991) The intact central nervous system of the newborn opossum in long-term culture: fine structure and GABA-mediated inhibition of electrical activity. J Exp Biol 161: 25–41

Suzue T (1984) Respiratory rhythm generation in the *in vitro* brain stem-spinal cord preparation of the neonatal rat. J Physiol, London 354: 173–183

Woodward SK, Treherne JM, Knott GW, Fernandez J, Varga ZM & Nicholls JG (1993) Development of connections by axons growing through injured spinal cord of neonatal opossum in culture. J Exp Biol 176: 77–88

Zou DJ (1994) Respiratory rhythm in the isolated central nervous system of newborn opossum. J Exp Biol 197: 201–13

Zou DJ, Treherne JM, Stewart RR, Saunders NR & Nicholls JG (1991) Regulation of GABAB receptors by histamine and neuronal activity in the isolated spinal cord of neonatal opossum in culture. Proc R Soc Lond Biol 246: 77–82

SIMULTANEOUS MEASUREMENTS OF CYTOSOLIC CALCIUM ION AND pH IN CULTURED SUPERIOR CERVICAL GANGLION CELLS OF RAT

K. Yoshizaki,[1] K. Ohtomo,[1] K. Fukuhara,[1] T. Kawaguchi,[1] and J. Kawaguchi[2]

[1] Akita University
College of Allied Medical Science
Akita 010, Japan
[2] Department of Pathology
Iwate Medical University
Morioka 020, Japan

1. INTRODUCTION

The postganglionic nerves from the superior cervical ganglion (SCG) innervate the carotid body, controlling the blood supply to this organ (Fidone & Gonzalez, 1986; Pallot, 1987; Gomez-Niño et al, 1990; McDonald, 1981; Verna et al 1984). The sympathetic postganglionic nerves receive cholinergic synapses from the cervical preganglionic nerves. The rich blood supply to the carotid body chemoreceptors allows them to sense changes in blood concentrations of oxygen, carbon dioxide and protons. Protons are locally produced in this organ when ATPs are consumed for chemotransduction, and cytosolic calcium ion ($[Ca^{2+}]_i$) is one of the second messengers important for chemotransduction. Therefore, it is interesting to investigate the relationship between changes in $[Ca^{2+}]_i$ and intracellular pH (pH_i) in response to conditions affecting not only the carotid body, but also the SCG neurons.

Changes of $[Ca^{2+}]_i$ and pH_i come in direct relation with each other. Sato (1994) reported the effects of CO_2, acetate and lowering extracellular pH on $[Ca^{2+}]_i$ and pH_i in cultured glomus cells of the newborn rabbit carotid body, although simultaneous measurement of $[Ca^{2+}]_i$ and pH_i were not made.

In this study, we measured simultaneously both the changes in $[Ca^{2+}]_i$ and in pH_i of cultured SCG cells of rat in response to acetylcholine (Ach), transmitter released by preganglionic nerves, to ammonium chloride (NH_4Cl), affecting the pH environment of cells, and to a high concentration of potassium (HK), affecting the electrical activity of ganglionic neurons. The relationship between changes in $[Ca^{2+}]_i$ and in pH_i was examined and the meaning of differences in the time course of such changes is discussed.

Frontiers in Arterial Chemoreception, edited by Zapata *et al.*
Plenum Press, New York, 1996

2. METHODS

Cultures were made by usual methods (Yoshizaki et al, 1995). Briefly, Wistar rats were anesthetized with urethane (4 ml of 25% urethane soln/kg weight) given intraperitoneally. The SCGs were isolated, treated with collagenase (3 mg/ml) for 15 to 30 min at 37°C, washed several times with culture medium and fragmented mechanically. Clusters consisting of several cells were plated on culture dishes with coverglass bottom and were cultured in a 5% CO_2 incubator at 37°C for up to 5 days. The culture medium was minimum essential medium (MEM; Gibco) supplemented with 10% fetal bovine serum (Gibco), 6.0 $mg{\cdot}ml^{-1}$ glucose, 50 $U{\cdot}ml^{-1}$ penicillin G (Sigma), 50 $\mu g{\cdot}ml^{-1}$ streptomycin (Sigma), 0.1 $\mu g{\cdot}ml^{-1}$ nerve growth factor (Sigma) and 2.2 $g{\cdot}l^{-1}$ $NaHCO_3$ (pH 6.8–7.2).

Cultured cells were loaded simultaneously with dual dyes, Fura-2/AM (10 μM) and BCECF/AM (1 μM) in a modified Krebs solution (NS (mM): NaCl 111; sodium glutamate 14,7; $NaHCO_3$ 25.6; KCl 4,7; $CaCl_2$ 2.2; $MgCl_2$ 1.1; glucose 5.6; HEPES 5; pH 7.4 at 37°C) in a 5% CO_2 incubator at 37°C for 1 to 2 h. Primary culture clusters of SCG cells, allowed to survive from < 5 up to 12 weeks, were used for all measurements of this study.

Simultaneous measurements of $[Ca^{2+}]_i$ and pH_i from cells loaded with dual dyes were made at room temperature using a microscopic fluorometer (Ratio Vision Real Time Digital Fluorescence Analyzer, Carl Zeiss/Attofluor) with an inverted microscope and an ICCD camera connected to a personal computer, for analysis and recording. The fluorescence dyes were excited from a mercury lamp alternatively at wavelengths of 334 and 380 for Fura-2 and also of 460 and 488 nm for BCECF, selected with band pass filters. Fluorescence emissions from single cultured cells were recorded at a wavelength of 520 nm. Alternate fluorescences of Fura-2 and BCECF were measured at intervals of 500 ms. The results of single measurement of $[Ca^{2+}]_i$ changes induced by stimulants, tested in cells loaded with only Fura-2, were similar to those in cells loaded simultaneously with dual dyes. The same was checked for BCECF measurements. That Fura-2 emission is independent from pH and that BCECF emission is independent from $[Ca^{2+}]_i$ have been previously reported (Shibuya et al, 1991). The ratios of fluorescence intensities were obtained, but calibrations into real concentrations were not intended, because we need only to assess changes of $[Ca^{2+}]_i$ and pH_i and the differences in their time courses.

Agents used in this study were Fura-2/AM, BCECF/AM (Dojin, Japan), HEPES (Nakarai Chem Inc., Japan), acetylcholine (Ach; Daiichi-seiyaku, Japan), atropine (Iwaki-seiyaku, Japan) and methoxyverapamil (D-600; Research Biochemicals Inc).

3. RESULTS

The changes of cytosolic $[Ca^{2+}]_i$ and pH_i in response to stimulants exhibited by completely isolated cells were sometimes different from each other and from those obtained in clustered cells. Cultured SCG cells studied within 40 days in culture showed similar responses to 20 mM Ach, while cells cultured for over 60 days responded to HK (30 mM), but not to Ach. Therefore, for this study, we analyzed the data obtained only from clusters consisting of several cells within 40 days in culture.

The typical pattern of changes in $[Ca^{2+}]_i$ evoked by 20 mM Ach (Fig 1) consists of a fast rise (within 5 seconds) to a peak and a gradual decline. For longer culture periods, cells exhibit longer declines. Washing with a normal solution after applying Ach sometimes brought a positive rebound. Atropine (2 μM), a muscarinic antagonist, blocked in

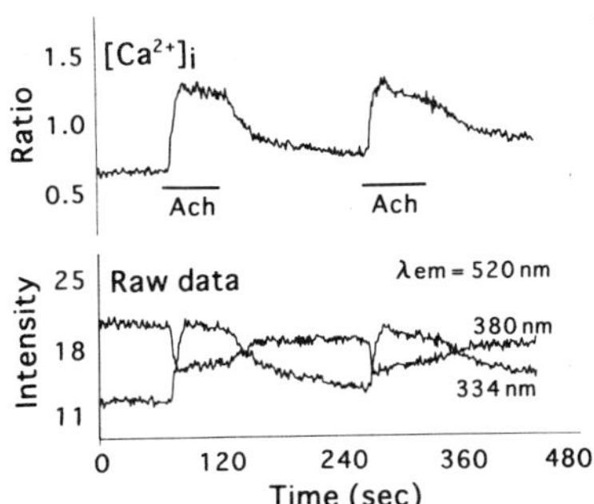

Figure 1. Typical changes in $[Ca^{2+}]_i$ induced by Ach (20 mM) in 19 days cultured SCG cells, loaded only with Fura-2/AM. Ratios (upper record) derived from fluorescence intensities (lower records).

part the response to 20 mM Ach, except for the initial peak (Fig 2A). Methoxyverapamil (D–600; 5 μM), an L–type Ca^{2+} channel blocker, inhibited part of the response to 20 mM Ach (Fig 2B). The effect of Ach on pH_i was not affected by D–600 (Fig 2B). Ammonium chloride (10 mM) transiently increased $[Ca^{2+}]_i$ and HK (30 mM) induced a large $[Ca^{2+}]_i$ increase (Fig 3). On the other hand, the pH_i declined when Ach (20 mM) or HK (30 mM) were applied. On the contrary, the pH_i rose rapidly when NH_4Cl (10 mM) was applied (Fig 3).

The latencies for changes in $[Ca^{2+}]_i$ and in pH_i from beginning of stimulation were different. These differences were assessed by means of magnification in time scale of the original recordings. Figure 4 shows on expanded time scale the effects induced by Ach, NH_4Cl and HK. On response to either Ach or HK, the appearance of $[Ca^{2+}]_i$ changes preceded that of pH_i changes. Contrarily to the above, NH_4Cl evoked first the appearance of changes in pH_i and then that of changes in $[Ca^{2+}]_i$ levels. Furthermore, after washout of NH_4Cl, a sudden fall in pH_i was observed while $[Ca^{2+}]_i$ went slowly up.

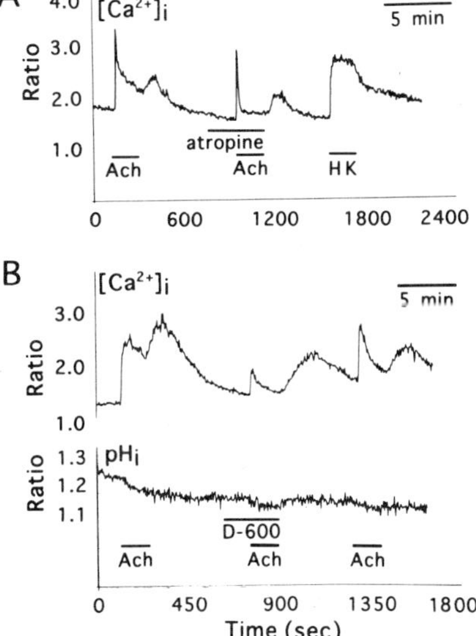

Figure 2. A. Changes in $[Ca^{2+}]_i$ induced by Ach (10 mM) and by a high concentration of K^+ (HK; 30 mM) in 40 days cultured SCG cells. Atropine (2 μM) blocked partially the response to Ach. Cells loaded only with Fura-2/AM. **B.** Simultaneous changes in $[Ca^{2+}]_i$ and in pH_i induced by Ach (10 mM) in 13 days cultured SCG cells. Methoxyverapamil (D-600, 5 μM) blocked partially the $[Ca^{2+}]_i$ increase induced by Ach, but did not reverse the pH_i decrease induced by Ach.

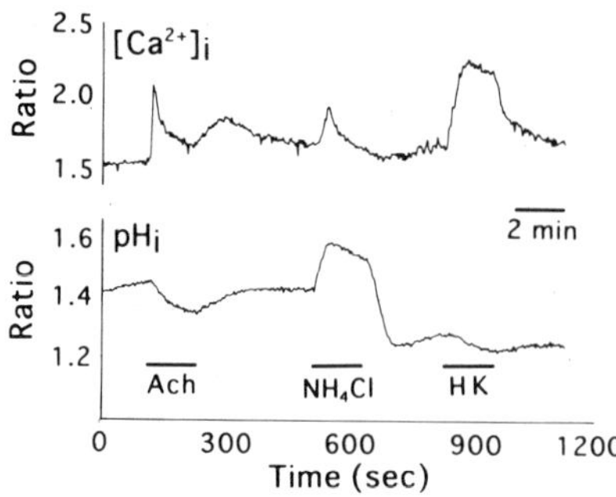

Figure 3. Simultaneous changes in $[Ca^{2+}]_i$ and in pH_i induced by Ach (10 mM), NH_4Cl (10 mM) and HK (30 mM) in 30 days cultured SCG cells. Cells loaded with a mixture of Fura-2/AM and BCECF/AM for 90 min.

4. DISCUSSION

The present study was designed to correlate the simultaneous changes in $[Ca^{2+}]_i$ and pH_i observed in cultured SCG cells in response to Ach, NH_4Cl and HK, applied as stimulants of ganglionic neuron activity.

In sympathetic ganglia, Ach released from the nerve endings of preganglionic fibers acts as a neurotransmitter on postganglionic neurons. The cultured SCG cells respond to Ach by releasing intracellular Ca^{2+} as a second messenger. Increase of $[Ca^{2+}]_i$ induced by Ach, for the most part, resulted considerably from activation of muscarinic receptors, because atropine blocked the Ach effect. The influx of calcium was induced through L–type Ca^{2+} channels, because D-600 inhibited the increase of $[Ca^{2+}]_i$ induced by Ach. The Ca^{2+}entry may activate a Ca^{2+}-induced Ca^{2+} release system (Kuba, 1994; Yoshizaki et al, 1995).

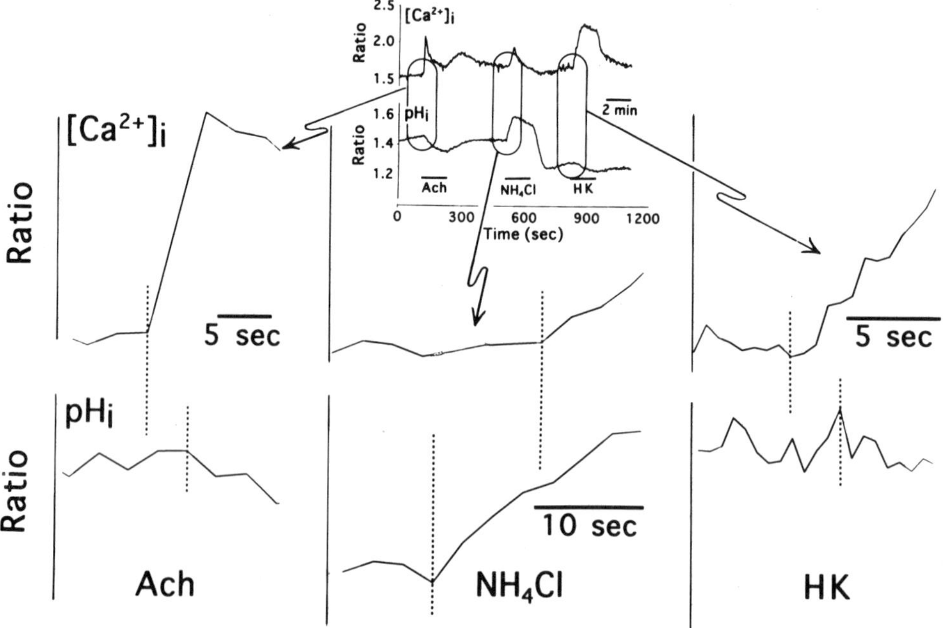

Figure 4. Magnification in time scale of simultaneous changes in $[Ca^{2+}]_i$ and $[H^+]_i$ in response to Ach (left), NH_4Cl (middle) and HK (right). Upper insert, original recording.

Extracellular HK depolarizes neurons and excites them, thus leading to the $[Ca^{2+}]_i$ increase observed in cultured SCG cells. Exposure to NH_4Cl, a weak base (pK'= 9.5), causes a large influx of NH_3 which results in intracellular alkalinization (Drapeau & Nachshen, 1988; Gillespie & Greenwell, 1988; Szatkowski & Thomas, 1989). When washing NH_4Cl solution, the cells acidified immediately, and gradually returned to the initial basal level of pH_i.

In this study, the simultaneous measurements of $[Ca^{2+}]_i$ and pH_i changes revealed that, in response to Ach and HK, $[Ca^{2+}]_i$ changes occurred earlier than pH_i changes. Drapeau and Nachshen (1988) reported that Ca^{2+} entry did not affect pH_i and its recovery. However, several reactions or acceleration steps must be intercalated between Ca^{2+} entry and $[Ca^{2+}]_i$ increase, during which biological energy may be consumed. This results possibly in the production of protons as by-products and the consequent change of pH_i. In general, cells have the regulatory system to maintain pH_i within normal range, but when a high amount of protons is produced, the buffering capacity of cells may be transiently surpassed, and pH_i may be reduced. Therefore, it is reasonable that pH_i may become lower after a $[Ca^{2+}]_i$ increase evoked by Ach or HK. Vaughan-Jones et al (1983) have reported H^+-release from Ca^{2+} binding proteins induced by increased levels of $[Ca^{2+}]_i$.

On the other hand, when NH_4Cl was applied to SCG cells, pH_i level changed first, followed by a transient rise in $[Ca^{2+}]_i$. Furthermore, the washout of NH_4Cl caused and abrupt fall of pH_i, after which the $[Ca^{2+}]_i$ level went up. Drapeau and Nachshen (1988) suggested that a Na^+-H^+ antiporter is the primary regulator of pH_i. Borle and Bender (1991) described that activation of Na^+-H^+ antiporters may be responsible for the transient rise of $[Ca^{2+}]_i$ level and/or Ca^{2+} influx through the Na^+-Ca^{2+}antiporter activated by the rise in $[Na^+]_i$. It may be speculated that when the cell environment is acidified or alkalinized and a change of pH_i occurs, some pH regulators activate Ca^{2+}influx, open Ca^{2+}-channels or release Ca^{2+} from Ca^{2+} stores. Gonzalez et al (1994) and also Sato (1994) proposed that cytosolic acidification may mediate the $[Ca^{2+}]_i$ increase induced in mammalian glomus cells by acidosis.

In conclusion, simultaneous measurements of changes of $[Ca^{2+}]_i$ and pH_i from rat cultured SCG cells reveal that time differences in the appearances of $[Ca^{2+}]_i$ and pH_i changes in response to Ach, HK and NH_4Cl. In response to Ach and HK, $[Ca^{2+}]_i$ changes occurred faster than pH_i changes, while in response to applied NH_4Cl, pH_i level changed first and then was followed by a transient rise in $[Ca^{2+}]_i$ level.

5. REFERENCES

Borle AB & Bender C (1991) Effects of pH on $[Ca^{2+}]_i$ Na^+_i and pH_i of MDCK cells: Na^+-Ca^{2+} and Na^+-H^+ antiporter interactions. Am J Physiol 261: C482-C489

Drapeau P & Nachshen DA (1988) Effects of lowering intracellular and cytosolic pH on calcium fluxes, cytosolic calcium levels and transmitter release in presynaptic nerve terminals isolated from rat brain. J Gen Physiol 91: 305–315

Fidone, SJ & Gonzalez C (1986) Initiation and control of chemoreceptor activity in the carotid body. In: Fishman AP (ed) Handbook of Physiology, The Respiratory System, vol II. Bethesda, MD: Am Physiol Soc. pp 247–312

Gillespie JL & Greenwell JR (1988) Changes in intracellular pH and pH regulating mechanisms in somitic cells of the early chick embryo: A study using fluorescent pH-sensitive dye. J Physiol, London 405: 385–395

Gomez-Niño A, Cheng GF, Yoshizaki, K, Gonzalez C, Dinger B & Fidone, SJ (1990) Regulation of the release of dopamine and norepinephrine from rabbit carotid body. In: Eyzaguirre C, Fidone, SJ, Fitzgerald RS, Lahiri S & McDonald DM (eds) Arterial Chemoreception. NY: Springer-Verlag. pp 92–99

Gonzalez C, Almaraz L, Obeso A & Rigual R (1994) Carotid body chemoreceptors: From natural stimuli to sensory discharge. Physiol Rev 74: 829–898

Kuba K (1994) Ca^{2+}-induced Ca^{2+} release in neurones. Jpn J Physiol 44: 613–650

McDonald DM (1981) Peripheral Chemoreceptors. Structure-function relationships of the carotid body. In: Hornbein TF (ed) Regulation of Breathing. Part I. NY: Dekker. pp 105–319

Nachshen DA & Drapeau P (1988) The regulation of cytosolic pH in isolated presynaptic nerve terminals from rat brain. J Gen Physiol 91: 289–303

Pallot DJ (1987) The mammalian carotid body. Adv Anat Embryol Cell Biol 102: 1–91

Sato M (1994) Effects of CO_2, acetate and lowering extracellular pH on cytosolic Ca^{2+} and pH in cultured glomus cells of the newborn rabbit carotid body. Neurosci Lett 173: 159–162

Shibuya I, Matsuyama K, Tanaka K & Doi K (1991) A microfluorometric method for simultaneous measurement of changes in cytosolic free calcium concentration and pH in single cardiac myocytes. Jpn J Physiol 41: 341–350

Szatkowski MS & Thomas RC (1989) The intrinsic intracellular H^+ buffering power of snail neurones J Physiol, London 409: 89–101

Vaughan-Jones RD, Lederer WJ & Eisner DA (1983) Ca^{2+} ion can affect intracellular pH in mammalian cardiac muscle. Nature 301: 522–524

Verna A, Barets A & Salat C (1984) Distribution of sympathetic nerve endings within the rabbit carotid body: a histochemical and ultrastructural study. J Neurocytol 13: 849–865

Yoshizaki K, Hoshino T, Sato M, Koyano H, Nohmi M, Hua SY & Kuba K (1995) Ca^{2+}-induced Ca^{2+} release and its activation in response to a single action potential in rabbit otic ganglion cells. J Physiol, London 486: 177–187

33

RELEASE OF ACETYLCHOLINE FROM THE *IN VITRO* CAT CAROTID BODY

Robert S. Fitzgerald[1,2,3] and Machiko Shirahata[1,4]

[1] Department of Environmental Health Sciences
[2] Department of Physiology
[3] Department of Medicine
[4] Department of Anesthesiology/Critical Care Medicine
The Johns Hopkins Medical Institutions
Baltimore, Maryland 21205

1. INTRODUCTION

Fidone and his colleagues (1976), using pyrolysis gas chromatography/mass fragmentometry, have measured the amount of acetylcholine (ACh) contained in the carotid bodies of cats. Hellström (1977) used similar techniques in rats. Indeed, a substantial amount of data suggests that ACh is synthesized and stored in the carotid body, and plays a significant role in the excitation of the carotid body in response to hypoxia (Eyzaguirre et al, 1983; Fidone and González, 1986, for reviews).

In several presentations to this Society (Fitzgerald & Shirahata, 1990; 1993; Fitzgerald et al, 1994) and elsewhere (Fitzgerald & Shirahata, 1992; 1994; Fitzgerald et al, 1995a,b), we have shown the carotid body's decreased neural output in response to perfusions of hypoxic Krebs Ringer bicarbonate solutions (KRB) when cholinergic blockers were included in the perfusate. Further, the classical criteria which are generally accepted as establishing a substance as a neurotransmitter in a neural process have been met by ACh, except for the "release" or "collectibility" of ACh. Metz (1969), using a bioassay, measured the amount of ACh released from the dog carotid bodies perfused with hypoxic/hypercapnic blood, though the techniques used in that study have been challenged. To our knowledge no chemical determination of the amount of ACh released from the carotid bodies of cats under varying conditions of stimulation has ever been reported.

The present study was intended to measure with High Pressure Liquid Chromatography (HPLC) the amount of ACh released from the cat carotid body perfused *in vitro*.

Frontiers in Arterial Chemoreception, edited by Zapata *et al.*
Plenum Press, New York, 1996

2. METHODS

2.1. Preparation

Cats (3–4 kg) were anesthetized with sodium pentobarbital (32 mg/kg). After 2 injections of tetramonoisopropyl pyrophosphortetramide (isoOMPA; 3 mg/kg) - an irreversible inhibitor of butyrylcholinesterase, both carotid bodies were perfused *in situ* with a solution of KRB containing 300 μM neostigmine and 1 mM isoOMPA. They were then removed and cleaned in KRB having the same concentrations of cholinesterase blockers. The carotid bodies were placed in a small water-jacketed (35–36°C) chamber (700 μl) and perfused at 0.047 ml/min with culture medium containing 300 μM neostigmine and 1 mM iso OMPA (PO_2 = 235 mm Hg; PCO_2 = 26.4 mm Hg; pH = 7.467) for 30 min.

2.2. Protocol

Carotid bodies were first perfused at 47 μl/min with hyperoxic KRB containing 30 μM neostigmine with KRB (PO_2 = 250 mm Hg; PCO_2 = 24.2 mm Hg; pH = 7.446) for 16 minutes. Perfusate from the chamber over the last four minutes was collected in filtering (0.2 μm diameter) vials. The perfusate was then shifted to a hypoxic/hypercapnic KRB (PO_2 = 46 mm Hg; PCO_2 = 65.3 mm Hg; pH = 7.251). Perfusate from the chamber was collected in four minute samples: 0–4'; 4–8'; 8–12'. All samples were centrifuged and stored at -80°C until analysis.

2.3. HPLC Analysis of Samples

KRB perfusate samples were measured in a Bioanalytical Systems High Pressure Liquid Chromatograph. The mobile phase was a solution of 30 mM sodium phosphate buffer containing the bactericidal Kathon. Flow was 1 ml/min. The pump was run at 2800–2900 PSI. The volume of filtered perfusate injected was 50 μl. The sample passed through a pre-column immobilized enzyme reactor (IMER) to remove most of the choline. It then proceeded through the analytical column where the ACh flowed more rapidly than the remaining choline. Finally in the last IMER the ACh was broken down into choline and then into betaine and H_2O_2. The H_2O_2 was detected by the electrochemical detector (-0.5 V) run at 2 nA full scale (the detector is capable of being run at 0.1 nA full scale). The amount of H_2O_2 is directly proportional to the amount of ACh.

2.4. Quantitation

Standards of known amounts of ACh were made up in KRB to quantitate the carotid body perfusates. KRB samples were also run to determine background noise at the retention time of the standards and samples. To quantitate data was sent from the electrochemical detector both to a strip chart recorder for direct write out (semi-quantitative), and to a computer (Packard Bell 840681/Force 205; 486SX) for processing with software (Bioanalytical Systems "Chromgraph"; quantitative). In this experiment the mean slope of the standard curve (picomoles/area in arbitrary units) was 1 picomole/78,508.

3. RESULTS

Figure 1 is a computer-generated chromatogram of a 50 μl sample of KRB.

Figure 2 is a computer-generated chromatogram of one of three standards used to create the curve. A 50 μl sample of KRB containing 0.720 picomoles (pmoles) was injected at time 0. The initial deviations are the solvent front or void volume passing through the columns. When the instrument is set with the above parameters, the ACh peak characteristically begins at about 240 s, reaches a peak maximum at 266 s, and is completed at about 300 s. A tolerance of 5% in time of peak maximum is allowed.

Figure 3 is taken from Experiment 4; a sample from the final four minutes of perfusion with a hyperoxic KRB (PO_2= 250 mm Hg; PCO_2= 24.2 mm Hg; pH= 7.446). The area recorded (24,069) corresponds to 0.316 pmoles ACh.

Figure 4 is taken from Experiment 4; a sample from minutes 0–4 of a perfusion of hypoxic/hypercapnic KRB (PO_2= 46 mm Hg; PCO_2= 65.3 mm Hg; pH= 7.251). The area (65,430) corresponds to 0.831 pmoles ACh. The peak which has a maximum at about 210 is frequently seen at the initiation of a hypoxic or hypoxic/hypercapnic challenge; it is as yet unidentified.

Figure 5 is taken from Experiment 4; a sample from minutes 4–8 of a perfusion of hypoxic/hypercapnic KRB (PO_2, etc. values as in 3.4). The area (65,508) corresponds to 0.853 pmoles ACh.

Figure 6 is taken from Experiment 4; a sample from minutes 8–12 of a perfusion of hypoxic/hypercapnic KRB (PO_2, etc, values as in 3.4). The area (79,313) corresponds to 1.029 pmoles ACh.

4. DISCUSSION

To our knowledge this is the first report of a chemically determined *release* of ACh from the carotid body of any species.

Metz (1969), using a bioassay, reported that the venous outflow from the isolated dog carotid body perfused with heparinized-eserinized blood (pH= 7.19; PCO_2= 87.1 Torr; PO_2= 42.6 torr) yielded 2807 pg/ml. This report received controversial acceptance due to some of the techniques involved in gathering the data. Fidone and his colleagues (Fidone et al, 1976; 1977) measured endogenous ACh levels in the cat carotid body, the effect of carotid sinus denervation on these levels, and the kinetics of choline uptake along with the autoradiographic localization of the high affinity component of this uptake process. They found about 11.5 pmoles of ACh per carotid body. We have found that during a 12 min perfusion with hypoxic/hypercapnic KRB the *in vitro* carotid body released 1.356 pmoles of ACh per carotid body. This represents about 12% of the stores measured by Fidone and his colleagues. Metz (1969) found that the dog carotid body perfused with a hypoxic/hypercapnic mixture of blood for 30 minutes at 1.2 ml/min released 2807 pg/ml. Under the conditions of our experiment the cat carotid body yielded 1320 pg/ml. These preliminary data indicate:

a. that very small amounts of acetylcholine can be measured with this technique.
b. that the cat carotid body releases acetylcholine in measurable amounts.
c. that the amount released increases under conditions which produce a significant increase in neural activity from the carotid body, hypoxia plus hypercapnia.
d. that acetylcholine release may well be involved in the excitation of the carotid body under these conditions.
e. that the "Cholinergic Hypothesis" needs further testing.

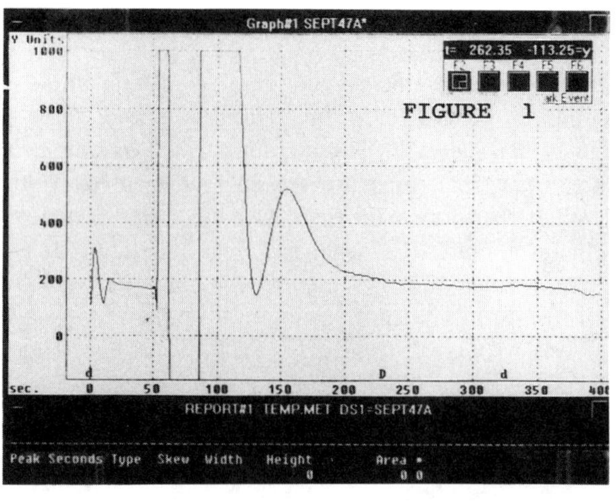

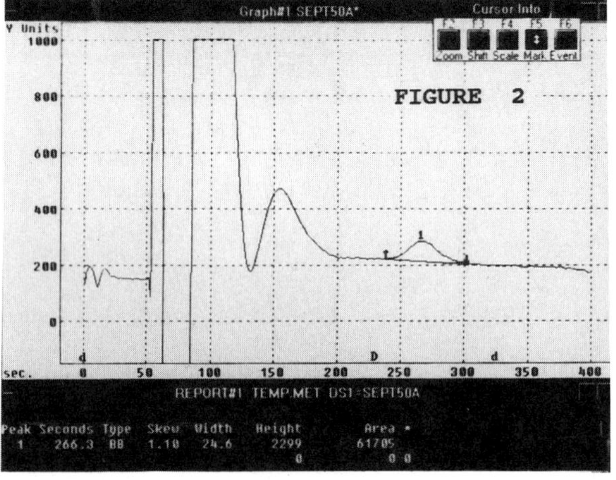

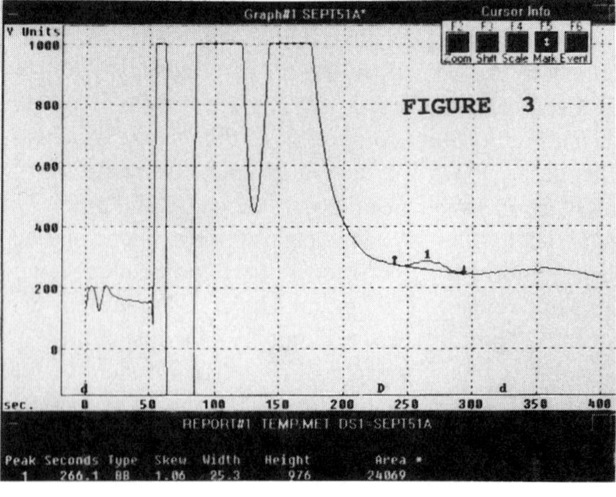

Figures 1-3. See text for description.

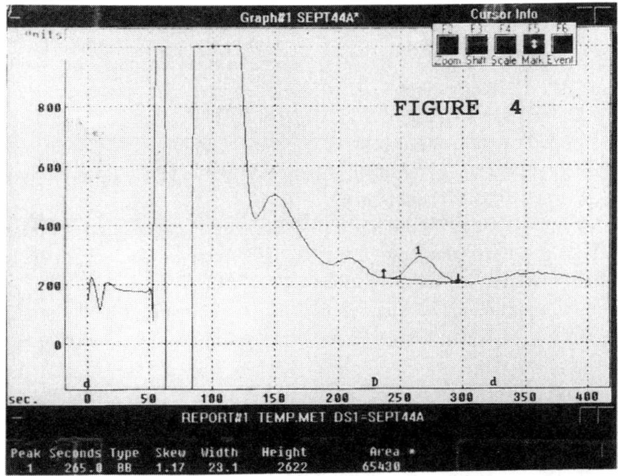

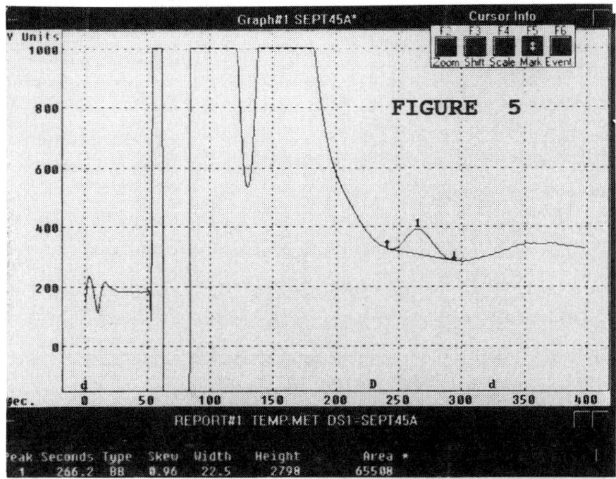

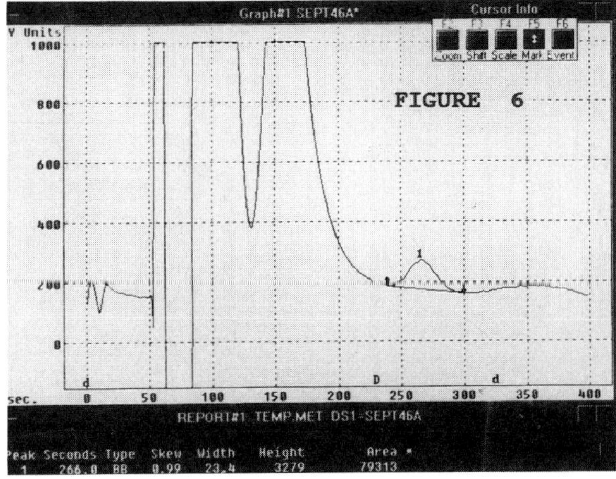

Figures 4-6. See text for description.

5. REFERENCES

Eyzaguirre C, Fitzgerald R, Lahiri S & Zapata P (1983) Arterial chemoreceptors. In: Shepherd J & Widdicombe JG (eds) Handbook of Physiology. Sect 2: The Cardiovascular System. Vol 3: Peripheral Circulation and Organ Blood Flow. Bethesda, MD: Amer Physiol Soc. pp 557–622

Fidone S & González C (1986) Initiation and control of chemoreceptor activity in the carotid body. In: Cherniack NS & Widdicombe JG (eds) Handbook of Physiology. Sect 3: The Respiratory System. Vol 2: Control of Breathing. Bethesda, MD: Amer Physiol Soc. pp 247–312

Fidone S, Weintraub S, Stavinoha W (1976) Acetylcholine content of normal and denervated cat carotid bodies measured by pyrolysis gas chromatography/mass fragmentometry. J Neurochem 26:1047–1049

Fidone S, Weintraub S, Stavinoha W, Stirling C & Jones L (1977) Endogenous acetylcholine levels in cat carotid body and the autoradiographic localization of a high affinity component of choline uptake. In: Acker H, Fidone S, Pallot D, Eyzaguirre C, Lübbers DW & Torrance RW (eds) Chemoreception in the Carotid Body. Berlin: Springer-Verlag. pp 106–113

Fitzgerald RS & Shirahata M (1990) The role of acetylcholine in carotid body chemotransduction of hypoxia. In: Eyzaguirre C, Fidone S, Fitzgerald RS, Lahiri S & McDonald D (eds) Arterial Chemoreception. New York: Springer-Verlag. pp 124–130

Fitzgerald RS, Shirahata M (1992) Carotid body chemotransduction. In: Honda Y, Miyamoto Y & Konno K (eds) Control of Breathing and Its Modeling Perspective. New York: Plenum Press. pp 441–445

Fitzgerald RS, Shirahata M (1993) Carotid body neurotransmission. In: Data PG, Acker H & Lahiri S (eds) Neurobiology and Cell Physiology of Chemoreception. New York: Plenum Press. pp 131–136

Fitzgerald RS, Shirahata M (1994) Acetylcholine and carotid body excitation during hypoxia an the cat. J Appl Physiol 76: 1566–1574

Fitzgerald RS, Shirahata M, Ide T & Schofield B (1994) Cholinergic aspects of carotid body chemotransduction. In: O'Regan RG, Nolan P, McQueen DS & Paterson DJ (eds) Arterial Chemoreceptors, Cell to System. New York: Plenum Press. pp 213–216

Fitzgerald RS, Shirahata M & Ide T (1995a) Cholinergic dimensions to carotid body chemotransduction. In: Semple SJG, Adams L & Whipp BJ (eds) Modelling and Control of Ventilation. New York: Plenum Press. pp 303–308

Fitzgerald RS, Shirahata M, Ide T, Lydic R (1995b) The cholinergic hypothesis revisited - an unfinished story. Biol Signals 4: 298–303

Hellström S (1977) Putative neurotransmitters in the carotid body. Mass fragmentographic studies. Adv Biochem Psychopharmacol 16: 257–263

Metz B (1969) Release of acetylcholine from the carotid body by hypoxia and hypoxia plus hypercapnia. Respir Physiol 6: 386–394

34

RELEASE OF ACETYLCHOLINE FROM CULTURED CAT AND PIG GLOMUS CELLS

Machiko Shirahata, Yumiko Ishizawa, Ayuko Igarashi and Robert S. Fitzgerald

Department of Environmental Health Sciences
The Johns Hopkins Medical Institutions
Baltimore, Maryland

1. INTRODUCTION

It is generally accepted that neurotransmitters play an essential role in the carotid body chemotransduction. Although roles of each transmitter are in debate, substantial evidence suggests that in cats acetylcholine (ACh) is involved in an excitatory step in the carotid body chemotransduction. The presence of choline acetyl transferase, an ACh-synthesizing enzyme, in glomus cells of cats has been known (Wang et al, 1989). Cholinergic receptors are localized on glomus cells (Dinger et al, 1985, 1986; Chen et al, 1981) and possibly on the carotid sinus nerve (Fitzgerald & Shirahata, 1990). Exogenously applied ACh provokes a fast and clear increase in carotid sinus nerve chemoreceptor discharge (Eyzaguirre et al, 1983; Fidone et al, 1990). Further, perfusion of the carotid body with cholinergic blockers inhibits hypoxia-mediated elevation in chemoreceptor neural activity (Fitzgerald & Shirahata, 1994). However, little is known about the release of ACh from glomus cells. This study was designed to obtain basic information as to the release pattern of ACh from cultured glomus cells.

2. METHODS

2.1. Cell Culture

Carotid body cells were cultured as previously described with a slight modification (Shirahata et al, 1994). Carotid bodies were harvested from adult cats and pigs which were euthanized with an overdose of pentobarbital or bleeding under deep anesthesia. The tissue was dissociated with collagenase and trituration, plated on small wells (6 mm in diameter) coated with polylysine and basement membrane complexes, and cultured in a defined medium for several days in an incubator (5% CO_2/air, 37°C).

Frontiers in Arterial Chemoreception, edited by Zapata *et al.*
Plenum Press, New York, 1996

2.2. Immunocytochemistry

The cultured cells were fixed with S.T.F.™ (Streck Laboratories, Inc) for overnight, and the cell membranes were permeabilized with 100% methanol for 5 min. Cells were incubated with either monoclonal (Boehringer Mannheim) or polyclonal antibody to choline acetyl transferase (Chemicon) overnight at 4°C. Standard ABC techniques are applied using VECTASTAIN^R *Elite* ABC kits for rat or rabbit antibodies to bind anti-choline acetyl transferase.

2.3. Measurement of ACh

For sample collection, cells were washed with Krebs containing 300 μM neostigmine and 1 M tetraisopropylpyrophosphor amide, and incubated in the same Krebs (5% CO_2/air, 37°C). Thirty minutes later, the solution was changed to 70 μl of Krebs containing 30 μM neostigmine and the incubation was continued for 30 min. The wells were placed in a small chamber through which a humidified mixed gas (either 5% CO_2/air or 5% CO_2/argon) was continuously supplied. Temperature of the chamber was controlled between 35 and 38°C, and PO_2 in the chamber was continuously monitored. Fifteen to sixty minutes later, samples of solutions (60 μl) were withdrawn. Subsequently, the cells were incubated in the culture medium containing 30 μM of neostigmine (5% CO_2/air, 37°C). One hour later, the cells were washed with Krebs containing 30 μM neostigmine and 70 μl of the same Krebs was added. Exposure to the second gas and the sample collection was the same as the first exposure. Samples were filter-centrifuged, and stored at -80°C until measurement.

ACh was measured with high pressure liquid chromatography (Bioanalytical Systems, Inc). The mobile phase consisted of 50 mM disodium phosphate hydrogen (pH 8.5). The analytical components of the high pressure liquid chromatography were a pre-column immobilized enzyme reactor (IMER), a polymeric analytic column, and an acetylcholinesterase/choline oxidase IMER. Separation was carried out at a flow rate of 1 ml/min and a pressure of 2800–3100 psi. Standard solutions of ACh were prepared in Krebs solution before injection. ACh was detected at a potential of +0.5 V with an amperometric detector. Data were acquired and analyzed with softwares (INJECT, CHROMGRAPH, Bioanalytical system) and a PC-based computer.

3. RESULTS

Cultured glomus cells of cats and pigs contained choline acetyl transferase (Fig 1).

We have tested 13 wells from 5 cats and 8 wells from 2 pigs as to the release of ACh. ACh was detected in most cases (Fig 2 and Tables 1 and 2). The amount measured varied extensively among wells, but hypoxia appeared to increase the release of ACh (Table 2).

4. DISCUSSION

The present study showed that ACh is synthesized in the cultured glomus cells and the release of ACh is measurable. The measured values were extremely variable. Particularly, ACh was not detected in 12 out of 21 wells during normoxia, but in 9 out of these 12

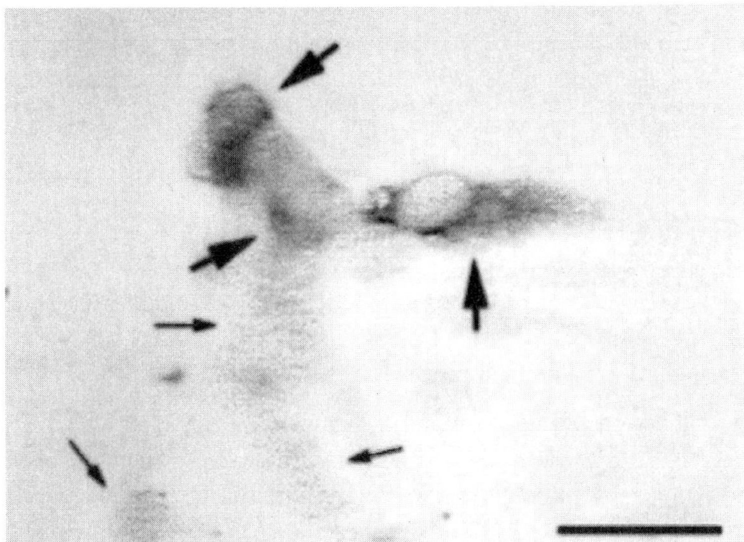

Figure 1. Carotid body cells from a pig were cultured in a defined medium for 4 days. Choline acetyl transferase (ChAT) was visualized using 3-amino-9-ethylcarbazole (Vector) as a chromogen. Large arrows indicate cells stained for ChAT. Small arrows indicate negative cells. Bar, 20 μm.

wells ACh was detected during hypoxia. The results suggest that glomus cells were functional, but the basal release of ACh was low. On the other hand, in three wells ACh was detected during normoxia (between 116 and 1441 fmoles), but not during hypoxia. We do not have a clear explanation of these unexpected results, but variable amounts of ACh among wells may reflect the number of viable glomus cells in the wells. In this study we did not check the viability of the glomus cells. It is possible that some cells might have died during experiments. It is important in future studies to assess the viability of cells in the course of experiments. Checking the presence of ChAT in all cells tested would be also necessary.

5. ACKNOWLEDGMENTS

This work was supported by grants HL50712 and HL47044.

Table 1. ACh secretion from cultured glomus cells

Species	Exposure time (min)	n	ACh secretion (mean ± SEM; fmoles/well)			
			Normoxia		Hypoxia	
cat	15	2	284	(0)*	0	(2)
	30	6	455 ± 281	(3)	324 ± 221	(2)
	60	5	1503 ± 973	(1)	7463 ± 7053	(0)
pig	30	4	314 ± 181	(2)	762 ± 404	(2)
	60	4	529 ± 529	(3)	426 ± 319	(2)

* ACh not detected in some wells. Numbers of those wells shown in parentheses. Amount of ACh in those wells assumed 0 fmole for calculation of mean values.

A

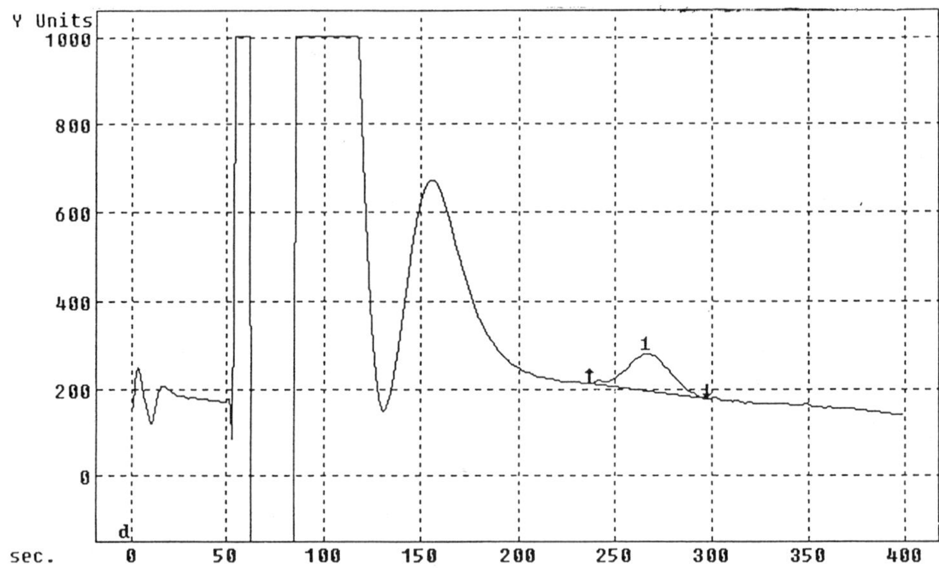

B

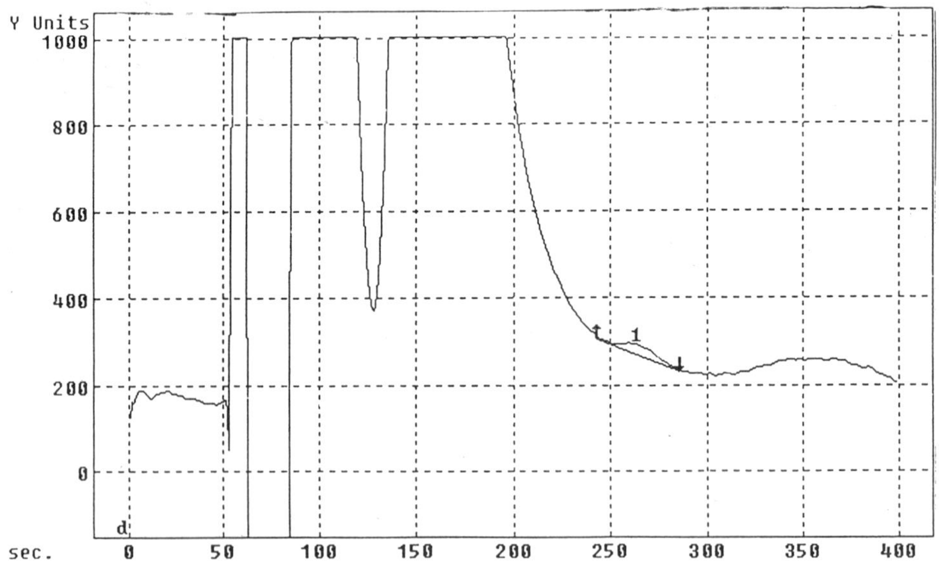

Figure 2. Acetylcholine secretion from cultured cat glomus cells. Chromatograms of (A) an ACh standard solution in Krebs (720 fmoles), (B) a sample of the solution which was collected from a well with glomus cells after 60 min of normoxia. Approximately 180 fmoles were detected.

Table 2. Patterns of ACh secretion during hypoxic exposure compared with normoxic exposure

Species	Exposure time (min)	Number of wells		
		Increase	No change	Decrease
cat	15	0	0	2*
	30	4 (3)	1†	1*
	60	3 (1)	0	1
pig	30	4 (2)	0	0
	60	2 (3)	2†	0

* ACh not detected during hypoxia in these wells.
† ACh was not detected during both normoxia and hypoxia in these wells.
( ) Numbers of wells in which ACh was not detected during normoxia.

6. REFERENCES

Chen I, Mascorro JA & Yates RD (1981) Autoradiographic localization of alpha-bungarotoxin-binding sites in the carotid body of the rat. Cell Tissue Res 219: 609–618

Dinger B, Gonzalez C, Yoshizaki K & Fidone S (1985) Localization and function of cat carotid body nicotinic receptors. Brain Res 339: 295–304

Dinger BG, Hirano T & Fidone SJ (1986) Autoradiographic localization of muscarinic receptors in rabbit carotid body. Brain Res 367: 328–331

Eyzaguirre C, Fitzgerald RS, Lahiri S & Zapata P (1983) Arterial chemoreceptors. In: Shepherd JT & Abboud FM (eds) Handbook of Physiology, Section 2: The Cardiovascular System. Bethesda, MD: American Physiological Society. pp 557–621

Fidone SJ, Gonzalez C, Obeso A, Gomez-Niño A & Dinger B (1990) Biogenic amines and neuropeptide transmitters in carotid body chemotransmission: experimental findings and perspectives. In: Sutton JR, Coates G & Remmers JE (eds) Hypoxia: The Adaptations. Philadelphia, PA: Decker. pp 116–126

Fitzgerald RS & Shirahata M (1990) The role of acetylcholine in the chemoreception of hypoxia by the carotid body. In: Eyzaguirre C, Fidone SJ, Fitzgerald RS, Lahiri S & McDonald DM (eds) Arterial Chemoreception. New York: Springer-Verlag. pp 124–130

Fitzgerald RS & Shirahata M (1994) Acetylcholine and carotid body excitation during hypoxia in the cat. J Appl Physiol 76: 1566–1574

Shirahata M, Schofield B, Chin BY & Guilarte TR (1994) Culture of arterial chemoreceptor cells from adult cats in defined medium. Brain Res 658: 60–66

Wang ZZ, Stensaas LJ, Dinger B & Fidone SJ (1989) Immunocytochemical localization of choline acetyltransferase in the carotid body of the cat and rabbit. Brain Res 498: 131–134

35

ACETYLCHOLINE ELEVATES INTRACELLULAR Ca^{2+} VIA MUSCARINIC AND NICOTINIC RECEPTORS IN RAT CAROTID BODY TYPE I CELLS

Leonardo L. T. Dasso, Keith J. Buckler, and Richard D. Vaughan-Jones

University Laboratory of Physiology
University of Oxford
Oxford, United Kingdom

1. INTRODUCTION

Acetylcholine (ACh) has been proposed to act as an excitatory neurotransmitter on sensory nerve endings (reviewed in Fidone & González, 1986) in the carotid body. However, several facts undermine this hypothesis, particularly the species-dependence of its effects and the apparent absence of cholinergic receptors on afferent terminals of the carotid sinus nerve. In contrast, both nicotinic and muscarinic receptors abound in type I and type II cells (Dinger et al, 1985, 1986). Consequently, although the evidence for a post-synaptic role for ACh is questionable, there is good evidence for a pre-synaptic role, which would account for the high ACh-sensitivity of the discharge frequency of the sinus nerve (Monti-Bloch & Eyzaguirre, 1980). We have therefore investigated the effects of ACh on Ca^{2+} signalling in freshly isolated single type I cells.

2. METHODS

Enzymic isolation of type I cells and fluorimetric $[Ca^{2+}]_i$ determinations using Indo-1 were essentially as described (Buckler & Vaughan-Jones, 1993). Changes in $[Ca^{2+}]_i$ were calculated as the difference between the peak $[Ca^{2+}]_i$ value elicited by exposure to a pharmacological agent and the mean resting $[Ca^{2+}]_i$ value determined prior to the exposure. Statistical significance of the results was assessed by two-tailed Student's paired *t*-test.

Ca^{2+} influx was monitored using the method of Mn^{2+} quench of Fura-2 fluorescence (Merritt et al, 1989). Fluorescence was excited alternately at 380 and 360 nm and measured at 510 nm. Quenching of the 360 nm fluorescent signal reflected Mn^{2+} entry into the cytoplasm.

Frontiers in Arterial Chemoreception, edited by Zapata *et al.*
Plenum Press, New York, 1996

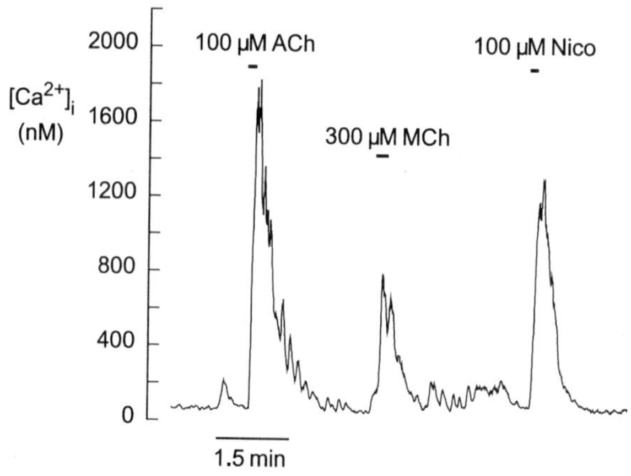

Figure 1. Effect of acetylcholine (ACh), methacholine (MCh) and nicotine (Nico) on $[Ca^{2+}]_i$ in a single type I cell in Ca^{2+}-containing medium.

3. RESULTS

3.1. Studies in 2.5 mM Ca^{2+} Containing Medium

Fifty-five percent of the cells (n = 182) responded to ACh (1–300 μM) with a rapid elevation of $[Ca^{2+}]_i$ (Fig 1). Maximal responses were typically obtained with 10–100 μM ACh. The average peak value of the elevation in $[Ca^{2+}]_i$ evoked by 100 μM ACh was 798 ± 76 nM above basal (n = 89). The responses evoked by ACh were partially abolished by the muscarinic antagonist atropine (1 μM) (67 ± 9% inhibition, n = 4) or the nicotinic antagonist mecamylamine (1 μM) (53 ± 2% inhibition, n = 3). The simultaneous presence of both antagonists completely abolished the elevations of $[Ca^{2+}]_i$ elicited by ACh (n = 3) (not shown).

Maximal methacholine (MCh) concentrations (300 μM) raised $[Ca^{2+}]_i$ to 672 ± 87 nM, n = 39, above basal (Figs 1, 2). Other muscarinic agonists: muscarine (10–100 μM) (n = 59), oxotremorine (100 μM) (n = 77) and oxotremorine M (100 μM) (n = 7) evoked similar $[Ca^{2+}]_i$ rises. When cells were challenged with 300 μM MCh for longer than 1–2 min, the $[Ca^{2+}]_i$ response was biphasic: $[Ca^{2+}]_i$ levels rapidly peaked (634 ± 215 nM above basal, n = 6) and then declined to a sustained and elevated plateau (108 ± 19 nM, $p < 0.003$ *vs* basal (89 ± 14 nM) (n = 6) (Fig 2A). Nicotine (100–500 μM) or the nicotinic agonist DMPP (100 μM) also led to $[Ca^{2+}]_i$ elevations. 100 μM nicotine evoked maximal elevations of $[Ca^{2+}]_i$ (701 ± 80 nM) (n = 42) (Fig 1). Exposure to nicotine for more than 1–2 min, caused $[Ca^{2+}]_i$ to rise (683 ± 161 nM) (n = 18) and then decline (Fig 2B) to resting levels which were indistinguishable from those observed before application of nicotine. Responses to MCh and nicotine were abolished by atropine (1 μM) (n = 4) and mecamylamine (1 μM) (n = 7), respectively (not shown).

The distribution of muscarinic and nicotinic responses was assessed by exposing ACh-responding cells to MCh (300 μM) and to nicotine (100 μM). A majority of cells (63%) responded to both agonists, while 9% responded only to MCh and 29% only to nicotine (n = 35).

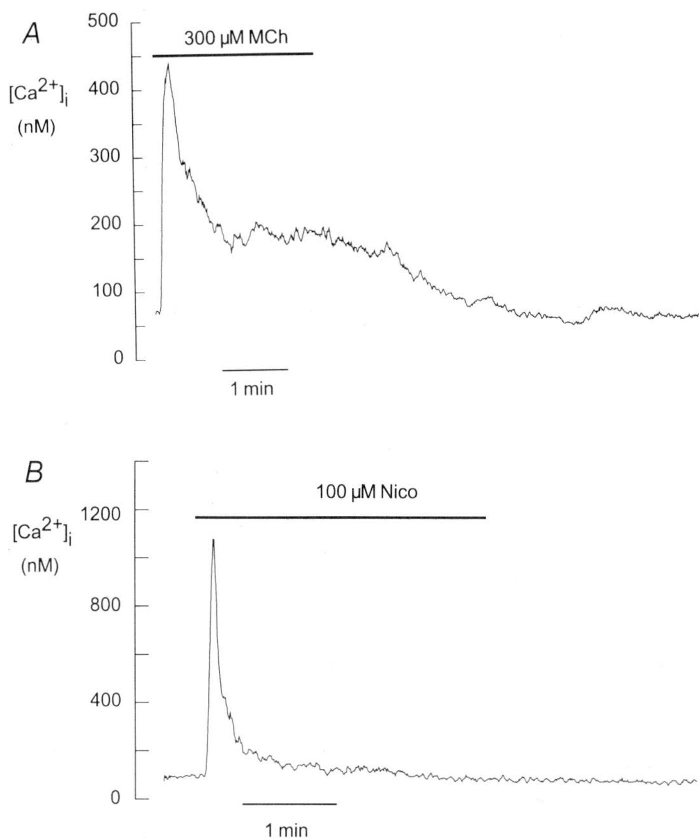

Figure 2. Effect of MCh (A) and nicotine (B) on $[Ca^{2+}]_i$.

3.2. Studies in Ca^{2+}-Free Medium

In Ca^{2+}-free medium (no $CaCl_2$ added and containing 1 mM EGTA), muscarinic agonists evoked a transient increase in $[Ca^{2+}]^i$ (Fig 3A) (n = 35). In general, muscarinic responses were of lesser amplitude in Ca^{2+}-free medium: $[Ca^{2+}]_i$ transients decreased single exponentially ($t_{1/2}$ = 2.3 ± 0.6 min, n = 4) with increasing pre-incubation time in Ca^{2+}-free medium, typically disappearing completely within 5–15 min (not shown). It is noteworthy that in Ca^{2+}-free medium, resting $[Ca^{2+}]_i$ also declined single-exponentially with $t_{1/2}$ = 1.2 min (not shown).

In the absence of $[Ca^{2+}]_o$, nicotine failed to elevate $[Ca^{2+}]_i$ (n = 5) (Fig 3B).

3.3. Muscarine-Evoked Ca^{2+} Influx

$[Ca^{2+}]_o$ influx can be followed by replacing Ca^{2+} by Mn^{2+} in the extracellular medium and monitoring quenching of the fluorescent signal caused by excitation of Fura-2 at the isosbestic wavelength (360 nm) (Merritt et al, 1989). Muscarine (100 µM) increased dramatically the rate of quenching of intracellular Fura-2 fluorescence (n = 3) (not shown), indicating that it increased divalent cation entry.

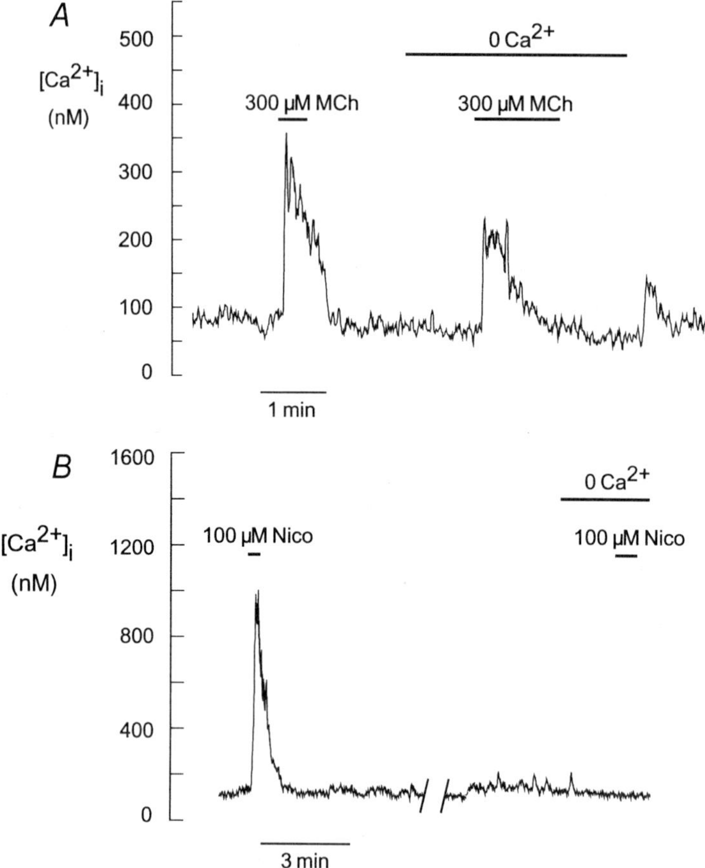

Figure 3. Effects of MCh (A) and nicotine (B) on $[Ca^{2+}]_i$ in Ca^{2+}-free medium.

4. DISCUSSION

Fifty-five percent of type I cells responded to ACh with increases in $[Ca^{2+}]_i$. ACh-evoked $[Ca^{2+}]_i$ rises were due to activation of muscarinic receptors (9%), nicotinic receptors (29%) or both (63%). Nicotinic responses were abolished in the absence of $[Ca^{2+}]_o$, consistent with the notion that nicotinic receptors depend on $[Ca^{2+}]_o$ to elevate $[Ca^{2+}]_i$ (Sargent, 1993). In contrast, muscarinic agonists increased $[Ca^{2+}]_i$ in Ca^{2+}-free medium, indicating that the response involves Ca^{2+} release from internal stores. This is the first demonstration that type-I cells possess agonist-releasable intracellular Ca^{2+}-stores. Muscarinic responses in Ca^{2+}-free medium were transient, *i.e.*, the plateau was absent, suggesting that muscarinic agonists evoke Ca^{2+}_o influx. This suggestion is supported by the dramatic muscarine-evoked increase in Mn^{2+} influx. This Ca^{2+} influx pathway may be triggered by depletion of intracellular stores. Ca^{2+} release-activated Ca^{2+} channels (CRACs) have been demonstrated in many non-excitable cells (Putney, 1990) and also recently in neuroblastoma (Mathes & Thompson, 1994) and cerebellar granule cells (Simpson et al, 1995). The amplitude of muscarinic responses in Ca^{2+}-free medium was dependent on the duration of pre-incubation in Ca^{2+}-free medium, suggesting a progressive depletion of the

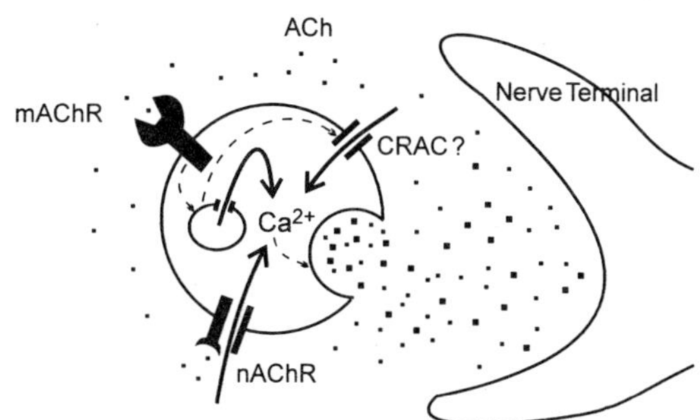

Figure 4. ACh (▪) raises $[Ca^{2+}]_i$ via activation of muscarinic (mAChR) and nicotinic (nAChR) autoreceptors. This $[Ca^{2+}]_i$ elevation may modulate release of neurotransmitters (*eg*, dopamine (■) or ACh itself).

MCh-sensitive intracellular stores. This depletion was surprisingly rapid, suggesting that these stores are very labile in $[Ca^{2+}]_o$-free conditions. The time course of store depletion was very similar to the time course of the decline in resting $[Ca^{2+}]_i$, suggesting a causal link between the two processes. The physiological role of cholinergic receptors in type I cells remains to be elucidated. ACh is released by type I cells during carotid body stimulation (Eyzaguirre & Zapata, 1984; Wang et al, 1989). Cholinergic receptors are found exclusively on type I and type II cells (Dinger et al, 1985; 1986). Chemotransduction of physiological stimuli in type I cells is presently thought to involve a rapid rise in $[Ca^{2+}]_i$ through voltage-operated Ca^{2+} channels (Buckler & Vaughan-Jones, 1994), which promotes neurosecretion (Ureña et al, 1994). In view of these data, our results suggest that ACh may activate autoreceptors on type I cells to evoke changes in $[Ca^{2+}]_i$ and thereby modulate neurotransmitter release (Fig 4). Cholinergic receptors may also be involved in the efferent control of the chemosensory discharge. The coexistence of both nicotinic and muscarinic receptors in type I cells, which bind the same endogenous ligand, but rely on different sources of Ca^{2+}, suggests that these different receptor subtypes may be involved in the regulation of different Ca^{2+}-dependent processes in these cells.

5. ACKNOWLEDGMENTS

This work was supported by the Wellcome Trust.

6. REFERENCES

Buckler KJ & Vaughan-Jones RD (1993) Effects of acidic stimuli on intracellular calcium in isolated type I cells of the neonatal rat carotid body. Pflügers Arch 425: 22–27

Buckler KJ & Vaughan-Jones RD (1994) Effects of hypoxia on membrane potential and intracellular calcium in rat neonatal carotid body type I cells. J Physiol, London 476: 423–428

Dinger B, González C, Yoshizaki K & Fidone S (1985) Localization and function of cat carotid body nicotinic receptors. Brain Res 339: 295–304

Dinger B, Hirano T & Fidone SJ (1986) Autoradiographic localization of muscarinic receptors in rabbit carotid body. Brain Res 367: 328–331

Eyzaguirre C & Zapata P (1984) Perspectives in carotid body research. J Appl Physiol 57: 931–957

Fidone SJ & González C (1986) Initiation and control of chemoreceptor activity in the carotid body. In: Cherniack NS & Widdicombe JG (eds) Handbook of Physiology, Sect. 3: The Respiratory System, Vol. II, Chapter 9. Bethesda, MD: Amer Physiol Soc. pp 247–312

Mathes C & Thompson SH (1994) Calcium current activated by muscarinic receptors and thapsigargin in neuronal cells. J Gen Physiol 104: 107–121

Merritt JE, Jacob R & Hallam TJ (1989) Use of manganese to discriminate between calcium influx and mobilization from internal stores in stimulated human neutrophils. J Biol Chem 264: 1522–1527

Monti-Bloch L & Eyzaguirre C (1980) A comparative physiological and pharmacological study of cat and rabbit carotid body chemoreceptors. Brain Res 193: 449–470

Putney JW (1990) Capacitative calcium entry revisited. Cell Calcium 11: 611–624

Sargent PB (1993) The diversity of neuronal nicotinic acetylcholine receptors. Annu Rev Neurosci 16: 403–443

Simpson PB, Challis RAJ & Nahorski SR (1995) Divalent cation entry in cultured rat cerebellar granule cells measured using Mn^{2+} quench of Fura 2 fluorescence. Eur J Neurosci 7: 831–840

Ureña J, Fernandez-Chacon R, Benot AR, Alvarez de Toledo GA & Lopez-Barneo J (1994) Hypoxia induces voltage-dependent Ca^{2+} entry and quantal dopamine secretion in carotid body glomus cells. Proc Natl Acad Sci USA 91: 10208–10211

Wang ZZ, Stensaas LJ, Dinger B & Fidone SJ (1989) Immunocytochemical localization of choline acetyltransferase in the carotid body of the cat and rabbit. Brain Res 498: 131–134

THE PRESYNAPTIC COMPONENT OF A CHOLINERGIC MECHANISM IN THE CAROTID BODY CHEMOTRANSDUCTION OF HYPOXIA IN THE CAT

Robert S. Fitzgerald,[1,2,3] Machiko Shirahata,[1,4] and Yumiko Ishizawa[1]

[1] Department of Environmental Health Sciences
[2] Department of Physiology
[3] Department of Medicine
[4] Department of Anesthesiology/Critical Care Medicine
The Johns Hopkins Medical Institutions
Baltimore, Maryland 21205

1. INTRODUCTION

In the past we have shown that cholinergic blockers given together or singly could greatly reduce the carotid body's response to a perfusion of hypoxic Krebs Ringer bicarbonate solution (KRB) (Fitzgerald & Shirahata, 1994; Fitzgerald et al, 1995). The operating model in those studies was transmission in the superior cervical ganglion. That is, the Type I cell of the carotid body was analogous to the presynaptic neuron; it contained acetylcholine (ACh). In fact the Type I cell has been identified as the source of ACh in several different studies. The synthesizing enzyme, choline acetyltransferase (ChAT), has been located there (Ballard & Jones, 1972; Wang et al, 1989). Fidone et al (1977) have located the high affinity sodium-dependent choline uptake transporter in the Type I cells. They have also reported that carotid bodies which had been denervated contained as much ACh as their intact counterparts (Fidone et al, 1976), suggesting that the extensive innervation in the carotid body and the very few ganglia reported to be there contribute an immeasurably small amount of ACh. And we (Goldberg et al, 1978) analyzed the carotid sinus nerve directly to find no appreciable amount of ACh in it.

The postsynaptic neuron in the above model was the sensory neuron apposed to the ACh-containing Type I cell. The data generated by the above-cited experiments were consistent with such a model. We also reported data consistent with the presence of M1 and M2 muscarinic receptors in the carotid body (Fitzgerald et al, 1995). In the superior cervical ganglion the postsynaptic M2 receptor is responsible for the slow inhibitory postsynaptic potential which tends to make the postsynaptic neuron less excitable. Hence, if

Frontiers in Arterial Chemoreception, edited by Zapata *et al.*
Plenum Press, New York, 1996

blocked, one would anticipate a larger postsynaptic response. When gallamine -an M2 receptor blocker- was included in the hypoxic perfusate, neural output from the carotid body was greater than under the no-blocker conditions. We interpreted the larger response to the hypoxic perfusate when gallamine was included as being consistent with the presence of a postsynaptic M2 receptor; *i.e.*, an M2 receptor on the neuron apposed to the Type I cell.

However, the data could be fit into other models as well. Dinger et al (1986) have reported ^{3}H-QNB binding sites -indicative of muscarinic receptors- on the Type I cells. In some systems where acetylcholine (ACh) is excitatory, presynaptic M2 receptors function to modulate the further release of ACh (Baker & Brown, 1992). If some of the sites reported by Dinger and his colleagues (1986) are M2 receptors and if ACh is an excitatory neurotransmitter in the carotid body, then blocking them would promote an even greater release of ACh, and generate a larger response. This, too, could be an interpretation of our data.

In the present set of on-going experiments we have sought to impede the release of ACh from the Type I cell. There are several ways in which this could be accomplished theoretically: (a) Impede the release of ACh from the vesicles into the synaptic cleft by interrupting the operation of a protein, mediatophore, located in the membrane of the presynaptic neuron; (b) Prevent the packaging of ACh in the presynaptic vesicles; (c) Inhibit the synthesizing enzyme, ChAT; (d) Reduce the availability of acetyl CoA; (e) Reduce the availability of choline (Fig 1).

2. METHODS

2.1. Preparation

Cats (3.5–4.5 kg) were anesthetized with pentobarbital sodium (30 mg/kg ip). They were prepared for selective perfusion of the carotid body as previously described in detail (Fitzgerald & Shirahata, 1994). In brief a stopcock-containing loop was inserted into one common carotid artery. The lingual artery was fitted with a cannula having a variable resistance; the remaining vessels were ligated except for the external and common carotid arteries around which snares were placed. A water-jacketed catheter was connected to the loop. When a perfusion was to be made, the snares around the common and external carotid arteries were drawn tight, the stopcock turned and the perfusion was made with outflow via the lingual artery and the vasculature of the carotid body. Upon completion of the perfusion the stopcock was returned to its original position and the carotid body was once again perfused with its own arterial blood.

Figure 1. Biosynthesis, storage, and release of ACh in neural tissue. Cytosolic glucose is the source of carbon atoms for the genesis of pyruvate which proceeds into the mitochondrion where it becomes acetyl CoA. Citrate is the acetyl carrier from the mitochondrion; it is cleaved by citrate lyase into oxaloacetate and acetyl CoA, destined for the synthesis of ACh. Choline must come from the extracellular compartment via the high affinity, sodium-dependent uptake transporter. Choline can be the substrate for ChAT in three different locations: membrane, vesicles, cytosol. Newly synthesized ACh proceeds into four different pools; the two forms of releasable ACh are sometimes called "depot" ACh. This is the ACh used for transmission. ACh is stored in vesicles perhaps through a mechanism involving the exchange of protons. It is released when the vesicle unites with the membrane protein, mediatophore.

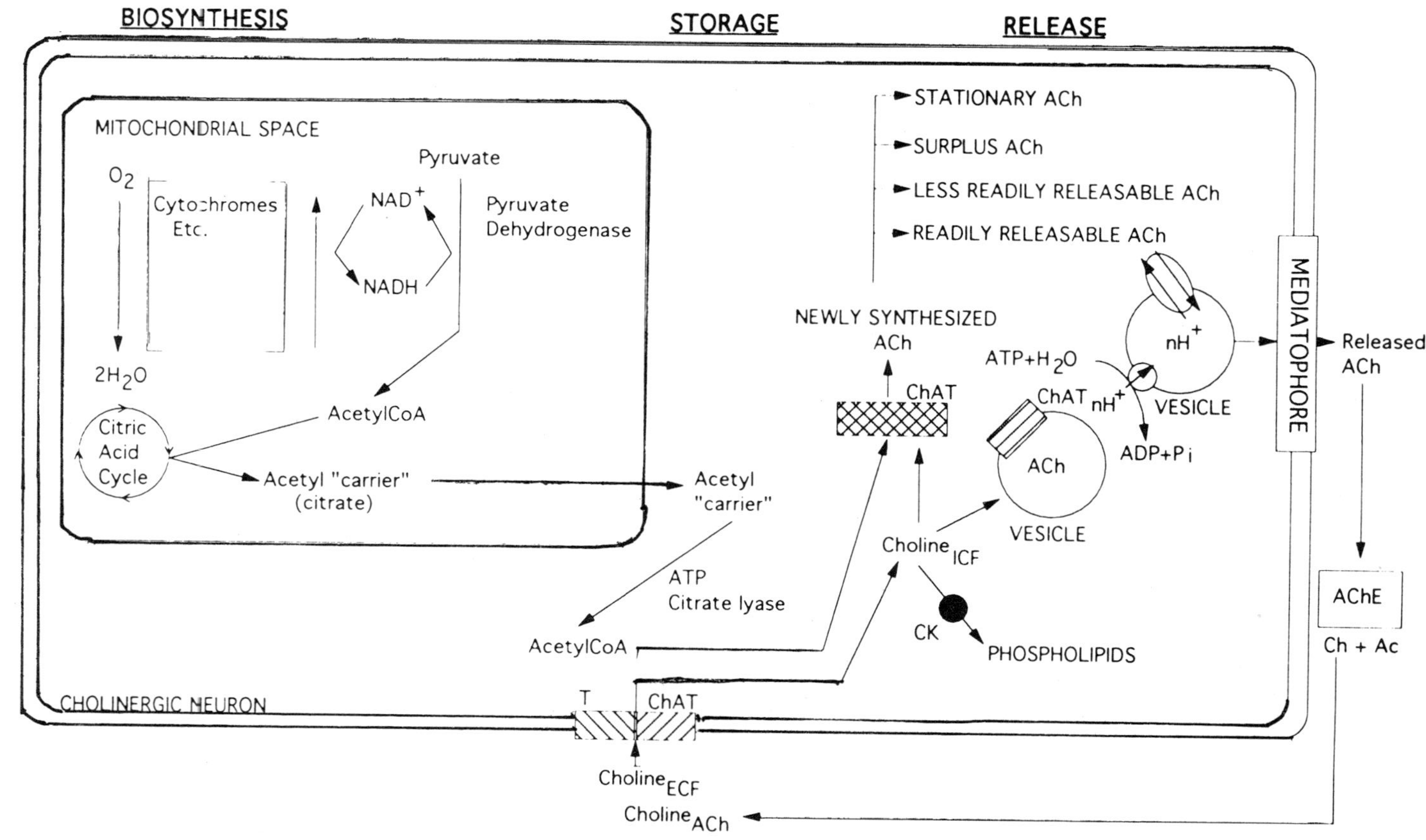
BIOSYNTHESIS
STORAGE
RELEASE
MITOCHONDRIAL SPACE
O_2
Cytochromes Etc.
$2H_2O$
Pyruvate
NAD^+
NADH
Pyruvate Dehydrogenase
AcetylCoA
Citric Acid Cycle
Acetyl "carrier" (citrate)
Acetyl "carrier"
ATP
Citrate lyase
AcetylCoA
CHOLINERGIC NEURON
T
ChAT
$Choline_{ECF}$
$Choline_{ACh}$
STATIONARY ACh
SURPLUS ACh
LESS READILY RELEASABLE ACh
READILY RELEASABLE ACh
NEWLY SYNTHESIZED ACh
ChAT
$Choline_{ICF}$
CK
PHOSPHOLIPIDS
$ATP+H_2O$
ChAT
nH^+
ACh
VESICLE
nH^+
VESICLE
ADP+Pi
MEDIATOPHORE
Released ACh
AChE
Ch + Ac

Neural output from the carotid body was recorded from the whole carotid sinus nerve, minus the baroreceptors which were thermally and mechanically manipulated to destroy the mechanoreceptor endings.

2.2. Protocol

After one hour recovery from surgery the animal was paralyzed and artificially ventilated. Blood gas values were adjusted with changes in ventilation and/or the administration of sodium bicarbonate. A challenge to the carotid body consisted of a perfusion of Krebs Ringer bicarbonate solutions (KRB) for varying lengths of time depending on the agent. The KRB was rendered either hypoxic by equilibrating it with 6% O_2/5% CO_2 or hyperoxic by equilibrating it with 95% O_2/5% CO_2.

3. RESULTS

3.1. Inhibiting Mediatophore, the Membrane Protein That Mediates the Direct Release of Vesicular ACh (Fig 2)

Assuming that ACh is an excitatory neuroagent in the carotid body, we first tried to determine if cetiedil (alpha-cyclohexyl-3-thienylacetic acid 2-(hexahydro-1H-azepin-1-yl)ethyl ester, citrate salt) had an effect in the carotid body which could be interpreted as a reduction in the release of ACh. We have begun this investigation using high doses of the agent (250 and 500 μM), and observed a very rapid decline in carotid sinus nerve activity to 50% of the maximum at 80 sec after beginning the perfusion of hypoxic KRB containing 250 μM cetiedil, and to pre-infusion levels of activity at 120 s. The higher dose reduced the response to hypoxic KRB to 50% of the maximum in 50 s, and to pre-infusion levels at 80 s. These effects were readily reversible upon re-exposure of the carotid body to its own arterial blood for from three to five minutes.

3.2. Inhibiting the Packaging of ACh in Vesicles (Fig 3)

Vesamicol (L-trans-2-(4-phenylpiperidin)cyclohexanol [L-AH5183]) inhibits the evoked quantal release of ACh from a wide range of intact preparations (Bahr & Parsons, 1986). Using graded doses of vesamicol we have observed what appears to be a dose-related depression in the response to hypoxic KRB. This depression was not significant at a concentration of 50 μM; it was so at 90 s when 100 μM was used. And at higher concentrations the depression was observed within 30–40 s.

3.3. Inhibiting ChAT

There is no known inhibitor of ChAT that is potent, specific, stable, and crosses cellular membranes. Some of the analogs of styrylpyridine are potent inhibitors, but are also inhibitors of acetylcholinesterase (AChE). The two styrylpyridines that inhibit ChAT *in vivo* without causing inhibition of AChE (naphthylvinyl pyridine and 4-chlorostilbazole) are also the least potent, therefore requiring large doses in the *in vivo* situation. In other systems such doses have caused side effects that make the results difficult to interpret in terms of ChAT inhibition. Halogenated analogs of the substrates have been helpful in

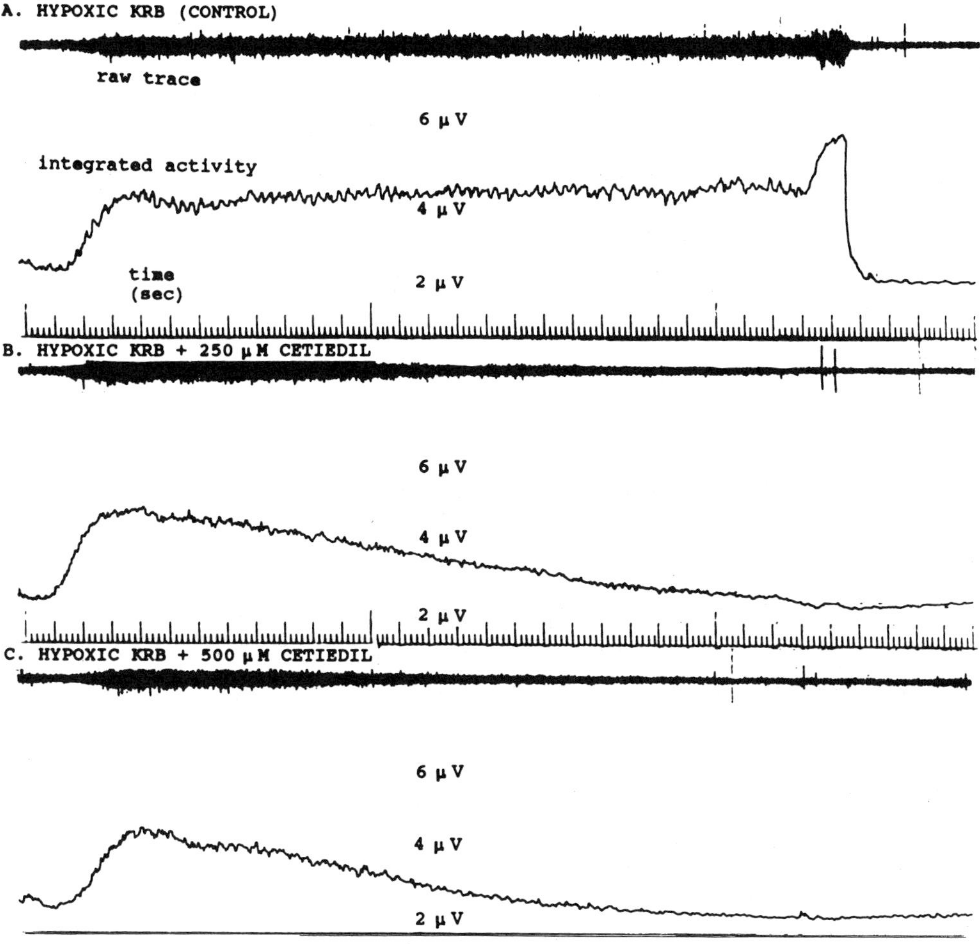

Figure 2. Polygraph tracing of the neural response (μV) from the carotid body to hypoxic KRB and to hypoxic KRB containing either 250 or 500 μM cetiedil.

studying mechanisms of the enzyme in isolation, but *in vivo* are unstable, probably would not penetrate readily into cells, and are likely to be nonspecific (Haubrich, 1976).

3.4. Inhibiting the Availability of Acetyl CoA

The carbon atoms of Acetyl CoA used in the synthesis of ACh have been shown to derive from cytosolic glucose. After becoming pyruvate these carbon atoms go into the mitochondria where via the citric acid cycle they become citrate and are transported out of the mitochondrion. At this point citrate lyase breaks down the citrate into Acetyl CoA and oxaloacetate. Inhibiting citrate lyase prevents acetyl CoA from entering into the synthesis of ACh. Several reports in different systems have demonstrated that hydroxycitrate is an inhibitor of citrate lyase. The most recent report of Burton and his colleagues (Burton et al, 1995) demonstrated that 2 and 4 mM hydroxycitrate in the solution perfusing the brain-stem of neonatal rats reduced the phrenic nerve output in 2 minutes or less. To date we

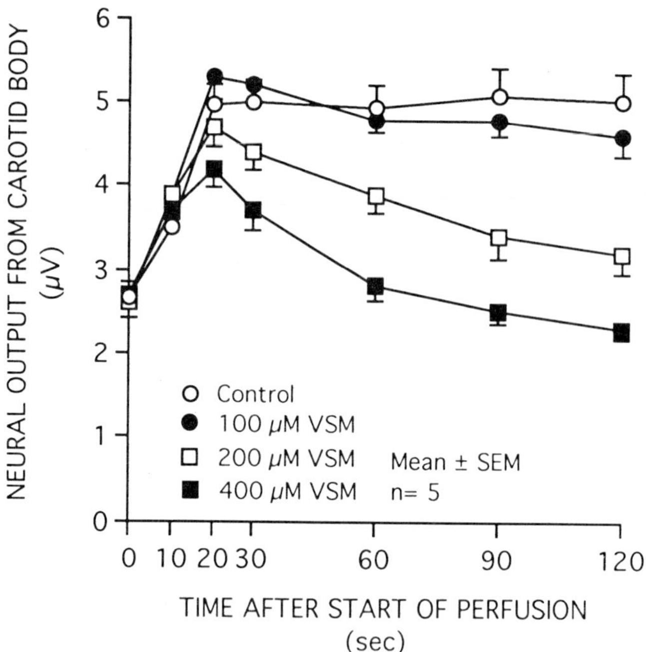

Figure 3. Summary of the neural response (μV) from the carotid body to hypoxic KRB, and to hypoxic KRB containing either 100, 200, or 400 μM vesamicol.

have found a five minute perfusion of hypoxic KRB containing 3 mM hydroxycitrate to be ineffective in reducing the response of the carotid body to the hypoxic perfusate.

3.5. Altering the Availability of Choline

The synthesis and release of ACh is essentially dependent on the presence of extracellular choline. Perfusing the carotid body with hypoxic KRB which contained 30 μM choline produced a response which was 20–25% greater than that produced by the hypoxic choline-free perfusate. Conversely 30 μM hemicholinium-3 (HC-3), an inhibitor of the high affinity choline uptake transporter in cholinergic neurons and presumably in the Type I cell of the carotid body, reduced the response of the carotid body to the hypoxic perfusate (Fig 4).

4. DISCUSSION

We must emphasize that these studies are in progress. Hence, our results with cetiedil and with vesamicol are still very tentative. When perfusing the brainstem of the neonatal rat *in vitro* with cetiedil solutions, Burton and his colleagues used concentrations of 177, 885, and 1770 μM (Burton et al, 1994). The two higher concentrations produced a rapid significant depression of phrenic nerve output. We chose intermediate concentrations assuming that the more extensive vasculature of the carotid body would deliver the agent to the susceptible locus on the Type I cell with greater efficiency than a perfusate

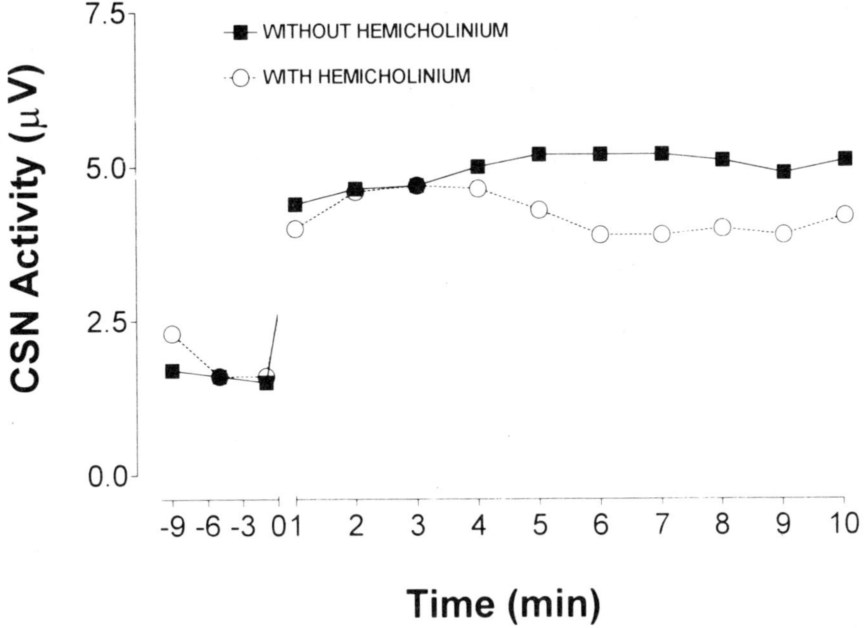

Figure 4. Neural response (μV) from the carotid body perfused first for 10 min with hyperoxic/normocapnic KRB either free from or containing 30 μM hemicholinium. At time 0 a second perfusion was immediately initiated. The effect of hemicholinium took about 5 min to manifest itself.

passing over the surface of the brainstem. We saw a very impressive reduction 40 s after the neural activity had reached its maximum response to the hypoxic KRB. Hence, it is quite conceivable that significantly lower doses perfused over 1–2 min will also reduce the response to hypoxic KRB.

With vesamicol we are also currently changing the design to study the effects of lower concentrations perfused over longer periods. We will also use the D-enantiomer of vesamicol as a control for any non-specific effects. The D-enantiomer is reportedly 25 times less effective than the L-enantiomer.

If one assumes that ACh is an excitatory neurotransmitter in the carotid body and that there appears to be some parallels between the carotid body and the superior cervical ganglion with respect to cholinergic neural transmission, the effect of choline on the neural activity from the carotid body was not particularly surprising. For Birks & MacIntosh (1961) found that if choline was absent from the extracellular fluid of the cat, then the release of ACh from the stimulated, perfused *in situ* superior cervical ganglion was reduced. Further, they found that adding choline to the Locke's solution perfusing the ganglion could maintain ACh turnover at a high level as long as stimulation continued. Collier & MacIntosh (1969) found that in the superior cervical ganglion perfused with physiological concentrations of choline, the rate of choline transport was faster when the tissue was depolarized by electrical stimulation than it was in non-depolarized tissue. And the rate of synthesis of ACh is higher in an active ganglion than in a resting ganglion. Others have made similar observations (Haubrich & Chippendale, 1977; O'Regan & Collier, 1981; Sacchi et al, 1978).

Addition of HC-3 to the perfusion medium slows the synthesis of ACh in the ganglion with a resulting depletion of transmitter-destined ACh and a reduction in ACh release (Birks & MacIntosh, 1961). Our brief perfusions of 30 μM HC-3 have to date clearly depressed the response to hypoxic KRB; these depressions have been readily reversible upon returning the carotid body to its own arterial blood.

The results reported above must be considered as "work-in-progress". But taken as they are, they suggest a significant excitatory role for ACh in the neural output from the cat's carotid body perfused *in situ* with hypoxic KRB.

5. ACKNOWLEDGMENTS

Supported by HL 50712 and HL 47044.

6. REFERENCES

Bahr BA & Parsons SM (1986) Demonstration of a receptor in *Torpedo* synaptic vesicles for the acetylcholine storage blocker L-trans-2-(4-phenyl[3,4-^{3}H]-piperidine)cyclohexanol. Proc Natl Acad Sci USA 83: 2267–2270

Baker D & Brown DH (1992) Direct measurement of acetylcholine release in guinea-pig trachea. Am J Physiol 263: L142-L147

Ballard KJ & Jones, JV (1972) Demonstration of choline acetyltransferase activity in the carotid body of the cat. J Physiol, London 227: 87–94

Birks R & MacIntosh FC (1961) Acetylcholine metabolism of a sympathetic ganglion. Can J Biochem Physiol 39: 787–827

Burton MD, Nouri K, Baichoo S, Samuels-Toyloy N & Kazemi H (1994) Ventilatory output and acetylcholine: perturbations in release and muscarinic receptor activation. J Appl Physiol 77: 2275–2284

Burton MD, Nouri M & Kazemi H (1995) Acetylcholine and central respiratory control: perturbations of acetylcholine synthesis in the isolated brainstem of the neonatal rat. Brain Res 670: 39–47

Collier B & MacIntosh FC (1969) The source of choline for acetylcholine synthesis in a sympathetic ganglion. Can J Physiol Pharmacol 47: 127–135

Dinger BG, Hirano T & Fidone SJ (1986) Autoradiographic localization of muscarinic receptors in rabbit carotid body. Brain Res 367: 328–331

Fidone S, Weintraub S & Stavinoha W (1976) Acetylcholine content of normal and denervated cat carotid bodies measured by pyrolysis gas chromatography/mass fragmentometry. J Neurochem 26: 1047–1049

Fidone S, Weintraub S, Stavinoha W, Stirling C & Jones L (1977) Endogenous acetylcholine levels in cat carotid body and the autoradiographic localization of a high affinity component of choline uptake. In: Acker H, Fidone S, Pallot D, Eyzaguirre C, Lübbers DW & Torrance RW (eds) Chemoreception in the Carotid Body. Berlin: Springer-Verlag. pp 106–113

Fitzgerald RS & Shirahata M (1994) Acetylcholine and carotid body excitation during hypoxia in the cat. J Appl Physiol 76: 1566–1574

Fitzgerald RS, Shirahata M & Ide T (1995) Cholinergic dimensions to carotid body chemotransduction. In: Semple SJG, Adams L & Whipp BJ (eds) Modelling and Control of Ventilation. New York: Plenum Press. pp 303–308

Goldberg AM, Lentz AP & Fitzgerald RS (1978) Neurotransmitter mechanisms in the carotid body: absence of ACh in the carotid sinus nerve. Brain Res 140: 374–377

Haubrich DR (1976) Choline acetyltransferase and its inhibitors. In: Goldberg AM & Hanin I (eds) Biology of Cholinergic Function. New York: Raven Press. pp 239–268

Haubrich DR & Chippendale TJ (1977) Regulation of acetylcholine synthesis in nervous tissue. Life Sci 20: 1465–1478

O'Regan S & Collier B (1981) Effect of increasing choline, *in vivo* and *in vitro* on the synthesis of acetylcholine in a sympathetic ganglion. J Neurochem 36: 420–430

Sacchi O, Consolo S, Peri G, Prigioni I, Landinsky H & Perri V (1978) Storage and release of acetylcholine in the isolated cervical ganglion of the rat. Brain Res 151: 443–456

Wang ZZ, Stensaas LJ, Dinger B & Fidone SJ (1989) Immunocytochemical localization of choline acetyltransferase in the carotid body of the cat and rabbit. Brain Res 498: 131–134

LOCALIZATION OF NICOTINIC ACETYLCHOLINE RECEPTORS IN CAT CAROTID BODY AND PETROSAL GANGLION

Yumiko Ishizawa, Robert S. Fitzgerald, Machiko Shirahata, and Brian Schofield

The Johns Hopkins Medical Institutions
Baltimore, Maryland

1. INTRODUCTION

How the carotid body converts hypoxic stimuli into neural activity remains largely unknown. Several neurotransmitters, which have been demonstrated in type I cells in the carotid body, are still candidates for primary neurotransmitter(s) of chemotransduction.

Our previous pharmacological studies using adult cats have shown that cholinergic blockers, including mecamylamine, and atropine reduced the increased neural output from the carotid body during hypoxic perfusion (Fitzgerald & Shirahata, 1994). A nicotinic blocker, mecamylamine by itself also reduced hypoxic excitation of carotid sinus nerve activities in dose-related fashion (Fitzgerald et al, in press). We thus hypothesized that acetylcholine (ACh) was playing an excitatory role in carotid body chemotransduction in the cat.

However, where ACh is playing an excitatory role has not been elucidated. Although α-bungarotoxin binding sites and muscarinic antagonist binding sites have been reported to be expressed on the carotid body cells (Dinger et al, 1981, 1986; Chen & Yates, 1984), their roles remain unclear. Nicotinic receptors (nAChR) other than α-bungarotoxin binding sites, which have been reported to be abundantly expressed both in the central nervous system and the peripheral nervous system (McGehee & Role, 1995), could also be playing important roles in chemotransduction. The purpose of the present study was to identify and localize nAChR in the carotid body cells and in the petrosal ganglion neurons.

2. METHODS

2.1. Cell Culture

Adults cats of either sex were used in this study. We used the culture procedures which we developed previously to culture the carotid body cells (Shirahata et al, 1994).

Briefly, both carotid bodies and petrosal ganglia were excised from anesthetized adult cats. The tissues were incubated with 0.1–0.2% collagenase and then gently triturated. The cell suspension was divided into the wells which were previously treated with poly-D-lysine (Sigma) and diluted basement membrane complex (Matrigel, Collaborative Biomedical Products).

A chemically defined culture medium which has been used to culture hippocampal neurons was used (Brewer et al, 1993). The basic nutrient solution was Neurobasal™ (GIBCO/BRL), which was supplemented by B-27 supplement (GIBCO/BRL), L-glutamine, and 7s-nerve growth factor. The cells were cultured for 3 to 7 days and fixed with S.T.F.™ (Streck Tissue Fixative; Streck Laboratories, Inc).

2.2. Tissue Preparation

To prepare frozen tissue sections we perfused carotid bodies and petrosal ganglia with S.T.F.™ through the common carotid arteries. Then the tissues were removed and kept in the fixative for 6–12 hours. After the tissues were frozen in embedding medium, 8–16 μm sections were cut in a cryostat.

2.3. Immunocytochemistry

The monoclonal antibodies to nAChR α4 subunits (mAb299) and β2 subunits (mAb290) were used to detect immunoreactivity of nAChR. The monoclonal antibodies to tyrosine hydroxylase (TH) and glial fibrillary acidic protein (GFAP) were also used to identify type I and type II cells in the carotid body, respectively.

The tissue sections and cultured cells were incubated with the monoclonal antibodies to α4 and β2 subunits for 2–3 hours at room temperature and with the antibodies to TH and GFAP for 1 hour at room temperature. We applied standard ABC technique to both tissue sections and cultured cells. As chromogen 3-amino-9-ethylcarbazole and 3,3'-diaminobenzidine (VECTOR) were used.

3. RESULTS

In the cultured carotid body cells, α4 subunits of nAChR were expressed in both single cells (Fig 1) and the cells in clusters. The α4 -subunit immunoreactive cells were not stained for GAFAP, suggesting they are type I cells or a subgroup of type I cells. β2 subunits of nAChR seem to be absent or only very weakly expressed in cultured carotid body cells. In the tissue sections of the carotid body, some of the cells in glomeruli were stained for α4 subunits, but there was no appreciable immunoreactivity for β2 subunits in the carotid body.

The α4 subunits of nAChR were expressed in the cell bodies of petrosal ganglion neurons in both tissue sections and culture. Some of the nerve fibers in the petrosal ganglion appeared to be positive for α4 subunits. β2 subunits were negative or very weakly expressed in petrosal ganglion neurons in both tissue and culture.

We applied the same monoclonal antibodies to α4 and β2 subunits to superior cervical ganglion sections, in which mRNA of α4 and β2 subunits have been demonstrated in the rat. Some of the superior cervical ganglion neurons showed the immunoreactivity of α4 subunits, but the immunoreactivity of β2 subunits seemed to be absent.

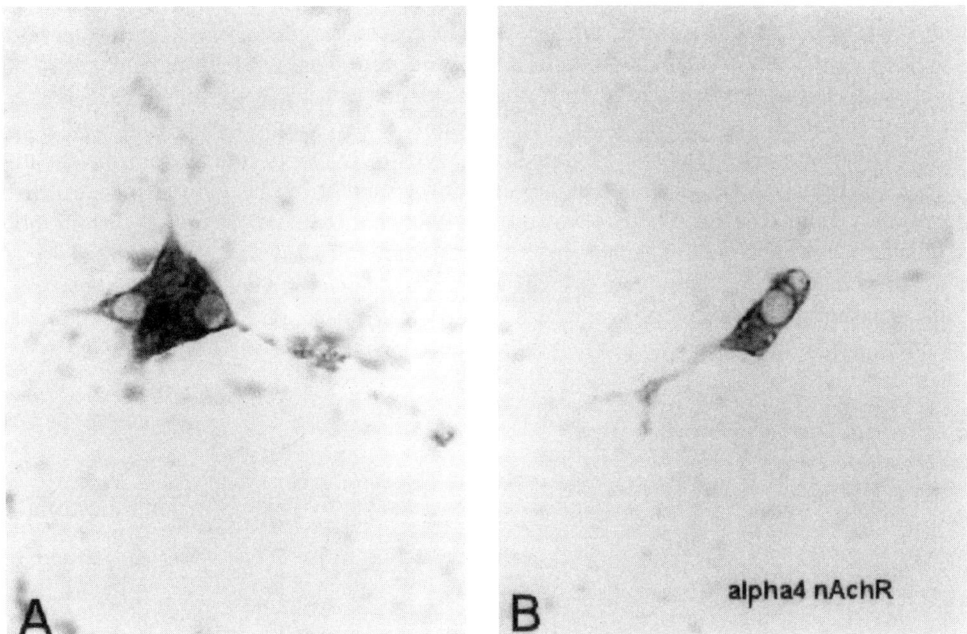

Figure 1. Carotid body cells cultured for 6 days. α4 subunit of nAChR was immunostained with the ABC technique. The cell bodies as well as processes were stained for α4 subunits.

4. DISCUSSION

Although early biochemical studies have shown a dominant role of α4 and β2 in the central nervous system and α3 and β4 in the peripheral nervous system, recent data indicate a significant variety of nAChR (McGehee & Role, 1995). The expression of α4 subunit in the carotid body cells and the petrosal ganglion neurons suggests that those cells express α4-containing nAChR, whose mRNA has recently been demonstrated in the rat superior cervical ganglion (Klimaschewski et al, 1994). Since the α subunits α2, α3,and α4 form distinct ACh-activated channels when expressed in combination with β2 or β4 (McGehee & Role, 1995), it is possible that the carotid body and petrosal ganglion have β4 subunits, or the other combination including α2 or α3.

Since α-bungarotoxin binding sites have previously been shown in type I cells, our present finding of α4 subunit on type I cells indicates the multiplicity of nAChR subtypes in the carotid body, which has been well described in chick ciliary ganglion neurons (Conroy & Berg, 1995). Recently McGehee et al (1995) reported that both α-bungarotoxin binding sites, which have low affinity for nicotine, and nAChR with high-affinity for nicotine are present on presynaptic neurons in lumbar sympathetic ganglion. They also suggested that high-affinity nicotine binding sites may play a compensatory role for α-bungarotoxin binding sites based on the experiment using α7 antisense treated culture (McGehee, 1995). In the carotid body physiological roles of nAChR might be associated with individual subtypes as well.

In our culture conditions, α4 subunits of nAChR were expressed in type I cells and in the petrosal ganglion neurons, which is consistent with our findings in tissue sections.

Recently we have reported that the expression of proteins in type I cells, such as tyrosine hydroxylase and neuron specific enolase, seemed to change over 2-week culture period (Ishizawa et al, 1995). The expression of nAChR has also been reported to be changed in PC12 cells and in M10 cells following various treatment in culture (Rogers et al, 1992; Zhang et al, 1995). The nAChR might be susceptible to culturing procedures as well as to culture conditions. The changes in expression of nAChR in our culture thus need to be investigated. However, the observed expression of α4 subunit in our culture indicates that the primary cultured carotid body cells and petrosal ganglion neurons can be a useful tool to elucidate further cellular mechanisms of chemotransduction.

In conclusion, localization of α4 subunit of nAChR in type I cells and in the petrosal ganglion neurons supports our hypothesis that ACh is an excitatory neurotransmitter in chemotransduction. Further studies on pre- and postsynaptic roles of ACh are needed.

5. ACKNOWLEDGMENTS

The antibodies to nAChR subunits were generously provided by Dr. Jon Lindstrom.

6. REFERENCES

Brewer GJ, Torricelli JR, Evege EK & Price PJ (1993) Optimized survival of hippocampal neurons in B27-supplemented Neurobasal, a new serum-free medium combination. J Neurosci Res 35: 567–576

Chen IL & Yates RD (1984) Two types of glomus cell in the rat carotid body as revealed by α-bungarotoxin binding. J Neurocytol 13: 281–302

Conroy WG & Berg DK (1995) Neurons can maintain multiple classes of nicotinic acetylcholine receptors distinguished by different subunit compositions. J Biochem Mol Biol 270: 4424–4431

Dinger B, González C, Yoshizaki K & Fidone S (1981) Alpha-bungarotoxin binding in cat carotid body. Brain Res 205: 187–193

Dinger BG, Hirano T & Fidone SJ (1986) Autoradiographic localization of muscarinic receptors in rabbit carotid body. Brain Res 367: 328–331

Fitzgerald RS & Shirahata M (1994) Acetylcholine and carotid body excitation during hypoxia an the cat. J Appl Physiol 76: 1566–1574

Fitzgerald RS, Shirahata M & Ide T (1996) Further cholinergic aspects of carotid body chemotransduction of hypoxia in the cat. J Appl Physiol (In press)

Ishizawa Y, Schofield B, Chou CL & Shirahata M (1995) Changes in protein expression of cultured cat glomus cells. ISOTT95 Satellite Symposium: Adaptation to Hypoxia. IV.3

Klimaschewski L, Reuss S, Spessert R, Lobron C, Wevers A, Heym C, Maelicke A & Schröder H (1994) Expression of nicotinic acetylcholine receptors in the rat superior cervical ganglion mRNA and protein level. Mol Brain Res 27: 167–173

McGehee DS & Role LW (1995) Physiological diversity of nicotinic acetylcholine receptors expressed by vertebrate neurons. Annu Rev Physiol 57: 521–546

McGehee DS, Heath MJ, Gelber S, Devay P & Role LW (1995) Nicotinic enhancement of fast excitatory synaptic transmission in CNS by presynaptic receptors. Science 269: 1692–1696

Rogers SW, Mandelzys A, Deneris ES, Cooper E & Heinemann S (1992) The expression of nicotinic acetylcholine receptors by PC12 cells treated with NGF. J Neurosci 12: 4611–4623

Shirahata M, Schofield B, Chin BY & Guilarte TR (1994) Culture of arterial chemoreceptor cells from adult cats in defined medium. Brain Res 658: 60–66

Zhang X, Gong Z-H, Hellström-Lindahl E & Nordberg A (1995) Regulation of α4 β2 nicotinic acetylcholine receptors in M10 cells following treatment with nicotinic agents. NeuroReport 6: 313–317

EFFECT OF ACETYLCHOLINE ON INTRACELLULAR CALCIUM OF CAROTID BODY CELLS OF ADULT CATS

Machiko Shirahata,[1,2] Robert S. Fitzgerald,[1,3,4] and James S. K. Sham[4]

[1] Department of Environmental Health Sciences
[2] Department of Anesthesiology/Critical Care Medicine
[3] Department of Physiology
[4] Department of Medicine
The Johns Hopkins Medical Institutions
Baltimore, Maryland 21205

1. INTRODUCTION

Recent studies of neuronal nicotinic acetylcholine receptors (nAChRs) have begun to reveal an important role of the presynaptic nAChRs for controlling release of neurotransmitters in the central and peripheral nervous system (McGehee & Role, 1995; McGehee et al, 1995). In the carotid body application of nicotine release catecholamines (Obeso et al, 1987; Dinger et al, 1985; Gomez-Nino et al, 1990). The nicotine-induced release of dopamine depends on the presence of extracellular calcium (Obeso et al, 1987). Further, the presence of α-bungarotoxin binding sites on glomus cells have been shown in rats and cats (Dinger et al, 1985; Chen et al, 1981), and ACh-induced inward currents have been observed in rat glomus cells (Wyatt & Peers, 1993). Nicotinic AChRs are the class of the ligand-gated cation channels. Calcium permeability of nAChRs is much greater than muscle-type nAChR. Among them α7 subunit-containing nAChRs (α-bungarotoxin sensitive receptors) are the most permeable to Ca^{2+} among ligand-gated channels (Role, 1996; McGehee & Role, 1995). This high calcium flux not only contributes to the total currents through nAChRs. The resultant increase in intracellular calcium also influences the dynamics of neurotransmitter release. In this study we examined the effect of ACh on intracellular calcium concentration in order to understand the role of presynaptic nAChRs of the carotid body.

2. METHODS

2.1. Cell Culture

Carotid body cells were cultured as previously described (Shirahata et al, 1994) with slight modifications. In short, carotid bodies were harvested from adult cats which were deeply anesthetized with pentobarbital (30–40 mg/kg, ip, then 50 mg/kg iv). Both carotid bodies were dissociated with collagenase (0.1–0.2 %, Sigma, type XI) and gentle trituration. The cells were divided into 10–15 wells. Each well consisted of a glass coverslip and a plastic cloning cylinder (Speciality Media). Wells were placed in a regular 30 mm culture dish, and the cells were cultured in a 5% CO_2/air incubator at 37° C using a defined medium up to two weeks.

2.2. Measurement of $[Ca^{2+}]_i$

$[Ca^{2+}]_i$ was measured with microfluorometric methods using Indo-1 (Molecular-probes, Inc.). The dye loading was performed by exposure of cells for 1 hour to Indo-1 (1 μM) in the 5% CO_2/air incubator at 37°C. Subsequently, a coverslip with cells was pasted to a bottom of a recording chamber with silicon glue. The recording chamber was heated with circulating water at 37°C. The chamber was mounted on an inverted microscope (TMD, Nikon), and the cells were superfused with a 1:1 mixture of Dulbecco's modified Eagle's medium and Ham's F12 medium (DMEM/F12, Sigma) for 45 min to wash out excess Indo-1. During the experiments the cells were continuously superfused with Krebs solution with or without chemical agents. Indo-1 in the cells was repeatedly excited at a wavelength of 395 nm (for 35 ms at every 2 s). Two wavelengths of emission light (405 nm, F_{405}; 495 nm, F_{495}) were collected from a restricted microscope field, which contained a small cluster of the carotid body cells. PC based computer and PClamp software were used for acquisition of the data. $[Ca^{2+}]_i$ was calculated with a following equation (Grynkiewicz et al, 1985) using Lotus 1–2–3 (Novell Inc.): $[Ca^{2+}]I = K_d \times \beta \times (R - R_{min}) / (R_{max} - R)$, where $R = (F_{405} - F_{405,bg}) / (F_{495} - F_{495,bg})$, $\beta = F_{min} / F_{max}$, and K_D of Indo-1 is 288 nM. F_{max} and F_{min} were obtained by exposing the cells to Tyrode solutions containing 10 mM $[Ca^{2+}]_i$ or 10 mM EGTA. Both Tyrode solutions included calcium ionophore (A23187; Calbiochem-Novabiochem Corp). Background signals ($F_{405,bg}$, $F_{495,bg}$) were measured by quenching Indo-1 with $MnCl_2$.

Krebs solutions and DMEM/F12 were equilibrated with 5% CO_2/16% O_2/79% N_2, and the same gas was supplied on the top of the superfusate in the recording chamber. All solutions were superfused using a peristaltic pump (Minipuls 3, Gilson) at a rate of 2 ml/min.

3. RESULTS

3.1. Dose-Response Relationship

Control Krebs solution was changed to Krebs containing ACh (1, 3, 10, or 100 μM) for 2 min. Most clusters were exposed to ACh more than once. A lower concentration was used first and twenty to thirty minutes were allowed between the challenges. On exposure of ACh $[Ca^{2+}]_i$ increased quickly. The maximal level was sustained at low concentrations of ACh (1 or 10 μM), but at the higher concentration the maximal level decayed. Removal

Table 1. Dose-dependent effect of ACh on increase in $[Ca^{2+}]_i$ of clusters of chemoreceptor cells

Dose (μM)		1	3	10	100
$[Ca^{2+}]_i$ (nM)	Mean	16	16	68	152
	SEM	6	9	13	14
	N	6	3	7	7

of ACh returned $[Ca^{2+}]_i$ to the control level. The responses differed among clusters. Nevertheless, the $[Ca^{2+}]_i$ response to ACh appeared dose-dependent (Table I).

3.2. Effects of Nicotine and Pilocarpine

Effects of nicotine, a nicotinic agonist of ACh, and pilocarpine, a muscarinic agonist, were tested to determine if they mimicked the effect of ACh. Clusters were exposed to 100 μM of ACh, nicotine, or pilocarpine for 45 sec. Increases in $[Ca^{2+}]_i$ by these agents were 124 ± 30, 123 ± 28, 24 ± 9, respectively (Mean ± SEM; n = 5).

3.3. Source of Calcium

To investigate if increase in $[Ca^{2+}]_i$ is due to the influx of Ca^{2+} from extracellular space or due to the release of Ca^{2+} from intracellular storage sites, ACh was administered in nominally Ca^{2+}-free Krebs, or Krebs containing caffeine. The clusters were exposed to these Krebs for 90 sec before superfusion of ACh (45 sec). The response to ACh during Ca-free Krebs and Krebs with caffeine was significantly attenuated. Mean inhibition of ACh responses during Ca^{2+}-free and caffeine-containing are 80 ± 12% (Mean ± SEM; n= 5) and 31 ± 13% (n= 7), respectively.

3.4. Involvement of L-Type Calcium Channels

The possibility that L-type calcium channels are involved in $[Ca^{2+}]_i$ response was tested. The clusters were exposed to Krebs containing 10 μM nifedipine for 90 sec before superfusion of ACh (45 sec). The effect of ACh was depressed to 67 ± 6% of control. The response of the cluster to Krebs containing 100 mM K^+ with or without nifedipine was also examined. Effect of high K was greatly attenuated by nifedipine (24 ± 7% of control; n= 4). Some clusters did not respond to high-K Krebs, suggesting a lack of functional voltage-gated calcium channels. However, ACh still increased $[Ca^{2+}]_i$.

4. DISCUSSION

This study demonstrated that cultured cat carotid body cells increase $[Ca^{2+}]_i$ by virtue of the nicotinic, not the muscarinic, effects of ACh. Recent studies have shown that neuronal nAChRs are highly permeable to Ca^{2+} with the permeability ratio of Ca^{2+} to Na^+ ranging from 1 to 20 depending on the subunits of the neuronal nAChRs. The EC_{50} of ACh in the peripheral nervous system are between 35 and 133 μM (McGehee & Role, 1995; Role, 1996). A rapid decay of the nicotinic receptor currents (desensitization) is often observed. All these characteristics of neuronal nAChRs are well fitted to the $[Ca^{2+}]_i$

response to ACh in chemoreceptor cells. The mechanisms responsible for the ACh-mediated increase in $[Ca^{2+}]_i$ in chemoreceptor cells are complex. The increase appears to be due mainly to the influx of extracellular Ca^{2+} through nAChRs. This view is consistent with the observation that nicotine-induced dopamine release from the carotid body was inhibited by a nominally calcium-free environment (Obeso et al, 1987). However, caffeine partially depressed the increase in $[Ca^{2+}]_i$, suggesting the contribution of intracellular storage sites to this increase. Another possible mechanism accounting for the ACh-induced increase in $[Ca^{2+}]_i$ is an ACh-induced depolarization of glomus cells and activation of voltage-gated calcium channels, followed by the influx of calcium ions. Other reports have indicated that ACh depolarizes glomus cells (Hayashida & Eyzaguirre, 1979; Wyatt & Peers, 1993). The fact that nifedipine attenuated ACh response indicates the contribution of L-type calcium channels to the increase in $[Ca^{2+}]_i$ by ACh. On the other hand, some clusters did not respond to high-K, suggesting the absence of functional voltage-gated calcium channels. These cells, however, still responded to ACh. Thus, ACh increases $[Ca^{2+}]_i$ even without the involvement of voltage-gated calcium channels. Determination of subunits of nAChRs that are responsible for increasing $[Ca^{2+}]_i$ needs further study. Nonetheless, our data, taken together with other studies, suggest that the nAChRs on glomus cells may play a significant role in regulating the release of neurotransmitters from these cells.

5. ACKNOWLEDGMENTS

This work was supported by grants HL 47044, HL 50712, and HL 52652.

6. REFERENCES

Chen I, Mascorro JA & Yates RD (1981) Autoradiographic localization of alpha-bungarotoxin-binding sites in the carotid body of the rat. Cell Tissue Res 219: 609–618

Dinger B, Gonzalez C, Yoshizaki K & Fidone S (1985) Localization and function of cat carotid body nicotinic receptors. Brain Res 339: 295–304

Gomez-Nino A, Dinger B, Gonzalez C & Fidone SJ (1990) Differential stimulus coupling to dopamine and norepinephrine stores in rabbit carotid body type I cells. Brain Res 525: 160–164

Grynkiewicz G, Poenie M & Tsien R (1985) A new generation of Ca^{2+} indicators with greatly improved fluorescence properties. J Biol Chem 260: 3440–3450

Hayashida Y & Eyzaguirre C (1979) Voltage noise of carotid body type I cells. Brain Res 167: 189–194

McGehee DS & Role LW (1995) Physiological diversity of nicotinic acetylcholine receptors expressed by vertebrate neurons. Annu Rev Physiol 57: 521–546

McGehee DS, Heath MJS, Gelber S, Devay P & Role LW (1995) Nicotine enhancement of fast excitatory synaptic transmission in CNS by presynaptic receptors. Science 269: 1692–1696

Obeso A, Fidone S & Gonzalez C (1987) Pathways for calcium entry into type I cells: Significance for the secretory response. In: Ribeiro JA & Pallot DJ (eds) Chemoreceptors in Respiratory Control. London: Croom Helm. pp 91–97

Role LW (1996) Diversity in primary structure and function of neuronal nicotinic acetylcholine receptor channels. Current Opinions Neurobiol 2: 254–262

Shirahata M, Schofield B, Chin BY & Guilarte TR (1994) Culture of arterial chemoreceptor cells from adult cats in defined medium. Brain Res 658: 60–66

Wyatt CN, Peers C (1993) Nicotinic acetylcholine receptors in isolated type I cells of the neonatal rat carotid body. Neuroscience 54: 275–281

39

DOPAMINE EFFLUX FROM THE CAROTID BODY DURING HYPOXIC STIMULATION

P. Zapata, R. Iturriaga, and J. Alcayaga

Laboratory of Neurobiology
Catholic University of Chile
Santiago, Chile

1. INTRODUCTION

The carotid bodies of cats are known to contain high levels of dopamine (DA), persisting even after complete denervation of these organs (Zapata et al, 1969; Mir et al, 1982; Fitzgerald et al, 1983). Thus DA appears to be concentrated in glomus cells, characterized by their chromaffin reaction, abundance in dense-core granules and formaldehyde-induced fluorescence (see Eyzaguirre & Zapata, 1984). Since the DA content and the number of dense-core granules are reduced in direct proportion to the severity and duration of hypoxia in rats (Hanbauer & Hellström, 1978; Hansen, 1981), and radiolabeled DA effluxes from rabbit and cat carotid bodies —in parallel with the frequency of carotid chemosensory discharges (f_x)— are also proportional to the intensity of hypoxic superfusions (Fidone et al, 1982; Rigual et al, 1986), the idea that DA serves as the glomus cell to sensory nerve endings transmitter during hypoxia is highly attractive (see Gonzalez et al, 1994).

On the other hand, exogenous DA applied to cat carotid bodies superfused *in vitro* transiently reduces f_x, this inhibitory effect being reversed into excitation after repeated exposure to this substance (Zapata, 1975). Similarly, intra-arterial and iv injections of DA also produce transient chemosensory inhibition of cat carotid bodies *in situ*, an effect reversed into delayed excitation to high doses of DA only after blockade of D_2 dopaminoceptors (Docherty & McQueen, 1978; Llados & Zapata, 1978). Thus, although endogenous DA is released from the carotid body subjected to hypoxic stimulation, exogenous DA mostly inhibits chemosensory discharges.

If DA would serve as a mediator of hypoxic stimulation of the carotid body, one should expect: a) a close temporal relation between the increases of DA efflux and f_x during hypoxia, ii) a high correlation between the intensities of DA efflux and chemosensory excitation, and iii) the maintenance of a given relationship between DA efflux and chemosensory excitation upon repeated exposure to hypoxic challenges of the same intensity.

Frontiers in Arterial Chemoreception, edited by Zapata *et al.*
Plenum Press, New York, 1996

2. METHODOLOGICAL CONSIDERATIONS

Measurements of [^{3}H]-DA effluxes from the carotid body require collecting samples of superfusate taken along several minutes, thus precluding the study of its temporal correlation with f_x changes. Fortunately, voltammetric and amperometric methods for detection of catecholamines (CAs) with carbon fiber electrodes (Gonon et al, 1984; Marsden et al, 1988) are now available to study the time course of DA efflux from the carotid body. Thus, Donnelly (1993) found that the peak of the chemosensory response to severe hypoxia preceded the peak of the electrochemical signal by 60 or more seconds in the rat carotid body superfused *in vitro*. But Buerk et al (1995), using gold electrodes, recorded faster DA effluxes in the cat carotid body perfused and superfused *in vitro*.

The studies mentioned above made use of a slow amperometric method, consisting in the application of a continuous fixed potential slightly above the oxidation potential of DA and the recording of the resulting oxidation current. A major disadvantage of this method is that compounds having similar structures exhibit similar oxidation potentials; thus, DA, its metabolite DOPAC, noradrenaline, adrenaline and ascorbic acid, which oxidize at comparable potentials, cannot be differentiated. Covering carbon electrodes with Nafion, a polysulphonated derivative of teflon which is permeable to DA but not to DOPAC or ascorbic acid, reduces considerably their sensitivity to DOPAC and ascorbic acid (Gerhardt et al, 1984). Another way to identify an electroactive compound is by determining the ratio between its oxidation and reduction currents. Thus, the ox:red ratios for ascorbic acid and cyanide are close to 0.0, because these compounds are almost irreversibly oxidized, while DA shows characteristic red:ox ratios of 0.4–0.7, depending on the carbon electrode tip area and number of Nafion covers (Gerhardt et al, 1984).

Therefore, to study the correlation between CA effluxes and chemosensory discharges during hypoxia, we choose a high-speed chronoamperometric system (IVEC-10, Medical System Corp., NY), allowing the simultaneous recording of oxidation and reduction currents at a rate of 5 Hz, while f_x was continuously recorded from the whole carotid sinus nerve. Carotid bodies excised from pentobarbitone anesthetized cats, after which they were superfused (Alcayaga et al, 1993) or perfused-superfused (Iturriaga et al, 1991) *in vitro* with a modified Tyrode's solution with pH 7.40 at 37.5°C, and equilibrated with 20% O_2 under control conditions. Hypoxia was induced by switching to solutions equilibrated with 100% N_2. Nafion coated carbon fibers were gently impaled into the carotid bodies and a potential of +0.55 V, with respect to the reference Ag/AgCl electrode, was applied for 100 ms at a rate of 5 Hz, and averaged and displayed at 1 Hz.

We did not attempt to discriminate between efflux of DA and that of other CAs from the carotid body. However, most of the electroactive signals measured would correspond to DA, since their red:ox ratios were similar to those obtained during the electrode calibration with DA (red:ox = 0.4–0.7). Effluxes of CAs evoked by hypoxic challenges (PO_2 reductions from 125 to 20 Torr) were expressed as ΔCA effluxes over baseline and were computed from the changes of the oxidation currents recorded by the carbon electrodes.

3. CORRELATIONS BETWEEN CA EFFLUX AND CHEMOSENSORY RESPONSE

Figure 1 shows concomitant CA effluxes and chemosensory responses evoked by hypoxic superfusions of a carotid body. The peak in f_x in response to the first stimulus

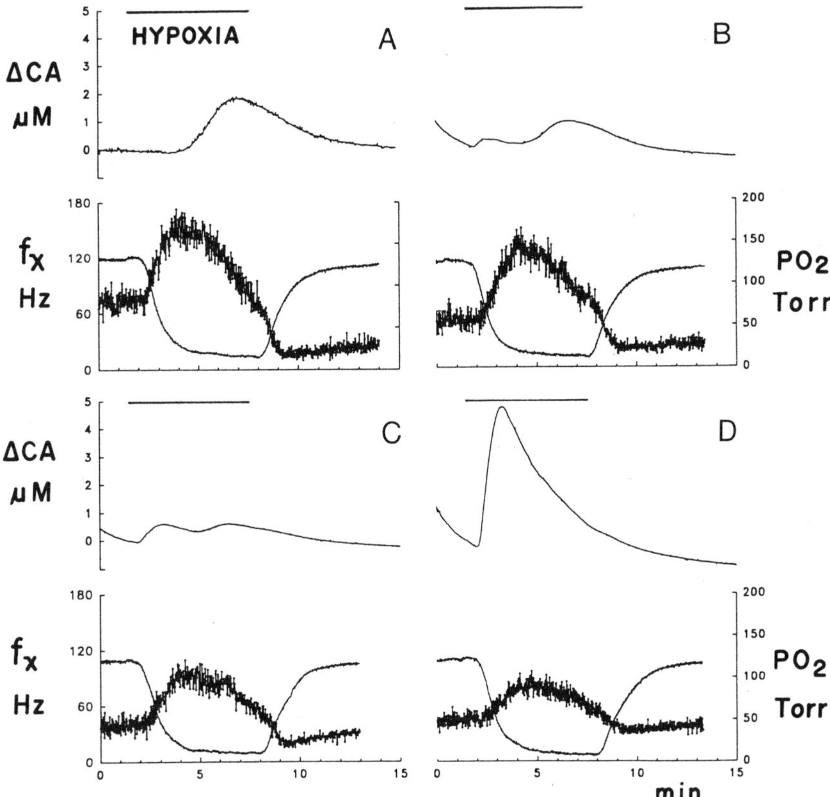

Figure 1. Effects of hypoxia on CA efflux and chemosensory activity of one carotid body. Superfusion with Tyrode's solution equilibrated with 20% O_2 in control conditions; hypoxic superfusions (upper horizontal traces) by switching to Tyrode's solution equilibrated with 100% N_2. ΔCA, catecholamine efflux (upper panels; left ordinates). f_x, frequency of chemosensory discharge (oscillating recordings in lower panels; left ordinates). PO_2, partial pressure of oxygen (smooth recordings in lower panels; right ordinates) of superfusate within the channel, measured by O_2 needle electrode through polarographic sensor. Preparation not previously exposed to exogenous DA (A) and after applying DA-HCl 22 μg (B), 30 μg (C) and 46 μg (D).

was reached after about 2 min, but the maximal CA efflux was reached after about 5 min, at a time when f_x was declining (Fig 1A). In 8 carotid bodies, we observed that the intervals between solutions switching and peak chemosensory responses (154.0 ± 14.5 s) were clearly shorter than those to reach maximal CA effluxes (370.1 ± 35.7 s). Furthermore, it must be noted that the amplitude of the electrochemical currents evoked by repeated hypoxic superfusions of similar intensity show progressive attenuation, in spite of the maintenance of peak f_x's in response to such stimuli.

We have also studied the effect of exogenous DA on the following CA effluxes and chemosensory responses to hypoxic superfusions (Fig 1B-D). If DA is taken up by glomus cells and then released to excite chemosensory nerve endings, we would expect an augmented CA efflux in response to the hypoxic challenge and a concomitantly higher chemosensory excitation. However, CA effluxes elicited by hypoxic superfusions after administering DA exhibit two apparent components: a fast one —only observed after recent exposure to exogenous DA— and a slow one -of similar time-course to those of

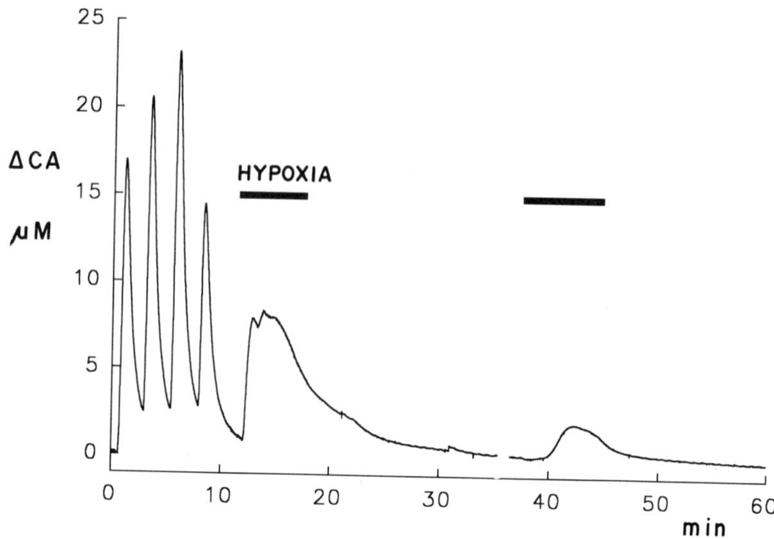

Figure 2. Effects of hypoxia, preceded by four intrastream injections of DA-HCl 15 μg each one, on catecholamine efflux (ΔCA). Superfusion with Tyrode's solution equilibrated with 20% O_2 in control conditions; hypoxic superfusions (upper horizontal traces) by switching to Tyrode's solution equilibrated with 100% N_2.

preparations not previously exposed to exogenous DA. While the slow component shows clear reduction in amplitude upon repeated exposures to hypoxia, the fast component is enhanced by repeated applications of exogenous DA.

Figure 2 illustrates the effects of four intrastream injections of DA applied at 4 min intervals, followed by two hypoxic superfusions separated by 18 min. The first of these challenges induced a prompt and intense release of DA from the carotid body, while the second one induced a markedly reduced and slower ΔCA efflux.

In confirmation of previous observations in cat carotid bodies superfused *in vitro* (Zapata, 1975), the initial injections of DA in the perfused-superfused preparation of the cat carotid body resulted in inhibition of chemosensory discharges. Figure 3 shows the electrochemical signals and chemosensory responses induced by three successive injections of DA into the perfusing line, followed by perfusion with hypoxic saline. Only the first DA injection reduced f_x, after which the preparation became desensitized to further DA injections. The expanded insert in the upper panel allows us to observe that the CA overflow elicited by the hypoxic perfusion was delayed with respect to the fast chemosensory response, recorded in the lower panel.

4. CONCLUSIONS

Our experiments confirm that hypoxia releases DA from the cat carotid body superfused *in vitro* and demonstrate that the same occurs from the carotid body perfused-superfused *in vitro*. Since this last preparation exhibits faster chemosensory responses, it seems to be more appropriate for discerning temporal correlations.

If DA would serve as an excitatory transmitter between glomus cells and chemosensory nerve endings, we should expect a close temporal relationship between DA release

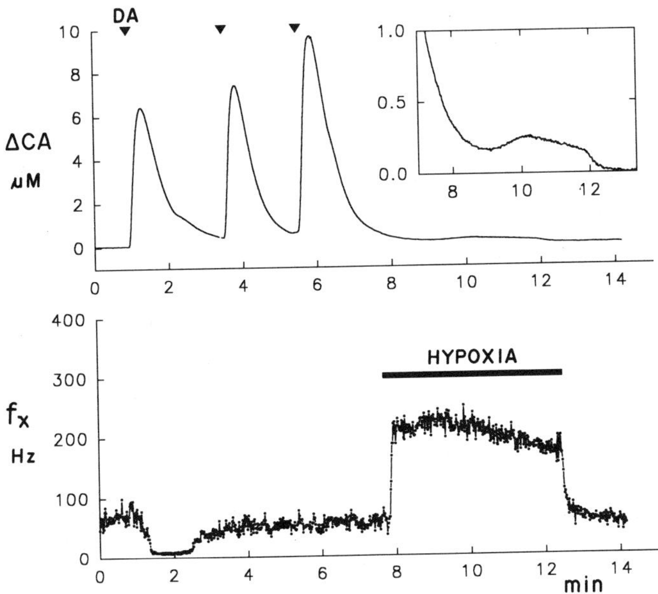

Figure 3. Effects of three consecutive intrastream injections of DA-HCl 100 μg (arrowheads) followed by hypoxia on one carotid body. ΔCA, catecholamine efflux (upper panel). Inset, enlargement of CA efflux recording. f_x, frequency of chemosensory impulses (lower panel). Perfusion and superfusion with Tyrode's solution equilibrated with 20% O_2 in control conditions. Hypoxic perfusion (horizontal trace) by switching to solution equilibrated with 100% N_2.

and chemosensory excitation. However, our results show that the hypoxic challenges evoked fast increases in f_x, but delayed and prolonged CA effluxes. These delayed CA overflows are of similar time-course than those elicited by severe hypoxia in the rat carotid body superfused *in vitro*, as reported by Donnelly (1993). The delayed CA efflux may be explained by a lengthy diffusion distance between the CA source (*i.e.*, conglomerate of glomus cells) and the tip of the electrode placed at the surface of the organ (see Buerk et al, 1995, for discussion).

Despite of the above, pre-loading of the carotid body with exogenous DA significantly shortened the latency and augmented the rate of rise of CA effluxes, without modifying the latency and rate of rise of chemosensory responses. It appears that exogenous DA —recently incorporated to carotid body tissues— is rapidly released when the organ is subsequently exposed to hypoxia, but this DA pool is also rapidly exhausted by repeated or prolonged hypoxic challenges. It is known that the efflux of incorporated radiolabeled DA from carotid body tissues is very fast (Gonzalez et al, 1987).

It must be noted that the hypoxia-induced DA release from the carotid body —either unexposed or exposed to exogenous DA— is rapidly reduced in amount upon repeated exposure to hypoxia. This results in a clear dissociation between the maximal frequencies of chemosensory discharges attained and the peak releases of DA from the stimulated carotid body. That DA efflux into the superfusate rapidly declines is already known from experiments performed in rabbit carotid bodies (Roumy et al, 1988).

In summary, the unsatisfactory and changing time correlation between electrochemical signals of DA release from the carotid body and its changes in chemosensory activity, and the changing correlation between the intensities of both parameters upon repeated hypoxic stimuli of the same strength are not compatible with the proposal that DA released from glomus cells serves as the excitatory transmitter between these cells and chemosensory nerve endings.

5. ACKNOWLEDGMENTS

Work supported by grant FONDECYT 1930645.

Thanks are due to Mrs Carolina Larrain for her valuable help during performance of the experiments, and in the preparation of illustrations.

6. REFERENCES

Alcayaga J, Sanhueza Y & Zapata P (1993) Thermal dependence of chemosensory activity in the carotid body superfused *in vitro*. Brain Res 600: 103–111

Buerk DG, Lahiri S, Chugh D & Mokashi A (1995) Electrochemical detection of rapid DA release kinetics during hypoxia in perfused-superfused cat CB. J Appl Physiol 78: 830–837

Docherty RJ & McQueen DS (1978) Inhibitory action of dopamine on cat carotid chemoreceptors. J Physiol, London 279: 425–436

Donnelly DF (1993) Electrochemical detection of catecholamine release from rat carotid body *in vitro*. J Appl Physiol 74: 2330–2337

Eyzaguirre C & Zapata P (1984) Perspectives in carotid body research. J Appl Physiol 57: 931–957

Fidone S, Gonzalez C & Yoshizaki K (1982) Effects of low oxygen on the release of dopamine from the rabbit carotid body *in vitro*. J Physiol, London 333: 93–110

Fitzgerald RS, Garger P, Hauer MC, Raff H & Fechter L (1983) Effect of hypoxia and hypercapnia on catecholamine content in cat carotid body. J Appl Physiol 54:1408–1413

Gerhardt GA, Oke AF, Nagy G, Moghaddam B & Adams RN (1984) Nafion-coated electrodes with high selectivity for CNS electrochemistry. Brain Res 290: 390–395

Gonon F, Buda M & Pujol JF (1984) Treated carbon fibre electrodes for measuring catechols and ascorbic acid. In: MARSDEN CA (ed) Measurement of neurotransmitter release in vivo. New York: Wiley. pp 153–171

Gonzalez E, Rigual R, Fidone SJ & Gonzalez C (1987) Mechanisms for termination of the action of dopamine in carotid body chemoreceptors. J Auton Nerv Syst 18: 249–259

Gonzalez C, Almaraz L, Obeso A & Rigual R (1994) Carotid body chemoreceptors: from natural stimuli to sensory discharges. Physiol Rev 74: 829–898

Hanbauer I & Hellström S (1978) The regulation of dopamine and noradrenaline in the rat carotid body and its modification by denervation and by hypoxia. J Physiol, London 282: 21–34

Hansen JT (1981) Chemoreceptor nerve and type A glomus cell activity following hypoxia, hypercapnia or anoxia: a morphological study in the rat carotid body. J Ultrastruct Res 77: 189–198

Iturriaga R, Rumsey WL, Mokashi A, Spergel S, Wilson DF & Lahiri S (1991) *In vitro* perfused-superfused cat carotid body for physiological and pharmacological studies. J Appl Physiol 70: 1393–1400

Llados F & Zapata P (1978) Effects of dopamine analogues and antagonists on carotid body chemosensors *in situ*. J Physiol, London 274: 487–499

Marsden CA, Joseph MH, Kruk ZL, Maidment NT, O'Neill RD, Schenk JO & Stamford JA (1988) *In vivo* voltammetry - Present electrodes and methods. Neuroscience 25: 389–400

Mir AK, Al-Neamy K, Pallot DJ & Nahorski SR (1982) Catecholamines in the carotid body of several mammalian species: effects of surgical and chemical sympathectomy. Brain Res 252: 335–342

Rigual R, Gonzalez E, Gonzalez C & Fidone S (1986) Synthesis and release of catecholamines by the cat carotid body in vitro: effects of hypoxic stimulation. Brain Res 374: 101–109

Roumy M, Armengaud C, Ruckebusch M, Sutra JF & Leitner L-M (1988) Fate of the catecholamine stores in the rabbit carotid body superfused in vitro. Pflügers Arch 411: 436–441

Zapata P (1975) Effects of dopamine on carotid chemo- and baroreceptors *in vitro*. J Physiol, London 244: 235–251

Zapata P, Hess A, Bliss EL & Eyzaguirre C (1969) Chemical, electron microscopic and physiological observations on the role of catecholamines in the carotid body. Brain Res 14: 473–496

CATECHOLAMINE SECRETION FROM GLOMUS CELLS IS DEPENDENT ON EXTRACELLULAR BICARBONATE

J. M. Panisello and D. F. Donnelly

Department of Pediatrics
Sections of Critical Care and Respiratory Medicine
Yale University School of Medicine
New Haven, Connecticut 06520

1. INTRODUCTION

Although an exact understanding of the mechanism of hypoxic transduction in the carotid body has remained elusive, it is generally accepted that the glomus cells play an essential role. These cells synthesize and store neurotransmitters, particularly catecholamines, in dense cored vesicles and release them during hypoxic stimulation. One major theory of hypoxic transduction proposes that hypoxia directly inhibits a K^+ current leading to depolarization, calcium influx through voltage-dependent channels and enhanced catecholamine secretion secondary to the influx of calcium. Catecholamine, in turn, causes nerve excitation (González et al, 1994).

Within this model, anion currents are not directly implicated as being important for transduction during hypoxia. However, several observations suggest that anions play an essential role in carotid body function. In particular, Shirahata and Fitzgerald (1991) observed a loss of sensitivity to hypoxia during *in vivo* perfusion of the cat carotid body with a solution lacking bicarbonate. Furthermore, using patch clamp recording, Stea and Nurse (1991) demonstrated a major decrease in glomus cell resistance by bicarbonate, suggesting that bicarbonate modulates ion channels or is itself a current carrying ion. The present work was undertaken to address two questions: 1) does bicarbonate/CO_2 alter the secretory response of the glomus cell to hypoxia, 2) if it does, what is the mechanism.

2. METHODS

Carotid bodies were harvested from anesthetized rats, age 18–25 days, along with a portion of the sinus nerve. After a brief exposure to a dilute solution of collagenase/trypsin, the organ was carefully cleaned and mounted in a perfusion chamber on the stage of

Frontiers in Arterial Chemoreception, edited by Zapata *et al.*
Plenum Press, New York, 1996

an inverted microscope. It was superfused with heated (32°C), Ringer's saline (mM: 125 NaCl, 3 KCl, 24 $NaHCO_3$, 1.25 NaH_2PO_4, 1.2 $CaCl_2$, 1.2 $MgSO_4$ and 10 glucose) equilibrated with 20% O_2–5% CO_2 balance N_2 (~150 Torr). The PO_2 next to the organ was measured with a platinum wire electrode covered with a butyl acetate membrane and polarized to -0.8 V. Single-fiber nerve activity was recorded using a suction electrode that was applied to the cut end of the sinus nerve. Unit activity was discriminated with a window discriminator, and the logic pulse output was counted by a computer. Tissue catecholamine was measured using voltammetry and a carbon fiber electrode. The electrode was constructed from a single 5–10 μ carbon fiber which was insulated in a glass pipette with only the tip exposed. The tip was covered with Nafion (perfluorinated ion-exchange resin) and the electrode was polarized to 160 mV with respect to a Ag/AgCl ground electrode. This potential is slightly above the oxidation potential for dopamine, as determined in a previous study (Donnelly, 1993). The electrode was calibrated before and after the experiment by saline perfusion with and without dopamine (2 μM).

Four experimental series were performed. In the first, the carotid body was initially superfused with HEPES saline (mM: 140 NaCl, 3 KCl, 10 HEPES, 2 $CaCl_2$ and 10 glucose) and the response to hypoxia (1 min duration, 0 Torr at nadir) was elicited. The superfusate was switched to HCO_3^- saline and the response to hypoxia was elicited at 1, 15 and 30 min into the HCO_3^- perfusion period. In the second experiment, the response to hypoxia was elicited in HEPES saline. The perfusate remained in HEPES saline but the pH was reduced from 7.4 to 6.5 for 15 min. In the presence of acid HEPES, the response to hypoxia was again elicited. In the third experiment, we tested the effect of DIDS (Cl/HCO_3^- exchanger blocker) on hypoxia. In the fourth experiment, we tested the effect of 9-AC (anion channel blocker) on hypoxia. In cases where the pH was changed or where the solutions were changed from HEPES to HCO_3^-, the catecholamine calibration was performed in both solutions.

Baseline and peak levels of nerve activity and free tissue catecholamine were measured for each of the trials and analyzed using ANOVA with repeated measures, followed by paired *t*-tests when appropriate.

3. RESULTS

3.1. Experiment 1: Effect of HCO_3^- on the Hypoxia Response

Carotid bodies were superfused with HEPES saline for > 15 min. In response to hypoxia, nerve activity increased from 1.4 ± 0.4 Hz (n= 8) at baseline to 29.3 ± 3.2 Hz ($p<0.001$), as shown in Figure 1. Free tissue catecholamine (CAT) increased from 0.2 ± 0.1 μM to 6.3 ± 2 μM at peak during hypoxia. After allowing the carotid bodies to rest for 15 min, the perfusate was switched to HCO_3^- saline. After 1 min of HCO_3^-, the baseline nerve activity increased to 2.2 ± 0.5 Hz ($p<0.05$), but the peak nerve response to hypoxia was not significantly different from that observed during HEPES (36 ± 3.8 Hz, p= 0.06). In contrast to the nerve response, peak CAT response to hypoxia was significantly elevated after 1 min of HCO_3^- perfusion (16.9 ± 2.3 μM, $p<0.001$).

Longer perfusion times in HCO_3^- saline did not enhance further the CAT response to hypoxia (Fig 1). At 15 min into HCO_3^-, peak CAT was 11.8 ± 2.9 μM, and at 30 min peak CAT was 10.5 ± 1.9 μM. Both values were significantly higher than that recorded during HEPES superfusion.

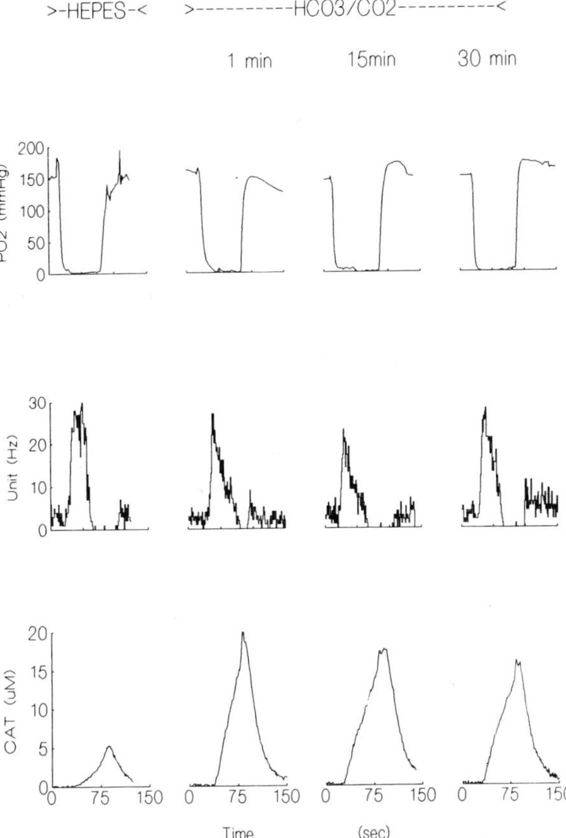

Figure 1. Effect of HCO_3^- on the catecholamine secretory response to hypoxia of the glomus cell. Top: PO_2 (mm Hg), middle: Single fiber nerve activity (Hz) and bottom: Free tissue catecholamine (CAT) (μM). Note the rapid HCO_3^- enhancement of CAT secretion in response to hypoxia, only after 1 min into HCO_3^- perfusion.

3.2. Experiment 2: Effect of pH on CAT Secretion

To test whether intracellular acidification by HCO_3^- accounted for the enhanced secretion in HCO_3^-, the response to hypoxia was observed in normal HEPES and following 15 min perfusion with acid (pH 6.5) HEPES, as illustrated in Figure 2. Peak nerve activity in response to hypoxia in normal HEPES was 17.1 ± 2.8 Hz and this increased to 24.2 ± 4.2 Hz during perfusion with acid HEPES ($p < 0.05$). However, peak CAT response was not significantly different in normal and acid HEPES (6.5 ± 1.2 and 5.6 ± 1.4 μM, respectively, n= 7).

3.3. Experiment 3: Effect of HCO_3^-/Cl^- Exchanger

After eliciting the response to hypoxia in HEPES saline, the exchanger blocker, DIDS (100–150 μM) was applied to the carotid bodies prior exposing to HCO_3^- saline. After switching to HCO_3^- in the continued presence of DIDS, the response to hypoxia was again tested. As shown in Figure 3, DIDS did not affect the bicarbonate enhancement of the CAT response. In HEPES, peak CAT during hypoxia was 8.3 ± 2.1 μM, and this increased to 18.2 ± 3.4 μM in HCO_3^- in the presence of DIDS ($p < 0.01$, n= 11). As a further test of the DIDS effect, the drug was washed out for 15 min using HCO_3 saline. The CAT response after DIDS washout was not different than in the presence of the drug; peak CAT was 18.9 ± 3.4 μM after washout.

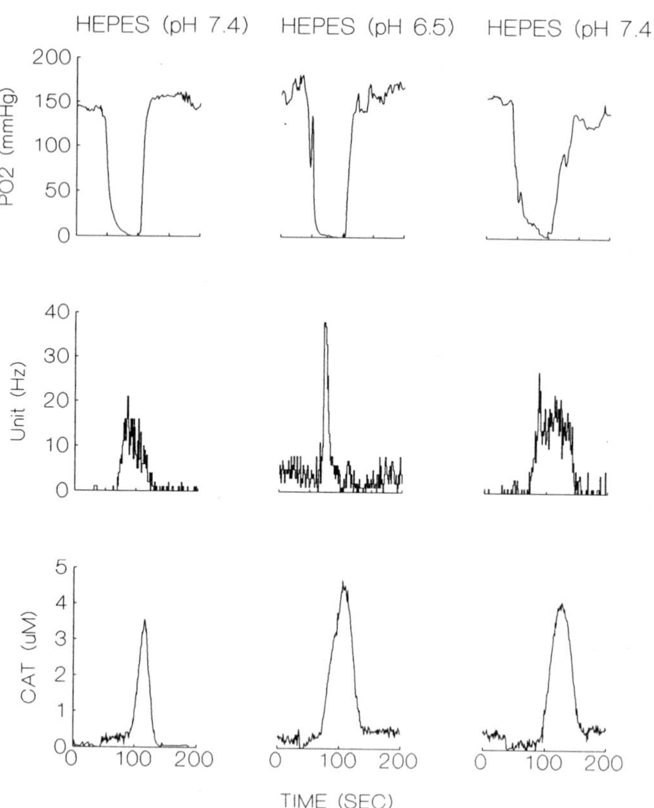

Figure 2. Effect of intracellular acidification. Carotid bodies were perfused at different pH in HEPES saline. Top: PO_2 (mm Hg), middle: Single fiber nerve activity (Hz) and bottom: Free tissue catecholamine (CAT) (μM). Acidification does not improve CAT secretion to hypoxia. In contrast, peak nerve activity is significantly increased.

3.4. Experiment 4: Effects of the Anion Channels

In contrast to DIDS, 9-AC had a major effect on the CAT response. The response to hypoxia was elicited in the presence of HCO_3^-, before and during perfusion with 9-AC (1.5–5 mM), as illustrated in Figure 4. The drug caused a reduction in the nerve response to hypoxia from 27.6 ± 7.4 Hz to 6.9 ± 2.2 Hz in the presence of 9-AC ($p < 0.05$), and the inhibition was reversed in the washout period (peak nerve = 26.2 ± 8.7 Hz, n= 8). CAT response to hypoxia was also dramatically reduced by 9-AC, decreasing from 25.5 ± 5.8 μM to 5.3 ± 1.6 μM in the presence of 9-AC ($p < 0.01$). After washout, the peak CAT during hypoxia increased to 16.7 ± 4.3 μM.

4. CONCLUSIONS

The main conclusion from this work is that catecholamine secretion in the carotid body is considerably enhanced in the presence of bicarbonate/CO_2 as compared to HCO_3^-/CO_2-free saline for the same stimulus. The mechanism for this enhancement is probably

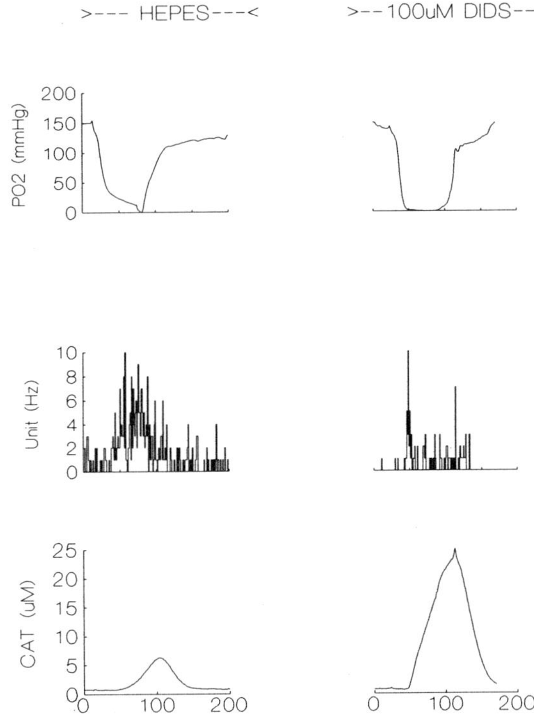

Figure 3. Effect of HCO_3^-/Cl^- exchanger. Carotid bodies alternatively perfused with HEPES, DIDS in HCO_3^- saline and HCO_3^- washout (washout not shown). Top: PO_2 (mm Hg), middle: Single fiber nerve activity (Hz) and bottom: Free tissue catecholamine (CAT) (μM). DIDS did not block the HCO_3^- dependent secretory response of the glomus cells.

not due to intracellular acidification in the presence of HCO_3^- but is likely related to an anion current in the glomus cells. Surprisingly, the nerve response to hypoxia was much less affected by switching from HEPES to HCO_3^-. Although the reason for the smaller affect on the nerve is presently obscure, it may have to do with a safety factor in glomus cell/nerve transmission as suggested by González et al (1994) when considering a similar observation obtained in low calcium solutions.

As noted in the introduction, HCO_3^-/CO_2 has been implicated as having important modulatory effects on the carotid body response to hypoxia. In some observations, HCO_3^--free perfusion virtually eliminated the nerve response to hypoxia (Shirahata & Fitzgerald, 1991), but in other work, HEPES saline reduced the speed of response to hypoxia but did not reduce the magnitude (Iturriaga et al, 1991). Previous work in our laboratory implicated indirectly a role for HCO_3^- in modulating catecholamine secretion. Our initial experiments on catecholamine secretion used carotid bodies which were maintained in HEPES saline, before and during the experiment. Peak catecholamine levels during brief anoxia were only 2–3 μM (Donnelly, 1993), but, in later work in which HCO_3^- was used, much higher values for tissue catecholamine were observed (Donnelly & Doyle, 1994). The present results confirm and extend these observations on the enhancement affect of HCO_3^- on catecholamine secretion, by not only demonstrating the effect on the same carotid body but by showing that the enhancement occurs within the first min of HCO_3^- perfusion.

We initially considered that the HCO_3^- enhancement was likely due to an intracellular acidification due to activation of a HCO_3^-/Cl transporter, an exchanger which is present and active in glomus cells (Buckler et al, 1991). However, two observations argue against this conjecture. First, acidification of HEPES saline to 6.5 failed to significantly enhance

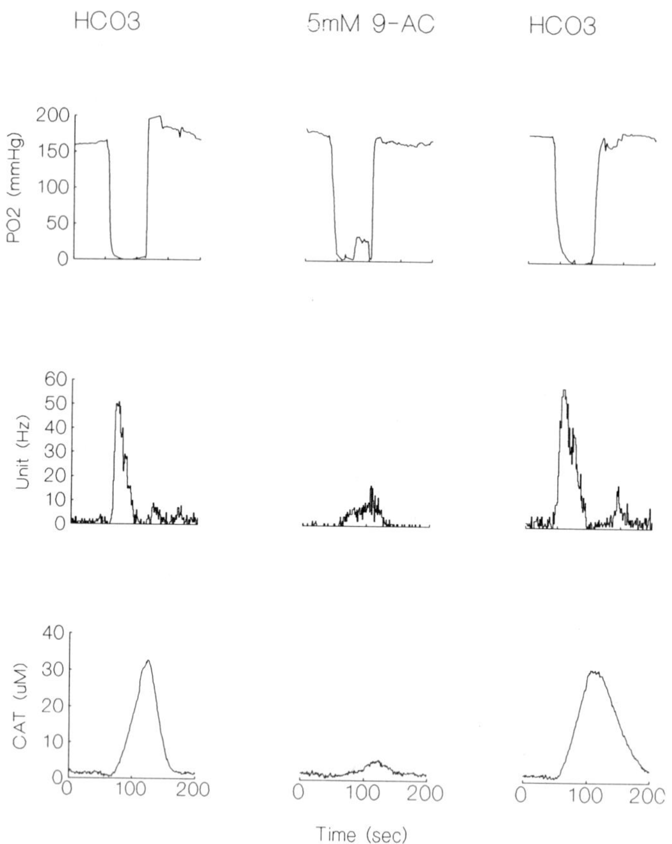

Figure 4. Effect of the anion channel. Carotid bodies alternatively perfused with HCO_3^-, 9-AC in HCO_3^- solution and then in HCO_3^- washout. Top: PO_2 (mm Hg), middle: Single fiber nerve activity (Hz) and bottom: Free tissue catecholamine (CAT) (μM). Note the severe decrease of CAT and nerve response to hypoxia.

the hypoxia-induced catecholamine release. At most, the exchanger would be expected to acidify the cell by 0.1–0.2 pH units and perfusion with HEPES at 6.5 would be expected to acidify the cell by ~ 0.7 pH units (Buckler et al, 1991). Second, treatment with DIDS failed to block the HCO_3^- enhancement of catecholamine secretion, again suggesting that acidification through a HCO_3^--dependent exchanger was not the reason for the enhanced secretion.

In contrast, the results strongly suggest that an anion current may be mediating the response. Stea and Nurse (1991) demonstrated that glomus cell membrane resistance was much lower in the presence of HCO_3^-, suggesting that HCO_3^- activated a conductance or could itself carry an ion current. This complemented earlier work showing that glomus cells have a large-conductance anion current which is sensitive to the anion channel blocker, 9-AC (Stea & Nurse 1989). In the present study, we found that 9-AC significantly reduced the magnitude of hypoxia-induced catecholamine secretion in the presence of HCO_3^-, suggesting an important role for an anion channel in the functioning of glomus cells.

We conclude that HCO_3^-/CO_2 greatly enhances the catecholamine response to hypoxia of rat carotid body, *in vitro*, and this enhancement is likely due to modulation of Cl/HCO_3^- currents and not to alteration in pH.

5. REFERENCES

Buckler K, Vaughan-Jones RD, Peers C, Lagadic-Gossmann D & Nye P (1991) Effects of extracellular pH, PCO_2 and HCO_3^- on intracellular pH in isolated type-I cells of the neonatal rat carotid body. J Physiol, London 444: 703–721

Buckler K, Vaughan-Jones RD, Peers C & Nye P (1990) Intracellular pH and its regulation in isolated type I carotid body cells of the neonatal rat. J Physiol, London 436: 107–129

Donnelly DF (1993) Electrochemical detection of catecholamine release from rat carotid body, *in vitro*. J Appl Physiol 74: 2330–2337

Donnelly DF & Doyle TP (1994) Developmental changes in hypoxia-induced catecholamine release from rat carotid body, *in vitro*. J Physiol, London 475: 267–275

González C, Almaraz L, Obeso A & Rigual R (1994) Carotid body chemoreceptors: from natural stimuli to sensory discharges. Physiol Rev 74: 829–898

Iturriaga R & Lahiri S (1991) Carotid body chemoreception in the absence and presence of CO_2-HCO_3^-. Brain Res 568: 253–260

Shirahata M & Fitzgerald RS (1991) The presence of CO_2/HCO_3^- is essential for hypoxic chemotransduction in the *in vivo* perfused carotid body. Brain Res 545: 297–300

Stea A & C A Nurse (1989) Chloride channels in cultured glomus cells of the rat carotid body. Am J Physiol 257: C174-C181

Stea A & Nurse CA (1991) Contrasting effects of HEPES *vs*. HCO_3^--buffered media on whole-cell currents in cultured chemoreceptors of the rat carotid body. Neurosci Lett 132: 239–242

CHRONIC HYPOXIA ENHANCES EXPRESSION OF CATECHOLAMINE BIOSYNTHESIZING ENZYMES IN RAT CAROTID BODY

Bernard Hannhart,[1] Amal Moftaquir,[2] Aida Bairam,[3] and Marie-Jeanne Boutroy[2]

[1] INSERM-Unité 14, Laboratoire de Physiopathologie Respiratoire CO 10, 54511 Vandoeuvre-lès-Nancy, France
[2] INSERM-Unité 272, Université Henri Poincaré Nancy 1, 24 rue Lionnois, BP 3069, Nancy, France
[3] Centre de Recherche HSFA, 10 rue de l'Espinay Université Laval, Québec, G1L 3L5, Québec, Canada

1. INTRODUCTION

Catecholamines, dopamine and norepinephrine, are present in a significant amount in the carotid body of many animal species (Fidone et al, 1980; Fitzgerald et al, 1983). Dopamine is synthesized in glomus cells since the presence of the rate limiting enzyme in catecholamine synthesis, tyrosine-hydroxylase (TH), has been clearly demonstrated. Moreover, hypoxia is known to increase dopamine release (Fidone et al, 1982), norepinephrine content (Hanbauer et al, 1981; Verna et al, 1993), and activity of TH in carotid body, and to induce the expression of TH-mRNA (Czyzyk-Krzeska et al, 1992). However, the presence of epinephrine in the carotid chemoreceptors remains controversial probably because of the difficulty in detecting small amounts of this substance.

According to the prominent activity of catecholamines in the hypoxic carotid body, we hypothesize that the biosynthesizing enzyme responsible for the metabolism of norepinephrine into epinephrine, the phenylethanolamine-N-methyltransferase (PNMT), should also be expressed in the cells of the chemoreceptors and should be stimulated by hypoxia as TH does.

Using a specific and sensitive double immunocytochemical technique (Léon et al, 1992), we tried to identify the presence of TH and PNMT in normoxia and their regulation by chronic hypoxia in rat carotid body. To avoid a potential counteractive effect of hypocapnia caused by hyperventilation in hypoxia, we maintained normocapnia during the chronic exposure to hypoxia.

Frontiers in Arterial Chemoreception, edited by Zapata *et al.*
Plenum Press, New York, 1996

2. METHODS

Twelve male Wistar rats weighing 180 to 200 g were maintained in a normobaric environmental chamber for 15 days at an average barometric pressure of 740 Torr. Six of them were exposed to isocapnic hypoxia (inspired PO_2 = 56–60 Torr and PCO_2 = 21–22 Torr), and six were kept in room air (controls). Carotid bodies were excised in pairs from the anesthetized animals (Nesdonal®, 25–30 mg/kg) while breathing the same gas mixture. Throughout the dissection, the animal was maintained alive. The carotid body was rapidly cleaned from surrounding tissues and fixed by immersion (4 to 5 h) in a fixative solution (4% phosphate buffered para-formaldehyde; 0.1 M; pH = 7.2), and frozen and stored at -80°C until cutting. Serial sections of 10 µm were done and dried onto gelatine chrome alum-subbed slides.

Immuno-labeling was performed by indirect immuno-fluorescence (Léon et al, 1992). Double labeling was done with anti-TH and anti-PNMT antibodies on the same sections. Secondary antibodies were preabsorbed and conjugated with fluorescein isothiocyanate or rhodamine. Examination was done with a Leica universal microscope equipped for epifluorescence. For each carotid body pair, at least 16 sections, situated in the middle of the piece, were examined. All cells positively labeled for TH were counted, as were the cells double positive for TH and PNMT. Due to wide variations in cell numbers depending on the inter individual variations in volume of carotid bodies, the number of double positively labeled TH and PNMT cells was expressed as a percentage related to the number of cells positively labeled only for TH.

Data statistical analysis was performed by Chi^2 test.

3. RESULTS

Immuno-labeling for TH was weaker in controls than in hypoxic group. Presence of PNMT was observed in two out of six cases in the control group and in five out of six cases in the hypoxic group. All cells immunoreactive for PNMT showed also TH fluorescence. A percentage of double immuno-labeled cells for PNMT and TH compared to cells labeled only for TH was calculated in each group. Results showed 19.7% of PNMT positive in hypoxic group against only 3.3% in the controls (Fig 1). This difference was statistically significant ($p < 0.001$).

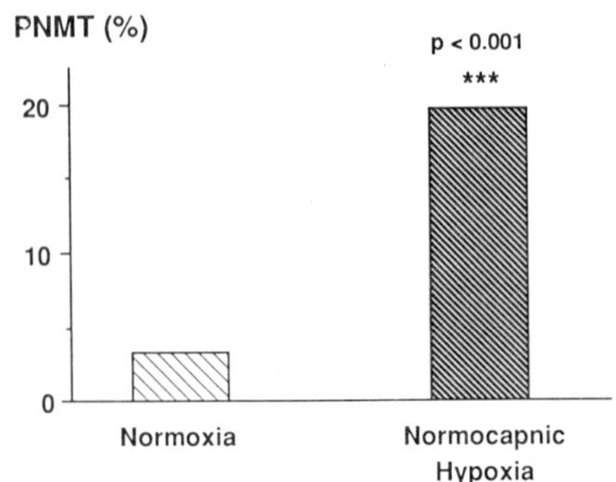

Figure 1. Percentage of cells positively immuno-labeled for PNMT + TH related to TH alone, in rat carotid body.

4. DISCUSSION

In the present study, we detected PNMT in a few normoxic rat carotid bodies. Bolme et al (1977) failed to detect any PNMT in cat carotid body maybe because either of a species difference or because their technique was not sufficiently sensitive. However, we found PNMT in only two control animals, which suggests that carotid body is not systematically able to synthesize epinephrine in normoxia. PNMT could have been induced by the experimental stress.

The experimental setup was optimal to reveal the effects of hypoxia: a) the conditions were similar for both control and hypoxic groups; b) since hypocapnia seems to be also determinant of catecholamines content and enzyme activity, we chose to maintain isocapnia during hypoxic exposure; c) carotid body excision was carried out in alive animals, while they were breathing the respective experimental gas mixture.

Hypoxia is known to be a potent stimulus for catecholamines synthesis in the carotid body. It acts directly by stimulation on the synthesizing enzymes. This effect has been well demonstrated only for TH (González et al, 1981) but we show in the present study, for the first time, that also PNMT expression appears to be regulated by chronic hypoxia.

These observations do not exclude a possible depletion in epinephrine during long-lasting hypoxia as found by Mills and Slotkin (1975) after 90-min hypoxia. Indeed, hypoxic stimulation of synthesis can occur with an increase in release or degradation of epinephrine. Moreover, immediate effects of acute hypoxia could differ from the effect of chronic exposure. Dynamics of these changes require further investigations.

In conclusion, the increased number of cells intensively immunoreactive with PNMT in the hypoxic carotid body in rat argues for the possibility that the expression of not only TH but also other catecholamines biosynthesizing enzymes, such as PNMT, is modulated by chronic isocapnic hypoxia.

5. REFERENCES

Bolme P, Fuxe K, Hokfelt T & Goldstein M (1977) Studies on the role of dopamine in cardiovascular and respiratory control: central versus peripheral mechanisms. Adv Biochem Psychopharmacol 16: 281–290

Czyzyk-Krzeska MF, Bayliss DA, Lawson EE & Millhorn DE (1992) Regulation of tyrosine hydroxylase gene expression in the rat carotid body by hypoxia. J Neurochem 58: 1538–1546

Fidone SJ, González C & Yoshizaki K (1980) Putative neurotransmitters in the carotid body: the case for dopamine Fed Proc 39: 2636–2640

Fidone SJ, González C & Yoshizaki K (1982) Effects of low oxygen on the release of dopamine from the rabbit carotid body *in situ*. J Physiol, London 333: 93–110

Fitzgerald RS, Garger P, Hauer MC, Raff H & Fechter L (1983) Effect of hypoxia and hypercapnia on catecholamine content in cat carotid body. J Appl Physiol 54: 1408–1413

González C, Kwok Y, Gibb JW & Fidone SJ (1981) Physiological and pharmacological effects on TH activity in rabbit and cat carotid body. Am J Physiol 240: R38-R43

Hanbauer I, Karoum F, Hellström S & Lahiri S (1981) Effects of hypoxia lasting up to one month on the catecholamine content in rat carotid body. Neuroscience 6: 81–86

Léon C, Grant NJ, Aunis D & Langley K (1992) Expression of cell adhesion molecules and catecholamine synthesizing enzymes in the developing rat adrenal gland. Dev Brain Res 70: 109–121

Mills E & Slotkin TA (1975) Catecholamine content of the carotid body in cats ventilated with 8–40% oxygen. Life Sci 16: 1555–1562

Verna A, Schamel A & Pequignot JM (1993) Long-term hypoxia increases the number of norepinephrine-containing glomus cells in the rat carotid body: A correlative immunocytochemical and biochemical study. J Auton Nerv Syst 44: 171–177

42

INTRACELLULAR Ca^{2+} DEPOSITS AND CATECHOLAMINE SECRETION BY CHEMORECEPTOR CELLS OF THE RABBIT CAROTID BODY

Ana Obeso, Asunción Rocher, José Ramón López-López, and Constancio González

Departamento de Bioquímica y Biología Molecular y Fisiología
Facultad de Medicina, Universidad de Valladolid
47005 Valladolid, Spain

1. INTRODUCTION

The pivotal role of intracellular free $[Ca^{2+}]$ fluctuations in the control of cellular functions such as contraction and secretion, including the release of neurotransmitters, was recognized many decades ago (see Rubin, 1982). More recently, the list of cellular functions triggered or modulated by the levels of $Ca^{2+}{}_i$ has grown enormously. Additional functions regulated by $[Ca^{2+}]_i$ include neuronal excitability, synaptic plasticity, gene expression, cellular metabolism, cell division and differentiation, and programmed cell dead (Miller, 1991; Clapham, 1995). Paralleling the growth in this list of Ca^{2+}-controlled functions, a multiplicity of cellular mechanisms aimed at maintaining resting free $[Ca^{2+}]_i$ in the range of 100 nM for most cells has been described, allowing increases in $Ca^{2+}{}_i$ levels that are specific in their magnitude, time course and spatial distribution, according to the cell function activated (Toescu, 1995).

Since Ca^{2+} cannot be metabolized, cells regulate their cytoplasmic levels of free Ca^{2+} through numerous binding proteins and influx and efflux mechanisms (Fig 1). Ca^{2+} influx to cell cytoplasm from the extracellular *milieu* occurs via voltage or receptor operated channels or via yet ill-defined capacitative pathways; the Na^+/Ca^{2+} exchanger can also produce in some circumstances net influx of Ca^{2+} (Miller, 1991; Clapham, 1995). Ca^{2+} efflux to the extracellular space occurs against electrochemical gradients, and thereby the pumping out of Ca^{2+} is directly (Ca^{2+} pump) or indirectly (Na^+/Ca^{2+}) coupled to the hydrolysis of ATP.

In addition to the extracellular space, there are intracellular stores, represented primarily by the smooth endoplasmic reticulum, capable of accumulating Ca^{2+} at very high concentrations (mM range) via specific Ca^{2+} ATPases (Fig 1). The smooth endoplasmic

Frontiers in Arterial Chemoreception, edited by Zapata *et al.*
Plenum Press, New York, 1996

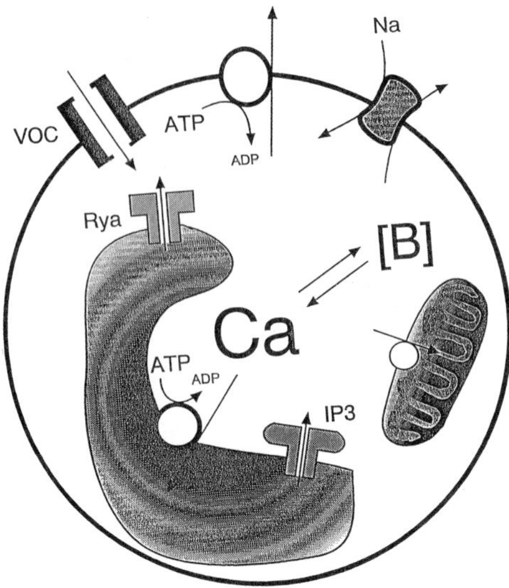

Figure 1. Model for the regulation of cellular calcium homeostasis. See text for an explanation.

reticulum of many cells may possess two specific mechanisms capable of mobilizing the accumulated Ca^{2+} in response to adequate signals, the inositol 1,4,5-triphosphate receptors (IP_3R) that on IP_3 binding are ensambled to produce a Ca^{2+} channel, and the ryanodine receptor-channel complex (RyR) equally permeant to Ca^{2+} (Pozzan et al, 1994; Simpson et al, 1995). Many extracellular signals, hormones and neurotransmitters, possess receptors in the plasma cell membrane that activate phospholipase C leading to the genesis of IP_3 in the cell interior and to the release of Ca^{2+} from the endoplasmic reticulum via the IP_3R (Clapham, 1995); the RyR are activated by local increases in free Ca^{2+}_i produced by Ca^{2+} entering via plasma cell membrane (López-López et al, 1995), and represent the substrate for the long time known process of Ca^{2+}-induced Ca^{2+} release (Simpson et al, 1995). Therefore, the endoplasmic reticulum may function as a sink or as a source for free cytoplasmic Ca^{2+} in different functional states of the cells, and additionally the sink or source function of the endoplasmic reticulum might vary from cell to cell, depending on the degree of expression of the repertoire of the molecules involved in the endoplasmic reticulum handling of Ca^{2+} (Simpson et al, 1995). At cytoplasmic levels of free Ca^{2+} higher than 500 nM (Clapham, 1995), *i.e.*, during cell activation, mitochondria may accumulate Ca^{2+}, thereby functioning as effective sinks to reduce cytoplasmic free Ca^{2+} concentration. Finally, many cytosolic constituents including proteins, and small organic molecules can bind Ca^{2+} ions contributing to modulate local levels of cytoplasmic free Ca^{2+} (Clapham, 1995; Toescu, 1995). The proteins with the capacity to bind Ca^{2+} may in turn acquire catalytic activities when their binding sites are occupied by the regulating ion.

In the carotid body (CB) chemoreceptor cells, our knowledge on the role of Ca^{2+} in cell signalling is rather restricted (see Gonzalez et al, 1994). It was only in 1968 that Eyzaguirre and Zapata showed the Ca^{2+} dependency of carotid sinus nerve (CSN) discharges elicited by hypoxia, acidity or flow interruption. In 1975, again Eyzaguirre's group (Eyzaguirre et al, 1975) reported that acetylcholine was incapable of generating action potentials in the CSN in Ca^{2+}-free solutions. Some years later, a few ultrastructural studies showed the appearance of omega exocytotic profiles and/or coated pits and vesicles in chemoreceptor cells of rat CBs incubated in Ca^{2+}-containing (but not in Ca^{2+}-free) rich K^+_e solutions or in the presence of the Ca^{2+} ionophore A23187, concluding that exocytosis was Ca^{2+}_e-dependent (Gronblad et al, 1980). Consistent with that, it was later shown that the release of dopamine (DA) elicited by hypoxia and high K^+_e was Ca^{2+}_e-dependent in >95% (Fidone et al, 1982; Almaraz et al, 1986; Obeso et al, 1992). More recently, three different laboratories (González et al, 1993; López-Barneo et al, 1993; Buckler & Vaughan-Jones, 1994) have used fluorescent dyes to measure $[Ca^{2+}]_i$ in isolated chemoreceptor cells, and have consistently found that more than 95% of the $[Ca^{2+}]_i$ rise produced by hypoxia is due to Ca^{2+} entering from the extracellular space. In the case of acidic stimulation the Ca^{2+}_e dependence of the release of DA was approximately 80% (Obeso et al, 1992) and the Ca^{2+}_i signal was reduced by a similar percentage in Ca^{2+}-free media (Buckler & Vaughan-Jones, 1993). At variance with those findings, Biscoe and Duchen (1990) reported that up to 40% of the hypoxic Ca^{2+}_i rise was due to Ca^{2+} entering the cytoplasm from intracellular stores, and Biscoe et al (1989) could not detect a rise in free Ca^{2+}_i during acidic stimulation. In addition, Lahiri et al (1995) have recently communicated that the anoxic CSN discharge was better preserved in Ca^{2+}-free media containing thapsigargin than in its absence, concluding that Ca^{2+} from intracellular deposits seems to contribute to the anoxic chemoreception.

2. METHODS

Using an *in vitro* preparation of the rabbit CB whose catecholamine deposits have been labeled by prior incubation of the organs with their natural precursor ^{3}H-tyrosine (Fidone & Gonzalez, 1982), we have studied the significance of intracellular Ca^{2+} stores as possible sources of Ca^{2+} for the secretory response, and as possible buffers (sinks) for the Ca^{2+} entering the cell cytoplasm during stimulation. The tools used in the experiments include: ATP and bradykinin as possible generators of IP_3, and thereby as possible activators of the IP_3R; ryanodine at submicromolar concentration and caffeine as activators of the RyR; thapsigargin as a blocker of the reticulum ATPase; ruthenium red as a blocker of the mitochondrial Ca^{2+} uniporter; and, ionomycin as a Ca^{2+} ionophore that allows rapid equilibration of Ca^{2+} throughout cellular membranes. The experiments have been performed in Ca^{2+}-containing and in Ca^{2+}-free solutions. The effects of the drugs have been tested on their ability to trigger a secretory response in basal normoxic conditions, to test for a role of intracellular Ca^{2+} stores as sources of Ca^{2+} for the secretory response, and on their ability to modify the intensity and time course of the secretory response elicited by hypoxia and high K^+_e. In this way, we have tested for the capacity of the intracellular stores to act as sources of Ca^{2+}, or as sinks of the Ca^{2+} entering from the extracellular space.

It should be noted that most of the experiments have been performed sampling the incubating solutions for their analyses in ^{3}H-catecholamine (^{3}H-CA) content every 2 min, thereby providing a high sensitivity of the overall procedures capable of detecting <6 fmol of labelled CA (<200 cpm), which after correction for the specific activity of ^{3}H-CA in the cells, represents approximately 120 fmol of total CA release, or an amount equivalent to the basal release/2 min in normoxic conditions. During stimulation (hypoxia, high K^+_e) the release increases markedly, and consequently the sensitivity of the radioisotopic method to detect the effect of a drug on the stimulus induced release decreases.

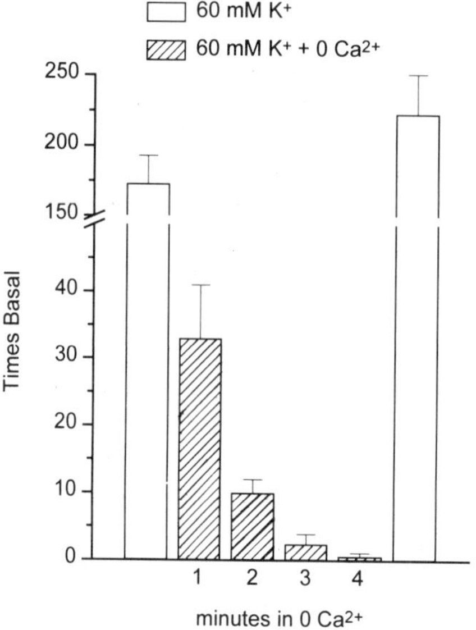

Figure 2. Time course of the disappearance of high external K^+ induced release of ^{3}H-catecholamines upon removal of calcium from the extracellular space. Empty bars: release response in Ca^{2+}-containing solutions at the beginning and the end of the experiments. Slashed bars: release response after incubation in Ca^{2+}-free solutions for the indicated periods. Release response (ordinate) is expressed as times basal release in normal K^+ solutions.

3. RESULTS AND DISCUSSION

Figure 2 shows the time course of extracellular Ca^{2+} washing out. In designing these experiments, the advantage that the release induced by high external K^+ is almost totally dependent on Ca^{2+} entering from the extracellular space was taken. Therefore, the minimum time of incubation in Ca^{2+} free medium required to abolish high K^+_e induced release would be equivalent to the time required to wash out Ca^{2+} ions from the incubating vial and the CB extracellular space. As shown in Figure 2, one min of incubation in 0 Ca^{2+} reduced markedly the release response, after 4 min in 0 Ca^{2+} the release was practically abolished, and on reintroduction of Ca^{2+} the release response recovered completely. In a similar experiment using hypoxic stimulation (2% O_2-equilibrated solutions, 2 min), the time course of inhibition was comparable; in fact, after 4 min in 0 Ca^{2+} the release induced by hypoxia was completely abolished. These experiments confirm previously reported findings with longer times of incubation in Ca^{2+} free solutions (*e.g.* Obeso et al, 1992), and suggest that intracellular Ca^{2+} stores do not play a significant role in mediating the secretory response to hypoxia, unless chemoreceptor cells have an unusually fast-emptying intracellular Ca^{2+} deposits. On the other hand, the present findings are consistent with observations of Fidone (see Fidone et al, 1977) and Torrance (1977) showing that the half-time for bicarbonate and sucrose wash out, respectively, was close to half a minute.

Next we performed a series of experiments aimed at mobilizing intracellular Ca^{2+} stores. In a first group of experiments we tested for the ability of ATP to mobilize Ca^{2+} stores. In a recent study, Spergel & Lahiri (1993) showed that ATP and analogs, but not adenosine, were able to increase CSN discharges in a dose-dependent manner, concluding that the CB expresses surface P_2 type ATP receptors. Since P_2 receptors are coupled to β type phospholipase C, it should be expected that their activation will lead to the formation of IP_3 and activation of IP_3R. ATP at 100 and 1500 μM did not affect the basal normoxic release of DA either in Ca^{2+} containing or in Ca^{2+} free solutions suggesting that the ATP receptors responsible for the activation of CSN discharges are located in a structure different from chemoreceptor cells. Bradykinin, a potent mobilizer of Ca^{2+} from intracellular deposits and potent secretagogue in chromaffin cells (Augustine & Neher, 1992), was also without effect on the basal release of ^{3}H-CA from the CB, suggesting that chemoreceptor cells do not possess bradykinin receptors or that the endoplasmic reticulum Ca^{2+} stores are really small. The same was true for the rest of the agents tested including ionomycin in Ca^{2+}-free solutions.

In conclusion, the participation of endoplasmic reticulum and mitochondria as sources of Ca^{2+} capable of altering the secretory response of chemoreceptor cells appear to be of secondary importance, implying that chemoreceptor cells must rely almost exclusively on plasma membrane mechanisms to maintain their Ca^{2+} homeostasis. Although the precise identity of the Ca^{2+} stores sites is not fully clear, it appears that the smooth endoplasmic reticulum (SER) may be the principal place where the intracellular Ca^{2+} ATPase is located and thereby the SER could be the main place where Ca^{2+} is stored (Pozzan et al, 1994). If this is the case in chemoreceptor cells our findings would correlate with the apparently rear SER profiles present in the cells that appear to be located mainly in the processes of chemoreceptor cells (Verna, 1975; McDonald, 1981). It should be mentioned that papers consistent with our conclusion have been presented in this Symposium. Thus, He et al (1996) communicated that endothelin I increases up to five times the normoxic basal levels of IP_3, and therefore it should be expected that IP_3R of the endoplasmic reticulum represents the target of the IP_3 formed. Although the cellular element in which the increase of IP_3 had occurred was not identified, it was shown that endothelin I did not affect the basal release of CA or the Ca^{2+}_i levels in chemoreceptor cells, but still endothelin I was effective in potentiating the release of DA and the Ca^{2+}_i rise produced by hypoxia. Those findings imply that chemoreceptor cells possess endothelin receptors, and therefore it could be expected that IP_3 has increased in chemoreceptor cells. Therefore, the lack of effect on the basal release of CA and Ca^{2+}_i would imply that the cellular deposits of Ca^{2+} sensitive to IP_3 are really small. The effects observed during stimulation would be produced via voltage-dependent Ca^{2+} channels, as it is the case in other systems. These pieces of information urge to explore the dynamics of intracellular Ca^{2+} stores in a more direct manner and to correlate the data with other functions of the chemoreceptor cells, besides the release of neurotransmitters.

4. ACKNOWLEDGMENTS

Supported by Spanish DGICYT Grant PB92/0267.

5. REFERENCES

Almaraz L, Gonzalez & Obeso A (1986) Effects of high potassium on the release of [^{3}H]dopamine from the cat carotid body *in vitro*. J Physiol, London 379: 293–307

Augustine GJ & Neher E (1992) Calcium requirements for secretion in bovine chromaffin cells. J Physiol, London 450: 247–271

Biscoe TJ & Duchen MR (1990) Responses of type I cells dissociated from the rabbit carotid body to hypoxia. J Physiol, Lond 428: 39–59

Biscoe TJ, Duchen MR, Eisner DA, O'Neill SC & Valdeolmillos M (1989) Measurements of intracellular Ca^{2+} in dissociated type I cells of the rabbit carotid body. J Physiol, London 416: 421–434

Buckler KJ & Vaughan-Jones RD (1993) Effects of acidic stimuli on intracellular calcium in isolated type I cells of the neonatal rat carotid body. Pflügers Arch 425: 22–27

Buckler KJ & Vaughan-Jones RD (1994) Effects of hypoxia on membrane potential and intracellular calcium in rat neonatal carotid body type I cells. J Physiol, London 476: 423–428

Clapham DE (1995) Calcium signaling. Cell 80: 259–268

Eyzaguirre C & Zapata P (1968) A discussion of possible transmitter or generator substances in carotid body chemoreceptors. In: RW Torrance (ed) Arterial Chemoreceptors. Oxford: Blackwell. pp 213–251

Eyzaguirre C, Fidone S & Nishi K (1975) Recent studies on the generation of chemoreceptor impulses. In: MJ Purves (ed) The Peripheral Arterial Chemoreceptors. London: Cambridge Univ Press. pp 175–194

Fidone S & Gonzalez C (1982) Catecholamine synthesis in rabbit carotid body *in vitro*. J Physiol, London 333: 69–79

Fidone S, Weintraub S, Stavinoha W, Stirling G & Jones L (1977) Endogenous acetylcholine levels in cat carotid body and the autoradiographic localization of a high affinity component of choline uptake. In: H Acker, S Fidone, D Pallot, C Eyzaguirre, DW Lübbers & RW Torrance (eds) Chemoreception in the Carotid Body. Berlin: Springer-Verlag. pp 106–113

Fidone S, Gonzalez C & Yoshizaki K (1982) Effects of low oxygen on the release of dopamine from the rabbit carotid body *in vitro*. J Physiol, London 333: 93–110

Gonzalez C, Lopez-Lopez JR, Obeso A, Rocher A & García-Sancho J (1993) Ca^{2+} dynamics in chemoreceptor cells: an overview. Adv Exp Med Biol 337: 149–156

Gonzalez C, Almaraz L, Obeso A & Rigual R (1994) Carotid body chemoreceptors: from natural stimuli to sensory discharges. Physiol Rev 74: 829–898

Grönblad M, Akerman KE & Eränkö O (1980) Exocytosis of amine-storing granules from glomus cells of the rat carotid body induced by incubation in potassium-rich media or media containing calcium and ionophore A23187. Adv Biochem Psycopharmacol 25: 227–233

He L, Chen J, Dinger B, Stensaas L & Fidone S (1966) Endothelin modulates chemoreceptor cell function in mammalian carotid body. Adv Exp Med Biol (This volume)

Lahiri S, Buerk DG, Osai S, Chugh D & Mokashi A (1995) Intracellular calcium store-dependent coupling between O_2 chemoreception and chemosensory discharge in the isolated perfused cat carotid body. J Physiol, London 487: 16P

Lopez-Barneo J, Benot JA & Ureña J (1993) Oxygen sensing and the electrophysiology of arterial chemoreceptor cells. News Physiol Sci 8: 191–195

López-López JR, Shacklock PS, Balke CV & Wier WG (1995) Local calcium transients triggered by single L-type calcium channel currents in cardiac cells. Science 268: 1042–1045

McDonald DM (1981) Peripheral chemoreceptors. Structure-function relationships of the carotid body. In: TF Hornbein (ed) Regulation of Breathing. Part I. New York: Marcel Dekker. pp 105–319

Miller RJ (1991) The control of neuronal calcium homeostasis. Prog Neurobiol 37: 255–285

Obeso A, Rocher A, Fidone S & Gonzalez C (1992) The role of dihydropyridine-sensitive Ca^{2+} channels in stimulus-evoked catecholamine release from chemoreceptor cells of the carotid body. Neuroscience 47: 463–472

Pozzan T, Rizzuto R, Volpe P & Meldolesi J (1994) Molecular and cellular physiology of intracellular calcium stores. Physiol Rev 74: 595–636

Rubin RP (1982) Calcium and Cellular Secretion. New York: Plenum

Simpson PB, Challiss RAJ & Nahorski SR (1995) Neuronal calcium stores: activation and function. Trends Neurosci 18: 299–306

Spergel D & Lahiri S (1993) Differential modulation by extracellular ATP of carotid chemosensory responses. J Appl Physiol 74: 3052–3056

Toescu EC (1995) Temporal and spatial heterogeneities of Ca^{2+} signaling: mechanisms and physiological roles. Am J Physiol 269: G173-G185

Torrance RW (1977) Discussion to paper: Fidone S, Weintraub S, Stavinoha W, Stirling G & Jones L: Endogenous acetylcholine levels in cat carotid body and the autoradiographic localization of a high affinity component of choline uptake. In: H Acker, S Fidone, D Pallot, C Eyzaguirre, DW Lübbers & RW Torrance (eds) Chemoreception in the Carotid Body. Berlin: Springer-Verlag. p 112

Verna A (1975) Contribution à l'étude du glomus carotidien du Lapin (*Oryctolagus cuniculus* L.) Recherches cytologiques, cytochimiques et expérimentales. Thesis. Bordeaux: Université de Bordeaux

43

DOPAMINE D_2 RECEPTOR mRNA ISOFORMS EXPRESSION IN THE CAROTID BODY AND PETROSAL GANGLION OF DEVELOPING RABBITS

Aida Bairam,[1] Charles Dauphin,[1] François Rousseau,[2] and Edouard W. Khandjian[2]

[1] Unité de Recherche en Néonatologie
[2] Unité de Recherche en Génétique Humaine et Moléculaire
Centre Hospitalier Universitaire de Québec
Centre de Recherche
Pavillon S.F.A., Québec, P.Q., Canada

1. INTRODUCTION

In the brain, dopamine (DA) D_2 receptors (D_2R) exist in two isoforms, referred to as D_2 short (D_{2S}) and D_2 long (D_{2L}), generated by alternative splicing of pre-messenger RNA. These two isoforms differ in their length by 29 amino acids inserted in the third intracytoplasmic loop of the receptors (Civelli et al, 1993). Both isoforms are detected in the same cell and their ratio has been shown to be tissue- and age-dependent (Mack et al, 1991).

Dopamine effects on carotid chemosensory activity are derived from the stimulation of DA D_2R which are present on carotid body cells and on carotid sinus nerve afferent endings (Gonzalez et al, 1994). Dopamine D_2R mRNA has been detected in the carotid bodies and petrosal ganglia of adult rats (Czyzyk-Krzeska et al, 1992), rabbits (Schamel & Verna, 1993) and cats (Gauda et al, 1994). The petrosal ganglion contains the perikarya of the carotid body's sensory innervation. However, it is not known whether D_2R mRNA isoforms are expressed in the carotid body and petrosal ganglion.

The aims of the present study were to evaluate the relative abundance of D_2R mRNA and its two isoforms in the carotid body and petrosal ganglion, and to identify changes in their expression in developing rabbits. Using reverse transcription-polymerase chain reaction (RT-PCR), we were able to detect the presence of mRNA of these receptors and estimate the expression ratios of both mRNA isoforms. Part of this work has been recently published elsewhere (Bairam et al, 1996b).

Frontiers in Arterial Chemoreception, edited by Zapata *et al.*
Plenum Press, New York, 1996

2. MATERIALS AND METHODS

2.1. Materials

Carotids bodies and petrosal ganglia of anesthesized rabbits aged ≤ 24 hours (40 pups), 10 days (30 pups), 25 days (25 pups) and ≤ 1 year (9 rabbits) were collected, frozen immediately, pooled for each age and stored at -80°C. Control cell lines and tissues used were: GH4C1 cell line which does not express D_2R mRNAs, GH4C1#19 that expresses only the D_{2S} mRNA (obtained from Dr P. Falardeau, Res. Ctr, Pavillon CHUL) and striata of newborn and adult rabbits.

2.2. RNA Extraction

Frozen organs were homogenized and cytoplasmic RNA was extracted and phenol purified. RNA was quantified after agarose gel electrophoresis followed by staining with ethidium bromide and comparison of the staining with different concentrations of standard 28S and 18S rRNA, and also by dot blot analyses and hybridization with ^{32}P-labelled 18S rRNA probe using as standard different quantities of rRNA.

2.3. RT-PCR reaction

Amplification of D_2R mRNAs target sequences by RT-PCR was done using specific oligodeoxynucleotide primers chosen based on GeneBank data for rat sequences. These primers were: D_{2S} and D_{2L} forward, 5'TCCTGTCCTTCACCATCTCCTGCCC-3' (residues 609–633) and reverse, 5'TGACTGGGAGGGATGGGGCTATACCG-3' (residues 920–945); D_2 common forward, 5'TGGGTCAGAAGGGAAGGCAGACAGGC-3' (residues 196–221) and reverse, 5'TTGTTGAGTCCGAAGAGCAGTGGG-3' (residues 631–654). The reverse primers were also used for reverse-transcription. Identical hybridization signals were obtained using these primers with RNA extracted from both adult rat and rabbit striata and from GH4C1 positive cell line but not from GH4C1 negative cell line. Briefly for RT-PCR, 1 μg of cytoplasmic RNA with appropriate primers was used to synthesize the specific first strand cDNA for each D_{2S} and D_{2L} and for the common D_2 mRNAs. The PCR reaction was for 35 cycles each composed of 1 min at 94°C (denaturation); 1 min at 58°C (annealing) for D_{2S} and D_{2L} and 56°C for the common segment D_2; 2 min at 72°C (primer extension), followed by a final extension step for 7 min at 72°C. RT-PCR was performed in duplicate using two RNA preparations. Those controls without RT did not yield any amplification products after hybridization.

2.4. Hybridization and Labeling

The short and long D_2R cDNA fragments of adult rabbit striata as well as the cDNA of the common segment generated by RT-PCR were ^{32}P-labelled using the random priming reaction. PCR products were separated by electrophoresis on 6% acrylamide gels in Tris-Borate-EDTA buffer (TBE), electrotransferred onto Hybond N+ membranes and fixed with 0.4 NaOH for 20 min, and hybridized overnight at 42°C in the presence of 5 x 10^5 cpm/ml of ^{32}P-labelled probe. The hybridization signals were quantified by exposing the membranes to phosphor-sensitive imaging plate type III-s (Phosphorimager, Fuji BAS 1000, Fuji Medical Systems USA Inc., Stanford, CT). Strong signals were detected as

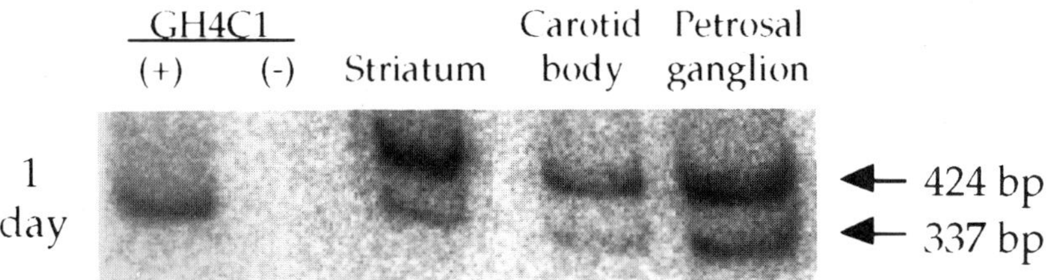

Figure 1. RT-PCR amplification of D_{2S} and D_{2L} mRNA isoforms in (+) and (-) GH4C1 cell lines and in the striatum, carotid body and petrosal ganglion of 1 day-old rabbits.

bands of 337 bp for D_{2S}, 424 bp for D_{2L} and 459 bp for the common segment, as calculated from the cDNA sequence data.

2.5. Data Analysis

For each age, the relative mean D_{2S}/D_{2L} ratio for each hybridization signal was obtained from different exposure times of the membranes after hybridization, while the relative signal intensity for the common D_2 was obtained after 30 min exposure.

3. RESULTS

3.1. DA D_{2S} and D_{2L} R mRNA Isoforms Expression

Both D_2R S and L mRNA isoforms were detected in rabbits at 1 day old in all organs studied as shown in Figure 1. They were also detected at all other ages and in all organs studied.

The D_{2L} R mRNA was found predominantly expressed in the striatum, in the carotid bodies and in the petrosal ganglia, but the relative D_{2S}/D_{2L} mRNA ratio appeared to differ between ages. These ratios (mean ± SEM) were: 0.42 ± 0.08, 0.44 ± 0.04, 0.29 ± 0.01 and 0.68 ± 0.17 for the carotid body; 0.72 ± 0.05, 0.43 ± 0.13, 0.25 ± 0.04 and 0.39 ± 0.09 for the petrosal ganglion; and 0.47 ± 0.10, 0.55 ± 0.10, 0.31 ± 0.01 and 0.44 ± 0.06 for the striatum, at 1, 10 and 25 days old and adult rabbits, respectively. In all organs, the lowest D_{2S}/D_{2L} ratio observed was at 25 days old.

3.2. DA D_2R mRNA Expression

Figure 2 shows the amplified products of a common segment reflecting the total amount of D_2 mRNA in the carotid body and petrosal ganglion at all ages. Membranes were exposed for 30 min to phosphor-sensitive imaging plate.

The intensity of the hybridized signal at 1 day-old was assumed to be equal to one. A difference of about 3-, 5- and 1.5- fold higher was observed for 10 and 25 days-old and for adult rabbits, respectively. The highest level of total D_2R mRNA was found at 25 day-old rabbits for the carotid body and petrosal ganglion as well as for the striatum.

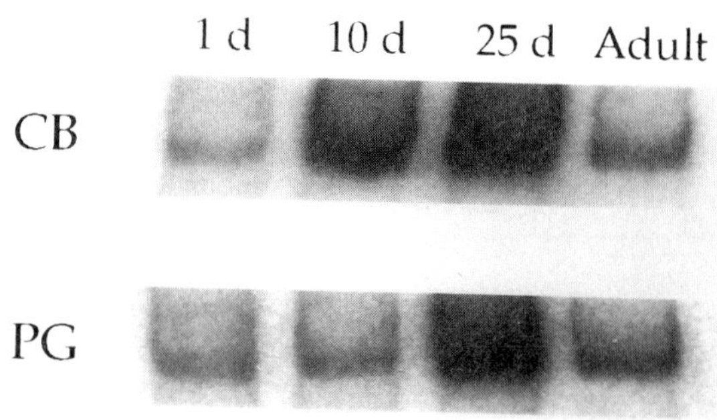

Figure 2. RT-PCR amplification for D_2 mRNA in carotid bodies and petrosal ganglia of developing rabbits.

4. DISCUSSION

This study shows that both DA D_2R S and L mRNA isoforms are expressed in the rabbit carotid bodies and petrosal ganglia from birth and that the level of the total D_2R mRNA expression is age-modulated.

The D_{2L} R mRNA isoform is found predominantly expressed in all organs tested. Although, the lowest D_{2S}/D_{2L} ratio observed is at 25 days-old in all organs studied, the highest levels of total D_2R mRNA are found at the same age suggesting that both the expression ratio of mRNA isoforms and the level of total D_2R mRNA vary during postnatal development. Dopamine metabolism in the carotid body of 25 day-old rabbits has been shown to be different compared to younger and adult rabbits (Bairam et al, 1996a). Thus, the age of 25 days seems to correspond to an important maturative step of the dopaminergic system in the rabbit carotid bodies. A similar pattern of age-related expression of DA D_2R mRNAs has been observed in pre- and postnatal rat brain (Xu et al, 1992). Although the two isoforms may have different affinities to DA antagonists (Castro & Strange, 1993) and may behave differently toward their coupling with G-protein (Montmayeur et al, 1993), it is still not known whether these isoforms induce different physiological responses when they are individually or concomitantly stimulated.

In the brain, DA D_2R located pre- and postsynaptically to dopaminergic neurons have been shown to behave differently, as the presynaptic receptors are autoreceptors regulating DA synthesis and release (Chesselet, 1984). And, it has been suggested that DA D_2R located on carotid body cells behave as autoreceptors (Czyzyk-Krzeska et al, 1992). It is not known if the function of these receptors is age dependent. However, we may suggest that the autoreceptor mechanism may not be fully developed in the early days of life because D_2R mRNA levels are lower in newborn as compared to growing rabbits.

Dopamine induces both inhibition and excitation of carotid chemosensory activity in different animal species, as shown by *in vivo* and *in vitro* studies (Gonzalez et al, 1994), and it seems that these effects are related to development (Marchal et al, 1992). The explanation of these data is still a debate. One proposal is that these DA effects may be due to a difference in the affinity to DA between pre- and postsynaptic receptors, and to the possibility of the presence of D_2R mRNA isoforms (Gonzalez et al, 1994). Our results may contribute to a better understanding of some of the contradictory data concerning DA effects on carotid body function.

5. REFERENCES

Bairam A, Marchal F, Cottet-Emard JM, Basson H, Pequignot JM, Hascoet JM & Lahiri S (1996a) Effects of hypoxia on carotid body dopamine content and release in developing rabbits. J Appl Physiol 80: 20–24

Bairam A, Dauphin C, Rousseau F & Khandjian EW (1996b) Expression of dopamine D_2 receptor mRNA isoforms at the peripheral chemoreflex afferent pathway in developing rabbits. Am J Respir Cell Mol Biol (In press)

Castro SW & Strange PG (1993) Differences in the ligand binding properties of the short and long versions of the D_2 dopamine receptor. J Neurochem 60: 372–375

Chesselet MF (1984) Presynaptic regulation of neurotransmitter release in the brain. Neuroscience 12: 347–375

Civelli O, Bunzow JR & Grandy DK (1993) Molecular diversity of the dopamine receptors. Annu Rev Pharmacol Toxicol 33: 281–307

Czyzyk-Krzeska MF, Lawson EE & Millhorn DE (1992) Expression of D_2 dopamine receptor mRNA in the arterial chemoreceptor afferent pathway. J Auton Nerv Syst 41: 31–40

Gauda EB, Shirahata M & Fitzgerald RS (1994) D_2-dopamine receptor mRNA in the carotid body and petrosal ganglia in the developing cat. Adv Exp Med Biol 360: 317–319

Gonzalez C, Almaraz L, Obeso A & Rigual R (1994) Carotid body chemoreceptors: from natural stimuli to sensory discharges. Physiol Rev 74: 829–898

Mack KJ, O'Malley KL & Todd RD (1991) Differential expression of dopaminergic receptor messenger RNAs during development. Dev Brain Res 59: 249–251

Marchal F, Bairam A, Haouzi P, Hascoet JM, Crance JP, Vert P & Lahiri S (1992) Dual responses of carotid chemosensory afferents to dopamine in the newborn kitten. Respir Physiol 90: 173–183

Montmayeur JP, Guiramand J & Borrelli E (1993) Preferential coupling between dopamine D_2 receptors and G-proteins. Mol Biol 7: 161–170

Schamel A & Verna A (1993) Localization of dopamine D_2 receptors mRNA in the rabbit carotid body and petrosal ganglion by *in situ* hybridization. Adv Exp Med Biol 337: 85–91

Xu S, Monsma FJ, Sibley DR & Creese I (1992) Regulation of D_{1A} and D_2 dopamine receptor mRNA during ontogenesis, lesion and chronic antagonist treatment. Life Sci 50: 383–396

44

DOMPERIDONE AS A TOOL TO ASSESS THE ROLE OF DOPAMINE WITHIN CAROTID BODY CHEMORECEPTION

P. Zapata, R. Iturriaga, and C. Larraín

Laboratory of Neurobiology
Catholic University of Chile
Santiago, Chile

1. DOPAMINE IN THE CAROTID BODY

The carotid bodies are composite receptors, *i.e.* hypoxia apparently acts upon glomus cells which are synaptically apposed to the sensory endings of primary afferent neurons, responsible for conveying the information to the medullary centers. Considerable effort has been directed to determine the transmitter(s) involved in signal transference between glomus cells and chemosensory nerve terminals. Dopamine is the putative transmitter that has received more attention, because of the following observations: *i*) glomus cells are characterized by their abundance in dense-core granules and strong formaldehyde-induced fluorescence, indicative of a high concentration of catecholamines (see Hess, 1975); *ii*) dopamine is the prevalent catecholamine in the carotid body of most species studied (see Fidone et al, 1983); *iii*) glomus cells possess the enzymes required for dopamine synthesis as well the transporter mechanisms for uptake of dopamine and its precursors (see Eyzaguirre & Zapata, 1984); *iv*) the dopamine content of the rat carotid body *in situ* is reduced in direct proportion to the severity and duration of hypoxia (Hellström et al, 1976; Hanbauer & Hellström, 1978); *v*) the dopamine content of the rabbit carotid body *in vitro* is reduced by hypoxic superfusates (Leitner, 1993); and *vi*) hypoxia induces dopamine release from rabbit and cat carotid bodies superfused *in vitro* (Fidone et al, 1982; Rigual et al, 1986; see also Zapata et al, 1996). These observations led to the proposal that dopamine may serve as the excitatory transmitter between glomus cells and chemosensory nerve terminals (see Gonzalez et al, 1994).

A crucial pharmacological test for accepting a substance as transmitter in a given synapse is the block of physiologically generated synaptic transmission after application of the selective antagonists to such substance. Since agonists and antagonists for D_1 receptors (mediated by activation of adenylate cyclase) proved to be without effects on carotid chemosensory activity (McQueen, 1984), studies have concentrated on the actions of D_2 antagonists. Domperidone, a highly selective D_2 antagonist (Laduron & Leysen, 1979),

Frontiers in Arterial Chemoreception, edited by Zapata *et al.*
Plenum Press, New York, 1996

proved to be an effective blocker of the actions exerted by exogenous dopamine upon carotid body chemoreceptors (Zapata & Torrealba, 1984).

If dopamine, released from glomus cells during hypoxic stimulation, mediates the excitation of chemosensory nerve endings, one should expect that hypoxia-induced chemosensory excitation would be reduced or abolished after blocking dopamine receptors. Therefore, we studied if the chemosensory excitation induced by hypoxic stimuli was affected by domperidone applied to carotid bodies *in situ* (Iturriaga et al, 1994) and *in vitro*.

2. DOMPERIDONE ACTIONS UPON CAROTID BODIES *IN SITU*

Experiments were performed in spontaneously breathing, pentobarbitone anesthetized cats, in which recordings of chemosensory impulse activity were obtained from the entire cut carotid (sinus) nerves, after interruption of the sympathetic innervation of the carotid bifurcations. Dose-response curves for the chemosensory effects induced by iv injections of dopamine hydrochloride (range 50 ng/kg to 20 μg/kg) revealed that the transient inhibitory effects exerted by dopamine were completely reversed by the iv administration of domperidone 50 μg/kg, the block being maintained for at least 4 h.

Intravenous injections of domperidone produced immediate and maintained increases in the basal frequency of chemosensory discharges. The frequency of chemosensory discharges established along the 5 min following domperidone administration was 129.5 ± 26.9% (mean ± SEM; n = 8)) higher than the mean frequency recorded along the 5 min preceding the injection ($p < 0.001$). This effect was not accompanied by changes in minute ventilatory volume or in the end tidal pressure of CO_2, since reflex effects were prevented by the section of both carotid nerves. An additional iv dose of domperidone (250 μg/kg) did not further modify the frequency of chemosensory discharges. However, in another series of experiments performed in pentobarbitone anesthetized cats with their carotid nerves intact, we observed that domperidone 50 μg/kg iv produced a small but significant increase in basal tidal ventilatory volume, which was not further increased by an additional dose of domperidone 250 μg/kg (N. Correa, C. Pérez & P. Zapata, unpublished observations). Since domperidone does not cross the blood-brain barrier (Laduron & Leysen, 1979), this ventilatory effect should be ascribed to an enhancement of peripheral chemosensory discharges.

Switching the breathing of cats from room air to pure O_2 for up to 30 s resulted in a deep decrease in chemosensory frequency. The minimal levels of chemosensory activity attained during these hyperoxic tests were not significantly different from those induced under control conditions. This is a proof that the enhanced rate of chemosensory discharges is dependent on the level of oxygenation of the animal.

The results shown above indicate that domperidone withdraws a tonic inhibitory control upon chemosensory activity exerted under normoxic eucapnic conditions. This low level of chemosensory discharges was probably due to a resting release of dopamine from glomus cells under normoxia.

Domperidone has also been reported to rise the ventilatory fluctuations of chemosensory discharges (Lahiri et al, 1985; Iturriaga et al, 1994), an index of enhanced chemoreceptor responsiveness to oscillations in respiratory gases.

The changes in carotid chemosensory frequency evoked by switching the breathing from room air to pure N_2 for brief periods were assessed initially during control conditions and then after domperidone administration, as illustrated in Figure 1. The 5 s tests of 100% N_2 breathing resulted in maximal frequencies of chemosensory discharges which

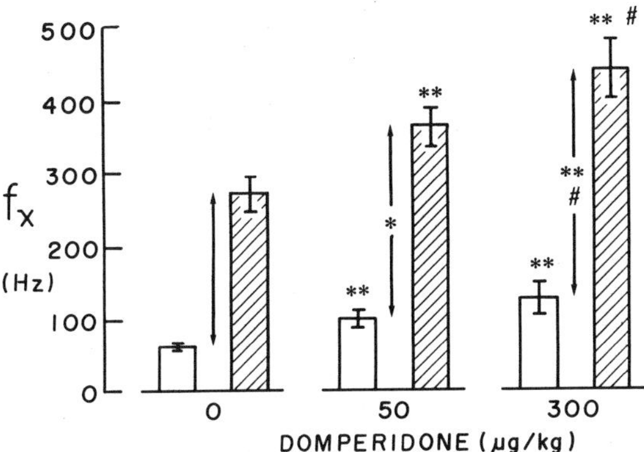

Figure 1. Summary of transient effects of 5-s periods of 100% N_2 inhalation on the frequency of carotid chemosensory discharges (f_x), tested during control condition and after iv administration of domperidone 50 and 300 µg/kg. Means ± SEM's of 8 carotid bodies *in situ*. Open bars, basal f_x; hatched bars, maximal f_x evoked by hypoxic tests; arrows, increase in f_x in response to hypoxia. Multiple comparisons by non-parametric Friedman tests (overall **p**'s = 6.1×10^{-5} for basal f_x, 4.7×10^{-7} for maximal f_x and 3.9×10^{-5} for Δf_x) followed by paired comparisons by Conover tests: *, $p < 0.01$ *vs* control; **, $p < 0.001$ *vs* control; #, $p < 0.01$ between both doses.

were 33.4 ± 8.5% (mean ± SEM; n = 8) higher than those attained in the controls, the maximal levels and the actual rises being significantly different ($p < 0.001$). An additional iv administration of domperidone 250 µg/kg, which did not significantly modify basal chemosensory activity, produced a further enhancement of chemosensory responses to hypoxic tests.

In spite of the above, the analysis of dose-response curves for chemosensory responses induced by iv injections of NaCN (range 0.5 to 100 µg/kg) revealed that while the calculated maximal frequency of chemosensory discharges was significantly higher after administration of domperidone, the calculated ED_{50} was not significantly different from controls (Iturriaga et al, 1994).

Thus, domperidone appears to turn off restraining dopaminergic controls on both the basal level of chemosensory activity observed under normoxia and the transient chemosensory responses to hypoxic stimuli recorded from cat carotid bodies studied *in situ*.

3. DOMPERIDONE ACTIONS UPON CAROTID BODIES *IN VITRO*

Experiments were also performed on carotid bodies excised from anesthetized cats and subsequently superfused *in vitro* with a modified Tyrode's solution, pH 7.40 at 37.5°C, and equilibrated with 20% O_2 under control conditions, while chemosensory activity was recorded from the entire carotid nerve.

Intrastream injections of domperidone 100 µg gave immediate and maintained increases in the basal frequency of chemosensory discharges (Figs 2 and 3). This suggests that the chemosensory activity generated from carotid bodies superfused *in vitro* with normoxic saline is also subjected to a tonic inhibitory control exerted by endogenous dopamine continuously released from glomus cells. That dopamine is continuously released from rabbit carotid bodies superfused *in vitro* with normoxic saline has been shown by Roumy et al. (1988).

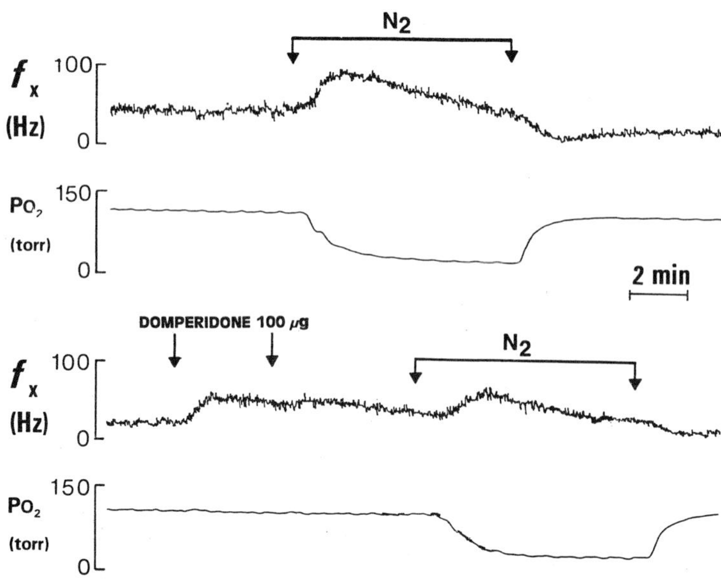

Figure 2. Carotid body superfused *in vitro*. Upper traces, changes in frequency of chemosensory discharges (f_x) in response to superfusions with 100% N_2-equilibrated saline before and after two intrastream injections of domperidone 100 μg. Lower traces, polarographic recordings of partial pressure of O_2 within the superfusing channel.

Switching the superfusate to Tyrode's solution equilibrated with 100% N_2 results in a prompt fall in the partial pressure of O_2 recorded in the superfusing channel close to the carotid body, followed shortly after by an increase in the frequency of chemosensory discharges, as illustrated in Figure 2. After application of domperidone, the hypoxic stimulus still evokes a chemosensory response, not significantly different from that recorded in control conditions.

Figure 3 illustrates the chemosensory responses to intrastream injections of NaCN recorded from another carotid body superfused *in vitro*. Such responses to cytotoxic hypoxia did not differ significantly in rise time and maximal frequency before and after administration of domperidone.

The results reported above clearly indicate that chemosensory responses to hypoxic stimuli are well preserved after dopaminergic blockade by domperidone.

It should be noted that the most common response of cat carotid bodies superfused *in vitro* to the initial intrastream injections of dopamine is a transient inhibition of chemosensory discharges, and that such inhibitory response is blocked by spiroperidol, another D_2 antagonist (Zapata, 1975).

4. REASSESSMENT OF THE ROLE OF DOPAMINE IN ARTERIAL CHEMORECEPTION

Our results indicate that domperidone produces a prolonged increase in the basal frequency of chemosensory discharges recorded from the cat carotid bodies *in situ* and *in vitro*. Such effect has been previously reported for preparations *in situ* (Zapata & Torre-

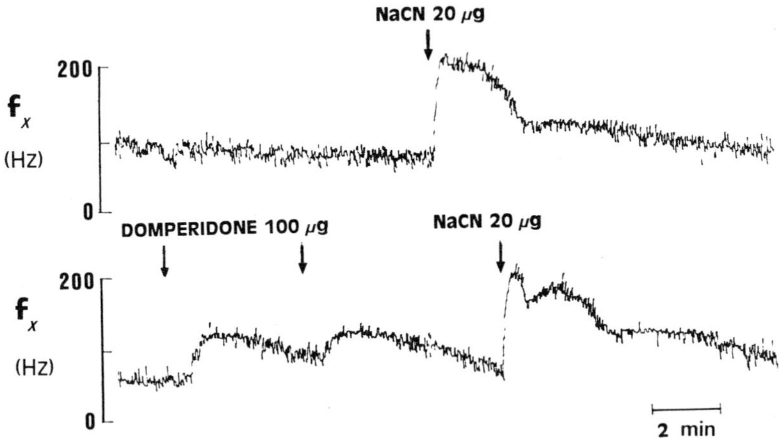

Figure 3. Carotid body superfused *in vitro*. Changes in frequency of chemosensory discharges (f_x) in response to intrastream injections of NaCN 20 μg before and after two intrastream injections of domperidone 100 μg.

alba, 1984; Lahiri et al, 1985; Iturriaga et al, 1994). Also, the present observations indicate that chemosensory responses to hypoxic stimuli are well preserved after dopaminergic blockade by domperidone. Thus, these observations do not agree with the idea that endogenous dopamine may serve as the excitatory transmitter between glomus cells and chemosensory nerve terminals when the carotid body is under normoxia or when it is stimulated by hypoxia.

Special attention should be given to the effects of exogenous dopamine on chemoreceptor activity. Dopamine inhibits the chemosensory discharges from cat carotid bodies *in situ* (Sampson et al, 1976; Nishi, 1977; Llados & Zapata, 1978; Docherty & McQueen, 1978; Lahiri & Nishino, 1980) and *in vitro* (Zapata, 1975), but in this last preparation the inhibitory response fades after several applications, giving way to excitatory responses to large doses of dopamine. In dogs, intracarotid and iv injections of low doses of dopamine cause chemosensory inhibition, while large doses induce inhibition preceded by excitation (Bisgard et al, 1979). In rabbits, intracarotid injections of dopamine produce chemosensory inhibition (Docherty & McQueen, 1979; Folgering et al, 1982), although preparations *in vitro* exhibit chemosensory excitation (Monti-Bloch & Eyzaguirre, 1980).

Chronic section of the carotid nerve in rabbits, leading to sensory denervation of their carotid bodies, reduces by two thirds the specific binding to ^{3}H-spiroperidol (Dinger et al, 1981) and by one third the specific binding to ^{3}H-domperidone (Mir et al, 1984). Thus, a fraction of D_2 receptors present in the carotid body should be located in sensory nerve endings, while the other fraction has been ascribed to dopamine autoreceptors in glomus cells. These receptors probably mediate the changes in the electrical properties of glomus cells shown by Matsumoto et al (1982) and by Goldman and Eyzaguirre (1984). The *in situ* hybridization method to localize the D_2 receptor mRNA confirmed its presence in glomus cells and in many perikarya of the petrosal ganglion (Czyzyk-Krzeska et al, 1992; Schamel & Verna, 1993; Gauda et al, 1994), which provides sensory innervation to the carotid body. In this case, domperidone antagonism of dopamine receptors in glomus cells will probably enhance dopamine release from those cells, while domperidone antagonism of dopamine receptors in chemosensory nerve endings will block dopaminergic transmission from glomus cells to sensory nerve endings. However, the results here reported indicate that domperidone —even in doses well above those that completely reverse D_2-mediated effects of exogenous dopamine- does not block chemosensory nerve activity, thus discarding dopamine as the excitatory transmitter between glomus cells and sensory nerve endings.

The enhanced chemosensory responsiveness to brief hypoxic tests observed in cats after domperidone treatment may explain the augmented ventilatory responses to hypoxic stimulation after domperidone treatment reported in chloralose anesthetized cats (Hsiao et al, 1989) and in awake goats (Kressin et al, 1986), provided that the innervation of the carotid bodies is kept intact.

It must be noted that an increased frequency of basal chemosensory impulses has also been observed in carotid bodies *in situ* after treating cats with other D_2 antagonists, such as butyrophenones (haloperidol and spiroperidol; Llados & Zapata, 1978) and benzamides (metoclopramide and sulpiride; Zapata et al, 1983).

The increase in chemosensory activity observed after applying a dopaminergic antagonist suggests that endogenous dopamine is exerting tonic inhibition within the chemoreceptor organ under conditions of eucapnic normoxia. This disinhibition of chemosensory discharges might also explain the enhanced chemoreceptor responsiveness to the normal arterial oscillations in O_2 and CO_2 pressures, observed after domperidone treatment. Thus, our present results rather confirm a restraining modulatory role for dopamine within the chemoreceptor process, as previously proposed (Zapata, 1975).

5. ACKNOWLEDGMENTS

Work supported by grant 193–0645 from the National Fund for Scientific and Technological Development (FONDECYT) and by the Research and Postgraduate Division of the University (DIPUC).

6. REFERENCES

Bisgard GE, Mitchell RA & Herbert DA (1979) Effects of dopamine, norepinephrine, and 5-hydroxytryptamine on the carotid body of the dog. Respir Physiol 37: 61–80

Czyzyk-Krzeska MF, Lawson EE & Millhorn DE (1992) Expression of D_2 dopamine receptor mRNA in the arterial chemoreceptor afferent pathway. J Auton Nerv Syst 41: 31–39

Dinger B, Gonzalez C, Yoshizaki K & Fidone S (1981) [^{3}H]Spiroperidol binding in normal and denervated carotid bodies. Neurosci Lett 21: 51–55

Docherty RJ & McQueen DS (1978) Inhibitory action of dopamine on cat carotid chemoreceptors. J Physiol, London 279: 425–436

Docherty RJ & McQueen DS (1979) The effects of acetylcholine and dopamine on carotid chemosensory activity in the rabbit. J Physiol, London 288: 411–423

Eyzaguirre C & Zapata P (1984) Perspectives in carotid body research. J Appl Physiol 57: 931–957

Fidone S, Gonzalez C & Yoshizaki K (1982) Effects of low oxygen on the release of dopamine from the rabbit carotid body *in vitro*. J Physiol, London 333: 93–110

Fidone SJ, Stensaas LJ & Zapata P (1983) Sites of synthesis, storage, release and recognition of biogenic amines in carotid bodies. In: Acker H & O'Regan RG (eds) Physiology of the Peripheral Arterial Chemoreceptors. Amsterdam: Elsevier. pp 21–44

Folgering H, Ponte J & Sadig T (1982) Adrenergic mechanisms and chemoreception in the carotid body of the cat and the rabbit. J Physiol, London 325: 1–21

Gauda EB, Shirahata M & Fitzgerald RS (1994) D_2-dopamine receptor mRNA in the carotid body and petrosal ganglia in the developing cat. Adv Exp Med Biol 360: 317–319

Goldman WF & Eyzaguirre C (1984) The effect of dopamine on glomus cell membranes in the rabbit. Brain Res 321: 337–340

Gonzalez C, Almaraz L, Obeso A & Rigual R (1994) Carotid body chemoreceptors: from natural stimuli to sensory discharges. Physiol Rev 74: 829–898

Hanbauer I & Hellström S (1978) The regulation of dopamine and noradrenaline in the rat carotid body and its modification by denervation and by hypoxia. J Physiol, London 282: 21–34

Hellström S, Hanbauer I & Costa E (1976) Selective decrease of dopamine content in rat carotid body during exposure to hypoxic conditions. Brain Res 118: 352–355

Hess A (1975) The significance of the ultrastructure of the rat carotid body in structure and function of chemoreceptors. In: Purves MJ (ed) The Peripheral Arterial Chemoreceptors. London: Cambridge Univ Press. pp 51–73

Hsiao C, Lahiri S & Mokashi A (1989) Peripheral and central dopamine receptors in respiratory control. Respir Physiol 76: 327–336

Iturriaga R, Larrain C & Zapata P (1994) Effects of dopaminergic blockade upon carotid chemosensory activity and its hypoxia-induced excitation. Brain Res 663: 145–154

Kressin NA, Nielsen AM, Laravuso R & Bisgard GE (1986) Domperidone-induced potentiation of ventilatory responses in awake goats. Respir Physiol 65: 169–180

Laduron PM & Leysen JE (1979) Domperidone, a specific *in vitro* dopamine antagonist, devoid of *in vivo* central dopaminergic activity. Biochem Pharmacol 28: 2161–2165

Lahiri S & Nishino T (1980) Inhibitory and excitatory effects of dopamine on carotid chemoreceptors. Neurosci Lett 20: 313–318

Lahiri S, Hsiao C, Zhang R, Mokashi A & Nishino T (1985) Peripheral chemoreceptors in respiratory oscillations. J Appl Physiol 58: 1901–1908

Leitner L-M (1993) Dopamine metabolism in the rabbit carotid body *in vitro*: effect of hypoxia and hypercapnia. Adv Exp Med Biol 337: 183–190

Llados F & Zapata P (1978) Effects of dopamine analogues and antagonists on carotid body chemosensors *in situ*. J Physiol, London 274: 487–499

Matsumoto S, Nakajima T, Uchida T, Ozawa H & Uchiyama J (1982) Effects of sodium cyanide, dopamine and acetylcholine on the resting membrane potential of glomus cells in the rabbit. Brain Res 239: 674–678

McQueen DS (1984) Effects of selective dopamine receptor agonists and antagonists on carotid body chemoreceptor activity. In: Pallot DJ (ed) The Peripheral Arterial Chemoreceptors. London: Croom Helm. pp 325–333

Mir AK, McQueen DS, Pallot DJ & Nahorski SR (1984) Direct biochemical and neuropharmacological identification of dopamine D_2-receptors in the rabbit carotid body. Brain Res 291: 273–283

Monti-Bloch L & Eyzaguirre C (1980) A comparative physiological and pharmacological study of cat and rabbit carotid body chemoreceptors. Brain Res 193: 449–470

Nishi K (1977) A pharmacologic study on a possible inhibitory role of dopamine in the cat carotid body chemoreceptor. In: Acker H, Fidone S, Pallot D, Eyzaguirre C, Lübbers DW, Torrance RW (eds) Chemoreception in the Carotid Body. Berlin: Springer-Verlag. pp 145–151

Rigual R, Gonzalez E, Gonzalez C & Fidone S (1986) Synthesis and release of catecholamines by the cat carotid body *in vitro*: effects of hypoxic stimulation. Brain Res 374: 101–109

Roumy M, Armengaud C, Ruckebusch M, Sutra JF & Leitner L-M (1988) Fate of the catecholamine stores in the rabbit carotid body superfused *in vitro*. Pflügers Arch - Eur J Physiol 411: 436–441

Sampson SR, Aminoff MJ, Jaffe RA & Vidruk EH (1976) Analysis of inhibitory effect of dopamine on carotid body chemoreceptors in cats. Am J Physiol 230: 1494–1498

Schamel A & Verna A (1993) Localization of dopamine D_2 receptor mRNA in the rabbit carotid body and petrosal ganglion by *in situ* hybridization. Adv Exp Med Biol 337: 85–91

Zapata P (1975) Effects of dopamine on carotid chemo- and baroreceptors *in vitro*. J Physiol, London 244: 235–251

Zapata P & Torrealba F (1984) Blockade of dopamine-induced chemosensory inhibition by domperidone. Neurosci Lett 51: 359–364

Zapata P, Serani A & Lavados M (1983) Inhibition in carotid body chemoreceptors mediated by D-2 dopaminoceptors: antagonism by benzamides. Neurosci Lett 42: 179–184

Zapata P, Iturriaga R & Alcayaga J (1996) Dopamine efflux from the carotid body during hypoxic stimulation. Adv Exp Med Biol 410: 261–266

45

ADENOSINE INCREASES THE cAMP CONTENT OF THE RAT CAROTID BODY *IN VITRO*

E. C. Monteiro,[1] P. Vera-Cruz,[2] T. C. Monteiro,[1] and M. A. Silva E Sousa[1]

[1] Department of Pharmacology
Faculty of Medical Sciences
New University of Lisbon, 1198 Lisbon, Portugal
[2] Higher Institute for Health Sciences
Monte da Caparica, Portugal

1. INTRODUCTION

The adenosine receptor involved in the excitatory effect of this nucleoside on respiration mediated through carotid body chemoreceptors has been characterised in *in vivo* experiments, and exhibits agonist (Monteiro & Ribeiro, 1987) and antagonist (Ribeiro & Monteiro, 1991) profiles which are compatible with the presence of an A_2 adenosine receptor subtype. The A_2 adenosine receptors have been defined on the basis of their ability to stimulate adenyl cyclase and cAMP production (Fredholm et al, 1994). The present work was undertaken to investigate *in vitro* the effect of adenosine on cAMP content of the rat carotid body.

2. METHODS

The experiments were performed with carotid bodies (CBs) isolated from male Wistar rats (380 ± 16 g) anaesthetised with urethane (1.5 g/Kg, ip), tracheostomised and breathing spontaneously. Under a dissecting scope the carotid bodies were removed *in vivo* from the carotid bifurcation and immediately placed in ice-cold 95% O_2/5% CO_2-equilibrated medium, for 15 min. Medium composition described by Pérez-García et al (1990) was (mM): NaCl 116; $NaHCO_3$ 24; KCl 5; $CaCl_2$ 2; $MgCl_2$ 1.1; HEPES 10; glucose 5.5; pH 7.42. After the pre-incubation period the CBs were placed in fresh 95% O_2/5% CO_2 medium containing the test drugs, for 30 min at 37°C in a metabolic shaker bath. After the incubation period, cyclic nucleotides were extracted from the CBs following the protocol described by Cunha et al (1994). Basically, CBs were immersed in ice-cold perchloric acid (3 M) for 10 min, homogenised and then kept at 0°C for 30 min with occasional swirling. After centrifugation at 12,000 g for 5 min (4°C) an aliquot (400 μl)

Frontiers in Arterial Chemoreception, edited by Zapata *et al.*
Plenum Press, New York, 1996

of the supernatant was neutralised at 0°C with a 4 M KOH solution containing 0.4 M Tris base, and the mixture was centrifuged again at 12,000 g for 2 min (4°C) to precipitate potassium perchlorate. An aliquot of the neutralised supernatant was collected and stored at -20°C until analysis. cAMP was assayed using a commercial kit (Amersham). The levels of cAMP are expressed as picomoles per CB. In each animal one carotid body was used as control.

2.1. Statistics

The data are presented as mean ± SEM values. The significance of the differences between the means was calculated by the unpaired Student's *t* test. Values of $p<0.05$ were considered to represent significant differences.

2.2. Drugs

Adenosine, 2-chloroadenosine, isobutylmethylxanthine and adenosine deaminase type VI (1,327 U/ml; EC 3.5.4.4) were from Sigma. CGS 21680 [2-p-(2-carboxyethyl)phenethylamino-5'ethylcarboxamido adenosine hydrochloride] was from RBI and erythro-9-(2-hydroxy-3-nonyl) adenine from Burroughs Wellcome Co. All solutions were made in incubation medium.

3. RESULTS

The basal cAMP levels quantified in 5 rat carotid bodies incubated under control conditions (95% O_2/5% CO_2-equilibrated medium, 37°C, for 30 min) were 4.9 ± 1.3 pmol/CB. Phosphodiesterase inhibition, obtained by the addition of isobutylmethylxanthine (IBMX 0,5 mM) to the incubation medium (95% O_2/5% CO_2 -equilibrated medium, 37°C, for 30 min), raised cAMP levels to 10.6 ± 1.8 pmol/CB (n=5).

The effect of adenosine on cAMP content of the carotid body was investigated in the presence of the adenosine deaminase inhibitor, erythro-9-(2-hydroxy-3-nonyl) adenine (EHNA), in order to prevent deamination of adenosine to its inactive metabolite inosine.

Carotid bodies were incubated in 95% O_2/5% CO_2 -equilibrated medium (37°C, for 30 min) containing IBMX (0.5 mM), EHNA (25 μM) and adenosine (1 mM) and the cAMP mean value obtained in 5 rats is illustrated in Figure 1.

Adenosine increases cAMP content of the carotid body to 40.5 ± 3.1 pmol/CB, which is significantly different from the value 25.8 ± 3.1 pmol/CB, quantified in the carotid bodies incubated with only EHNA and IBMX in the absence of adenosine.

It is also apparent from the results shown in Figure 1, that EHNA by itself increases the carotid body cAMP content from 10.6 ± 1.8 pmol/CB to 25.8 ± 3.1 pmol/CB.

Since adenosine has a high affinity for the nucleoside transporter system, and can modify cAMP levels acting intracellularly, a control experiment was performed with a stable adenosine analogue, 2-chloroadenosine (CADO). CADO is the non selective adenosine receptor agonist, with low affinity for the nucleoside transporter system (Jarvis et al, 1985). CADO shows in *in vivo* experiments approximately the same potency as adenosine, in terms of inducing respiratory stimulation mediated through carotid body chemoreceptors (Monteiro & Ribeiro, 1987).

As shown in Figure 2, CADO (1 μM) raised cAMP levels from 14.1 pmol/CB to 27 pmol/CB. The control value (14.1 pmol/CB) for the experiment with CADO was obtained

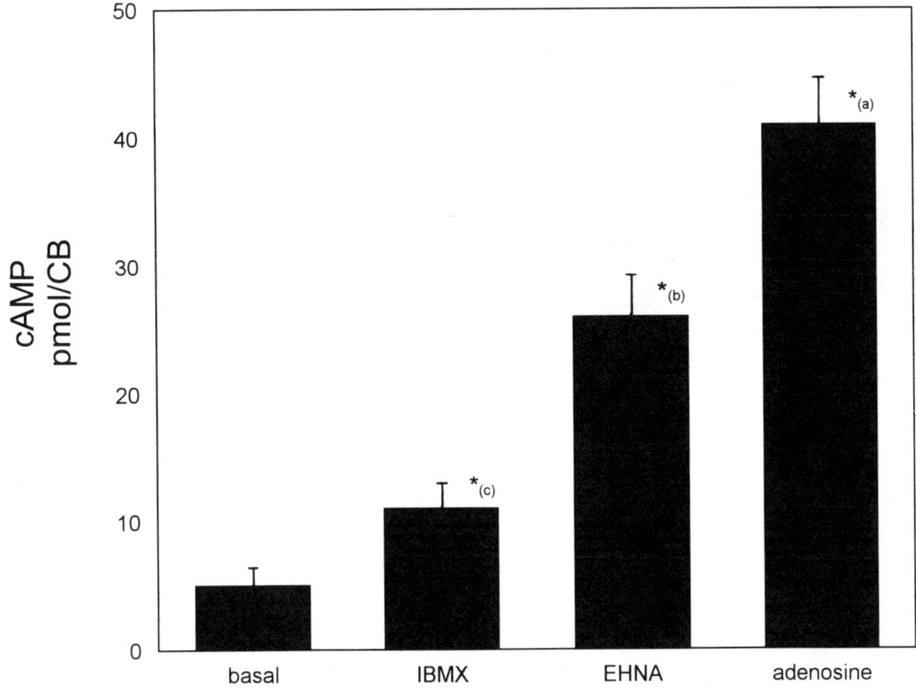

Figure 1. Effect of adenosine on cAMP content of rat carotid bodies. The carotid bodies were incubated with adenosine (1 mM) in the presence of IBMX (0.5 mM) and EHNA (25 μM). The IBMX and EHNA vertical bars correspond to the cAMP values quantified in carotid bodies incubated with IBMX (0.5 mM) alone or with IBMX (0.5 mM) in the presence of EHNA (25 μM) respectively. n = 5 for each group of experiments. * $p < 0.05$; unpaired Student's *t* tests corresponding to the differences between: a) adenosine and EHNA; b) EHNA and IBMX; c) IBMX and basal.

by incubating the carotid body with (95% O_2/5% CO_2- equilibrated medium (37°C, for 30 min), containing IBMX (0.5 mM) and adenosine deaminase (2 U/ml).

Since CADO is a non-selective adenosine receptor agonist the effect on the carotid body cAMP level of a selective A_{2a} adenosine receptor agonist, CGS 21680 (1 μM) (Fredholm et al, 1994) was also tested in one rat. In the control experiment the carotid body was incubated (95% O_2/5% CO_2- equilibrated medium, 37°C, for 30 min) with IBMX (0.5 mM) and adenosine deaminase (2 U/ml), and a value of 15.3 pmol/CB was determined. In the presence of CGS 21680 (1 μM) in the incubation medium the carotid body cAMP content was 29.7 pmol/CB.

4. DISCUSSION

The basal carotid body cAMP levels obtained in the present work (4.9 ± 1.3 pmol/CB) were higher than those of 0.59 pmol/CB described by Mir et al (1984) in rat carotid bodies incubated in the presence of IBMX but were inferior to the values, 45 pmol/pair CB, found by Hanbauer (1977) also in the rat. In the present work, incubation of the carotid bodies with IBMX for 30 min, increased cAMP level to about two times the

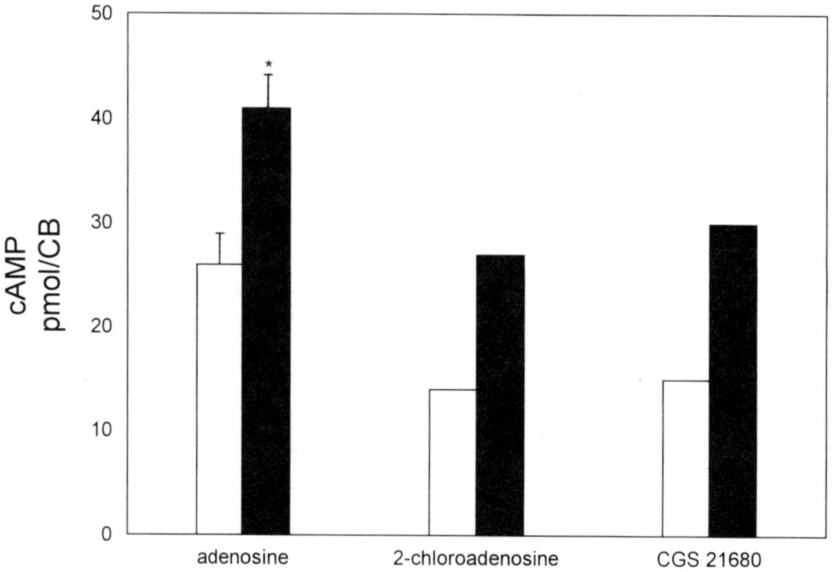

Figure 2. Comparison between the effects of adenosine (1 mM), 2-chloroadenosine (1 μM) and CGS 21680 (1 μM) on cAMP content of rat carotid bodies. Open bars correspond to control values obtained in carotid bodies incubated in the absence of test drugs. In all experiments the carotid bodies were incubated with IBMX (0.5 mM). EHNA (25 μM) was also present in the adenosine experiments (n=5) and adenosine deaminase (2 U/ml) in the experiments with adenosine analogues (n=1).

basal value. This result is comparable with the results described in the rabbit by Pérez-García et al (1990).

Inhibition of adenosine deaminase by EHNA caused a significant increase in carotid body cAMP content, indicating that endogenous adenosine is present in the carotid body and that the nucleoside at this level is metabolised by deamination. These results agree with the finding that *in vivo* EHNA mimics the excitatory adenosine effect on respiration mediated through carotid body chemoreceptors (Monteiro & Ribeiro, 1989).

In the present work it was observed that adenosine increased the cAMP content of the rat carotid body. This evidence supports the *in vivo* characterisation of an A_2 adenosine receptor subtype at the carotid body.

Since high doses of adenosine were used and this nucleoside has high affinity for the nucleoside uptake system, its effect on cAMP content could involve an intracellular mechanism instead of the activation of extracellular P_1 purinoceptors. However, the evidence that the stable adenosine analogue, 2-chloroadenosine, raised by 12.9 pmol/CB the carotid body cAMP content, mimicking the 14.8 ± 3.1 pmol/CB increment caused by adenosine, strongly supports the presence of an extracellular adenosine receptor positively coupled to the adenylyl cyclase/cAMP system.

Two subtypes of adenosine receptor A_{2a} and A_{2b} are defined as able to stimulate adenylyl cyclase. CGS 21680 is a 2-substituted adenosine analogue that discriminates well between A_{2a} and A_{2b} receptors, showing a very low (>100 μM) affinity to A_{2b} receptor subtype (Fredholm et al, 1994). Incubation of the carotid bodies with CGS 21680 caused, in the present work, an increase in cAMP content of about 14.4 pmol/CB. The intracarotid administration of CGS 21680, to anaesthetised and vagotomized rats breathing spontaneously, causes a dose-dependent increase in ventilation not present in the animals after bilateral section of the carotid bodies (Monteiro & Ribeiro, 1991).

From the results here described, it is concluded that the excitatory effect of adenosine on ventilation, probably involves the activation of an A_{2a} receptor present in the carotid body. A_{2a} receptor gene expression has recently been demonstrated at the carotid body (Weaver, 1993).

5. ACKNOWLEDGMENTS

The authors are grateful to Mrs Eunice Matos Silva for her skilful technical assistance, to the Department of Biology and Histology for the morphological preparations of the carotid bodies, and to the Department of Biochemistry for lending the β-liquid scintillation counter.

6. REFERENCES

Cunha RA, Milusheva E, Vizi ES, Ribeiro JA & Sebastião AM (1994) Excitatory and inhibitory effects of A_1 and A_{2A} adenosine receptor activation on the electrically evoked [^{3}H]acetylcholine release from different areas of the rat hippocampus. J Neurochem 63: 207–214

Fredholm BB, Abbracchio MP, Burnstock G, Daly JW, Harden TK, Jacobson KA, Leff P & Williams M (1994) Nomenclature and classification of purinoceptors. Pharmacol Rev 46: 143–156

Hanbauer I (1977) Molecular biology of chemoreceptor function: induction of tyrosine hydroxylase in the rat carotid body elicited by hypoxia. In: Acker H, Fidone S, Pallot D, Eyzaguirre C, Lübbers DW & Torrance RW (eds) Chemoreception in the Carotid Body. Berlin: Springer-Verlag. pp 114–121

Jarvis SM, Martin BW & Ng AS (1985) 2-chloroadenosine, a permeant for the nucleoside transporter. Biochem Pharmacol 34: 3237–3241

Mir AK, Pallot DJ & Nahorski SR (1984) Catecholamines: their receptors and cyclic AMP generating systems in the carotid body. In: Pallot DJ (ed) The Peripheral Arterial Chemoreceptors. London: Croom Helm. pp 311–323

Monteiro EC & Ribeiro JA (1987) Ventilatory effects of adenosine mediated by carotid body chemoreceptors in the rat. Naunyn-Schmiedeberg´s Arch Pharmacol 335: 143–148

Monteiro EC & Ribeiro JA (1989) Adenosine deaminase and adenosine uptake inhibitions facilitate ventilation in rats. Naunyn-Schmiedeberg´s Arch Pharmacol 340: 230–238

Monteiro EC & Ribeiro JA (1991) Characterization of the A_2 receptor involved in the excitatory action of adenosine on respiration through carotid body chemosensors. Portuguese Soc Pharmacol

Pérez-García MT, Almaraz L & González C (1990) Effects of different types of stimulation on cyclic AMP content in the rabbit carotid body: Functional significance. J Neurochem 55: 1287–1293

Ribeiro JA & Monteiro EC (1991) On the adenosine receptor involved in the excitatory action of adenosine on respiration: antagonist profile. Nucleosides & Nucleotides 10: 945–953

Weaver DR (1993) A_{2a} adenosine receptor gene expression in developing rat brain. Mol Brain Res 20: 313–327

ENDOTHELIN MODULATES CHEMORECEPTOR CELL FUNCTION IN MAMMALIAN CAROTID BODY

L. He, J. Chen, B. Dinger, L. Stensaas, and S. Fidone

Department of Physiology
University of Utah School of Medicine
Salt Lake City, Utah 84108

1. INTRODUCTION

The endothelins (ET-1, ET-2, ET-3), a family of unique 21 amino acid peptides, produce a transient vasodilation and protracted vasoconstriction in numerous vascular beds (see Rubanyi and Polokoff, 1994, for review). The synthesis and release of ETs was first described in cultured vascular endothelial cells, but later studies showed that ETs and specific ET receptor sites also exist in the peripheral and central nervous systems, suggesting that in addition to their role as local vasoactive agents, ETs may also function as neuropeptides (Greenberg et al, 1992; Rubanyi and Polokoff, 1994). The tissue distribution of ETs indicates that they frequently co-occur with two other potent vasoactive agents, atrial natriuretic peptide (ANP) and nitric oxide (NO). There are important interactions between these agents, and in some cases ETs are uniquely antagonistic to the physiological effects of NO and ANP (Rubanyi and Polokoff, 1994). Biochemical assessments of the signal transduction mechanisms employed by these agents have shown that the actions of ANP and NO result from increased cyclic GMP (cGMP) production and decreased cellular $[Ca^{2+}]_i$ (*e.g.*, see White et al, 1993), whereas the effects of ETs are mediated by elevated inositol phosphate (IPn), protein kinase C (PKc) and sometimes cAMP production, with consequent increases in $[Ca^{2+}]_i$ (Simonson & Dunn, 1990; Rubanyi & Polokoff, 1994).

Previous studies in our laboratory have demonstrated the existence of ANP in carotid body type I cells, and the involvement of cGMP in ANP-mediated inhibition of chemoreceptor activity (Wang WJ et al, 1993; Wang ZZ et al, 1991). Nitric oxide is another inhibitor of chemoreceptor activity, and we and others have localized nitric oxide synthase (NOS) to a plexus of fibers which innervate type I cell lobules and the carotid body vasculature (Wang ZZ et al, 1993; Prabhakar et al, 1993; Grimes et al, 1994; Hohler et al, 1994). Again, these studies have suggested that NO-dependent inhibition in the carotid body is mediated by the production of cGMP in type I cells (Wang ZZ et al, 1994,

Frontiers in Arterial Chemoreception, edited by Zapata *et al.*
Plenum Press, New York, 1996

1995). In the present study, we demonstrate that ET is also present in the carotid body, and that the application of ET *in vitro* potentiates chemoreceptor responsiveness to hypoxia, a finding similar to that recently published by McQueen et al. (1995a) using an *in vivo* preparation. Our results further suggest that the effects of ET are mediated by specific signaling mechanisms in type I cells, and that ET may be involved in physiological adjustments associated with exposure to chronic hypoxia. Finally, the data are consistent with the hypothesis that carotid body inhibition mediated by NO and ANP is counteracted by an opposing transduction pathway mediated by ET.

2. METHODS

For immunocytochemical studies, young adult male rats (180–200 g) were exposed to hypoxia in a hypobaric chamber at a barometric pressure approximately equivalent to 5500 m. The pressure was reduced incrementally over a four-day period and then maintained for ten additional days. Fresh food, water and litter were provided every three to four days. Following exposure, tissues from the chronically hypoxic rats as well as three control, age/weight-matched, male rats were removed under pentobarbital anesthesia (40 mg/Kg). Details of standard immunocytochemical procedures can be found elsewhere (Wang ZZ et al, 1993). Tissue sections were incubated with a rabbit-anti-endothelin antibody (Penninsula) specific for ET-1, ET-2 and ET-3.

Rabbit carotid bodies removed under pentobarbital anesthesia (35 mg/Kg) were used *in vitro* for evaluations of chemoreceptor activity recorded from the carotid sinus nerve (CSN), catecholamine (CA) release and cAMP determinations. Detailed descriptions of these techniques have been published previously (Wang WJ et al, 1991, 1993). For inositol phosphate (IPn) assays, rabbit carotid bodies were preincubated for 2 h (37°C) in 1 ml of modified Tyrode's solution containing 20 μCi of myo-[2–^{3}H]-inositol (0.3–0.6 μM). The carotid bodies were washed for 60 min in two changes of 100% O_2-equilibrated solution (37°C), preincubated for 15 min in solution containing 10 mM LiCl, and incubated for 30 min in selected concentrations of ET-1 (100% O_2-media containing 10 mM LiCl). Incubations were terminated in a mixture of chloroform/methanol (1:2), and the tissue homogenized in a glass-glass homogenizer. Following the addition of 2 ml chloroform and 1.0 ml water, the tubes were vortexed and phase-separated by centrifugation. The upper phase was removed and subjected to a stream of N_2 for 5 min to remove any traces of chloroform. The samples were added to columns of Doxex-1 x 8 resin (formate form) and washed with 10 ml of water, 15 ml of sodium tetraborate (5 mM) plus sodium formate (60 mM), and finally the labeled inositol phosphates were eluted with 1.0 M ammonium formate/0.1 M formic acid (1 x 2 ml). Aliquots were removed for determination of tritium in a liquid scintillation counter (Packard).

3. RESULTS

Immunocytochemical assessments of the normal rat carotid body revealed low levels of ET in the tissue (Fig 1A). While faint, ET-immunopositive cells were found throughout the carotid body parenchyma, virtually all chemoreceptor cell lobules and a high percentage (> 80%) of type I cells appeared to contain ET. ET-immunoreactivity was also observed in endothelial cells lining the larger blood vessels near to the periphery of the carotid body, but staining was not seen in the sinusoidal capillaries. Examination of tissue

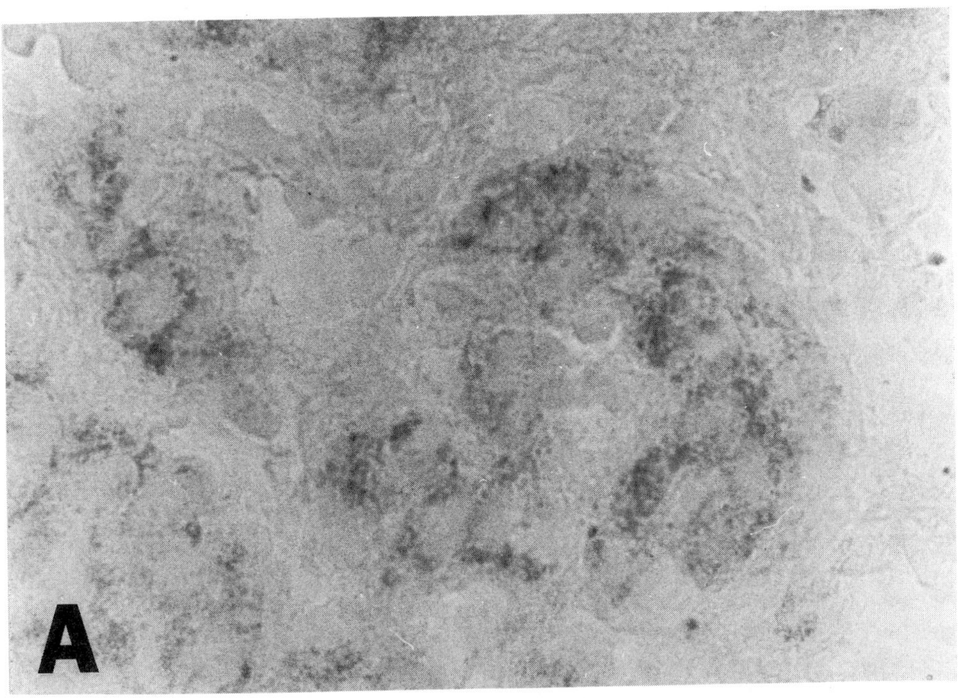

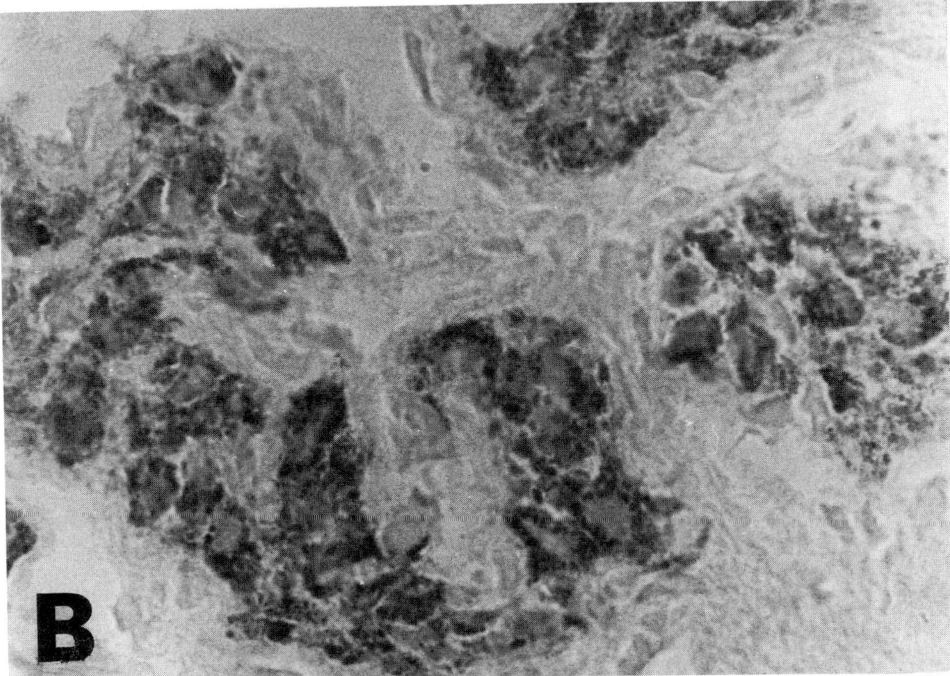

Figure 1. Endothelin-like immunoreactivity in rat carotid body. **A**. Reaction product in a normal animal is restricted to lobules of type I (glomus) cells. **B**. Staining is substantially more intense in type I cell lobules from a rat exposed to chronic (2 weeks) hypobaric hypoxia.

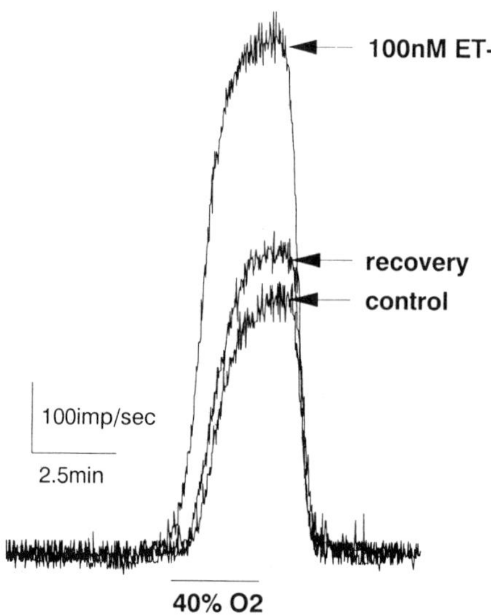

Figure 2. Endothelin-1 (ET-1, 100 nM) potentiates low O_2- (40%) evoked CSN activity recorded from a rabbit carotid body/carotid sinus nerve preparation superfused *in vitro*. ET-1 did not alter basal nerve activity (100% O_2 equilibrated media) during the 7.5 min superfusion period immediately prior to low O_2 stimulation.

sections at high magnification (not shown) revealed a granular reaction product in type I cells, consistent with the abundant dense-core vesicle population commonly found in these cells. Following a two-week exposure to hypobaric hypoxia, the level of ET-immunostaining in type I cells was substantially increased. As with normoxic carotid bodies, the storage of ET appeared to be uniform within the cytoplasm of type I cells, and the peptide was evident in virtually all lobules of chemosensory cells.

Figure 2 shows the effect of ET-1 (0.1 μM) on rabbit CSN activity recorded *in vitro* in a conventional superfusion chamber. This representative trace shows that ET-1 did not measurably alter basal chemoreceptor activity recorded in 100% O_2-equilibrated modified Tyrode's solution (pH 7.4). However, the response to a moderate hypoxic challenge (40% O_2 media) was significantly enhanced in the presence of ET-1. Following a 30 min superfusion in the absence of ET, the response to hypoxia returned to the previous control level. Other experiments in our laboratory have shown that ET-3 also enhances chemoreceptor activity in response to low O_2. In experimental trials using more severe hypoxia (*e.g.*, media equilibrated with 20% O_2), ET-1 and ET-3 increased chemoreceptor activity, but the percentage increase in CSN discharge was smaller, suggesting that ETs do not further elevate a maximal chemoreceptor response.

The data presented in Figure 3 show the effect of ET-1 (0.1 μM) on ^{3}H-catecholamine (^{3}H-CA; synthesized from ^{3}H-tyrosine) release from rabbit carotid bodies superfused *in vitro*. The results demonstrate that ET-1 potentiated (1.74-fold increase) CA release evoked by 10% O_2 media, but had no effect on basal release measured in solutions equilibrated with 100% O_2; thus, these results parallel the effects of ET on basal and low O_2-evoked CSN discharge. Additional experiments in our laboratory indicated that higher concentrations (1.0 μM) of ET-1 caused a further increase in low O_2-evoked ^{3}H-CA release, and that ET-3 likewise potentiated the release of this putative chemosensory transmitter.

Further experiments explored the possible role of cAMP and IPn as intracellular messengers mediating the effects of ET. Figure 4 shows assay data for these second messengers in rabbit carotid bodies following 10 min (cAMP) or 30 min (IPn) incubations, respectively, in the presence of selected concentrations of ET-1. The results demonstrate that both IPn and cAMP content in the carotid body are elevated by ET-1 at concentra-

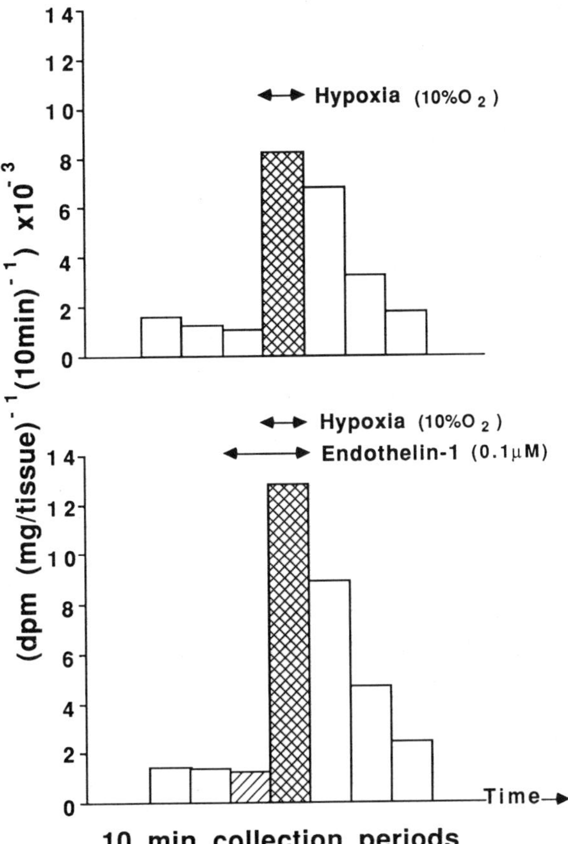

Figure 3. Catecholamine (CA) release from rabbit carotid bodies evoked by low O_2 (10%) superfusion media is increased in the presence of 100 nM ET-1. Addition of ET-1 to 100% O_2-equilibrated media did not alter basal CA release.

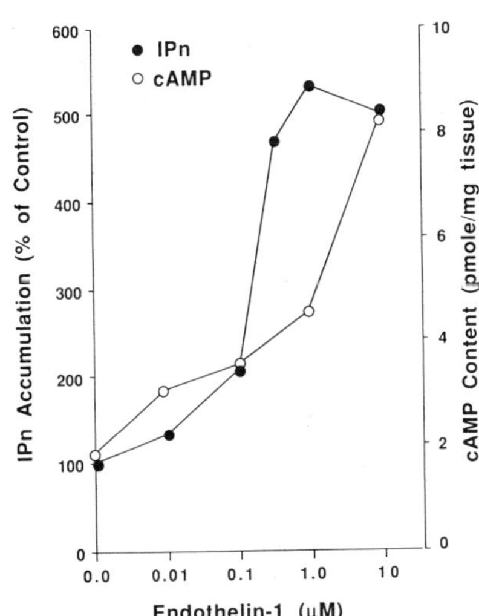

Figure 4. The effect of ET-1 on second messenger content in the rabbit carotid body. Submicromolar concentrations of the peptide increased inositol phosphate (IPn) and cyclic adenosine monophosphate (cAMP) levels in carotid bodies superfused with the peptide *in vitro* for 10 min (cAMP) or 30 min (IPn) incubation periods.

tions of 0.01 μM or higher. This concentration range includes 0.1 μM ET-1, which effectively enhanced both CSN discharge and CA release.

4. DISCUSSION

Since its discovery more than 10 years ago in cultured endothelial cells, numerous studies have documented the effects of ET in the cardiovascular, pulmonary and renal systems (see Rubanyi and Polokoff, 1994). A general conclusion drawn from these studies is that ET acts as an autocrine or paracrine factor which locally regulates cellular activity. Likewise, our investigations of the pharmacological effects of ET are consistent with this notion, in that they suggest that ET contained in type I cells amplifies the chemosensory cell response to hypoxic stimuli. Thus, we find that ET-1 potentiates both CA release from type I cells and low O_2-evoked chemoreceptor activity, but the peptide fails to alter basal nerve activity or CA secretion in O_2-saturated media. Specific receptor sites for ET have been localized to type I cells and the carotid body vasculature (Spyer et al, 1991; McQueen et al, 1995b). The signaling mechanisms which mediate chemosensory adjustments in the organ appear to involve the generation of IPn and cAMP. These findings are consistent with the actions of ETs in other tissues and cells (Abdel-Latif & Zhang, 1991; Rubanyi & Polokoff, 1994), and they suggest that in the carotid body increased $[Ca^{2+}]_i$ may be the ultimate mediator of the effects of ET. In preliminary experiments using Ca^{2+}-imaging techniques we have found that ET does not alter basal $[Ca^{2+}]_i$ in normoxic superfusion media, but it greatly enhances hypoxia-evoked Ca^{2+} responses. It is important to note that our ET-induced increases in IPn and cAMP were measured in 100% O_2-equilibrated media, when CSN activity and CA release are at basal levels. Thus, elevated levels of these second messengers are not of themselves sufficient to excite the chemoreceptor apparatus. These results are consistent with earlier studies which showed that large, forskolin-induced increases in cAMP do not augment either CSN activity nor CA release from normoxic carotid bodies (Wang WJ et al, 1991; Perez-Garcia et al, 1990).

Despite an intense research effort during the past decade, the precise physiological role of ETs in many biological systems remains elusive. Some investigators have suggested that because of their potent vasoconstrictor properties, ETs may contribute primarily to pathological events (Barnes, 1994; Rubanyi & Polokoff, 1994). Interestingly, in addition to their vasoactive properties, ETs also possess mitogenic activity, and have been implicated in the development of pulmonary hypertension associated with chronic hypoxic exposure, wherein smooth muscle and fibroblast proliferation are evident (Simonson & Dunn, 1990; Barnes, 1994). In the carotid body, our own immunocytochemical data suggest that ET levels are substantially increased following a two-week hypobaric exposure. Furthermore, our preliminary experiments indicate that ET receptor antagonists inhibit low O_2-evoked CSN activity recorded from superfused *in vitro* preparations of these chronically (hypobaric) hypoxic carotid bodies. In contrast, these ET antagonists do not alter low O_2-evoked responses from normal carotid bodies. These findings suggest that ET may play a significant physiological role in the chronically hypoxic carotid body. In this regard, previous studies have demonstrated increased CA storage in chronically hypoxic carotid bodies (Hanbauer et al, 1981) which also may be related to altered chemosensitivity (Tatsumi et al, 1995). The additional possible involvement of ETs in these chronic adjustments suggests that prolonged hypoxia may initiate a series of dynamic interactions between multiple neuroactive agents present in the carotid body, ultimately leading to a resetting of hypoxic chemosensitivity.

5. ACKNOWLEDGMENT

Supported by USPHS Grants NS12636 and NS07938. LH and JC made equal contributions to this work.

6. REFERENCES

Abdel-Latif AA & Zhang Y (1991) Species differences in the effects of endothelin-1 on myo-inositol trisphosphate accumulation, cyclic AMP formation and contraction of isolated iris sphincter of rabbit and other species. Invest Ophthal Vis Sci 32: 2432–2438

Barnes PJ (1994) Endothelins and pulmonary diseases. J Appl Physiol 77: 1051–1059

Greenberg DA, Chan J & Sampson HA (1992) Endothelins and the nervous system. Neurology 42: 25–31

Grimes PA, Lahiri S, Stone R, Mokashi A & Chug D (1994) Nitric oxide synthase occurs in neurons and nerve fibers of the carotid body. Adv Exp Med Biol 360: 221–224

Hanbauer I, Karoum F, Hellström S & Lahiri S (1981) Effects of hypoxia lasting up to one month on the catecholamine content in rat carotid body. Neuroscience 6: 81–86

Hohler B, Mayer B & Kummer W (1994) Nitric oxide synthase in the rat carotid body and carotid sinus. Cell Tiss Res 276: 559–564

McQueen DS, Dashwood MR, Cobb VJ, Bond SM, Marr CG & Spyer KM (1995a) Endothelin and rat carotid body: autoradiographic and functional pharmacological studies. J Auton Nerv Syst 53: 115–125

McQueen DS, Dashwood MR, Cobb VJ & Marr CG (1995b) Effects of endothelins on respiration and arterial chemoreceptor activity in anaesthetised rats. Adv Exp Med Biol 360: 289–291.

Perez-Garcia MT, Almaraz L & Gonzalez C (1990) Effects of different types of stimulation on cyclic AMP content in the rabbit carotid body: functional significance. J Neurochem 55: 1287–1293

Prabhakar NR, Kumar GK, Chang CH, Agani FH & Haxhiu MA (1993) Nitric oxide in sensory function of the carotid body. Brain Res 625: 16–22

Rubanyi GM & Polokoff MA (1994) Endothelins: Molecular biology, biochemistry, pharmacology, physiology and pathophysiology. Pharmacol Rev 46: 325–415

Simonson MS & Dunn MJ (1990) Cellular signaling by peptides of the endothelin gene family. FASEB J 4: 2989–3000

Spyer KM, McQueen DS, Dashwood MR, Sykes RM, Daly MdB & Muddle JR (1991) Localisation of [^{125}I]endothelin binding sites in the region of the carotid bifurcation and brain stem of the cat: possible baro- and chemoreceptor involvement. J Cardiovasc Pharmacol 17: S385–389

Tatsumi K, Pickett CK & Weil JV (1995) Decreased carotid body hypoxic sensitivity in chronic hypoxia: role of dopamine. Respir Physiol 101: 47–57

Wang W-J, Cheng G-F, Yoshizaki K, Dinger B & Fidone S (1991) The role of cyclic AMP in chemoreception in the rabbit carotid body. Brain Res 540: 96–104

Wang W-J, He L, Chen J, Dinger B & Fidone S (1993) Mechanisms underlying chemoreceptor inhibition induced by atrial natriuretic peptide in rabbit carotid body. J Physiol, London 460: 427–441

Wang Z-Z, He L, Stensaas LJ, Dinger BG & Fidone SJ (1991) Localization and *in vitro* actions of atrial natriuretic peptide in the cat carotid body. J Appl Physiol 70: 942–946

Wang Z-Z, Bredt DS, Fidone SJ & Stensaas LJ (1993) Neurons synthesizing nitric oxide innervate the mammalian carotid body. J Comp Neurol 336: 419–432

Wang Z-Z, Stensaas LJ, Bredt DS, Dinger B & Fidone SJ (1994) Localization and actions of nitric oxide in the cat carotid body. Neuroscience 60: 275 286

Wang Z-Z, Stensaas LJ, Dinger BG & Fidone SJ (1995) Nitric oxide mediates chemoreceptor inhibition in the cat carotid body. Neuroscience 65: 217–229

White RE, Lee AB, Shcherbatko AD, Lincoln TM, Schonbrunn A & Armstrong DL (1993) Potassium channel stimulation by natriuretic peptides through cGMP-dependent dephosphorylation. Nature 361: 263–266

EXPRESSION AND LOCALIZATION OF ENKEPHALIN, SUBSTANCE P, AND SUBSTANCE P RECEPTOR GENES IN THE RAT CAROTID BODY

E. B. Gauda[1] and C. R. Gerfen[2]

[1] Department of Pediatrics
Johns Hopkins Medical Institutions
Baltimore, Maryland 21287–3200
[2] Laboratory of Neurophysiology
National Institute of Mental Health
Bethesda, Maryland 20892

1. INTRODUCTION

Peripheral chemoreceptors in the carotid body sense changes in arterial oxygen, carbon dioxide tension and pH and play a critical role in modulating ventilation. The major components of the carotid body involved in chemoreception are the chemosensitive Type 1 cell which contains vesicles that store and release excitatory and inhibitory neurotransmitters, the supportive Type 2 cell, blood vessels and fibers from the carotid sinus nerve, the output from the carotid body. Dopamine, Met-enkephalin and substance P are three putative neurotransmitters/neuromodulators that have been identified in the carotid body (for review see Gonzalez et al, 1995).

Dopamine, the most abundant putative neurotransmitter found in the carotid body appears to function as an inhibitory neurotransmitter, attenuating carotid sinus nerve output similar to met-enkephalin (Iturriaga et al, 1994; McQueen & Ribeiro 1980). Evidence supports that dopamine binds to the D2-dopamine receptor subtype found on both the Type 1 cell and the carotid sinus nerve fibers, and met-enkephalin binds to the δ-opioid receptor (Dinger et al, 1981; Kirby & McQueen, 1986). The location of the δ-opioid receptor has not been determined. Substance P, on the other hand, is a major excitatory neuropeptide and has been extensively studied in several animal models (for review see Gonzalez et al, 1995). Immunocytochemical studies have demonstrated SP-immunoreactivity in the carotid body, and exogenously administered substance P agonist increase while antagonist decrease the afferent output of the carotid sinus nerve in response to hypoxia (Kusakabe et al, 1994; Prabhakar et al, 1984, 1989; Wharton et al, 1980). Because the specific substance P receptor antagonist, CP-96,345 markedly attenuates the chemosensory excitation to hypoxia, substance P is thought to bind to this G-protein coupled receptor, also known as the neurokinin 1 receptor (Prabhakar et al, 1993).

Chemosensitivity increases with postnatal maturation in several animal models including the newborn rat (Hertzberg et al, 1990; Carroll et al, 1993). Changes in the levels of neurotransmitters and corresponding receptors in the carotid body may in part account for changes in chemosensitivity with maturation. We have previously demonstrated that level of expression of the mRNAs in the Type 1 cell for tyrosine hydroxylase, the rate limiting enzyme for dopamine synthesis decreases, and the D2-dopamine receptor increases with development (Gauda et al, 1996). In order to extend those findings, the purpose of this study was to determine the presence and cellular location of the mRNAs encoding: 1) preproenkephalin, the gene that encodes met-enkephalin, 2) preprotachykinin A, the gene that encodes substance P, and 3) the neurokinin 1 receptor, the gene that encodes the substance P receptor in the carotid body, petrosal ganglion and superior cervical ganglion in the maturing rat.

2. METHODS

Time-dated, pregnant Sprague-Dawley rats were sacrificed on postnatal days 0 (n= 6), 7 (n= 5), 14 (n= 10), and 21 (n= 5). All animals were briefly anesthetized with 3% methoxyflurane and decapitated. The bifurcation of the carotid artery with the carotid body, superior cervical, nodose and petrosal ganglia were quickly removed *en bloc*, place in embedding media and then quick frozen on dry ice. Both tissue blocs were removed from the animals within 5 min of decapitation. The tissues were stored at -70°C until further processing.

2.1. In situ Hybridization

Tissue sections were cut in 12 micron sections on a cryostat. Sections were thaw-mounted onto gelatin-chrome, alum-subbed slides. Slides were then post-fixed in 4% paraformaldehyde, acetylated in fresh 0.25% acetic anhydride in 0.1 M triethanolamine, dehydrated in ascending series of alcohols, delipidated in chloroform, and then rehydrated in a descending series of alcohols. Slides were air dried and then stored at -20°C.

Antisense ribonucleotide probes were used for detection of mRNAs for preproenkephalin (PPE), preprotachykinin A (PPT-A), and substance P receptor (SPR). The antisense probes were constructed from complementary DNAs (cDNA) for each of these genes by *in vitro* transcription. The cDNA for: 1) PPE was complementary to base pairs 51–987 of the rat gene (Yoshikawa et al, 1984), 2) PPT-A was 465 base pairs (exon 7) of the rat gene (Krause et al, 1987) and 3) SPR was complementary to base pairs 637–1224 of the rat gene (Hershey et al, 1991).

Probes were labeled with ^{35}S-UTP. 1.2–1.5 x 106 dpm of labeled probe was added to 100 µl of hybridization buffer (50% formamide, 600 nM NaCl, 80 mN Tris HCL, pH 7.5 4 mM EDTA, 0.1% sodium pyrophosphate, 0.2% sodium polyacrylate, 100 mM dithiothreitol) were applied to slides containing 8–10 sections per slide and then coverslipped. Hybridization was performed at 55°C overnight. The slides were then washed in 1xSSC (0.15 M sodium chloride/0.015 M sodium citrate, pH 7.2) at room temperature. After treatment with RNAase A (20 mg/ml) slides were then washed for 4 x 20 min at 60°C in 0.2xSSC, rinsed briefly in deionized water and air dried. Slides were then dipped in Kodak photographic emulsion, dried and exposed in the dark at -20°C for 4–8 weeks. Slides were then thawed and developed with Dektol (Kodak, NY) (1:1 with water, 2 min at 17°C, stopped for 1 min with 0.5% acetic acid, fixed for 2 min with Rapid Fix without hardener, rinsed for 20 min in water, counterstained with thionin, dehydrated through alcohols and xylenes, coverslipped with Permount.

2.2. Data Analysis

Slides were qualitatively analyzed for the presence or absence of silver grains over cells in the carotid body, nodose, petrosal or superior cervical ganglia.

3. RESULTS

Adult rat brain sections that were hybridized with radioactive antisense riboprobes complementary to the mRNAs encoding preproenkephalin (enkephalin), preprotachykinin A (substance P) and neurokinin 1 (substance P) receptor showed silver grains over selected neurons in the striatum without nonspecific binding in the white matter or cortical neurons.

All animals in each age group had the same pattern of expression for enkephalin, substance P and substance P receptor mRNAs in the petrosal, nodose, jugular and superior cervical ganglia and carotid body. Represented photomicrographs are shown from animals at 14 postnatal days (Fig 1). Enkephalin mRNA was present in few cells in the superior jugular ganglion and petrosal ganglion clustered around the XI cranial nerve (Fig 1A) It was also abundantly expressed in the majority of cells in the superior cervical ganglion and not detected in cells in the carotid body (Fig 1B). Similarly, substance P mRNA was abundantly expressed in cells in the nodose, petrosal and jugular ganglia (Fig 1C) but was not expressed in cells in the superior cervical ganglion or carotid body. Lastly, mRNA encoding the substance P receptor was not detected in the carotid body (Fig 1F) but was detected in many cells in the petrosal ganglion (Fig 1D) and few cells in the superior cervical ganglion (not shown).

4. DISCUSSION

Using *in situ* hybridization which is a sensitive method of detection, the present study demonstrates that the mRNAs encoding enkephalin, substance P and the substance P receptor are not present in the Type 1 cells in the carotid body, of the maturing rat. However, the mRNA for these genes are expressed in the petrosal ganglion which contains the cell bodies for the carotid sinus nerve.

The role of opioid peptides in chemotransmission has been most extensively studied in the cat and rabbit (for review see Gonzalez et al, 1995). In both these species, met-enkephalin has been shown to be the more abundant opioid peptide in the carotid body. It has been localized to Type 1 cells by immunohistochemistry and is co-localized with catecholamines in dense core vesicles (Gonzalez-Guerrero et al, 1993; Hansen et al, 1982; Varndell et al, 1982). Similar to dopamine, met-enkephalin is released from the carotid body during hypoxia (Hanson, 1986) and inhibits chemosensory discharge (McQueen & Ribeiro, 1980). Agonists to the δ-opioid receptor attenuate and antagonists to this receptor augment chemosensory discharge in response to hypoxia in the cat (Kirby & McQueen,

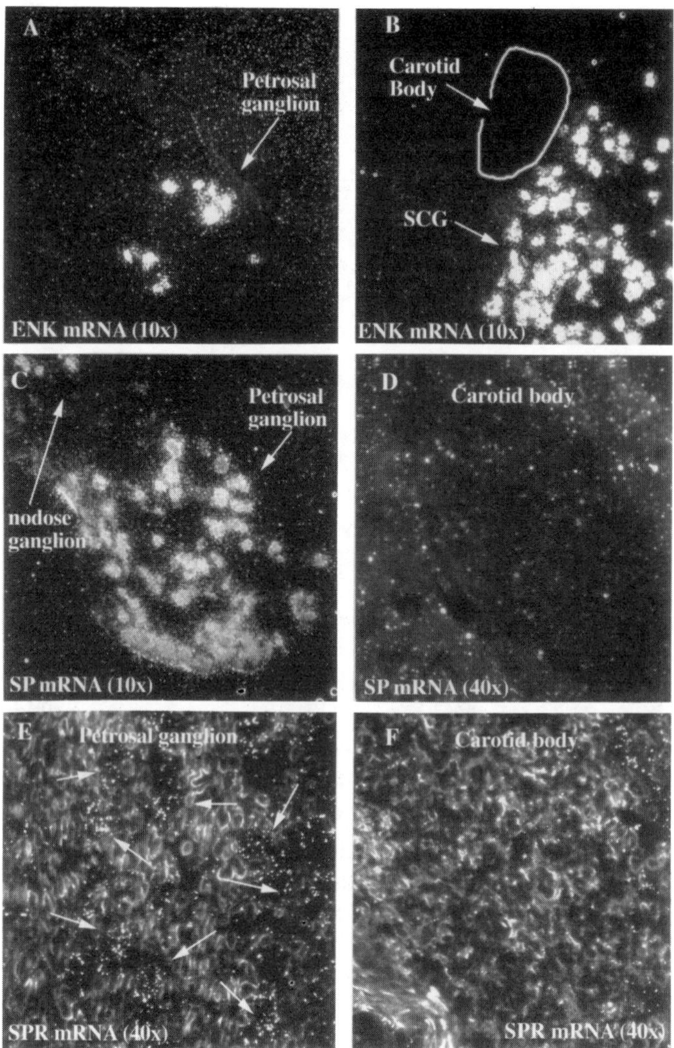

Figure 1. Dark field photomicrographs showing gene expression in the petrosal (A,E), nodose, superior cervical ganglia (B) and the carotid body (B,D,F) for preproenkephalin (ENK mRNA, panels A,B); preprotachykinin A (SP mRNA; panels C,D), and neurokinin 1 receptor (SPR mRNA, panels E,F). Silver grains appear as dense clusters of white dots. Expression is not seen for the various genes in the carotid body; panels B,D and F. Arrows in panel E are depicting gene expression in petrosal ganglion cells.

1986). Since we did not detect the mRNA for preproenkephalin, our data suggest that met-enkephalin and leu-enkephalin are not significant neuropeptides in the Type 1 cell of the rat. Thus, met or leu-enkephalin are probably not involved in alterating carotid sinus nerve output by being released presynaptically from Type 1 cells and binding postsynaptically to receptors on carotid sinus nerve fibers in response to natural stimuli. These peptides, however, may be involved in altering blood flow in the carotid body since the mRNA for this peptide was abundantly expressed in the superior cervical ganglion which contains the cell bodies for the ganglioglomerular nerve.

Substance P has also been extensively studied in the cat and immunocytochemistry studies have localized this neuropeptide to glomus cells and nerve fibers in the carotid body in this species (Kusakabe et al, 1994; Prabhakar et al, 1989). Furthermore, substance P has been measured in the carotid body of cat, rabbit and human, and is thought to be an important neuromodulator of hypoxic chemotransduction (for review see Gonzalez et al, 1995). Although pharmacology experiments in the rat suggest that endogenous substance P is released from the Type 1 cell in the rat and then binds to substance P receptors on the carotid sinus nerve (Cragg et al, 1994), our data suggest that substance P is probably not made in or released from Type 1 cells in the carotid body in this species. The mRNA encoding this tachykinin or its receptor was not detected in the Type 1 cell in the carotid body. Our data also suggest that the substance P-immunoreactivity found in the rat carotid body is most likely in parasympathetic and carotid sinus nerve fibers innervating the carotid body (Helke & Hill, 1988). In addition, neither do the binding sites for substance P appear to be on Type 1 cells. Although the mRNA encoding substance P receptor was found in petrosal ganglion cells, it has not been determined if the protein for this receptor is on carotid sinus nerve fibers innervating the carotid body.

In summary, evidence for the presence of neurotransmitters in the carotid body has been extrapolated from physiology experiments, visualized with immunocytochemistry or measured with biochemical assays. Radioligand binding studies, physiology experiments in addition to immunocytochemistry studies have also provided evidence for corresponding receptors and receptor location for many of the putative neurotransmitters in the carotid body. Now that the sequence for many of the genes for these neurotransmitters and receptors are known, more definitive localization experiments are being done to determine in what cells the neurotransmitters and corresponding receptors are made in the carotid body. By using *in situ* hybridization we have shown that the mRNA encoding two neuropeptides, enkephalin and substance P, and substance P receptor are not detected in cells in the carotid body, but are present in ganglion cells in the petrosal ganglion. In light of these findings, the role of substance P and Met-enkephalin in chemotransduction in the rat needs to be re-examined.

5. REFERENCES

Carroll JL, Bamford OS & Fitzgerald RS (1993) Postnatal maturation of carotid chemoreceptor responses to 0_2 and $C0_2$ in the cat. J Appl Physiol 75: 2383–2391

Cragg PA, Runold M, Kou YR & Prabhakar N (1994) Tachykinin antagonists in carotid body responses to hypoxia and substance P in rat. Respir Physiol 95: 265–310

Dinger B, Gonzalez C, Yoshizaki K & Fidone S (1981) ^{3}H-Spiroperidol binding in normal and denervated carotid bodies. Neurosci Lett 21: 51–55

Gauda EB, Bamford O & Gerfen CR (1996) Developmental expression of tyrosine hydroxylase, D2-dopamine receptor and substance P genes in the carotid body of the rat. Neuroscience (In Press)

Gonzalez C, Dinger BG & Fidone SJ (1995) Mechanisms of carotid body chemoreception. In: Dempsey JA, Pack AI (eds) Regulation of Breathing. New York: Dekker. pp 391–470

Gonzalez-Guerrero PR, Rigual R & Gonzalez C (1993) Opioid peptides in the rabbit carotid body: Identification and evidence for co-utilization and interactions with dopamine. J Neurochem 60: 172–1768

Hansen JT, Brokaw J, Christie D, Karasek M (1982) Localization of enkephalin-like immunoreactivity in the cat carotid and aortic body chemoreceptors. Anat Rec 203: 405–410

Hanson GR, Jones JF, Fidone S (1986) Physiological chemoreceptor stimulation decreases enkephalin and substance P in the carotid body. Peptides 7: 767–769

Helke CJ & Hill KM (1988) Immunohistochemical study of neuropeptides in vagal and glossopharyngeal afferent neurons in the rat. Neuroscience 26: 539–551

Hershey AD, Dykema PE, Krause JE (1991) Organization, structure and expression of the gene encoding the rat substance P receptor. Biol Signals 1: 143–149

Hertzberg T, Hellström S, Langercrantz H & Pequignot JM (1990) Development of arterial chemoreflex and turnover of carotid body catecholamines in the newborn rat. J Physiol, London 425: 211–225

Iturriaga R, Larrain C, Zapata P (1994) Effects of dopaminergic blockade upon carotid chemosensory activity and its hypoxia-induced excitation. Brain Res 663: 145–154

Kirby GC & McQueen DS (1986) Characterization of opioid receptors in the cat carotid body involved in chemosensory depression in vivo. Br J Pharmacol 88: 889–898

Krause JE, Chirgwin JM, Carter MS, Xu ZS & Hershey AD (1987) Three rat preprotachykinin mRNAs encode the neuropeptides substance P and neurokinin A. Proc Natl Acad Sci USA 84: 881–885

Kusakabe T, Kawakami T, Tanabe Y, Fujii S & Takenaka T (1994) Distribution of substance P-containing and catecholaminergic nerve fibers in the rabbit carotid body: an immunohistochemical study in combination with catecholamine fluorescent histochemistry. Arch Histol Cytol 57: 193–198

McQueen DS & Ribeiro JA (1980) Inhibitory actions of methionine-enkephalin and morphine on the cat carotid chemoreceptors. Br J Pharmacol 71: 297–305

Prabhakar NR, Runold M, Yamamoto Y, Lagercrantz H & Von Euler C (1984) Effect of substance P antagonist on hypoxia-induced carotid chemoreceptor activity. Acta Physiol Scand 121: 301–303

Prabhakar NR, Landis SC, Kumar GK, Mullikin-Kilpatrick D, Cherniack NS & Leeman SE (1989) Substance P and neurokinin A in the cat carotid body: Localization, exogenous effects and changes in content in response to arterial PO_2. Brain Res 481: 205–214

Prabhakar NR, Cao H, Lowe JA III & Snider RM (1993) Selective inhibition of the carotid body sensory response to hypoxia by the substance P receptor antagonist CP-96,345. Proc Natl Acad Sci USA 90: 10041–10045

Varndell IM, Tapia FJ, De Mey J, Rush RA, Bloom SR & Polak JM (1982) Electron immunocytochemical localization of enkephalin-like material in catecholamine-containing cells of the carotid body, the adrenal medulla, and in pheochromocytomas of man and other mammals. J Histochem Cytochem 30: 682–690

Wharton J, Polak JM, Pearse AGE, McGregor GP, Bryant MG, Bloom SR, Emson PC, Bisgard GE & Will JA (1980) Enkephalin-, VIP-and substance P-like immunoreactivity in the carotid body. Nature 284: 269–271

Yoshikawa K, Williams C & Sabol SL (1984) Rat brain preproenkekphalin mRNA: cDNA cloning, primary structure and distribution in the central nervous system. J Biol Chem 259: 14301–14308

48

NEUROPEPTIDE PROCESSING ENZYMES OF THE CAROTID BODY

Biochemical and Immunological Characterization of Carboxypeptidase Activity

Ganesh K. Kumar

Department of Biochemistry
Case Western Reserve University
Cleveland, Ohio 44106

1. INTRODUCTION

Several studies using immunocytochemical approaches have demonstrated that a variety of neuropeptides occur in the carotid body and that they are associated with nerve fibers or type I cells or blood vessels (Table 1). Furthermore, elegant electrophysiological studies showed that carotid body activity is augmented by exogenous administration of neuropeptides like substance P (McQueen, 1980; Prabhakar et al, 1989) and endothelins (Chen et al, 1994) whereas it is attenuated by enkephalins (Monti-Bloch & Eyzaguirre, 1985), and atrial natriuretic peptide (Wang et al, 1991). The occurrence of multiple neuropeptides and their exogenous effects on the activity of the carotid body suggest that they may be of importance in the sensory response of the carotid body.

It has been well established that neuropeptide hormones are formed as prepropeptides which undergo sequential proteolytic processing as outlined in Figure 1 to generate the biologically active forms. Prohormone convertase, an endopeptidase with trypsin-like specificity, cleaves the prepropeptide molecules at bi-basic amino acid residues generating the propeptide forms. In the ensuing step, a carboxypeptidase B-like enzyme removes the carboxy terminal arginine or lysine residue generating the active form of the neuropeptide with free carboxyl group.

It is not known whether the mammalian carotid body has the necessary enzyme machinery to synthesize neuropeptides. As a first step toward understanding the various features pertaining to the biosynthesis of neuropeptides in the chemoreceptor tissue, cell-free extracts from the cat carotid bodies were analyzed for neuropeptide processing carboxypeptidase activity using radio-labeled synthetic peptide substrate, appropriate activators, protease inhibitors and carboxypeptidase E polyclonal antibody. The results provide

Frontiers in Arterial Chemoreception, edited by Zapata *et al.*
Plenum Press, New York, 1996

Table 1. Neuropeptides found in the carotid body

Neuropeptides	Species	Cellular location	Physiological effect
Atrial natriuretic peptide (ANP)	Rabbit	Type I cells	Inhibition
Calcitonin gene related peptide (CGRP)	Human, Guinea pig, rat	Co-localized with SP, galanin; mostly nerve fibers	Not known
Endothelin	Rabbit, cat	Type I cells	Stimulation
Enkephalin	Cat, rabbit, rat, human	Type I cells, nerve fibers	Inhibition
Galanin	Human, rat, guinea pig	Co-localized with CGRP; nerve fibers	Not known
Secretoneurin	Rat	Type I cells	Not known
Substance P (SP)	Cat, rabbit, rat, human	Type I cells, nerve fibers	Stimulation
Neurokinin A	Cat	Type I cells, nerve fibers	Stimulation
Vasoactive intestinal polypeptide (VIP)	Cat	Nerve endings and ganglion cells	Not known

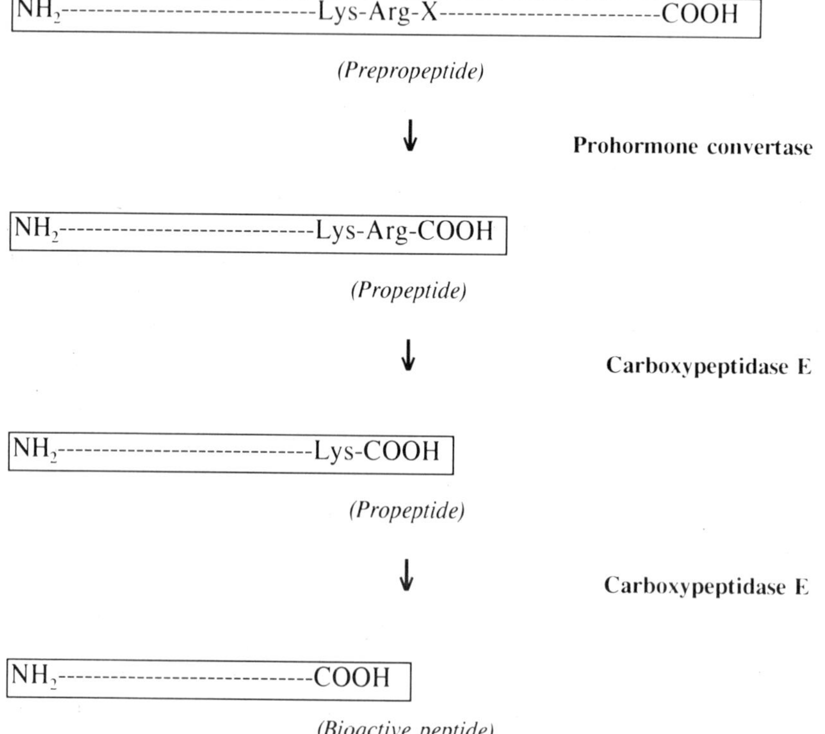

Figure 1. Illustration of proteolytic processing of bioactive peptide from precursor prepropeptide molecule.

evidence for the occurrence of carboxypeptidase-E like activity, one of the major neuropeptide processing enzymes, in the carotid body.

2. METHODS

2.1. Animal Preparation

Biochemical analyses were performed on tissues obtained from adult cats of either sex (n= 12). The animals were anaesthetized with sodium pentobarbital. The carotid bifurcation was isolated and carotid bodies were removed. The surrounding connective tissues were dissected out and the tissues were washed with physiological saline, frozen in liquid nitrogen and stored at -70°C until they were processed for enzyme analyses.

2.2. Preparation of Cell-Free Extract of the Carotid Body

For the studies of total cellular carboxypeptidases, the tissues were homogenized in 100 mM sodium acetate buffer, pH 5.6 containing 1 M NaCl and 1% Triton X-100 using a Dounce glass homogenizer and a sonicator. The homogenate was centrifuged at 50,000 x *g* for 30 min at 4°C and the pellet was extracted second time with the same buffer. The resultant supernatants were combined for enzyme analysis.

2.3. Assay of Carboxypeptidase E Activity

Carboxypeptidase E activity was assayed by the radiometric procedure as described by Rossier et al (1989). Briefly, aliquots (25 µl) of cell-free extracts or cellular fractions of the carotid body were pre-incubated at 4°C for 20 min with an equal volume of 0.1 M sodium acetate buffer, pH 5.6 containing 20 mg/ml of bovine serum albumin (incubation mixture). In parallel studies, to assess the effect of cobalt (activator) and guanidinoethylmercaptosuccinic acid (GEMSA; inhibitor) the cell-free extract was treated with incubation mixture containing either 4 mM cobalt chloride or 1 µM GEMSA. The reaction was started at 37°C by adding aliquots of the pre-incubated enzyme samples to 1.5-ml Eppendorf conical polypropylene tube containing radiolabeled substrate [^{3}H]Benzoyl-phe-ala-arg (0.02 µM) prepared in 0.1 M sodium acetate buffer, pH 5.6. The reaction was stopped after 10 min at 37°C with 680 µl of a mixture of acetonitrile: 0.25 M HCl (0.7:1 [V/V]). The content of the reaction tube was transferred to a scintillation vial, mixed with 4 ml of Econofluor, a water-immiscible scintillation fluid (NEN, Boston, MA) and counted in a Beckman Scintillation counter. The bottom, aqueous phase contained the unreacted hydrophilic substrate; the upper, organic phase contained the hydrophobic product, Benzoyl-phe-ala. Under the experimental condition, the contribution of radioactivity from the unreactive substrate was well below 200 cpm.

Carboxypeptidase E activity was calculated from the difference between the total carboxypeptidase activity in the presence of cobalt and the activity in the presence of GEMSA (Stack et al, 1984) and is expressed in femtomole of product formed per min per mg protein. The protein concentration was determined by the colloidal gold method (Stoscheck, 1987) using bovine serum albumin as the standard.

2.4. Immune-Blot Analysis of Carboxypeptidase E in Cell-Free Extract of the Carotid Body

Aliquots of the cell-free extract of the carotid body containing 0.5 to 1 μg of protein were transferred to nitrocellulose membranes using the Slot-blot apparatus (Bio-Rad Labs,) by the application of vacuum. Duplicate blots were probed with polyclonal antibody raised against peptide corresponding to the N-terminal region of carboxypeptidase E (Fricker et al, 1990). Following exposure of the nitrocellulose membranes to the primary antiserum, the bound antibody was detected by treatment with goat anti-rabbit antibody conjugated with alkaline phosphatase and the blue color developed in the presence of nitro blue tetrazolium hydrochloride and 5-bromo-4-chloro-3-indolyl phosphate.

3. RESULTS

The carboxypeptidase activity in the cell-free extract of the carotid body was analyzed by following the rate of hydrolysis of the synthetic substrate, Benzoyl-phe-ala-arg in the absence of any added metal ions. Carboxypeptidase activity of 130 femtomole per min per mg protein was observed in the cat carotid body which was completely inhibited by EDTA.

A four-fold stimulation of the carboxypeptidase activity was seen in the presence of 4 mM cobalt chloride. More than 90% of the hydrolysis, stimulated by cobalt, is inhibited by GEMSA (1 μM). The above observed stimulation of the carboxypeptidase activity by cobalt and its inhibition by GEMSA suggest that the stimulated activity may arise from carboxypeptidase E-like activity, a well studied member of the carboxypeptidase B gene family.

Carboxypeptidase E purified from pituitary has a pH optimum of 5.5. Therefore, the effect of pH on carboxypeptidase E-like activity of the carotid body was examined. Maximum enzyme activity was seen between pH 5 and pH 6 and was fully inhibited in the presence of GEMSA (1 μM).

In order to assess whether carboxypeptidase E-like activity of the carotid body is structurally similar to authentic EC 3.4.17.10 enzyme, immune-blot analysis of the cell-free extract was performed using a polyclonal antibody, directed against the N-terminal region of the pituitary carboxypeptidase E. A strong immunoreactivity was observed with the cell-free extract prepared from the cat. Also, similar immunoreactivity was also noted with the rabbit, rat and calf carotid bodies.

4. DISCUSSION

The major goal of the present study is to gain information pertaining to neuropeptide processing in the carotid body. It is well established that neuropeptides are synthesized ribosomally as prepropeptide precursor molecules and the biologically active form is then formed by the combined actions of a prohormone convertase with trypsin-like endopeptidase activity and a carboxypeptidase B-like activity cleaving the basic amino acids. In various systems, a variety of prohormone convertases and carboxypeptidases have been identified. The demonstration of the occurrence of one or more of these enzymes in the carotid body and their biochemical characterization is crucial to the understanding of neuropeptide processing in the chemoreceptor tissue.

Previously, the occurrence of trypsin-like activity in the cat carotid body has been reported (Kumar, 1996). As shown in the present study carboxypeptidase activity could be detected in the carotid body. Since a host of carboxypeptidases has been described the determination of the activation, inhibition and pH-activity profiles of the carboxypeptidase-like activity of the carotid body would facilitate in the identification of this enzyme to a specific carboxypeptidase. Based on the criteria of cobalt stimulation, GEMSA inhibition and the pH optimum of pH 5.5 carboxypeptidase-like activity of the carotid body has significant amount of carboxypeptidase E (also known as carboxypeptidase H) in addition to other carboxypeptidases. The identification of a pool of carboxypeptidase activity of the carotid body to carboxypeptidase E is further confirmed by the strong immunoreactivity of the carotid body extracts from cat, calf, rat and rabbit toward the antibody specific to the pituitary carboxypeptidase E.

The above results, thus, demonstrate that an enzyme, resembling carboxypeptidase E (EC 3.4.17.10), both in its activity profile and immunological properties, occurs in the mammalian carotid body and further lend support to the idea that the carotid body cells can process neuropeptide precursors to synthesize biologically active neuropeptides in response to the need of various cellular demands.

5. ACKNOWLEDGMENT

This investigation was supported by grant from National Institutes of Health, Heart, Lung and Blood Institute, HL-46462. The author thanks Dr Lloyd Fricker for the generous gift of carboxypeptidase E antibody.

6. REFERENCES

Chen J, He L, Dinger B & Fidone SJ (1994) Endothelin-1 activates chemosensory type I cells and potentiates the hypoxic response in rabbit carotid body. Soc Neurosci Abst 20: 1352

Fricker LD, Das B & Angeletti RH (1990) Identification of the pH-dependent membrane anchor of carboxypeptidase E (EC 3.4.17.10). J Biol Chem 265: 2476–2482

Kumar GK (1996) Peptidases of the peripheral chemoreceptors: Biochemical, immunological, *in vitro* hydrolytic studies and electron microscopic analysis of neutral endopeptidase-like activity of the carotid body. Brain Res (In press)

McQueen DS (1980) Effects of substance P on carotid chemoreceptor activity in cats. J Physiol, London 302:31–47

Monti-Bloch L & Eyzaguirre C (1985) Effects of methionine-enkephalin and substance P on the chemosensory discharge of the cat carotid body. Brain Res 338: 297–307

Prabhakar NR, Landis SC, Kumar GK, Mullikin-Kilpatrick D, Cherniack NS & Leeman SE (1989) Substance P and neurokinin A in the cat carotid body: localization, exogenous effects and changes in content in response to arterial PO_2. Brain Res 481: 205–214

Rossier J, Barres E, Hutton JC & Bicknell RJ (1989) Radiometric assay for carboxypeptidase H (EC 3.4.17.10) and other carboxypeptidase B-like enzymes. Anal Biochem 178: 27–31

Stack G, Fricker LD & Snyder SH (1984) A sensitive radiometric assay for enkephalin convertase and other carboxypeptidase B-like enzymes. Life Sci 34: 113–121

Stoscheck CM (1987) Protein assay sensitive at nanogram levels. Anal Biochem 160: 301–305

Wang ZZ, He L, Stensaas LJ, Dinger BG & Fidone SJ (1991) Localization and *in vitro* actions of atrial natriuretic peptide in the cat carotid body. J Appl Physiol 70: 942–946

COEXISTENCE OF NEUROPEPTIDES IN THE AMPHIBIAN CAROTID LABYRINTH

An Application of Double Immunolabelling in Combination with a Multiple Dye Filter

Tatsumi Kusakabe,[1] Tadashi Kawakami,[2] and Toshifumi Takenaka[2]

[1] Department of Anatomy and
[2] Department of Physiology
Yokohama City University School of Medicine
Yokohama 236, Japan

1. INTRODUCTION

The amphibian carotid labyrinth has arterial chemoreceptor and baroreceptor functions analogous to those of the mammalian carotid body and carotid sinus (Ishii et al, 1966). In addition, it has been suggested that the carotid labyrinth functions in controlling the blood flow to the internal and external carotid arteries (Kusakabe et al, 1987). We have observed several neuropeptide-containing nerve fibers in the carotid labyrinth, and suggested that the peptidergic innervation may participate in the function of the labyrinth (Kusakabe et al, 1991). In the carotid labyrinth, the coexistence of substance P (SP) with calcitonin gene-related peptide (CGRP) was first supposed from two adjacent sections (Kusakabe et al, 1991). Later, this speculation was clarified using the double-labelling method with an individual filter system (Kusakabe et al, 1993, 1994). It is now necessary to consider whether this coexistence is in a single axon within a bundle, or whether the two immunoreactivities originate from separate neurons in the same bundle. To clarify this, the precise coexistence of SP, CGRP, vasoactive intestinal polypeptide (VIP), neuropeptide Y (NPY), and galanin (GAL) was examined using a combination of double immunofluorescence labelling and a multiple dye filter system.

2. MATERIALS AND METHODS

The carotid labyrinths of bullfrogs, *Rana catesbeiana*, were fixed by perfusion and cryostat sections were processed for indirect double-labelling immunofluorescence as described previously (Kusakabe et al, 1994). In brief, the sections were first incubated with rat anti-SP (Chemicon), and then incubated with rabbit antiserum directed against either CGRP, GAL (Cambridge), VIP, or NPY (Incstar). Then they were incubated with a mixture of antisera containing rhodamine-conjugated goat anti-rat IgG (Cappel) and FITC-conjugated goat anti-rabbit IgG (Cappel). The immunostained sections were examined with a Zeiss Axiomat microscope equipped with a dual band filter set (Chroma Tecnol) for simultaneous viewing of both red and green fluorescent dyes.

3. RESULTS

Immunoreactivity of SP, CGRP, VIP, NPY, and GAL was recognized in nerve fibers distributed in the intervascular stroma of the carotid labyrinth, although there was a difference in the abundance of immunoreactive fibers as previously reported (Kusakabe et al, 1991, 1993, 1994, 1995).

When the sections double-labelled for SP and CGRP were examined with the multiple dye filter system, most SP immunoreactive fibers showed yellow fluorescence (Fig 1), which indicates the coexistence of SP and CGRP. A few fibers showed the immunoreactivity of SP but not CGRP (Fig 1). When the sections double-labelled for SP and VIP, and SP and NPY were observed in the same way, nearly one third of the former, and about half of the latter immunoreactive fibers showed yellow fluorescence. This indicates that approximately one third of the SP fibers contain VIP and one half contain NPY. These results are generally in agreement with those previously obtained with the individual filter system (Kusakabe et al, 1994). However, in high magnification images of about 10% of the yellowish fibers, there was a definite difference in localization between the fluorescence originating from rhodamine (SP fibers) and from FITC (VIP and NPY fibers), but it was clear that they are intertwined within a single nerve bundle (Figs 2, 3). The yellowish fields in Figures 2 and 3 indicate overlap between SP and VIP, and SP and NPY at different depths. This means that the coexistence suggested previously by the individual filter system may actually represent the phenomenon as described above. The distribution pattern of GAL fibers was different from that of SP fibers. Some GAL fibers were intertwined with SP fibers to form a nerve bundle (Fig 4), as previously demonstrated using a combination of double-labelling and image processing (Kusakabe et al, 1995).

4. DISCUSSION

The combination of double immunolabelling and a multiple dye filter system demonstrated new findings regarding the distribution pattern of peptidergic fibers in the carotid labyrinth, in addition to the previous findings shown by the individual filter system. In other words, combination method is able to discriminate two different fibers which run side by side. This method could be applied to various other organ systems as well.

In vascular systems, a number of physiological studies have suggested the vasoactive nature of SP, CGRP, VIP, and NPY in relation to vascular smooth muscles (Hallberg & Pernow, 1975; Heistad et al, 1980; Lundberg et al, 1982; Brain et al, 1985; Kline et al, 1988), although SP and CGRP are originally involved in sensory mechanisms (Iversen, 1982). Based on this, we have proposed that the target of these peptidergic fibers is the smooth muscles abundantly distributed in the intervascular stroma of the labyrinth, and that the vascular regulatory function may be modulated by the interaction of multiple

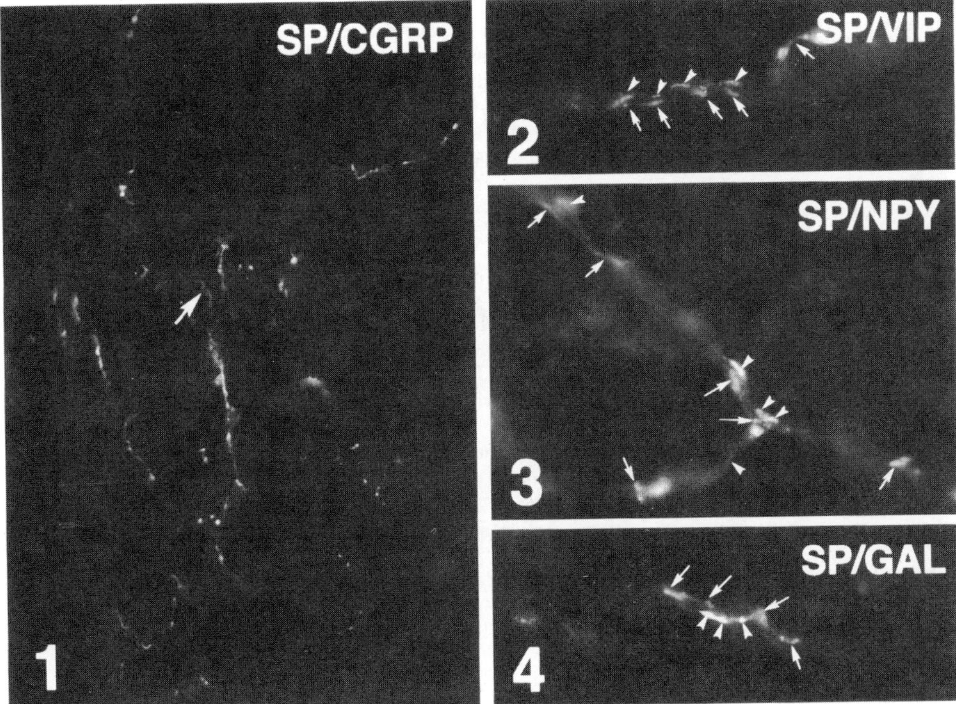

Figures 1-4. Halftone photographs of double-labelled immunofluorescent images of the bullfrog carotid labyrinth. In the original color image, most fibers show yellow fluorescence which indicates the coexistence of SP with CGRP. The arrow indicates an SP fiber without CGRP immunoreactivity. X250. High magnification images showing SP (arrows) and VIP, NPY, and GAL immunoreactive fibers (arrowheads). SP and VIP (Fig 2), SP and NPY (Fig 3), and SP and GAL (Fig 4) fibers are intertwined. X1000.

neuropeptides, although the possibility that these peptides also take part in the chemoreception in the carotid labyrinth cannot be ruled out.

5. ACKNOWLEDGMENTS

The present work was supported by grants-in-aid 04770053, 05670024, and 05770035 from the Ministry of Education, Science and Culture, Japan.

6. REFERENCES

Brain SD, Williams TJ, Tipping JR, Morns HO & McIntyre I (1985) Calcitonin gene-related peptide is a potent vasodilator. Nature 313: 54–56

Hallberg D & Pernow B (1975) Effect of substance P on various vascular beds in the dog. Acta Physiol Scand 93: 277–285

Heistad DUD, Marcus MI, Said SO & Gross PM (1980) Effect of acetylcholine and vasoactive intestinal peptide on cerebral blood flow. Am J Physiol 238: H73-H80

Ishii K, Honda K & Ishii K (1966) The function of the carotid labyrinth in the toad. Tohoku J Exp Med 88: 103–116

Iversen LL (1982) Substance P. Br Med Bull 38: 277–282

Kline LO, Kink T, Chit OW, Harvey S & Pang PUT (1988) Calcitonin gene-related peptide in the bullfrog, *Rana catesbeiana*: localization and vascular actions. Gen Comp Endocrinol 72: 123–129

Kusakabe T, Ishii K & Ishii K (1987) A possible role for the glomus cell in controlling vascular tone of the carotid labyrinth of *Xenopus laevis*. Tohoku J Exp Med 151: 395–408

Kusakabe T, Anglade P & Tsuji S (1991) Localization of substance P, CGRP, VIP, neuropeptide Y, and somatostatin immunoreactive nerve fibers in the carotid labyrinths of some amphibian species. Histochemistry 96: 255–260

Kusakabe T, Kawakami T, Tanabe Y, Fujii S, Bando Y & Takenaka T (1993) Coexistence of substance P and calcitonin gene-related peptide in the nerve fibers of the carotid labyrinth of the bullfrog *Rana catesbeiana*. Brain Res 603: 153–156

Kusakabe T, Kawakami T & Takenaka T (1994) Coexistence of substance P, neuropeptide Y, VIP, and CGRP in the nerve fibers of the carotid labyrinth of the bullfrog, *Rana catesbeiana*: a double-labelling immunofluorescence study in combination with alternative consecutive sections. Cell Tiss Res 276: 91–97

Kusakabe T, Kawakami T, Ono M, Hori H, Sawada H & Takenaka T (1995) Distribution of galanin-immunoreactive nerve fibers in the carotid labyrinth of the bullfrog, *Rana catesbeiana*: comparison with substance P-immuno-reactive fibers. Cell Tiss Res 281: 63–67

Lundberg JM, Terenis L, Hökfelt T, Martling CR, Tatemoto K, Mutt V, Polak J, Bloom S & Goldstein M (1982) Neuropeptide Y (NPY)-like immuno-reactivity in peripheral noradrenergic neurons and effects of NPY on sympathetic function. Acta Physiol Scand 116: 477–480

SECRETONEURIN

A Novel Carotid Body Peptide

D. S. McQueen,[1] U. Eder,[2] M. Timm,[3] H. Winkler,[2] M. R. Dashwood,[3] and S. M. Bond[1]

[1] Department of Pharmacology
University of Edinburgh Medical School
Edinburgh EH8 9JZ, United Kingdom
[2] Institute of Pharmacology
University of Innsbruck
A-6020 Innsbruck, Austria
[3] Department of Physiology
Royal Free Hospital Medical School
London, NW3 2PF, United Kingdom

1. INTRODUCTION

Secretoneurin (SN) is a 33 amino acid peptide formed by proteolysis from secretogranin II (chromogranin C) which is widely distributed in endocrine and neural tissue where it is stored in large dense-cored vesicles (see Kirchmair et al, 1993; Marksteiner et al, 1993). SN has been found in various parts of the brain, including the nucleus tractus solitarii —a region where chemoreceptor afferents terminate— and it is stored in C-fibre afferent neurons (Kirchmair et al, 1994). The association of SN with chromaffin tissue and with small diameter sensory nerves led us to hypothesise that SN is present in the carotid body, and we performed experiments in rats to test this hypothesis.

2. METHODS

Experiments were performed on male Wistar rats (body weight range 270–450 g) which were anaesthetised with pentobarbitone (60 mg·kg^{-1} ip, supplemented iv as required) for removal of tissues and for ventilatory and neural studies.

Frontiers in Arterial Chemoreception, edited by Zapata *et al.*
Plenum Press, New York, 1996

2.1. Measurement of SN/SN-Like Material in Rat Carotid Bodies by Radioimmunoassay

The right carotid sinus nerve was cut under halothane anaesthesia (2% in oxygen) in each of six rats. Eight days later both carotid bodies were dissected from the anaesthetised animals, weighed, rapidly frozen and stored at -70°C. Individual carotid bodies were subsequently thawed in 150 μl distilled water, ultrasonicated for 10 s, boiled for 10 min, then freeze-dried overnight. The lyophilised material was analysed by radioimmunoassay using an antibody raised against synthetic SN (secretogranin II 154–186). In the RIA the antibody reacts with free SN, but also with the precursor (secretogranin II) and intermediate breakdown products (Kirchmair et al, 1993). However, in neuroendocrine tissues (with the exception of the adrenal medulla), secretogranin II is proteolytically processed to a high degree with significant amounts of SN being present (Leitner et al, 1996).

2.2. Identification of SN Immunoreactivity in Rat Carotid Bodies by Immunocytochemistry

Anaesthetised rats were perfused via the left ventricle with 50 ml phosphate buffered ice-cold saline PBS, pH 7.4, followed by 250 ml 4% paraformaldehyde in PBS. The carotid bifurcation was dissected, stored in cold fixative for a further 2 h, then transferred to 20% sucrose in PBS at 4°C for 24 h. The tissues were subsequently quick-frozen and stored at -70°C. Serial sections (10 μm) were cut in a cryostat, -20°C, and thaw-mounted onto gelatinized microscope slides. SN-like immunoreactivity was identified using a specific antibody to SN (Marksteiner et al, 1993) by standard immunohistochemistry using the Vectastain ABC method (Vector Laboratories, Peterborough, UK) and controls were established by incubating in the absence of primary antibody. Sections were visualised on an Olympus Vanox microscope and photographed.

2.3. Measurement of Ventilation and Chemoreceptor Discharge in Anaesthetised Rats

Ventilation was measured by a pneumotachograph, and in some experiments chemoreceptor discharge was also recorded from the peripheral end of the sectioned left carotid sinus nerve (for details see McQueen et al, 1989). Drugs were injected into a cannulated femoral vein, and arterial blood pressure measured via a catheter in a femoral artery. Arterial blood samples were taken for determining pH, P_aO_2, and P_aCO_2. SN was injected either 20 s before onset of a stimulus (hypoxia, cyanide) or during a stimulus (at 150 s of a 180 s hypoxic challenge).

3. RESULTS

3.1. Radioimmunoassay for SN and SN-Like Material

RIA showed the presence of SN/SN-like immunoreactivity in the carotid bodies; the mean (± SEM) level of SN was 8.5 ± 1.6 fmol per intact carotid body; corresponding to a tissue content of 170 fmoles SN·mg^{-1}, given the carotid body's mean wet weight of 0.05 mg. Chronically denervated carotid bodies contained 13.8 ± 3.1 fmol per carotid body,

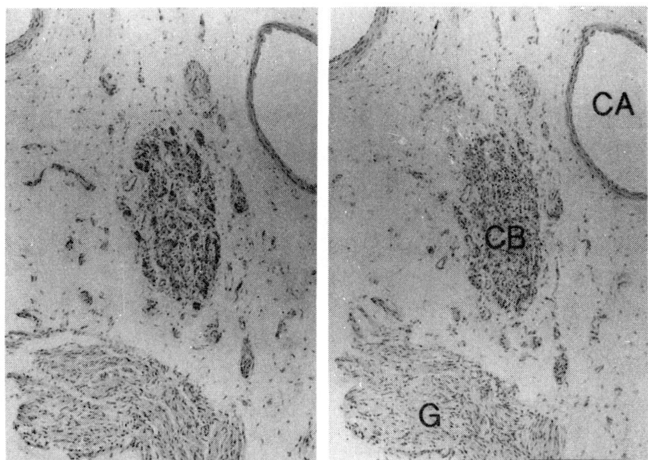

Figure 1. Left panel: section of rat carotid bifurcation showing positive SN-LI (dark areas) within the cells of the carotid body. Right panel: adjacent control section incubated in the absence of primary antibody. Tissues stained in Mayer's haemotoxylin. CA = carotid artery; CB = carotid body, G = ganglion. Calibration bar = 250 μm. SN-LI is associated with type 1 cells; there is no vascular or neural staining.

which was not significantly different from the levels in the contralateral intact carotid bodies (P>0.05, Wilcoxon test; n=6).

3.2. Immunocytochemistry for SN Immunoreactivity

The specific antibody for SN reacted with cells, probably type 1 although detailed histology was not undertaken, in the rat carotid body (see Fig 1). There was no reaction with blood vessels.

3.3. Effects of SN on Ventilation and Chemoreceptor Discharge

Low doses of SN (0.3–8 pmoles injected iv as a bolus either 15 s before induction of hypoxia, or during hypoxia) had no effect on spontaneous ventilation, nor on the reflex hyperventilation evoked by steady-state hypoxia (10% O_2 for 3 min, mean P_aO_2 35 ± 2 mm Hg; see Fig 2).

There was also no effect on mean arterial blood pressure, nor on arterial blood pH or gas tensions (mean pH 7.40 ± 0.01, PCO_2 43 ± 0.3, PO_2 70 ± 2 mm Hg before; corresponding values 3 min after SN: pH 7.38 ± 0.02, PCO_2 41 ± 3.5 and PO_2 80 ± 3.4 mm Hg; n=5). Chemoreceptor discharge, expressed in terms of basal activity, was 110 ± 11% (n=6) when averaged over the 30 s period immediately following the injection of 8 pmoles SN.

Higher doses of SN caused a slight but significant dose-related increase in chemoreceptor discharge (138 ± 9% after 80 pmoles SN, n=6, P<0.05) and a concomitant small increase in mean BP (see results from an individual experiment in Fig 2). In contrast to the lack of effect of SN on ventilation during normoxia or hypoxia, the hyperventilation caused by sodium cyanide (0.6–2.0 μmoles iv) was potentiated by SN, even in low doses, as illustrated in Figure 3. Recordings of chemoreceptor discharge confirmed that the short-lasting chemoexcitation evoked by cyanide was potentiated after SN, whereas the sustained increase in discharge associated with steady-state hypoxia was not significantly

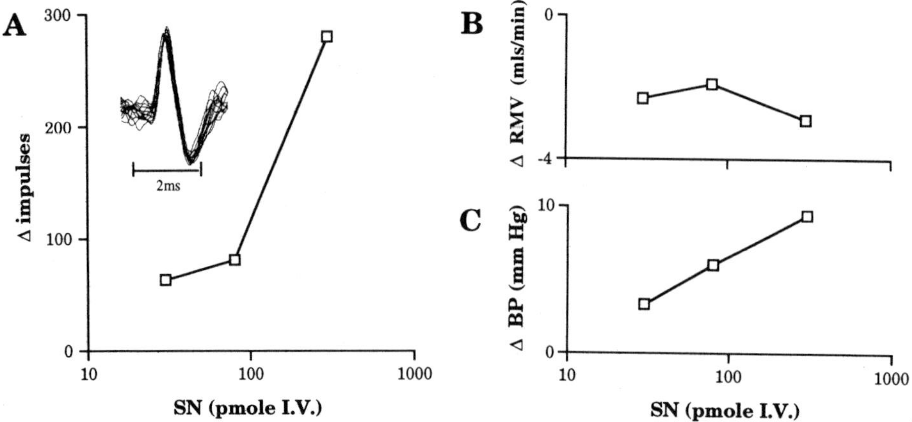

Figure 2. Data from a single experiment illustrating: A. Chemoreceptor discharge (recorded from a single unit, 10 superimposed sweeps shown in the inset panel; mean basal activity on air: 1.7 ± 0.2 impulses·s^{-1}); B. The changes in ventilation (breathing air), and C. Mean BP during the 30 s period post-SN. Higher doses of SN caused a slight dose-related increase in discharge and a rise in BP, but ventilation did not increase.

affected. As an example, the discharge following NaCN 2.0 μmoles averaged 47.6 before and 80.2 impulses·s^{-1} after SN 80 pmoles, while the discharge during steady-state 10% O_2 was 22.9 before and 27.7 impulses·s^{-1} in the 30 s period after SN 80 pmoles iv.

4. DISCUSSION

We have confirmed that SN or SN-like material is present in the rat carotid body, in amounts similar to those reported in the rat hippocampus, amygdala, thalamus and sub-

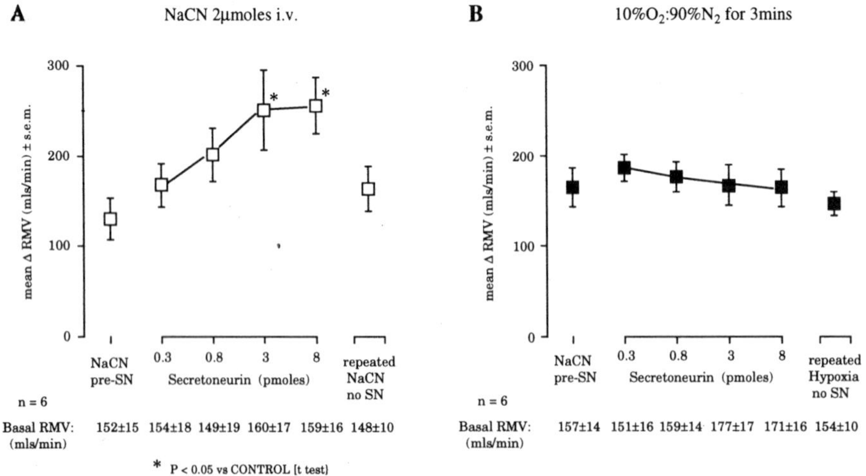

Figure 3. A. Hyperventilation evoked by sodium cyanide before and 20 s after iv injection of SN in various doses. B. Effect of SN (injected iv 150 s earlier) on hyperventilation evoked by ventilating the animal with 10% O_2. Data shown as mean ± SEM, n=6. Basal values listed below the graphs.

stantia nigra (Marksteiner et al, 1993), and the peptide appears to be localised to cells —there was no detectable binding to blood vessels. The fact that chronic denervation of the carotid body did not affect SN levels significantly demonstrates that the peptide is located within the carotid body, as confirmed by the immunocytochemistry, although we can not preclude the possibility that low levels may also be present in nerve terminals in the glomus. Measuring levels of SN in the petrosal ganglion would be informative.

Exogenous SN had no appreciable effect on ventilation in anaesthetized rats breathing either 10% O_2 or air, but it potentiated cyanide-induced hyperventilation. Evidence from recording chemoreceptor discharge in the carotid sinus nerve showed that SN caused slight dose-related increases in basal discharge, evidently insufficient to affect ventilation significantly, and confirmed that responses to cyanide were potentiated by prior administration of SN. The potentiation of cyanide's chemoexcitatory action may relate to the intense nature of this stimulus. These preliminary findings are compatible with SN having a role in arterial chemoreception, and knowing that SN causes release of dopamine in the rat striatum (Agneter et al, 1995), one could speculate that the effects of this peptide on chemoreceptor discharge might involve release of dopamine within the rat carotid body. However, the present study involving bolus iv injection of the peptide —in doses that may not be appropriate— and looking for rapid changes in ventilation or chemoreceptor discharge in anaesthetised animals may not reveal the peptide's physiological actions, particularly if they are exerted over a longer time scale.

In conclusion, there is sufficient evidence to add SN to the list of peptides that are found in the carotid body. In common with these other peptides, the mechanisms involved in secretoneurin's actions and their physiological role(s), particularly in relation to chemotransduction in the carotid body, remain to be established.

5. REFERENCES

Agneter E, Sitte HH, Stocklehiesleitner S, Fischer-Colbrie R, Winkler H & Singer EA (1995) Sustained dopamine release induced by secretoneurin in the striatum of the rat - a microdialysis study. J Neurochem 65: 622–625

Kirchmair R, Hogue-Angeletti R, Gutierrez J, Fischer-Cobrie R & Winkler H (1993) Secretoneurin - a neuropeptide generated in brain, adrenal medulla and other endocrine tissue by proteolytic processing of secretogranin II (chromogranin C). Neuroscience 53: 359–365

Kirchmair R, Marksteiner R, Troger J, Mahata M, Donnerer J, Amann R, Fischer-Colbrie R, Winkler H & Saria A (1994) Human and rat primary C-fiber afferents store and release secretoneurin, a novel neuropeptide. Eur J Neurosci 6: 861–868

Leitner B, Fischer-Colbrie R, Scerzer G & Winkler H (1996) Secretogranin II: Relative amounts and processing to secretoneurin in various rat tissues. J Neurochem (In Press)

Marksteiner J, Kirchmair R, Mahata SK, Mahata M, Fischer-Colbrie R, Hogue-Angeletti R, Saria A & Winkler H (1993) Distribution of secretoneurin, a peptide derived from secretogranin II, in rat brain : an immunocytochemical and radioimmunological study. Neuroscience 54: 923–944

McQueen DS, Ritchie IM & Birrell GJ (1989) Arterial chemoreceptor involvement in salicylate-induced hyperventilation in rats. Br J Pharmacol 101: 715–721

CARBON MONOXIDE EXCRETION, NOT OXYGEN SECRETION?

R. W. Torrance

St John's College
Oxford, United Kingdom

1. INTRODUCTION

Carbon monoxide (CO) is now thought to be involved in transmission between cells, perhaps even in the carotid body (Prabhakar, 1994), and in other, quite different, processes as well (Coburn & Forman, 1987). But that was not always thought to be so. And thereby hangs a tale.

2. INDIFFERENT GASES

I hope to show that diffusion pure and simple is sufficient to account for O_2 intakes which have been actually observed by the Pike's Peak Expedition. The principle according to which the diffusion can be estimated takes as its starting point the assumption that an essentially indifferent gas like carbon monoxide must pass through the alveolar epithelium by diffusion alone - an assumption that has never been questioned by anybody. It is assumed further that when a small proportion of CO is allowed to pass into the blood, the gas will combine practically instantaneously with the haemoglobin and the CO pressure in the blood can be taken as 0 (Krogh, 1914).

Around the turn of this century, it was still hotly debated whether O_2 gets into the blood simply by diffusion down a partial pressure gradient from the alveolar air to the pulmonary capillary blood, or whether, rather, it is actively secreted into the blood in the lungs. The answer is particularly important in the chronic hypoxia of high altitude, for secretion would make the arterial oxygen tension greater than the alveolar ($P_aO_2 > P_AO_2$) and so O_2 transport would be increased.

3. OXYGEN AT ALTITUDE

During the Pike's Peak Expedition of 1911 to study acclimatisation to high altitude in Colorado (Douglas et al, 1913), Haldane did not try to measure P_aO_2 directly in arterial blood

Frontiers in Arterial Chemoreception, edited by Zapata *et al.*
Plenum Press, New York, 1996

samples when he was testing for O_2 secretion. Instead, he refined (Douglas & Haldane, 1912) his earlier indirect method (Haldane & Lorrain Smith, 1895) for determining P_aO_2. Subjects breathed a mixture of O_2 and CO until they reached equilibrium and then the HbCO in their blood was measured, If *in vivo* the amount of HbCO, relative to the amount of HbO_2, was exactly what would be expected from the *in vitro* reactions of blood with mixtures of O_2 and CO, Haldane held that there was no evidence for anything but simple diffusion of gases between the alveolar air and the pulmonary capillary blood. But if there was more HbO_2 relative to HbCO than work *in vitro* suggested, one of two things had happened: either O_2 had been pushed into the blood - O_2 secretion had occurred - or else CO had been pushed out - it had been "actively excluded", to use Haldane's expression. The problem then was to decide which of the two gases had not been pushed, so that gas could be regarded as a reference gas for judging what had happened to the other gas. At that time, there was not an adequate direct method for measuring the PO_2 of arterial blood samples. Haldane, like Marie Krogh, thought of CO as a physiologically indifferent gas: "apart from its one property of combining with haemoglobin, it behaves as a physiologically indifferent gas like nitrogen or hydrogen" (Douglas & Haldane, 1912). He believed that CO does not occur naturally in the body, and so he could not conceive that a mechanism for its active excretion had evolved. This was his fundamental assumption when he devised his indirect method.

4. PIKE'S PEAK

Haldane used his refined method on the Pike's Peak Expedition (Douglas et al, 1913) and it did not give any evidence of O_2 secretion, either at sea level or immediately on arrival on the peak (4300 m), but after a few days at altitude, it showed that the amount of HbO_2, relative to HbCO, had increased. Haldane argued from this that the hypoxia of altitude had caused O_2 secretion to develop, and he regarded that as the principal conclusion of the expedition.

5. *CERRO DE PASCO*

Ten years later, Barcroft et al (1923) measured P_aO_2 directly in arterial blood samples taken from men at altitude and found that P_aO_2 did not increase, relative to alveolar P_AO_2, with time at altitude. This was direct evidence that O_2 secretion does not develop: it contradicted Haldane's conclusion. But if one accepts both the measurements of Barcroft et al (1923) and the measurements of Douglas et al (1913) and also accepts Haldane's argument that one or other of the two gases, O_2 and CO, was pushed, one must conclude that it was not O_2 that was pushed: Barcroft had tested for that directly. So Barcroft had established O_2 as a reference gas for judging what happens to CO, and therefore it emerged that what Haldane had shown was that, after a few days at altitude on Pike's Peak, CO came to be "actively excluded" from the body, and not that O_2 came to be secreted into the body. And CO came to be excluded on Pike's Peak presumably because of the repeated exposure of the body to CO that was required in the method of Douglas & Haldane (1912).

6. ACCLIMATISATION TO CO BY EXCRETING CO

That conclusion was not then drawn, but around that time Haldane did recognise that his body acclimatised to exposure to CO. After he had been repeatedly exposed to

CO, he found that 0.06% CO was no more noxious to him than 0.04% CO had been when he was not acclimatised. He explained that change by supposing that he had developed O_2 secretion in response to the hypoxia that CO poisoning had caused. Then Esther Killick (1948) used Haldane's method quite specifically to study acclimatisation to CO. She found that repeated exposure to CO does evoke either O_2 secretion or CO excretion, and she thought it more likely that it was CO excretion that had developed. But she could not then do what clearly she recognized to be the crucial direct experiment of measuring PO_2 in samples of arterial blood, a procedure that is now quite routine in many laboratories, but regrettably, has still not yet been applied to solving Killick's problem.

7. CO A NATURAL PRODUCT

There still remained the difficulty that CO was believed not to occur naturally in the body. But Sjöstrand (1951) suggested that CO is formed during the breakdown of Hb in the body. And then some 10 years later, a stream of papers (Coburn & Forman, 1987) established that CO is formed when a haem ring is broken open in the catabolism of Hb. Ten ml of CO is formed in that way each day in a man and it causes 1% of the Hb of his blood to be HbCO and so be blocked from transporting O_2 during normal life. And there is more HbCO in haemolytic anaemia and presumably also in the haemolysis of the newborn. Quite apart from this, it is now being suggested that CO, like nitric oxide, another free radical gas, is involved in transmissions between cells, even in the carotid body! (Prabhakar, 1994). CO simply is not an indifferent gas.

8. CO TRANSPORT AROUND THE BODY

The demonstration that CO is formed naturally in the body raises the question of how CO is transported in the body. An output through the lungs of 10 ml/day gives a concentration of 10^{-6} in the alveolar gas, or a PCO of 10^{-6} Atm. But the presence of 1% HbCO in the blood implies that P_aCO is much higher than P_ACO -it is more nearly 10^{-5} Atm. That large difference indicates that equilibrium is not reached for CO between blood and air in the lungs. But so far as transport by the blood from the tissues to the lungs is concerned, the high affinity of Hb for CO, and its low saturation with CO of only 1%, give rise to a tiny a-v PCO difference. Tissue PCO seems to be set principally by the PCO difference needed to carry CO from the blood in the lungs into the alveolar gas by diffusion, rather than by transport to the lungs in the blood in combination with Hb (Torrance, 1995). The lack of PCO equilibrium between blood and gas occurs in a situation in which CO movement is not helped by such ingenuities as the Bohr Shift and the Bohr Integral that help P_aO_2 to be very near to P_AO_2. The situation during CO excretion is much nearer to that present when the lung diffusing capacity for CO, D_LCO, is being measured, though of course CO is moving in the opposite direction in excretion. During D_LCO measurement, only about 10% of the PCO difference between gas and blood is eroded in 1 sec, the time a red bood cell spends in a pulmonary capillary, whereas, in the same length of time in normal life, well over 90% of the PO_2 difference is eroded. But also one probably should not suppose that 1% HbCO gives off CO into the plasma anywhere near so instantaneously in normal life as Marie Krogh assumed that Hb took on CO from the alveolar air during her measurements of D_LCO (American Thoracic Society, 1995).

These considerations indicate that the single CO tension that permeates the whole of the tissues of the body as a consequence of the great affinity of Hb for CO, could be little reduced by changing the blood dissociation curve for CO. But if some fraction of the output of CO were actively helped across the blood-gas barrier by active excretion, the pulmonary capillary PCO would be reduced by the same fraction, and tissue PCO should be reduced by nearly the same fraction. And that is what the data suggest happens.

9. HAEM PROTEINS AND CO

The very different affinities of Hb for O_2 and for CO are appropriate for the two quite distinct functions of Hb in transporting both of these two quite different gases, one of which, O_2, is needed by the tissues and the other of which is poisonous to them. Were the affinity of Hb for CO no more than that for O_2, there would be a quite definite a-v PCO difference - 200 times as great - and that would raise tissue PCO.

In the tissues it is different. Haem-end-oxidases, from Warburg's *Atmungsferment* and onwards to cytochrome a-a_3 and beyond, can be inhibited by CO. But their affinity for CO is less than their affinity for O_2 and therefore CO does not impede their uptake of O_2.

There are interesting consequences of the differences that exist between the relative affinities of haemproteins for O_2 and CO, and the molecular biologists have got the differences explained at a molecular level. It is nice to see how the differences may fit together at the level of the transport of gases around the body. Hb is adapted to transporting CO as well as O_2 in the body: its reactions with CO are normally an advantage at the low PCO of the body, even though the internal combustion engine may make them lethal.

10. CO *NOT* AN INDIFFERENT GAS

The idea that it can be established that a substance like CO, which reacts vigorously with one substance Hb, does not react with any other substance in the body, was wrong. And the argument that it is inconceivable that the body has mechanisms that react with substance that it has never experienced in its evolution, is disproved by nearly every new drug that is synthesised. Excretory mechanisms of the kidney, for example, deal with categories of substances, not with individual substances. When Haldane invoked the concept that CO is an indifferent gas, he got caught out because he made observations with low concentrations of CO at equilibrium. O_2 secretion destroyed Haldane's reputation in many peoples eyes. But Marie Krogh got away with regarding CO as an indifferent gas because she used such huge concentrations of CO that she swamped the mechanisms that Haldane revealed; or else she did not cause them to develop.

Of course, if Barcroft had claimed in 1923 that he had proved the existence of active excretion of CO before CO had been shown to be a natural product, or if Haldane had done that, they would have been laughed out of court for proposing a ridiculous mechanism that did not fit in with current ideas of how the body works. Haldane was tempted by O_2 secretion because it did fit in with his cherished ideas.

11. REFERENCES

American Thoracic Society (1995) Single-breath carbon monoxide diffusing capacity (Transfer Factor). Am J Crit Care Med 152: 2185–2198

Barcroft J, Binger CA, Bock AV, Doggart JH, Forbes HS, Harrop G, Meakins JC & Redfield AC (1923) Observations on the effect of high altitude on the physiological processes of the human body, carried out in the Peruvian Andes, chiefly at Cerro de Pasco. Phil Trans Roy Soc London 211B: 351–480

Coburn RF & Forman HJ (1987) Carbon monoxide toxicity. In: Cherniack NS & Widdicombe JG (eds) Handbook of Physiology, Sect 3, Respiratory System, Vol IV, Bethesda, Md: Amer Physiol Soc. pp 439–456

Douglas CG & Haldane JS (1912) The causes of absorption of oxygen by the lungs. J Physiol, London 44: 305–354

Douglas CG, Haldane JS, Henderson Y & Schneider EC (1913) Physiological observations made on Pike's Peak, Colorado, with special reference to adaptation to low barometric pressures. Phil Trans Roy Soc, London 203B: 185–318

Haldane JS & Lorrain Smith J (1896) The oxygen tension of arterial blood. J Physiol, London 20: 497–517

Killick EM (1948) The nature of the acclimatisation occurring during repeated exposure of the human subject to atmospheres containing low concentrations of carbon monoxide. J Physiol, London 107: 27–44

Krogh M (1914) The diffusion of gases through the lungs of man. J Physiol, London 49: 271–300

Prabhakar NR (1994) Neurotransmitters in the carotid body. Adv Exp Med Biol 360: 57–69

Sjöstrand T (1951) Endogenous formation of carbon monoxide. Acta Physiol Scand 16: 137–141

Torrance RW (1995) Oxygen secretion - or carbon monoxide excretion rather? J Physiol, London 487: 204P-205P

CARBON MONOXIDE AND CAROTID BODY CHEMORECEPTION

Jeffrey L. Overholt,[1] Gary R. Bright,[2] and Nanduri R. Prabhakar[1]

[1] Department of Physiology and
[2] Department of Anatomy
Case Western Reserve University
Cleveland, Ohio 44106

1. INTRODUCTION

It is being increasingly recognized that endogenously generated carbon monoxide (CO) functions as a chemical messenger in the nervous system. CO is released during the breakdown of heme to biliverdin by the enzyme heme oxygenase (HO). Two isoforms of HO have been identified: HO-1 is an inducible form and is found predominantly in spleen and liver; HO-2 is constitutive and is widely distributed in brain and nervous tissues (Verma et al, 1993). We have recently reported that HO-2 is present in the carotid bodies where it is found primarily in the glomus cells (Prabhakar et al, 1995). More importantly, we showed that zinc protoporphyrin-9 (ZnPP-9), an inhibitor of HO, increased chemoreceptor activity, suggesting that endogenous CO is inhibitory to carotid body (CB) activity. In the present study we assessed cellular mechanisms by which endogenous CO modulates CB activity. It is generally accepted that Ca^{2+}-dependent neurotransmitter release from glomus cells plays an important role in transduction of a hypoxic stimulus by the CB. Therefore, we tested the idea that endogenous CO exerts its effects on carotid body sensory activity in part by regulating cytosolic calcium ($[Ca^{2+}]_I$) in glomus cells. To test this possibility we monitored $[Ca^{2+}]_I$ and ion channel activities in glomus cells in response to ZnPP-9, an inhibitor of CO synthesis.

2. METHODS

Experiments were performed on glomus cells derived from carotid bodies of adult male rabbits euthanized with CO_2. Individual glomus cells were dissociated from carotid bodies by enzymatic digestion (trypsin, collagenase and DNAse). Single cells were obtained by gentle trituration during the incubation. Following the incubation, cells were maintained at 37°C (fluorescence ratio imaging) or room temperature (patch clamp) and used within 8 hours.

For measurements of cytosolic calcium, cells were plated on glass cover slips that were pre-treated with a cell adhesive (Cell-Tak, Collaborative Biomedical Products) and placed in 3 ml of serum free DMEM medium containing 5 μM fura-2. Following incubation at 37°C for 60 min, they were washed with serum free medium and allowed to recover for 15 min. The coverslip was placed in a gas tight, temperature regulated (37 ± 1°C) cell chamber and superfused with a solution composed of (mM): NaCl (110), KCl (5), $MgCl_2$ (0.5), $CaCl_2$ (2.2), sucrose (54), glucose (5.5) and HEPES (5). Fluorescence ratio imaging was used to quantitate $[Ca^{2+}]_I$ as previously described (Bright et al, 1996). Images were collected every 10 seconds.

Membrane currents were recorded from cells using the whole cell configuration of the patch clamp technique. Pipettes were made from borosilicate glass capillary tubing, and had resistances of 4–5 MΩ. Currents were elicited from a holding potential of -80 mV, filtered at 5 kHz and sampled at a frequency of 10 kHz. Current-voltage (IV) relations were elicited from steps to test potentials over the range of -50 to +70 mV in 10 mV increments. For recording K^+ currents the intracellular solution contained (mM): K-Glut (120), KCl (20), MgATP (5), TrisGTP (0.1), EGTA (5) and HEPES (5); and the extracellular solution contained (mM): NaCl (140), KCl (5.4), $CaCl_2$ (2.5), $MgCl_2$ (0.5), HEPES (5.5) and glucose (11). To isolate Ca^{2+} currents, K^+ and Na^+ currents were eliminated by using K^+ and Na^+-free intra and extracellular solutions with the following compositions: CsCl (130), TEA-Cl (20), MgATP (5), TrisGTP (0.1), EGTA (5) and HEPES (5); NMGCl (140), CsCl (5.4), $BaCl_2$ (10), HEPES (10) and glucose (11), respectively.

In all experiments stock solutions of zinc protoporphyrin 9 (ZnPP-9; Porphyrin Products; Logan, UT) were prepared by dissolving in distilled H_2O adjusted to pH 11 with NaOH, brought to 10 ml with 100% ethanol and were added directly to the extracellular solutions (1/1000 dilution).

3. RESULTS

We tested the effects of ZnPP-9 on $[Ca^{2+}]_I$ in glomus cells using fluorescence imaging. Glomus cells were identified as cells that responded to a brief hypoxic challenge with an increase in $[Ca^{2+}]_I$. Exposure to 1–3 μM ZnPP-9 resulted in marked elevations of $[Ca^{2+}]_I$, however, a lower dose (0.1 μM) had no effect. Changes in $[Ca^{2+}]_I$ began after the 5th min of ZnPP-9 exposure, whereby 54 of the 99 cells tested responded with an increase in $[Ca^{2+}]_I$. The remaining 45 cells showed no change in $[Ca^{2+}]_I$.

To determine whether influx of extracellular Ca^{2+} is necessary for the observed increase in $[Ca^{2+}]_I$, we tested the effect of ZnPP-9 on $[Ca^{2+}]_I$ changes in cells treated in the absence of extracellular Ca^{2+}. Figure 1 shows that $[Ca^{2+}]_I$ did not increase in response to ZnPP-9 in the absence of extracellular Ca^{2+}. These observations demonstrate that the increase in $[Ca^{2+}]_I$ in response to ZnPP-9 is mediated by an influx of extracellular Ca^{2+}, presumably conducted via Ca^{2+} channels in the plasma membrane.

To further examine the involvement of membrane ion channels in this response, we tested the effect of ZnPP-9 on Ca^{2+} current in glomus cells. As with $[Ca^{2+}]_I$, the response varied: some cells responded with an increase in Ca^{2+} current (n=2) during application of ZnPP-9; while others responded with a decrease (n=3). In neither case (increase or decrease) did ZnPP-9 appear to shift the activation curve for the macroscopic Ca^{2+} current. This suggests that the ZnPP-9 induced increase in $[Ca^{2+}]_I$ via Ca^{2+} channels in glomus cells would require depolarization, possibly by decreasing K^+ conductance. To test this possibility we monitored K^+ current in glomus cells. Macroscopic K^+ current decreased in 4 of 5 cells tested during application of ZnPP-9.

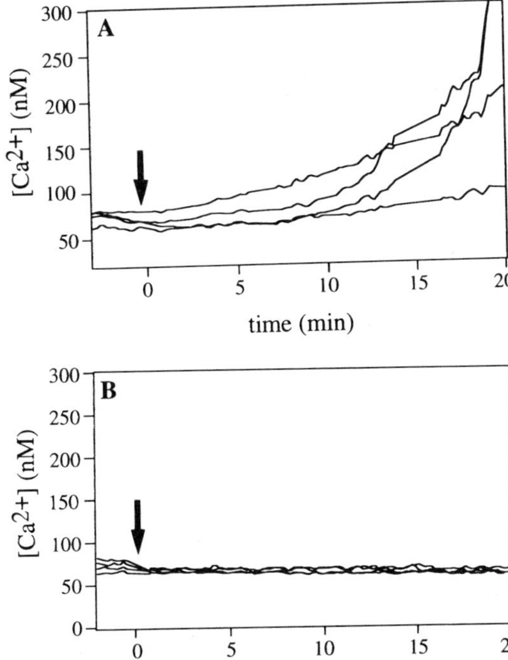

Figure 1. The effect of zinc protoporphyrin-9 (ZnPP-9; 1 μM) on cytosolic calcium in 4 glomus cells exposed to an extracellular solution before (A) and after removal (B) of Ca^{2+}. ZnPP-9 increased intracellular Ca^{2+} in 3 of 4 cells shown when the extracellular solution contained Ca^{2+}, this increase was abolished by removing Ca^{2+} from the extracellular solution.

4. DISCUSSION

The present results demonstrate that ZnPP-9 increases $[Ca^{2+}]_I$ in glomus cells. It is interesting that not all glomus cells responded to ZnPP-9. Previously we noted that HO-2 distribution is not uniform in all glomus cells (Prabhakar et al, 1995). Therefore, it is conceivable that the lack of ZnPP-9 effects in some glomus cells could be due to the absence of heme oxygenase in these cells and suggests that the effects of porphyrin are not due to non-specific toxic actions. The time course of the $[Ca^{2+}]_I$ increase was similar to that observed for the effect of ZnPP-9 on chemosensory activity in the CB (Prabhakar et al, 1995). Both were slow in onset and required minutes. This slow effect of ZnPP-9 is expected because porphyrins exert their influence by acting as a false substrate for heme oxygenase and this reaction requires minutes in *in vitro* biochemical assays. Taken together, these observations support the idea that the effects of ZnPP-9 are due to blockade of HO-2 leading to reduced endogenous CO production. Thus, these results suggest that, while the response is variable, endogenous CO can regulate $[Ca^{2+}]_I$ in glomus cells expressing HO-2.

The findings that elevation of $[Ca^{2+}]_I$ by Zn PP-9 could be blocked by removal of extracellular Ca^{2+} and Ca^{2+} currents could be augmented by ZnPP-9, demonstrate the involvement of Ca^{2+} channels. The finding that K^+ currents are inhibited by ZnPP-9 suggests that endogenous CO could maintain $[Ca^{2+}]_I$ at a low level by increasing K^+ current and hyperpolarizing the cell. Support for such a notion comes from Lopez-Lopez and Gonzalez (1992) who reported that exogenous CO decreases the hypoxia-induced inhibition of K^+ currents in glomus cells.

Lahiri et al (1993) recently showed that, at low doses, exogenous CO inhibits the CB chemosensory response. These observations, taken together with our previous study (Prabhakar et al, 1995), support the idea that endogenous CO is inhibitory to carotid body activity. The present results further support this idea and provide evidence that the effects of endogenous CO are in part due to it's action on glomus cells. In this scheme, CO generated by glomus cells acts back on the same or nearby glomus cells in an autocrine or paracrine manner. It is envisaged that CO is continuously generated during normoxia, because molecular oxygen is absolutely essential for synthesis of CO by HO (Maines, 1988). The low sensory discharge observed during normoxia might in part be due to the actions of CO on glomus cells where it prevents the release of excitatory transmitter(s) by maintaining low levels of $[Ca^{2+}]_I$. It follows that the increased sensory discharge during hypoxia might result in part from decreased CO production resulting in disinhibition. However, further studies are necessary to test these possibilities.

5. ACKNOWLEDGMENTS

Supported by NIH grants HL-07288, HL-52038, HL-02599 and HL-25830.

6. REFERENCES

Bright GR, Agani FH, Haque U, Overholt JL & Prabhakar NR (1996) Heterogeneity in cytosolic calcium responses to hypoxia in carotid body cells. Brain Res 706: 297–302

Lahiri S, Iturriaga R, Mokashi A, Ray DK & Chugh D (1993) CO reveals dual mechanisms of O_2 chemoreception in the cat carotid body. Respir Physiol 94: 227–240

Lopez-Lopez JR & González C (1992) Time course of K current inhibition by low oxygen in chemoreceptor cells of adult rabbit carotid body. Effects of carbon monoxide. FEBS Lett 299: 251–254

Maines MD (1988) Heme oxygenase: function, multiplicity, regulatory mechanisms, and clinical applications. FASEB J 2: 2557–2568

Prabhakar NR, Dinerman JL, Agani FH & Snyder SH (1995) Carbon monoxide: A role in carotid body chemoreception. Proc Natl Acad Sci USA 92: 1994–1997

Verma A, Hirsch DJ, Glatt CE, Ronnett GV & Snyder SH (1993) Carbon monoxide: A putative neural messenger. Science 259: 381–384

REGULATION OF NEURONAL NITRIC OXIDE SYNTHASE GENE EXPRESSION BY HYPOXIA

Role of Nitric Oxide in Respiratory Adaptation to Low pO_2

Nanduri R. Prabhakar, Shobha Rao, David Premkumar, Sean F. Pieramici, Ganesh K. Kumar, and Rajesh K. Kalaria

Departments of Physiology & Biophysics and Neurology
Case Western Reserve University
Cleveland, Ohio 44106

1. INTRODUCTION

Nitric oxide synthase (NOS) catalyzes the formation of nitric oxide (NO) in mammalian cells. Three isoforms of NOS have been isolated that include inducible (i), endothelial (e) and neuronal (n) NOS. We have previously reported the distribution of nNOS in carotid bodies as well as in brain stem neurons that process peripheral chemoreceptor inputs (Prabhakar et al 1993, 1995a). Physiological studies have further shown that endogenous NO modulates the ventilatory response to hypoxia by acting both at peripheral chemoreceptors and central neurons. Chronic hypoxia is known to trigger expression of several genes including erythropoietin (Goldberg et al, 1988); tyrosine hydroxylase (Czyzyk-Krzeska et al, 1994), *c-fos* protoncogene (Prabhakar et al, 1995b). The objective of the present study is to examine whether chronic hypoxia also regulates nNOS gene expression, and if so to assess the role of NO in ventilatory adaptations to hypoxia.

2. METHODS

2.1. Animal Preparation

Experiments were performed on adult rats of either sex (Sprague-Dawley) weighing between 200–250 g. Animals were exposed to hypobaric hypoxia at 0.4 Atm for 4, 12, or 24 h. Following which, they were anaesthetized (pentobarbital sodium; 40 mg/kg, ip) and nodose ganglion and cerebellum were removed, frozen in liquid nitrogen and stored at -80°C till further analysis. We chose cerebellum and nodose ganglion representing the central and peripheral neurons and they are known to contain highest amounts of NO synthase.

Frontiers in Arterial Chemoreception, edited by Zapata *et al.*
Plenum Press, New York, 1996

2.2. Measurements of mRNA and Western Blot Analysis

Messenger RNA encoding neuronal NOS was analyzed by reverse transcriptase polymerase chain reaction (RT-PCR). Tissues were homogenized and RNA was extracted by acid guanidinium/phenol method. The RNA was treated with RNase -free DNase 1 (Boehringer, Indianapolis, USA) for 1 h at room temperature to digest contaminated genomic DNA. For reverse transcription (RT), 3 μg of total RNA was added to a reaction mixture containing 5 mM MgCl, 1 mM of each deoxynucleoside-triphosphate, 2.5 μM of random hexamers, 50 mM KCl, 10 mM Tris-HCl (pH 8.3), RNase inhibitor 1 unit/μl and reverse transcriptase 2.5 units/μl. all reagents are from Perkin-Elmer. The total reaction volume (10 μl) was allowed to sit at room temperature for 10–15 min. and then incubated at 42°C for 30 min. The reaction was terminated by heating to 95°C for 5 min. and flash cooled and stored at -70°C until further analysis. 2 μl of reverse transcribed material (cDNA) was diluted with PCR buffer (50 mM KCl, 10 mM Tris-HCl, pH 8.3, 2 mM MgCl, 1.5 μM each sense and anti-sense primers, 1 μCi pdCTP (300 Ci/mmol, NEN Dupont). The total reaction volume of this resulting mixture was 10 μl incubated with 0.3 units of Taq DNA polymerase (Perkin-Elmer Cetus) and overlaid with 50 μl of light mineral oil (Sigma). cDNA was amplified for 35 cycles with following cycle profile: denaturation at 94°C for 45 seconds; annealing at 56°C for 45 seconds; extension at 72°C for 1 min. 5 μl of the PCR product was taken and electrophoresed on 2.0% agarose gels. Gels were stained with ethidium bromide radioactive products were visualized following exposure of the dried gels to X-ray film and quantified using the phosphor imaging. The primer sequence of neuronal NOS (n NOS) and β-actin were as follows: n NOS (sense) 5'TTT AAG AAA TTG GCA GAG GCC GTC-3' and anti-sense 5'TTG AAT CGG ACC TTG TAG CTC TTT 3', and β-actin (sense) 5'CAG GTC CAG AGG ATG CCA T 3' and anti-sense 5' CGA CAT GGA GAA AAT CTG CAC 3'. In preliminary experiments, we found that the PCR and product amplification was linear (r = 0.90) up to 35 cycles with the primers. The cDNA templates, isotope label and number of PCR cycles were maintained to be equal for all samples. For immuno-blot analysis of NOS protein, pre-weighed tissues were added to two volumes of cold extraction buffer containing 50 mM Tris-HCl, pH 7.6, 20 mM EDTA, 2 mM phenylsulfonyl fluoride (PMSF), 1 μg/ml leupeptin. The samples were homogenized in a motorized rotor homogenizer and centrifuged at 10,000 X *g* for 15 min and the supernatants were combined with 1 volume of 2 X sample buffer, pH 8.0, boiled and soluble proteins analyzed by 10% Tris-Tricine gels and transferred to nylon membrane. Each lane contained an equal amount of protein 100 μg. The neuronal type of NOS was detected on immunoblots using an antibody specific for nNOS and ECL Western blotting detection reagents (Amersham). Quantification of the fragments was accomplished by densitometry.

2.3. Measurements of Nitric Oxide Synthase Activity

The enzyme activity was determined by monitoring the conversion of [^{3}H] arginine to [^{3}H] citrulline. Briefly, pre-weighed tissues were placed in 10 volumes (w/v) of ice-cold buffer having the following composition in mM: Tris-HCl (pH= 7.4) 50, EDTA 1, EGTA 1. Tissues were homogenized and centrifuged at 12,000 x *g* for 1 min at 4°C. Enzyme assays contained 100 μl of tissue supernatant and 50 μl of 100 nM of [^{3}H] arginine (62 Ci/mmol; 1 pmol of [^{3}H] arginine = 0.48 x 10^5 cpm and the counting efficiency was 60%). And 10 nM NADPH and 10 nM $CaCl_2$. After 60 min of incubation at room temperature, the reaction was terminated with 3 ml of 20 mM of Hepes (pH = 5.5) with 2 mM EDTA and applied to 1.0 ml columns of Dowex AG50WX8 (Na^+ form). [^{3}H] Citrulline was quantified by liquid scintillation spectroscopy of the 3 ml flow-through. Enzyme activity was expressed as picomoles of [^{3}H] citrulline/min/mg of protein.

2.4. Histochemistry of Nitric Oxide Synthase

Tissues removed from anesthetized animals were fixed in 4% paraformaldehyde, infiltrated with 30% sucrose in 0.1 M phosphate buffer. Cryostat sections, 10 micron thick, were cut and thaw mounted on gelatin-coated slides. To demonstrate NADPH-diaphorase reaction, sections were incubated in 0.1 M phosphate buffer, pH 7.4 containing 0.3% triton X-100, 0.1 mg/ml nitroblue tetrazolium and 1.0 mg/ml β-NADPH at 37°C for 60 min. Following the reaction, the sections were rinsed in phosphate buffer (pH 7.4), rinsed in distilled water and were air dried. After placing the cover slips, sections were examined under the microscope. As controls, sections were incubated with the oxidized form of NADP along with nitroblue tetrazolium, wherein no reaction product was seen.

2.5. Measurement of Respiration

Rats exposed to normoxia or to hypobaric hypoxia were anaesthetized with intraperitoneal injections of urethane (1.2 mg/kg). A femoral artery and vein were cannulated for measurements of arterial blood pressure and for systemic administration of fluids respectively. After tracheal intubation, animals were ventilated with a respirator. Phrenic nerve was dissected from C4-C5 regions, cut and desheathed. Efferent phrenic nerve activity was monitored as an index of respiratory output from central neurons. To avoid the interference of pulmonary stretch receptors with respiratory pump, all experiments were performed after bilateral resection of vagus nerves.

3. RESULTS

Exposure to hypobaric hypoxia increased nNOS mRNA expression in both cerebellum and nodose ganglion. Significant elevations in mRNA levels were seen after 12 h of hypoxia. Average increases were 12 and 2 fold in nodose ganglion and cerebellum, respectively. β-actin mRNA expression was unaffected by hypoxia in both tissues. To establish whether mRNA is translated to NOS protein, we performed immuno-blot analysis in cerebellar extracts. nNOS protein increased by 56% percent at 24 h of hypoxia. In nodose ganglion we examined the NOS protein expression by NADPH-diaphorase histochemistry, because immuno-blot analysis could not be performed owing to the relatively small size of the tissue. In normoxic controls, 42% of the cells were positive for NADPH-diaphorase, whereas ganglion from hypoxic animals had 96% NADPH-diaphorase positive cells. To assess whether increased NOS protein is functionally active, we monitored the enzyme activity by [^{3}H] citrulline assay in cerebellum and nodose ganglion. NOS activity in cerebellum and nodose ganglion was 84% and 92%, respectively, higher in hypoxic animals than the normoxic controls.

To elucidate the functional significance of increased NO, we monitored respiratory responses to acute 6% O_2 challenge in anaesthetized rats exposed to either normoxia (n = 5) or to hypobaric hypoxia for 24 h (n = 5). In response to 6% O_2, ventilation increased in both groups of animals. However, increased respiration was maintained during the entire period of 6% O_2 exposure in animals exposed to hypobaric hypoxia, but not to normoxia. After systemic administration of L-NNA (30–60 mg/kg), an inhibitor of NOS, hypoxia exposed animals could not maintain increased respiration with 6% O_2. Instead, severe respiratory depression, often leading to apnea was seen after the first minute of hypoxic exposure.

4. DISCUSSION

Chronic hypoxia activates expression of several genes. Present results demonstrate that hypoxia as short as 12 h activates nNOS gene and increases post-transcriptionally nNOS protein. Present results, however, differ from those reported on the effects of hypoxia on eNOS expression (McQuillian et al, 1994). Unlike nNOS, prolonged hypoxia seems to inhibit eNOS expression in endothelial cultures (McQuillian et al, 1994). Neuronal and eNOS are both products of distinct genes. It is likely that the effects of hypoxia may not be uniform on both genes, in that low pO_2 may stimulate one and inhibit the other. It is clear from the western blot-analysis and enzyme activity measurements, that NOS protein levels are not only elevated, but more importantly, enzyme is functionally active. It follows that NO generation in central and peripheral neurons is increased during chronic hypoxia. What might be the physiological significance of increased NO production in the neurons? Results from ventilatory measurements implicate NO in ventilatory adjustments during chronic hypoxia. The lack of ventilatory depression in response to 6% O_2 in animals exposed to hypobaric hypoxia suggests that these animals developed tolerance to low pO_2 environment. The fact that the same animals could not tolerate acute hypoxic challenge after systemic administration of NOS suggests that NO is associated with the development of tolerance to low pO_2 in animals exposed to hypobaric hypoxia. The mechanism(s) by which NO participates in ventilatory adaptation to chronic hypoxia, however, remains to be investigated. In summary, the present results demonstrate that prolonged hypoxia up-regulates nNOS mRNA and consequent post-transcriptional increases in NOS protein. The resulting increase in NO production may help the animals to develop tolerance to low pO_2 environment.

5. ACKNOWLEDGMENT

This investigation was supported by grants from National Institutes of Health - Heart, Lung and Blood Institute HL-52038, HL-02599 and HL-25830.

6. REFERENCES

Czyzyk-Krzeska MF, Furrnari BA, Lawson EE & Millhorn DE (1994) Hypoxia increases rate of transcription and stability of tyrosine hydroxylase mRNA in pheochromocytoma (PC12) cells. J Biol Chem 269:760–764

Goldberg M, Dunning S & Bunn HF (1988) Regulation of erythropoietin gene: Evidence that the oxygen sensor is a heme protein. Science 242: 1412–1415

McQuillian LP, Leung GK, Marsden PA, Kostyk SK & Kourembanas S (1994) Hypoxia inhibits expression of eNOS via transcriptional and post-transcriptional mechanisms. Am J Physiol 267: H1921-H1927.

Prabhakar NR, Kumar GK, Chang CH, Agani F & Haxhiu MA (1993) Nitric Oxide in the sensory function of the carotid body. Brain Res 625:16–22.

Prabhakar NR, Cherniack NS & Haxhiu MA (1995a) Inhibitory and excitatory effects of nitric oxide on respiratory responses to hypoxia. In: Trouth CO, Millis RM, Kiwull-Schone HF & Schlafke ME (eds) Ventral Brain Stem Mechanisms and Control of Respiration and Blood Pressure. Lung Biology in Health and Disease, vol 82. NY: Dekker. pp 393–404.

Prabhakar NR, Shenoy BC, Simonson MS & Cherniack NS (1995b) Cell selective induction and transcriptional activation of immediate early genes by hypoxia. Brain Res 697: 266–270.

54

COHERENCE OF CHEMOSENSORY DISCHARGES IN CATS' CAROTID NERVES

Cooperative Inputs or Redundant Afferences?

J. Alcayaga,[2] R. Iturriaga,[1] and P. Zapata[1]

[1] Laboratory of Neurobiology
Catholic University of Chile
Santiago, Chile
[2] Laboratory of Neurobiology
Faculty of Sciences
University of Chile, Santiago, Chile

1. INTRODUCTION

The study of neural coding involves the analysis of four formal aspects: the *referent* (relevant features of the input), the *transformation* (encoding process), the *transmission* (anatomical and physiological substrates of neural signaling) and the *interpretation* (re-coding by a higher-order set of neurons or decoding by an effector) (Perkel & Bullock, 1968). Much of this study has been experimentally attacked by recordings obtained from sensory systems, where the fidelity or reliability of the representation process may be easily assessed.

The fidelity of transmission with regard to the referent is usually studied by searching the reproducibility of sensory responses evoked by repeated identical stimuli. However, when rapid adjustments are required from the organism, this cannot wait for repetition of stimuli to take a decision. For this purpose, "much greater capacity, sensitivity, and flexibility are furnished by the use of impulses in parallel channels" (Perkel & Bullock, 1968, p 308). Simultaneous changes in the frequency of sensory discharges of two parallel channels provide a measure of the reliability of the information processed, *i.e.*, coherent discharges along two channels are mutually confirmatory that a stimulus has indeed occurred, how intense it was and how long it lasted.

An increase in synchronization of impulses among fibers might serve to encode intensity (Perkel & Bullock, 1968, p 283). Mean frequency of discharges during stimulating conditions might not be necessarily different from mean frequency during resting conditions, but the complete asynchrony (expected for independent random processes in each unit) will be converted into synchronized bursts evoked by stimuli. The simultaneous re-

Frontiers in Arterial Chemoreception, edited by Zapata *et al.*
Plenum Press, New York, 1996

cording of pairs of single chemosensory fibers of the same carotid nerve in cats reveals high degrees of coherence in their discharges, in response to hypoxic, hyperoxic and hypercapnic challenges (Goodman, 1974).

The fidelity of transmission with regard to the referent may also be searched by studying the coherence of impulse trains carried by homologous nerves in response to a single stimulus. Since both common carotids are derived from the brachycephalic (innominate) artery in the cat, this provides similar intensive and temporal characteristics for the chemical changes of the blood circulated through both carotid bodies, and thence an ideal situation for the study of this problem. Thus, we decided to make use of this preparation.

2. ANALYSIS

In four spontaneously breathing, pentobarbitone anesthetized cats, we recorded simultaneously the impulses in the chemosensory fibers of both carotid (sinus) nerves, to analyze their temporal correlations in terms of the frequencies of chemosensory discharges (f_χ) recorded along successive 1-s periods, and their activation ($\{df_\chi/dt\}_a$) and deactivation ($\{df_\chi/dt\}_d$) rates.

Resting levels of chemosensory activities of both carotid nerves during normoxic eucapnic ventilation were analyzed, as well as the concomitant chemosensory responses of both nerves to brief changes in the O_2 content of ventilatory gases and to i.v. injections of chemoexcitatory and chemodepressant agents.

3. RESTING LEVELS OF CHEMOSENSORY ACTIVITY

In three cats, similar basal levels of f_χ were recorded from both carotid nerves. In a fourth animal, the activity of one carotid nerve consisted of few chemosensory fibers, an indication that remaining fibers have been damaged during dissection of the nerve (excision of its epineurium).

Studies on the intensive and temporal correlations between carotid chemosensory activity and ventilatory parameters commonly rest upon the analysis of the mean frequencies of chemosensory units or entire carotid nerve discharges, derived from samplings taken along each ventilatory cycle. However, such analyses do not take into account the possibility that the variance of pulse intervals may also convey significant information in terms of sensory coding. This is the case of ventilatory fluctuations in chemosensory activity, which were observed closely in phase in both carotid nerves in two animals of our present study (Fig 1).

Furthermore, concomitant transient but deep depressions in the chemosensory activities of both carotid nerves were observed in all cats immediately after spontaneous gasps (augmented breaths), and they may contribute to determine the reduced tidal volumes observed after spontaneous gasps (Zuazo & Zapata, 1980).

The neural signals sent by the carotid bodies to the brain stem may provide a measure of statistical confidence about the null hypotheses, *i.e.*, that there are no changes in the chemical composition of the blood. For this representation to occur, minimal but physiologically relevant variations in the rate of chemosensory impulses (like ventilatory fluctuations) must be differentiated from the spontaneous variability in their interspike intervals (random or not random; see Donnelly et al, 1985). The assumption can be safely

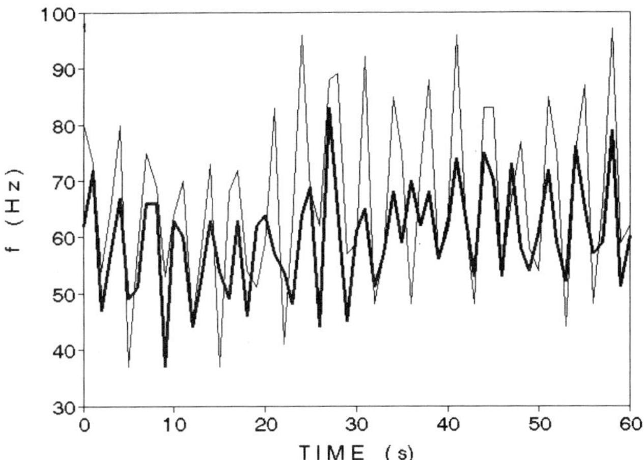

Figure 1. Ventilatory fluctuations in frequencies of chemosensory discharges (f) recorded simultaneously from both carotid nerves (heavy and light traces) of a cat breathing air spontaneously at 18 min^{-1}. Frequencies averaged for 1-s from counts taken along consecutive 100 μs periods.

made that the spontaneous variabilities in the generation of chemosensory discharges along two chemosensory units of the same carotid nerve must be mutually independent. On the contrary, coincident changes in the spontaneous rates of discharge of two chemosensory fibers may signal physiological changes in the chemical (or physical) composition of the blood. Thus, the spontaneous variations in impulse occurrence along each sensory unit will be buried into an apparently random noise when recording from the entire carotid nerve, while the physiological fluctuations will be more evident because of the temporal coincidence in the probability of such discharges between parallel channels. Similarly, minimal but temporally coherent variations in the instantaneous frequencies of discharges recorded from the two carotid nerves must also correspond to physiologically relevant changes in the intensive properties of the referent.

4. RESPONSES TO HYPOXIA AND HYPEROXIA

Brief exposures to hypoxia (breathing 100% N_2 for 5 s) increased f_χ in carotid nerves, with a high temporal correlation between frequency levels of paired nerves (r >0.97) (Fig 2A). In response to this hypoxic challenge, activation rates were more pronounced than deactivation rates, both rates of changes being highly correlated between both carotid nerves (Fig 2B). Prolonging hypoxic exposures to 10 s increased f_χ as well as $\{df_\chi/dt\}_d$, without statistically significant changes in $\{df_\chi/dt\}_a$. Figure 3A shows the time correlation between the changes in frequencies of both nerves in response to breathing 100% N_2 for 10 s.

The observation that the maximal f_χ's recorded from both carotid nerves were proportionally enhanced by prolonging N_2 tests from 5 s to 10 s, without modifying their activation rates, serves as further confirmation of the behavior of carotid chemoreceptors as proportional receptors (see Torrance et al, 1994).

The fact that while hypoxic reflex hyperventilation is abolished in cats acutely after bilateral resection of the carotid bodies (Smith & Mills, 1980), the ventilatory response of

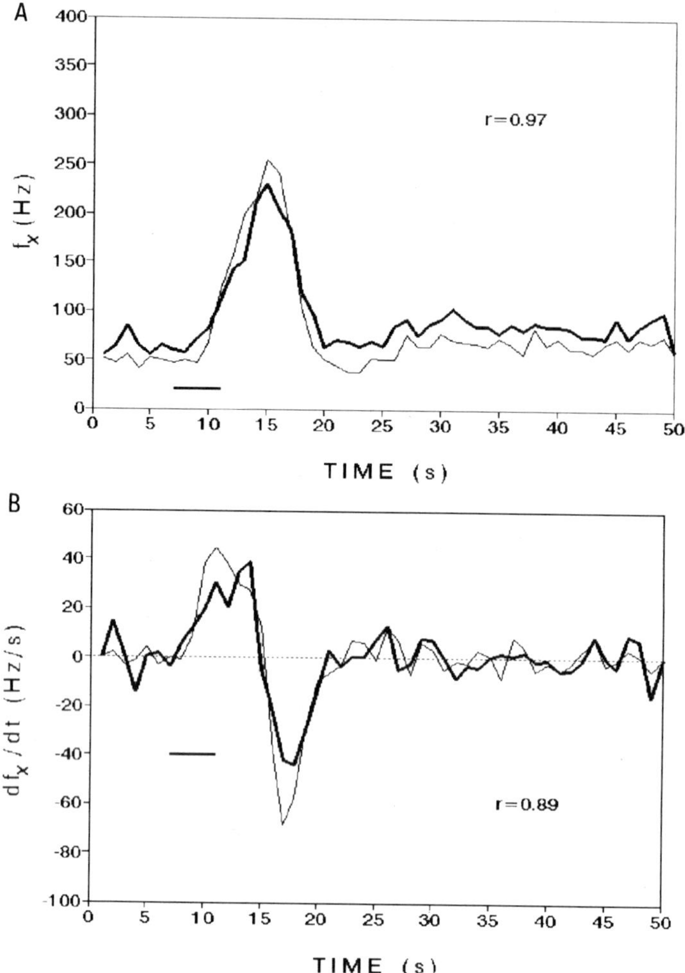

Figure 2. Changes in the frequencies of chemosensory discharges (f_χ) (**A**) and in the rates of change of those frequencies (df_χ/dt) (**B**) recorded from both carotid nerves (thin and thick lines) of one cat in response to 5 s hypoxic stimulation (breathing 100% N_2, horizontal lines). Insets, correlation coefficients. In B, activations (positive deflections) shortly after switching to 100% N_2 breathing, followed by deactivations (negative deflections) upon returning to air breathing.

cats to progressive isocapnic hypoxia is not modified by cutting one carotid nerve (Vizek et al, 1987) may be explained by present observations in terms that hypoxic-evoked coherent increases in f_χ carried by both carotid nerves will be treated as redundant inputs by the ventilatory controlling brain stem centers.

Brief exposures to hyperoxia (breathing 100% O_2 for 30 s) reduced f_χ, with a high correlation (p >0.90) between concomitant frequency levels recorded in both carotid nerves, as shown in Figure 3C. This means that both carotid bodies exhibit similar sensitivities and time reactions to changes in the PO_2 of the blood.

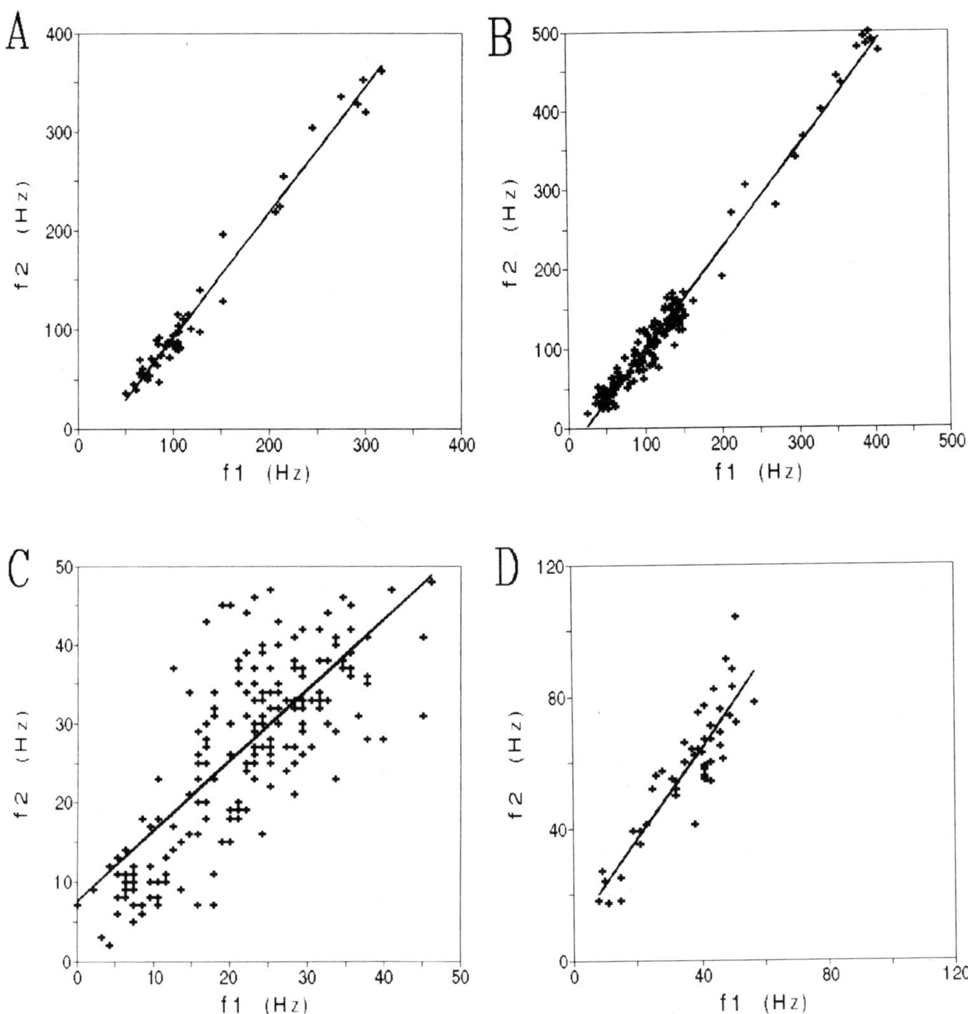

Figure 3. Correlative changes in frequencies of chemosensory discharges recorded simultaneously from both carotid nerves ($f1$ and $f2$) of same cats (A and B, same cat; C and D, another cat). Responses to: breathing 100% N_2 for 10 s (**A**), i.v. injection of NaCN 100 μg/kg (**B**), breathing 100% O_2 for 30 s (**C**), and i.v. injection of dopamine hydrochloride 20 μg/kg (**D**). Linear regression lines depicted as continuous lines. Hysteresis not evident along the temporal course of these responses.

5. RESPONSES TO NaCN AND DOPAMINE

Intravenous injections of NaCN (0.2–100 μg/kg) produced highly correlated dose-dependent increments in f_χ's recorded concomitantly from both carotid nerves (Fig 3B). Similarly, $\{df_\chi/dt\}_a$ and $\{df_\chi/dt\}_d$ increased in a dose-related manner. The ratio $\{df_\chi/dt\}_a/\{df_\chi/dt\}_d$ remained constant along the range of doses injected in most animals.

What is the purpose of having both carotid nerves conveying similar (redundant) profiles of chemosensory excitation to the brain stem? Dose-response curves for ventilatory effects evoked by i.v. injections of NaCN in pentobarbitone anesthetized cats show that while bilateral carotid neurotomy causes pronounced reductions in sensitivity and reactivity, unilateral carotid neurotomy produces mild reductions of one or both of these parameters in some cats, but not attaining statistical significance in the entire group of animals (Serani & Zapata, 1981). Thus, halving carotid afferences does not halve carotid mediated reflex effects. Then, the duplicated input carried by both carotid nerves is not simply additive.

Intravenous injections of dopamine hydrochloride (0.02–20 μg/kg) reduced f_{χ} bilaterally, chemosensory silences being reached with doses of about 0.2–0.5 μg/kg. The correlations between the reduced f_{χ}'s recorded from both carotid nerves (Fig 3D) remained constant within the dose range analyzed.

Intravenous injections of dopamine are known to produce transient ventilatory depression, which results from the sudden withdrawal of carotid chemosensory drive (Zapata & Zuazo, 1980). It was found that the first cycle of reduced tidal volume was shortly preceded by pronounced reduction or silencing of chemosensory discharges recorded from one carotid nerve. Furthermore, the depressant ventilatory responses to dopamine were not significantly modified by section of one carotid nerve, but they were abolished after sectioning both carotid nerves (Zapata & Zuazo, 1980). Thus, present observations may explain the intense (although transient) reduction in ventilation produced by dopamine as the result of the concomitant reduction or brief abolition of chemosensory impulses carried by both carotid nerves.

6. COHERENCE OF CHEMOSENSORY DISCHARGES PROPAGATED ALONG BOTH CAROTID NERVES. REDUNDANCY OF AFFERENT PATHWAYS

Our results indicate that afferent discharges recorded simultaneously from both carotid nerves in response to chemical stimuli present quite coherent patterns: similar delays, maximal (or minimal) frequencies of discharges, durations of impulse trains above or below basal activities, activation and deactivation rates. Thus, the carotid nerves may be considered as replicated afferent pathways, conveying redundant information on the composition of the blood.

Redundancy of afferent channels is an essential feature of systems characterized by a high safety factor. It implies that no one neuron is crucial to the operation of the system. The homogeneity of the afferent activity carried by the chemosensory fibers contained within each carotid nerve (Goodman, 1974) must be interpreted as redundant information and results in a high safety factor for the afferent branch intervening in the chemical regulation of ventilation. The additional redundant information carried by both carotid nerves (as shown in the present report) duplicates this safety factor and signals the physiological importance of the process involved.

7. COOPERATIVENESS OF CHEMOSENSORY INPUTS WITH REGARD TO VENTILATORY REGULATION

It has been observed that unilateral intracarotid administration of dopamine, to transiently reduce or silence the discharges of only one carotid nerve, results in minimal or absent depression of ventilation, while the same injection evokes consistent transient ventilatory depression when repeated after section of the contralateral carotid nerve (Zapata & Zuazo, 1980). Thus, respiratory controlling bulbar structures appear to disregard falls in f_χ arriving through one carotid nerve if the contralateral homologous nerve continues carrying a normal frequency of chemosensory discharges. However, in the absence of chemosensory impulses impinging through one carotid nerve, the same falls in f_χ arriving through the contralateral nerve are translated into transient depression of ventilation.

On the other hand, which is the ventilatory output resulting from concomitant changes in carotid chemosensory inputs? While studying the integrated phrenic activity evoked by submaximal electrical stimulation of either one or both carotid nerves in cats, Eldridge et al (1981) observed that the combined stimulation of both nerves resulted in an increase of ventilatory output of about two thirds of that predicted from a summing of the stimulations given by separate. Thus, an hypoadditive integration of concomitant carotid inputs was performed by the central ventilatory controller.

Since observations here reported show that both carotid nerves carry essentially similar chemosensory information, which will be the result of suppressing the activity of one of these nerves? In pentobarbitone anesthetized cats, the conduction blockade caused by applying lidocaine to one carotid nerve induces transient ventilatory depression, after which basal ventilation returns to levels not significantly different from those observed in previous control conditions (Eugenin et al, 1989). However, analysis of the dose-response curves for the ventilatory effects induced in these cats by i.v. injections of NaCN revealed a minimal reduction of sensitivity after unilateral carotid neurotomy, compared to the pronounced decrease following bilateral carotid neurotomy, whereas the reduction in tidal volume reactivity after unilateral carotid neurotomy approximately halved that induced by bilateral carotid neurotomy. Partly different results were observed in pentobarbitone anesthetized rats breathing gas mixtures which O_2 content varies between 21% and 8%, in which ventilation was not significantly decreased by unilateral carotid nerve section, in contrast with bilateral carotid nerve section which caused significant reductions in ventilation in all the conditions studied (Cragg & Khrisanapant, 1994). These observations indicate that a variable part of the information conveyed by both carotid nerves is treated as redundant input by brain stem structures involved in ventilatory regulation.

In summary, under physiological conditions, the ventilatory output to a given chemoreceptive stimulus rests upon central structures reading the ensemble averaged activity obtained simultaneously over the population of primary chemosensory inputs contained within both carotid nerves.

8. ACKNOWLEDGMENTS

This work was supported by the National Fund for Scientific and Technological Development (FONDECYT grant 193 0615) and the Research and Postgraduate Division of the Catholic University of Chile (DIPUC).

9. REFERENCES

Cragg PA & Khrisanapant W (1994) Is the second carotid body redundant? Adv Exp Med Biol 360: 297–299

Donnelly DF, Nolan WF, Smith EJ & Dutton RE (1985) Interspike interval dependency from arterial chemoreceptors. J Appl Physiol 59: 1566–1570

Eldridge FL, Gill-Kumar P & Millhorn DE (1981) Input-output relationships of central neural circuits involved in respiration in cats. J Physiol, London 311: 81–95

Eugenin J, Larrain C & Zapata P (1989) Correlative contribution of carotid and aortic afferences to the ventilatory chemosensory drive in steady-state normoxia and to the ventilatory chemoreflexes induced by transient hypoxia. Arch Biol Med Exp 22: 395–408

Goodman NW (1974) Some observations on the homogeneity of response of single chemoreceptor fibres. Respir Physiol 20: 271–281

Perkel DH & Bullock TH (1968) Neural coding. A report based on an NRP work session. Neurosci Res Program Bull 6: 221–348

Serani A & Zapata P (1981) Relative contribution of carotid and aortic bodies to cyanide-induced ventilatory responses in the cat. Arch Intl Pharmacodyn Thér 522: 284–297

Smith PG & Mills E (1980) Restoration of reflex ventilatory response to hypoxia after removal of carotid bodies in the cat. Neuroscience 5: 573–580

Torrance RW, Iturriaga R & Zapata P (1994) Effects of expiratory duration on chemoreceptor oscillations. Adv Exp Med Biol 360: 241–243

Vizek M, Pickett CK & Weil JV (1987) Interindividual variation in hypoxic ventilatory response: potential role of carotid body. J Appl Physiol 63: 1884–1889

Zapata P & Zuazo A (1980) Respiratory effects of dopamine-induced inhibition of chemosensory inflow. Respir Physiol 40: 79–92

Zuazo A & Zapata P (1980) Regulatory role of carotid nerve afferences upon the frequency and pattern of spontaneous gasp complexes. Neurosci Lett 16: 11–116

55

CAROTID CHEMOREFLEX

Neural Pathways and Transmitters

Hreday N. Sapru

Section of Neurological Surgery and Department of Pharmacology
New Jersey Medical School
Newark, New Jersey 07103

1. INTRODUCTION

Relatively little is known regarding the neural pathways mediating the respiratory responses to chemoreceptor stimulation and the transmitters involved in these pathways. Recently published information on this topic is presented in this short review.

2. CAROTID CHEMORECEPTOR PROJECTION SITE (CPS)

The chemoreceptor fibers from the carotid body and the baroreceptor fibers from the carotid sinus travel together in the carotid sinus nerve, which joins the glossopharyngeal nerve (Sapru & Krieger, 1977). It is generally believed that the chemoreceptor afferents make their first synapse in the nucleus tractus solitarius (NTS) at the same site where the baroreceptor afferents terminate (Jordan, 1994). However, the studies mentioned in this section indicate that the carotid body afferents in the rat do not project to the intermediate portion NTS where the baroreceptor afferents make their primary synapse. Instead, they project to a midline area in the commissural subnucleus of NTS. This midline area, tentatively designated as "chemoreceptor projection site (CPS)", is located in an area 0.5–0.75 mm caudal and 0.3–0.5 mm deep with respect to the *calamus scriptorius* (caudal most point of the 4th ventricle).

Microinjections of L-glutamate (88.5 mM/20–50 nl), which stimulates neuronal cell bodies but not fibers of passage, into the CPS elicited responses similar to those following carotid chemoreceptor stimulation (*i.e.*, increase in mean arterial pressure and minute ventilation). On the other hand, microinjections of glutamate into the intermediate portion of NTS (0.5 rostral, 0.5 lateral and 0.5 deep with respect to the *calamus scriptorius*) elicited responses (apnea, bradycardia and hypotension) which were reminiscent of either pulmonary J receptor activation (Sapru et al, 1981b) or baroreceptor stimulation (Sapru et al, 1981a; Sundaram et al, 1989; Urbanski & Sapru, 1988).

Frontiers in Arterial Chemoreception, edited by Zapata *et al.*
Plenum Press, New York, 1996

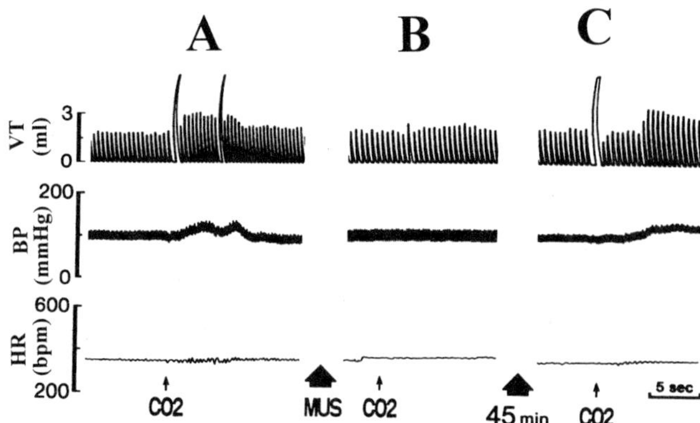

Figure 1. Inhibition of neurons in the CPS blocks carotid chemoreflex response. Identification of CPS by microinjections of glutamate (not shown). A: Control response to saline saturated with CO_2. Muscimol (140 pmole) microinjected into the CPS (large arrow between A and B). B: Carotid body stimulation failed to produce usual increase in ventilation. C: Response recovered within 45 min (From Vardhan et al, 1993).

Muscimol (a GABA receptor agonist) hyperpolarizes neuronal cell bodies, but does not affect fibers of passage, and renders them non-responsive to excitatory agents. Microinjections of muscimol (7 mM/ 20–50 nl) into the CPS abolished the responses to carotid body stimulation (Fig 1). On the other hand, the cardiovascular and respiratory effects produced by pulmonary J receptor stimulation were not blocked by microinjections of muscimol into the CPS (Vardhan et al, 1993; Chitravanshi et al, 1994).

Anatomical studies also showed that when horseradish peroxidase injections were restricted to the carotid body, densest labeling occurs in the commissural subnucleus of NTS (Finley & Katz, 1992; Claps & Torrealba, 1988).

3. CHEMOSENSITIVE NEURONS

Experiments on the identification of chemosensitive neurons in the CPS were carried out in anesthetized, paralyzed, artificially ventilated, bilaterally vagotomized, rats with a pneumothorax (Chitravanshi & Sapru, 1995a). Extracellular spontaneous action potentials of neurons were recorded using glass microelectrodes. A midline area in the commissural subnucleus of NTS (coordinates in mm: 0.3 rostral to 0.5 caudal, 0 to 0.5 lateral and 0.3 to 0.5 deep with respect to the *calamus scriptorius*) was explored.

Tracings from one chemosensory neuron are shown in Figure 2. Its firing showed no rhythmic relation with the PN bursts. After a brief tracheal administration of N_2, firing increased concomitantly with the increase in the frequency of PN bursts. N_2 administration causes cardiovascular and respiratory response by activating peripheral, but not central chemoreceptors, because bilateral section of carotid sinus nerves prevented these responses. When baroreceptors were activated by raising arterial pressure, no significant change was elicited in the firing of chemosensitive neurons.

Activity was also recorded from single neurons located in the intermediate portion of NTS (coordinates in mm with respect to the *calamus scriptorius*: 0.5 rostral, 0.5 lateral and 0.5 mm deep) where baroreceptor afferents are known to project. Neurons recorded from this region exhibited continuous firing with no correlation with the blood pressure

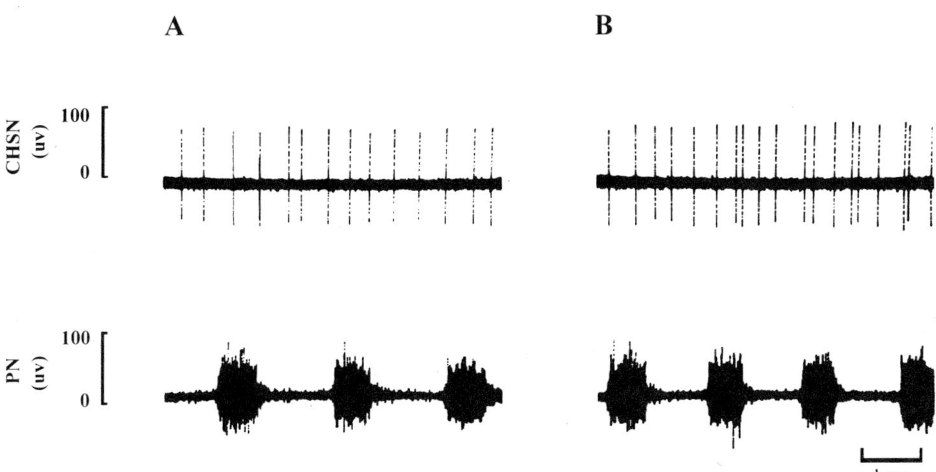

Figure 2. Effect of N_2 on the activity of a chemosensitive neuron (CHSN) in the commissural subnucleus of NTS (top trace). Bottom trace: Phrenic nerve (PN) activity. A: Control firing of CHSN at 2.5 spikes/sec, without apparent relationship with the PN bursts (at 38 bursts/min). B: Firing of CHSN increased to 4 spikes/sec and that of PN bursts to 48 bursts/min following tracheal administration of N_2 for 7 sec. (From Chitravanshi & Sapru, 1995).

pulses. The units which were excited by intravenous injection of phenylephrine (considered to be barosensitive) did not increase their firing after CO_2-saturated saline was injected near the carotid body. Thus, chemosensitive neurons are located primarily in the CPS encompassing the commissural subnucleus of NTS adjacent to the *calamus scriptorius*. The barosensitive neurons are located in a relatively more rostral and lateral region of NTS (Sundaram et al, 1989; Urbanski & Sapru, 1988).

4. PRE-CENTRAL RESPIRATORY PATTERN GENERATOR

In the cat, carotid chemoreceptor stimulation excites both Rα and Rβ respiratory neurons (Davies & Edwards, 1975; Lipski et al, 1977). The activity of Rα neurons is closely related to that of the PN and appears to arise from the central inspiratory drive. The activity of Rβ neurons arises partly from the central inspiratory drive and partly from an excitatory input via the vagus following lung inflation. These respiratory neurons are located in the NTS (2 mm rostral to the obex, 1.4–1.8 mm below the dorsal surface of the medulla). It has been suggested that chemoreceptor afferents synapse directly on respiratory neurons in this region of NTS (Davies & Edwards, 1975).

The demonstration of continuously firing chemosensitive neurons, devoid of any respiratory rhythm, in the commissural subnucleus of NTS of the rat may provide an alternative mechanism to the one described above, in which the chemosensitive neurons receive signals directly from the chemoreceptor afferents and transmit them to the respiratory neurons. In such a scenario, these chemosensitive neurons may constitute one of the integrating areas for respiration and serve as a pre-central pattern generator (pre-CPG). Although considerable progress has been made in elucidating the organization of respiratory neuronal pools (Bonham, 1995; Bianchi et al, 1995), the exact pathways and mechanisms of neurotransmission between the pre-CPG and the respiratory neurons remain to be established.

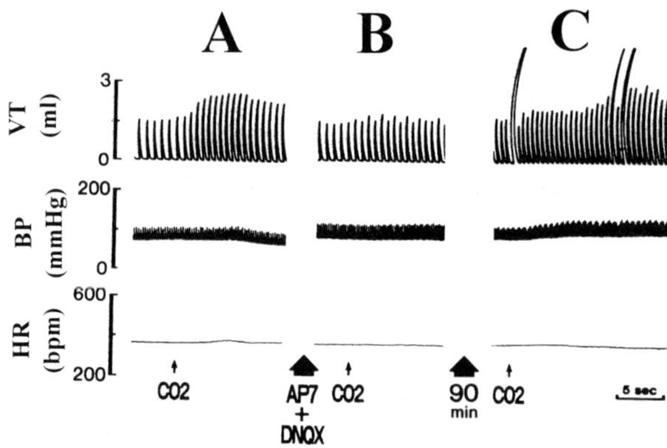

Figure 3. Blockade of EAA receptors in the CPS abolished the responses to carotid body chemoreceptor stimulation. The CPS site was identified by microinjections of glutamate (not shown). A: Control carotid chemoreceptor response to saline saturated with CO_2. AP-7 (1 mole) and DNQX (1 mole) were microinjected into this site sequentially within an interval of 1–2 min (large arrow between A and B). B: After waiting for 2–3 min, stimulation of carotid body on either side failed to produce the usual increase in ventilation. C: Responses to chemoreceptor stimulation recovered within 60–90 min (From Vardhan et al, 1993).

5. EAA RECEPTORS IN THE CPS

The excitatory amino acids (EAAs) used in this study included: glutamate, NMDA (N-methyl-D-aspartic acid) and AMPA (±-α-amino-3-hydroxy-5-methyl-isoxazole-4-propionic acid hydrobromide). DNQX (6,7-dinitro-quinoxaline-2,3-dione) and NBQX (1,2,3,4-tetrahydro-6-nitro-2,3-dioxo-benzo-quinoxaline-7-sulfonamide) were used as specific antagonists for non-NMDA receptors while AP-7 [D(-)-2-amino-7-phosphonoheptanoic acid] served as a specific antagonist for NMDA receptors.

Microinjections of EAAs into the CPS increased minute ventilation. When AP-7 and DNQX were microinjected into the CPS sequentially, within an interval of 5 min, the responses to subsequent stimulation of chemoreceptors were blocked. The responses to carotid body chemoreceptor stimulation recovered within 60–90 min (Fig 3). These results suggest that both NMDA and non-NMDA receptors in the CPS mediate the responses to chemoreceptor stimulation.

6. INSPIRATORY DRIVE TO THE PMN

The medullary inspiratory neurons are known to provide inspiratory drive to the phrenic motor nucleus (PMN) via monosynaptic projections (Ellenberger & Feldman, 1988). The neurotransmission in the PMN has been reported to be mediated primarily by non-NMDA receptors (Greer et al, 1991; Liu et al, 1990; McCrimmon et al, 1989). This conclusion is based on the results obtained mostly in an *in vitro* brainstem-spinal cord preparation isolated from neonatal (0–5 day old) rats. However, some components of respiratory networks may not be fully developed in neonatal rats, raising the possibility that the mechanism of neurotransmission in the PMN may be different in the adult animal. Therefore, an *in vivo* investigation was undertaken to identify the transmitter/receptor mechanisms in the PMN which are involved in the neurotransmission of inspiratory drive in anesthetized, bilaterally vagotomized, paralyzed, artificially ventilated, adult rats with a pneumothorax.

The spinal cord was exposed from C_1-T_1. All the dorsal and ventral rootlets at C_2-C_6 (except at C_3 segment) were sectioned. Therefore, the activity of the PN represented the output from the phrenic motoneurons located in the C_3 segment of the cervical cord.

Microinjections of L-glutamate into the PMN at C_3 segment increased the background discharge of the ipsilateral PN. No significant changes in the frequency of PN bursts occurred indicating that the neurons involved in respiratory rhythm generation are located in supraspinal structures. Microinjection of an NMDA receptor blocker (AP-7; 50 or 100 mM) into the PMN, decreased significantly the amplitude of PN bursts within 5–10 min. Similarly, microinjection of NBQX (a non-NMDA receptor blocker; 0.5 mM or 1 mM) into the PMN, significantly decreased the amplitude of the spontaneous PN bursts. However, microinjections of AP-7 or NBQX alone into the PMN did not completely abolish the spontaneous PN bursts. On the other hand, combined microinjections of AP-7 and NBQX into the PMN decreased the PN amplitude dramatically (Fig 4). Thus, unlike in the neonatal rat, both NMDA and non-NMDA receptors mediate the neurotransmission of inspiratory drive in the PMN of the adult rat.

7. EAA RECEPTORS IN THE PMN: ROLE IN CHEMOREFLEX

The transmitter/receptor mechanisms in the PMN that mediate carotid chemoreceptor responses were investigated in the *in vivo* model described in section 6 (Chitravanshi & Sapru, 1995b). The PMN at C_3 segment was identified by microinjecting NMDA (5 mM). Tracheal administration of N_2 produced a significant increase in the PN burst-fre-

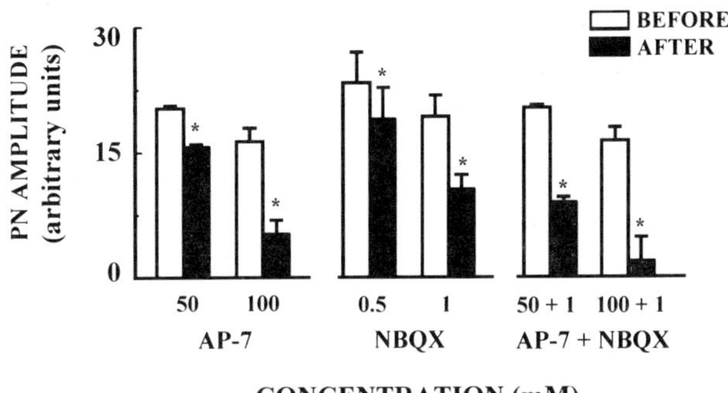

Figure 4. Effect of EAA-receptor antagonists on spontaneous PN bursts. First pair of bars (n = 10): microinjection of AP-7 (50 mM) into the PMN significantly reduced (22.7%; $p < 0.01$) spontaneous PN burst amplitude (SPNBA). Second pair of bars (n = 5): SPNBA was significantly reduced (67.9%; $p < 0.01$) by a microinjection of AP-7 (100 mM solution) into the PMN. Third pair of bars (n = 5): microinjections of NBQX (0.5 mM) into the PMN significantly reduced (18.5%; $p < 0.05$) the SPNBA. Fourth pair of bars (n = 8): microinjections of NBQX (1 mM) into the PMN significantly reduced (44.8%; $p < 0.01$) SPNBA. Fifth pair of bars (n = 5): combined microinjections of AP-7 (50 mM) and NBQX (1 mM) into the PMN reduced significantly (55.7% reduction; $p < 0.01$) SPNBA. Sixth pair of bars (n = 7): combined microinjections of higher concentrations of AP-7 (100 mM) and NBQX (1 mM) into the PMN significantly reduced (87.7 %; $p< 0.01$) SPNBA. No significant alterations in the frequencies of PN bursts were observed (From Chitravanshi & Sapru, in press).

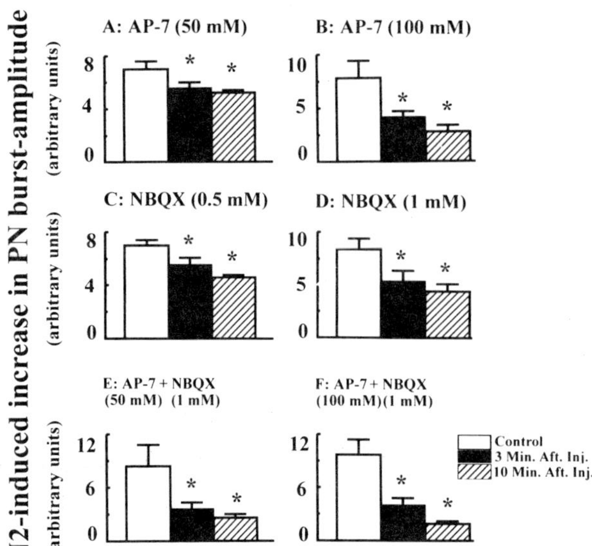

Figure 5. Effect of injections of EAA-receptor antagonists into the PMN on chemoreceptor responses. In each panel, n = 5. A: The N_2-induced increase in PN burst amplitude (PNBA) was significantly reduced ($p < 0.05$ in this and other groups of rats) by an injection of AP-7 (50 mM) into the PMN within 3–10 min. B: Similar effects were elicited by a higher concentration of AP-7 (100 mM). C & D: Effects of NBQX (0.5–1 mM) were similar to those shown in A and B. E: Combined injections of AP-7 (50–100 mM) and NBQX (1 mM) produced a drastic reduction of N_2-induced increase in PNBA.

quency and burst-amplitude. The PN burst amplitude (PNBA) was significantly increased after the tracheal inhalation of N_2. Microinjection of AP-7 (50 or 100 mM) into the PMN decreased the N_2-induced increase in PNBA. Similarly, the N_2-induced increase in PNBA was significantly reduced by an injection of a non-NMDA receptor antagonist (NBQX; 0.5–1 mM) into the PMN. However, microinjections of AP-7 or NBQX alone into the PMN did not abolish the PN responses to N_2-inhalation. On the other hand, blockade of NMDA as well as non-NMDA receptors in the PMN, by combined microinjections of AP-7 (50–100 mM) and NBQX (0.5–1 mM), drastically reduced N_2-induced increase in PNBA (Fig 5).

8. CARDIOVASCULAR RESPONSES TO CHEMORECEPTOR STIMULATION

In the rat, microinjections of glutamate into the caudal and rostral ventrolateral medulla elicit depressor and pressor responses, respectively (Willette et al, 1984). The former has been designated as "ventrolateral medullary depressor area" (VLDA), while the latter as "ventrolateral medullary pressor area" (VLPA). The pathways mediating the cardiovascular responses to chemoreceptor stimulation can be summarized as follows. As mentioned earlier, the chemoreceptor afferents make their primary synapse in the caudal portion of NTS (CPS) encompassing commissural subnucleus (Vardhan et al, 1993; Chitravanshi et al, 1994). Following the carotid chemoreceptor stimulation, an EAA (probably glutamate) is released in the CPS where both NMDA and non-NMDA receptors are activated (Vardhan et al, 1994). The secondary neurons mediating cardiovascular chemoreceptor responses in the CPS send glutamatergic projections to VLPA (Guyenet & Koshiya, 1995). Activation of VLPA neurons results in pressor and tachycardic responses characteristic of chemoreceptor activation.

9. SUMMARY

The chemoreceptor projection site encompasses a midline area (0–0.5 mm caudal, 0–0.5 mm lateral and 0.3–0.5 deep with respect to the *calamus scriptorius*) which includes the commissural subnucleus of NTS. The chemosensitive neurons located in this site fire tonically, without any rhythmic relation to the phrenic nerve bursts, and are not responsive to baroreceptor stimulation. These neurons may serve as a pre-central pattern generator for respiration.

The mechanisms which mediate respiratory responses (*i.e.*, PN responses) to carotid chemoreceptor stimulation are as follows. Activation of carotid chemoreceptors results in the release of an excitatory amino acid (probably glutamate) in the chemoreceptor projection site; both NMDA and non-NMDA receptors in this site mediate the responses to chemoreceptor stimulation. The chemosensitive neurons send projections (which have not been identified yet) to respiratory neurons. Unlike in the neonatal rat, the inspiratory drive to the phrenic motoneurons is mediated by both NMDA and non-NMDA receptors. The PN responses to chemoreceptor stimulation are also mediated by NMDA and non-NMDA receptors located in the phrenic motor nucleus.

Cardiovascular responses to chemoreceptor stimulation are mediated by neural pathways connecting the chemosensitive neurons to the rostral ventrolateral medullary pressor area. These projections are glutamatergic. Activation of the sympatho-excitatory neurons in the rostral ventrolateral medulla results in pressor and tachycardic responses characteristic of chemoreceptor activation.

10. ACKNOWLEDGMENTS

This work was supported in part by the following grants awarded to Dr HN Sapru: NIH (HL24347) and American Heart Association (NJ).

11. REFERENCES

Bianchi AL, Denavit-Saubie M & Champagnat J (1995) Central control of breathing in mammals: neuronal circuitry, membrane properties, and neurotransmitters. Physiol Rev 75: 1–45

Bonham A (1995) Neurotransmitters in the CNS control of breathing. Respir Physiol 101: 219–230

Chitravanshi VC, Kachroo A & Sapru HN (1994) A midline area in the nucleus commissuralis of NTS mediates the phrenic nerve responses to carotid chemoreceptor stimulation. Brain Res 662: 127–133

Chitravanshi VC & Sapru HN (1995a) Chemoreceptor-sensitive neurons in commissural subnucleus of nucleus tractus solitarius of the rat. Am J Physiol 268: R851-R858.

Chitravanshi VC & Sapru HN (1995b) NMDA as well as non-NMDA receptors in the phrenic motor nucleus mediate respiratory effects of carotid chemoreflex. Soc Neurosci Abstr 21: 642

Claps A & Torrealba F (1988) Carotid body connections: A WGA-HRP study in the cat. Brain Res 455: 123–133

Davies RO & Edwards Jr MW (1975) Medullary relay neurons in the carotid body chemoreceptor pathways of cats. Respir Physiol 24: 69–79

Ellenberger HH & Feldman JL (1988) Monosynaptic transmission of respiratory drive to phrenic motoneurons from brainstem bulbospinal neurons in rats. J Comp Neurol 269: 47–57

Finley JCW & Katz DM (1992) The central organization of carotid body afferent projections to the brainstem of the rat. Brain Res 572: 108–116

Greer JJ, Smith JC & Feldman JL (1991) Role of excitatory amino acids in the generation and transmission of respiratory drive in neonatal rat. J Physiol, London 437: 727–749

Guyenet PG & Koshiya N (1995) Working model of the sympathetic chemoreflex in rats. Clin Exp Hypertens 17: 167–179

Jordan D (1994) Central integration of chemoreceptor afferent activity. In: O'Regan RG, Nolan P, McQueen DS & Paterson DJ (eds) Arterial Chemoreceptors: Cell to System. New York: Plenum Press. pp 87–98

Lipski J, McAllen RM & Spyer KM (1977) The carotid chemoreceptor input to the respiratory neurons of the nucleus of tractus solitarius. J Physiol, London 269: 797–810

Liu G, Feldman JL & Smith J (1990) Excitatory amino acid-mediated transmission of inspiratory drive to phrenic motoneurons. J Neurophysiol 64: 423–436

McCrimmon DR, Smith J. & Feldman, JL (1989) Involvement of excitatory amino acids in neurotransmission of inspiratory drive to spinal respiratory motoneurons. J Neurosci 9: 1916–1921

Sapru HN & Krieger AJ (1977) Carotid and aortic chemoreceptor function in the rat. J Appl Physiol 42: 344–348

Sapru HN, Gonzalez ER & Krieger AJ (1981a) Aortic nerve stimulation in the rat: cardiovascular and respiratory responses. Brain Res Bull 6: 393–398

Sapru HN, Willette RN & Krieger AJ (1981b) Stimulation of pulmonary J receptors by an enkephalin-analog. J Pharmacol Exp Ther 217: 228–234

Sundaram K, Murugaian J, Watson M & Sapru HN (1989) M2 muscarinic receptor agonists produce hypotension and bradycardia when injected into the nucleus tractus solitarius. Brain Res 477: 358–362

Urbanski RW & Sapru HN (1988) Putative neurotransmitters involved in medullary cardiovascular regulation. J Auton Nerv Syst 25: 181–193

Vardhan A, Kachroo A, Sapru HN (1993) Excitatory amino acid receptors in commissural nucleus of the NTS mediate carotid chemoreceptor responses. Am J Physiol 264: R41-R50

Willette RN, Barcas PP, Krieger AJ & Sapru HN (1984) Vasopressor and depressor areas in the rat medulla: identification by microinjection of L-glutamate. Neuropharmacology 22: 1071–1079

AFFERENT INPUT FROM PERIPHERAL CHEMORECEPTORS IN RESPONSE TO HYPOXIA AND AMINO ACID NEUROTRANSMITTER GENERATION IN THE MEDULLA

Homayoun Kazemi,[1] John Beagle,[1] Timothy Maher,[2] and Bernard Hoop[1]

[1] Pulmonary and Critical Care Unit, Medical Services
Massachusetts General Hospital
Harvard Medical School
Boston, Massachusetts 02114
[2] Division of Pharmaceutical Sciences
Massachusetts College of Pharmacy and Allied Health Sciences
Boston, Massachusetts 02115

1. INTRODUCTION

The ventilatory response to acute hypoxia is biphasic with an initial hyperventilatory response followed by a fall in ventilation within a few minutes (roll-off) to levels above the pre-hypoxic values, but below the peak. The physiological sequence of events underlying the biphasic ventilatory response to hypoxia has not been completely elucidated. Different experimental approaches suggest that both local (*i.e.*, neurochemical activity) and global (*i.e.*, metabolic) mechanisms may very well be crucial during this transient phase of ventilatory hypoxic response. Numerous investigations (Bianchi et al, 1995; Weil, 1994), as well as work in our own laboratory (Kazemi et al, 1989; Hoop et al, 1990; Kazemi & Hoop, 1990), have directed attention to a possible central locus of the phenomenon in the ventrolateral medullary surface (VMS). The excitatory amino acid glutamate and the inhibitory amino acids γ-aminobutyric acid (GABA) and glycine appear to have special roles to play in the response. Namely, afferent stimuli from peripheral chemoreceptors lead to release of excitatory glutamate in the intermediate area of the VMS which cause the increase in central ventilatory output (Soto-Arape et al, 1995). Brain hypoxia also causes a rise in inhibitory GABA and glycine which then diminishes respiratory neuronal output.

The present study therefore addresses the hypothesis that hypoxia modifies the content of glutamate in the intermediate area of the VMS by afferent stimuli arising from pe-

Frontiers in Arterial Chemoreception, edited by Zapata *et al.*
Plenum Press, New York, 1996

ripheral chemoreceptors and of GABA and glycine by direct effect on brain cells, which then to a large extent determines the biphasic ventilatory response in hypoxia. To test this hypothesis, amino acid neurotransmitter content of microdialysates from respiratory-related nuclei in the medulla was measured during 30 minutes of hypoxic breathing (10% O_2). Specifically, we measured the time dependence of concentrations of selected amino acids in the intermediate area of the VMS during normoxia and during periods of hypoxia with a microdialysis technique which achieves spatial and temporal resolutions of 0.25 to 0.50 mm and 3 minutes, respectively.

2. METHODS

Fourteen male Sprague-Dawley rats (300–350 g) were anesthetized with continuous inhalation of 2.5% isoflurane. This level of anesthesia produced sustained cessation of responses to the cornea or footpad stimulation. Animals were ventilated mechanically through a cervical tracheostomy. Level of ventilation was adjusted as needed to maintain P_aCO_2 between 36 and 42 Torr. The abdominal aorta was cannulated for arterial pressure and blood gas tension monitoring. Body temperature was monitored and maintained at 37.5°C by an electrical heating pad.

To expose the ventrolateral medullary surface, the cephalad end of the trachea and the esophagus were reflected rostrally, and the musculature and bony surface between the tympanic bullae were removed. The exposed area extended laterally to the bullae and rostrally 2 to 3 mm above the point of exit of the sixth cranial nerve. The dura was opened and fixed to the bony edges. The underlying VMS remained covered by a pool of cerebrospinal fluid (CSF).

Bilateral vagotomy was performed. Phrenic nerve output on one side was measured as an index of central ventilatory drive and each animal acted as its own control. A phrenic nerve was exposed and connected to a bipolar AgCl electrode, and the electrode was grounded. The phrenic neurogram was amplified and monitored on an oscilloscope. Integrated neurograms were displayed on a pen chart recorder and acquired as digital files for subsequent analysis.

Concentric 1- or 2-mm by 0.5 mm diameter microdialysis probes were placed at depths of 1.25 to 2.00 mm in the intermediate chemosensitive area in the VMS under stereotaxic control with reference to coordinates taken from a standard neuroanatomy atlas of the rat (Paxinos & Watson, 1982) and perfused with artificial CSF at a rate of 1.6 μL/min using an infusion pump. For the intermediate area in the VMS the dialysis probe was placed at the level of the rostral rootlets of the 12th nerve approximately 4 mm caudal to the foramen cecum. Fused silica tubing with a dead volume of 0.44 μL/cm was used for dialysate collection. A 20-cm length was turned over in *ca.* 1 min at a flow rate of 1.6 μL/min. Artificial CSF was a 0.22 μm-filtered ten-fold dilution (electrochemical grade water) of a stock solution of 1450 mM NaCl, 27 mM KCl, 10 mM $MgCl_2$ ($6H_2O$), 12 mM $CaCl_2$ ($2H_2O$), and 20 mM Na_2HPO_4 equilibrated with 95% 0_2- 5% $C0_2$ to pH 7.35–7.40 and $PC0_2$ 36–42 Torr (Moghaddam & Bunney, 1989).

After approximately 1.5 h post surgery, to allow for stabilization, two 3- to 5-minute dialysate samples were collected to determine basal levels of amino acid concentrations in the VMS site. Three to six 3- to 5-minute consecutive dialysate samples were then collected over a 30-minute period in each of the animals. Contents of selected amino acids in dialysate samples were determined with high pressure liquid chromatography (HPLC) by comparison with an amino acid standard. All samples for HPLC analysis were derivatized according to the method of Donzanti and Yamamoto (1988).

One group of five animals (controls) was ventilated on an FIO_2 of 0.3 throughout the entire experiment. A second group of nine animals were first ventilated on an FIO_2 of 0.3 and then exposed to hypoxia at an FIO_2 of 0.1. Duration of a single experiment, from induction of anesthesia to collection of the final microdialysate sample was typically two to three hours. At the end of the experiment, animals were sacrificed with an overdose of KCl via the abdominal aorta, and remains were disposed of as prescribed by the Massachusetts General Hospital Subcommittee on Animal Care.

3. RESULTS

Phrenic nerve output showed a biphasic response during hypoxia. There was an initial rise in mean (± SEM) phrenic nerve output to 59 ± 14% above control level within the first 5 to 7 min of hypoxia, at which time mean PO_2 had fallen from 127 ± 5 to 39 ± 2 Torr. The initial rise in phrenic nerve output gradually declined to a new level (roll-off) after about 12 minutes of hypoxia but remained at a mean level of 31 ± 4% of control values while hypoxia was maintained.

Mean arterial blood pressure decreased from 105 ± 9 to 63 ± 10 Torr after 3 min of hypoxia and did not change thereafter. Since the animals were on controlled mechanical ventilation, mean arterial PCO_2 (35 ± 2 Torr), pH (7.29 ± 0.02), and HCO_3^- (17.8 ± 1.2 mM) remained unchanged.

Corresponding percent changes in dialysate concentrations of glutamate, GABA, and glycine during hypoxia are given in Table 1. Compared with normoxia, glutamate concentration tended to increase gradually during 18 minutes of hypoxia. At the same time, GABA concentration remained unchanged during 10 minutes of hypoxia and then increased significantly ($p < 0.05$; one-tailed two-sample t-test, n_1=10, n_2=5) to 93.0 ± 19.6% of normoxic levels by 18 minutes of hypoxia. In addition, glycine concentration changes tended to exhibit a biphasic behavior, first decreasing within 3 minutes of hypoxia and then increasing after 18 minutes of hypoxia.

4. DISCUSSION

The rationale for the present investigation is the considerable circumstantial evidence which suggests that neuronal membrane conductance and related respiratory neuronal activity is determined by a balance between generation of excitatory and inhibitory neurotransmitters in respiratory chemosensitive areas of the brainstem. Our basic hypothesis is that relative release of excitatory (*e.g.*, glutamate) and inhibitory (*e.g.*, GABA, glycine) neurotransmitters in the medulla determines the final neuronal output and command to respiratory muscles, and it is the interaction between these agents that ultimately determines the total ventilatory output during hypoxia.

This preliminary study describes changes in amino acid concentrations of microdialysate samples taken from within the intermediate chemosensitive area of the VMS during exposure of experimental animals to 10% O_2. A major feature of this study is *in vivo* microdialysis as a method of sampling local changes in amino acids in the brainstem chemosensitive areas during hypoxic challenge. As discussed in Methods above, artificial CSF is perfused through a dialysis probe at a rate of 1.6 μL/min. Diffusive exchange

Table 1. Mean (± SEM) percent changes in amino acid content during hypoxia, compared to normoxia

Minutes of Hypoxia	Glutamate	GABA	Glycine
3	7.0 ± 3.1	2.4 ± 0.5	-15.0 ± 6.1
10	4.2 ± 1.3	9.4 ± 2.4	9.2 ± 3.1
18	15.4 ± 5.1	93.0 ± 19.6*	18.0 ± 7.6

* $p < 0.05$ compared to normoxia.

across the permeable dialysis membrane allows estimation of extracellular amino acid content within a time resolution of minutes. Under these conditions, uptake efficiencies (recoveries) for amino acids is 10–20%. Brainstem site for placement of the dialysate collection probes is determined on the basis of responses in microinjection experiments.

We have employed an anesthetized rat model whose ventilation, pH, and PCO_2 are kept constant and whose central neuronal output is measured through the phrenic pneumogram. Ventilatory drive and the final output from the respiratory centers from the brain are a series of interactive processes and many pathways and nuclei in the midbrain and higher centers are involved. Impulses from the peripheral chemoreceptors are integrated in the NTS (Jordan, 1994). Recent neuroanatomical data also show connections between NTS and VMS before impulses go to the phrenic nerve (Mtui et al, 1993). Namely, neuronal input from the NTS is transmitted to the VMS, and the chemosensitive areas on the VMS have a significant controlling effect on the discharge of respiratory motoneurons. These results support our previous findings of the importance of the VMS in the ventilatory response to hypoxia and the fact that blocking glutamate on the VMS abolishes the hyperventilation of hypoxia (Kazemi et al, 1989; Soto-Arape et al, 1995). Specifically, application of the N-methyl-D-aspartate (NMDA) receptor blocker MK-801 directly on the ventral surface of the medulla on the intermediate area leads to depression of phrenic nerve output and no response to hypoxia, thus indicating the importance of central glutamate action in the ventilatory response to hypoxia. Furthermore, the effects of hypoxia on the brain, particularly the elevation of brain GABA in relation to phrenic nerve output, is a generalized brain response and, in turn, ventilatory output is depressed. Our results indicate that the specific site of action of GABA in generating the roll-off phenomenon appears to be in the intermediate area of the VMS. The VMS is an important area for the action of central amino acid neurotransmitters, as well as the NTS. As in the case with the baroreceptor reflex pathway (Sved & Gordon, 1994), conclusive evidence for glutamate as the primary excitatory agent is confounded by its dual role as neurotransmitter and metabolic precursor. It is, however, precisely this latter identity of glutamate as a GABA precursor which is unique to our hypothesis.

In summary, glutamate, GABA and glycine contents of microdialysates from the intermediate chemosensitive area increased during hypoxia. The increases in glutamate and GABA support our hypothesis that glutamatergic and GABAergic mechanisms in the intermediate region of the ventral medulla are responsible for the biphasic ventilatory response to acute hypoxia. Although our hypothesis restricts attention to the two biochemically closely related neurotransmitters, glutamic acid and γ-aminobutyric acid, it is clear that other important amino acid neurotransmitters and, in particular, glycine play a role in the biphasic response to hypoxia.

5. REFERENCES

Bianchi AL, Denavit-Saubie M & Champagnat J (1995) Central control of breathing in mammals: neuronal circuitry, membrane properties, and neurotransmitters. Physiol Rev 75: 1–45

Donzanti BA & Yamamoto BK (1988) An improved and rapid HPLC-EC method for the isocratic separation of amino acid neurotransmitters from brain tissue and microdialysis perfusates. Life Sci 43: 913–922

Hoop B, Masjedi RM, Shih VE & Kazemi H (1990) Brain glutamate metabolism during hypoxia and peripheral chemodenervation. J Appl Physiol 69: 147–154

Jordan D (1994) Central integration of chemoreceptor afferent activity. In: O'Regan RG, Nolan P, McQueen D & Paterson DJ (eds) Arterial Chemoreceptors: Cell to System. New York: Plenum. pp 87–98

Kazemi H & Hoop B (1990) Glutamic acid and γ-aminobutyric acid neurotransmitters in the central control of breathing. J Appl Physiol 70: 1–7

Kazemi H, Chiang CH & Hoop B (1989) Role of medullary glutamate in the hypoxic ventilatory response. In: Lahiri S (ed) Comroe Memorial Symposium: Chemoreceptors and Reflexes in Breathing. New York: Oxford Univ Press. pp 233–242

Moghaddam B & Bunney B (1989) Ionic composition of microdialysis perfusing solution alters the pharmacological responsiveness and basal outflow of striatal dopamine. J Neurochem 53: 652–654

Mtui EP, Anwar M, Gomez R, Reis DJ & Ruggiero DA (1993) Projections from the nucleus tractus solitarii to the spinal cord. J Comp Neurol 337: 231–252

Paxinos G & Watson C (1982) The Rat Brain in Stereotaxic Coordinates. Sydney: Academic Press

Soto-Arape I, Burton MD & Kazemi H (1995) Central amino acid neurotransmitters and the hypoxic ventilatory response. Am J Respir Crit Care Med 151: 1113–1120

Sved AF & Gordon FJ (1994) Amino acids as central neurotransmitters in the baroreceptor reflex pathway. News Physiol Sci 9: 243–246

Weil JV (1994) Invited editorial on "Ventilatory responses to CO_2 and hypoxia after sustained hypoxia in awake cats". J Appl Physiol 76: 2251–2252

AUGMENTED VENTILATORY RESPONSE TO SUSTAINED NORMOCAPNIC HYPOXIA FOLLOWING 100% O_2 BREATHING IN HUMANS

Y. Honda, H. Tani, A. Masuda, T. Kobayashi, T. Nishino, H. Kimura, S. Masuyama, and T. Kuriyama

Departments of Physiology, Anesthesiology and Chest Medicine
School of Medicine
Chiba University, and Chiba College of Allied Sciences
Wakaba-Ku, Chiba, Japan

1. INTRODUCTION

The presence of hyperoxic hyperventilation seems to have been well confirmed in humans by Becker et al (1995) when the $P_{ET}co_2$ is maintained at a normocapnic level. They also observed that augmented ventilation at higher than the control level still continued even 15 min after termination of hyperoxia, suggesting that a humoral agent might be involved to stimulate ventilation.

We have examined the effect of this possible chemical agent on sustained hypoxia. The time course of ventilation during sustained isocapnic hypoxia is now known to exhibit a biphasic profile: an initial rapid rise is followed by a gradual decline. This is called the biphasic hypoxic ventilatory depression (Biph HVD) (Easton et al, 1986). The effect of prior O_2 breathing on Biph HVD was another object to examine in the present study.

2. METHODS

Sixteen young college students participated in the study.

2.1. Experiment I: Measurement of Ventilatory Response

The subject breathed from a closed circuit on which a bypass tube to a CO_2 absorber, two small tubes to draw out respiratory air and to draw in N_2 or O_2 and two three-way stopcocks were incorporated. A thick paper screen was placed between the subject and the circuit during operation, so that the maneuver of administering the different gas mixture was not noticed by the subject. With the stopcocks disconnected from the closed

Frontiers in Arterial Chemoreception, edited by Zapata *et al.*
Plenum Press, New York, 1996

circuit, the subject breathed either room air or 100% O_2 for 10 min. Then for about 5 min he breathed room air during which time a rubber bag containing 10 l of 9% N_2 gas mixture was connected to the respiratory circuit. The subject then rebreathed this hypoxic gas mixture and arterial S_ao_2, measured by a pulse oximeter (S_po_2), was rapidly adjusted to 80% with normocapnic condition within 2–3 min and was maintained for 20 min. Ventilation, S_po_2, $P_{ET}o_2$ and $P_{ET}co_2$ were continuously maintained constant during this sustained normocapnic hypoxia. The hypoxic challenges with prior 10 min O_2 or air breathing were defined as +O_2 and -O_2 runs, respectively. Both runs were conducted in random order.

2.2. Experiment II: Chemical Analysis of Blood Plasma

Just before the beginning of a sustained hypoxia test in +O_2 and -O_2 runs, 10 ml of venous blood was withdrawn in 10 out of the 16 subjects. Plasma concentration of β-endorphin, adrenaline, noradrenaline, dopamine, serotonin, GABA, glutamine, glutamic acid and glycine were analyzed.

3. RESULTS

Figure 1 shows the time course of inspiratory minute ventilation ($\dot{V}_I$) during sustained hypoxia. Clearly, $\dot{V}_I$ in the +O_2 run significantly exceeds the level in the -O_2 run from 3rd min to the end of 20 min hypoxia. Augmented ventilation was accompanied with a significant increment of V_T but not of respiratory frequency. Although prior O_2 breathing induced augmented ventilation, the general profile in time course of ventilatory response appeared similar in both +O_2 and -O_2 runs, *i.e.*, Biph HVD pattern was similar. The

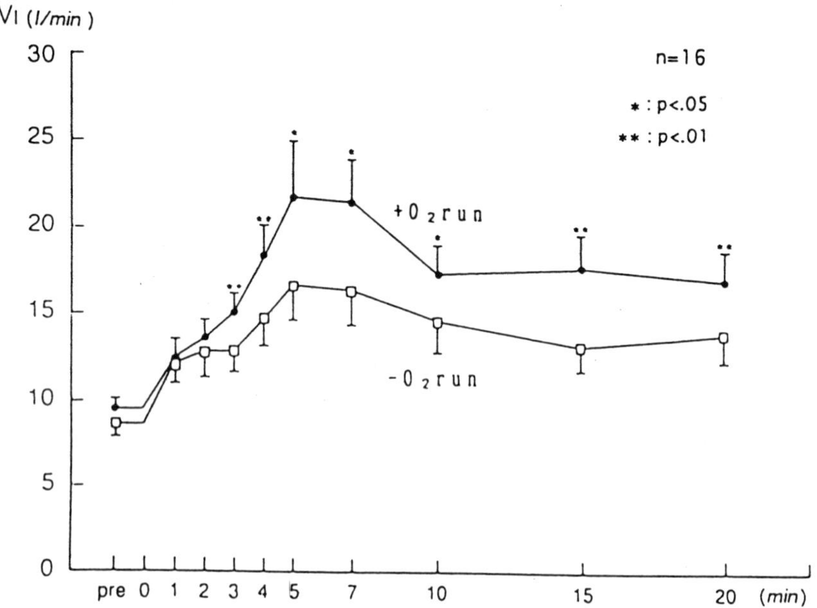

Figure 1. Time course of changes in inspiratory minute ventilation ($\dot{V}_I$). $\dot{V}_I$ in the +O_2 run significantly exceeded the $\dot{V}_I$ in the -O_2 run from the 3rd min hypoxia. The magnitude of both initial peak ventilatory increment and Biph HVD was observed to be almost the same in relative magnitude.

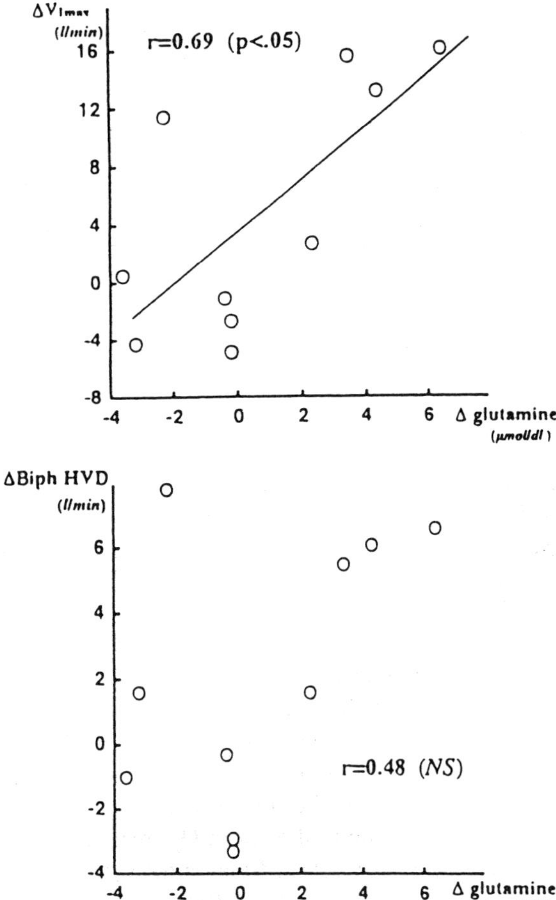

Figure 2. Relationship between maximal increment in hypoxic hyperventilation (top) and amount of Bip HVD (bottom) against plasma glutamine concentration in terms of the difference from $-O_2$ run to $+O_2$ run. The relationship between maximal increment of hypoxic ventilation and glutamine concentration is significant at 5% level whereas the amount of Biph HVD *vs* glutamine relationship does not attain significant level.

magnitude of Biph HVD was about 50% of the initial rapid increment in both runs. Therefore, ventilatory response of $+O_2$ run was shifted upwards in parallel with that of $-O_2$ run. When the resting $P_{ET}co_2$ level just before hypoxia challenge was compared in the two runs, $P_{ET}co_2$ in the $+O_2$ run was significantly lower than in the $-O_2$ run.

Among the 9 chemicals measured in blood plasma, a significant finding was observed only in glutamine in relation to the augmented hypoxic response. Fig 2 demonstrates the relationship between maximal $\dot{V}_I$ (top) and Bip HVD (bottom) against glutamine concentration in terms of difference from $-O_2$ to $+O_2$ run in all variables. A significant linear correlation was found in the former but not in the latter.

4. DISCUSSION

Miller and Tenney (1975) first reported in unanesthetized and carotid-deafferented cats that breathing 400–450 mm Hg P_Ao_2 induced a 16% elevation in ventilation with a significant P_Aco_2 depression. Subsequently, Gautier et al (1986) confirmed the presence of hyperoxic hyperventilation in conscious cats with carotid body denervation. They further found that anesthesia abolished this hyperpneic response. $P_{ET}co_2$, had however, significantly decreased already before, and even more after, carotid chemodenervation in these conscious cats. They reasoned that the enhanced ventilatory response after chemodenervation can be ascribed to a loss of hyperoxia-induced inhibitory afferent information from the carotid bodies. Both investigator groups also noted that hyperoxic hyperventilation developed gradually.

The presence of hyperoxic hyperventilation in humans was also confirmed by Becker et al (1995): breathing 50% O_2 while adjusting $P_{ET}CO_2$ to a normocapnic level resulted in as much as a 60% elevation in ventilation. They further observed that this hyperpneic influence still lasted even 15 min after termination of hyperoxia.

All these observations in cats and humans seem to indicate that some humoral agent(s) may be involved in the results. The present study further indicated that such an agent effectively augmented the ventilation during sustained hypoxia.

As presented in Fig 2, the increment in maximal hypoxic ventilation from $-O_2$ to $+O_2$ run was significantly correlated with the difference in plasma glutamine concentration between the two runs. Glutamine is known to be the most potent precursor of excitatory amino acid neurotransmitter glutamate (Hamberger et al, 1979; Kazemi & Hoop, 1991), which stimulates ventilation by altering neuronal excitability centrally. In addition, Li and Nattie (1995) recently demonstrated long-lasting augmented ventilation by stimulating the metabotropic glutamate receptors in the brain-stem retrotrapezoid nucleus (RTN) region which is claimed to be the most potent CO_2 chemosensitive area by this group (Nattie et al, 1991). Although the glutamate concentration measured in plasma was too small to assess a definite tendency and its actual concentration in the brain was unable to be measured, we assumed that the increment in plasma glutamine concentrations from $-O_2$ to $+O_2$ run might have reflected the increment of glutamate in the plasma as well as in the affected site of the brain. Based on this assumption, we speculated that the glutamine-glutamate system might be responsible, at least in part, for the augmented hypoxic hyperventilation induced by prior O_2 breathing.

Figure 1 demonstrated that, although prior O_2 breathing shifted the ventilation level upward, the general profile of Biph HVD appeared nearly unchanged. Both the relative magnitude of ventilation in the initial rapid increment and in the subsequent gradual decline were the same in both $-O_2$ and $+O_2$ runs. This may signify that the chemical agent possibly generated during O_2 breathing is different from the one induced by sustained hypoxia. Another possibility may be that the mechanism responsible for Biph HVD is a non-chemical process, such as the adaptation of chemoreceptor activities (Bascom et al, 1990). In any event, ventilatory stimulation generated by prior O_2 breathing appeared not directly related with the Biph HVD.

5. CONCLUSION

Prior O_2 breathing induced a marked augmentation of the ventilatory response to sustained normocapnic hypoxia. This augmentation appeared to be due to generation of chemical agent(s), possibly the same one that is produced during hyperoxic hyperventilation. The excitatory amino acid neurotransmitter glutamate was suspected to be involved in this process.

Although hypoxic hyperventilation was enhanced by preliminary O_2 breathing, the specific profile of biphasic hypoxic ventilatory depression was not modified in terms of feature of relative ventilatory magnitude.

6. REFERENCES

Bascom DA, Clements ID, Cunningham DA, Painter R & Robbins PA (1990) Changes in peripheral chemoreflex sensitivity during sustained isocapnic hypoxia. Respir Physiol 62: 161–176

Becker H, Polo O, McNamara SG, Berthon-Jones M & Sullivan CE (1995) Ventilatory response to isocapnic hyperoxia. J Appl Physiol 78: 696–701

Easton PA, Slykerman LJ & Anthonisen NR (1986) Ventilatory response to sustained hypoxia in normal adults. J Appl Physiol 61: 906–911

Gautier H, Bonora HM & Gaudy JH (1986) Ventilatory response of the conscious or anesthetized cat to oxygen breathing. Respir Physiol 65: 181–196

Hamberger AC, Chiang GH, Nylen ES, Scheff SW & Cotman CW (1979) Glutamate as a CNS transmitter. I. Evaluation of glucose and glutamine as precursors for the synthesis of preferentially released glutamate. Brain Res 168: 513–530

Kazemi H & Hoop B (1991) Glutamic acid and γ-aminobutyric acid neurotrasmitters in central control of breathing. J Appl Physiol 70: 1–7

Li A & Nattie EE (1995) Prolonged stimulation of respiration by brain stem metabotropic glutamate receptors. J Appl Physiol 79: 1650–1656

Miller MJ & Tenney SM (1975) Hyperoxic hyperventilation in carotid-deafferented cats. Respir Physiol 23: 23–30

Nattie EE, Li A & St John WM (1991) Lesions in retrotrapezoid nucleus decrease ventilatory output in anesthetized or decerebrate cats. J Appl Physiol 71: 1364–1375

58

ROLE OF CAROTID BODIES IN THE GUINEA-PIG

Patricia A. Cragg and Daryl O. Schwenke

Department of Physiology
University of Otago Medical School
Dunedin, New Zealand

1. INTRODUCTION

Guinea-pigs have a normal, possibly accentuated, hyperventilatory response to hypercapnia whereas that to hypoxia is delayed and extremely blunted (Blake & Banchero, 1985a,b; Alarie & Stock, 1988; Cragg & Menzies, 1992; Peebles & Cragg, 1995). Although these Guinea-pigs are low altitude dwellers, their breathing responses are typical of small mammals and humans adapted to high altitude (Monge & Leon-Velarde, 1991), where the adaptation is termed phenotypic because it requires prior exposure to long-term hypoxia. As Guinea-pigs originated some centuries ago from the high altitude habitats of South America, it is tempting to ask whether they have retained a genotypic adaptation to high altitude. The mechanism(s) responsible for the blunted ventilatory response to hypoxia in other mammals is controversial; much of the evidence indicates involvement of the carotid bodies (Bisgard & Neubauer, 1995).

Carotid bodies are peripheral arterial chemoreceptors (González et al, 1994) which in most mammals are the main, often the only, sensors of hypoxia; in some species there is a small contribution from the aortic bodies and other paraganglia. Carotid bodies are also sensitive to hypercapnia, although the predominant contribution to hyperventilation comes from central intracranial chemoreceptors. Cyanide, presumed to be via the production of a histotoxic hypoxia, also stimulates the carotid bodies. As the carotid bodies of Guinea-pigs are structurally and biochemically normal (Mir et al, 1982; Kummer et al, 1989), we have examined whether they are functionally operative by comparing the breathing responses to hypoxia, hypercapnia and cyanide before and after carotid body (CB) denervation.

2. METHODS

Guinea-pigs (albino females; ~100 days old; body wt. ~680 g; n = 18) were anesthetized with pentobarbitone (ip 30 mg/kg, then iv 15–30 mg/kg/h) and maintained at a body

Frontiers in Arterial Chemoreception, edited by Zapata *et al.*
Plenum Press, New York, 1996

temperature of 39°C with a thermostatically controlled heating pad. The trachea, femoral artery and femoral vein were cannulated. To measure ventilation the Guinea-pig was placed supine in a plethysmograph with cannulae exteriorized; the pressure changes in the plethysmograph were recorded with a Grass PT5A volumetric pressure transducer. Tidal gas was continuously monitored from a side-arm in the tracheal cannula with a Perkin-Elmer mass spectrometer sampling at 12 ml/min; the end-tidal values were taken as representative of alveolar PO_2 and PCO_2. Mean arterial blood pressure (MABP) was also continuously recorded with a Statham pressure transducer and heart rate (HR) was derived from the pulses. All signals were converted from analog to digital form by a MacLab/4e and displayed on a Macintosh LCIII computer.

In between tests a Guinea-pig breathed from the air surrounding the plethysmograph. Test gases were manufactured using rotameters and were mixed, humidified and delivered at a flow rate of ~2 L/min through a tube past the tracheal opening. In 9 Guinea-pigs 8% CO_2 was tested for 10 min and 40% CO_2 for 15 s (in a background of 21% O_2 plus N_2). In a further 9 Guinea-pigs hypoxia (6% O_2 for 5 min and 100% N_2 for 10 s), hyperoxia (100% O_2 for 15 s) and sodium cyanide (NaCN, 500 μg/kg) were tested. NaCN was given iv in a 0.1 ml aliquot followed by a 0.25 ml saline chaser administered rapidly (~1 s). Recovery periods of up to 15 min were allowed between tests. During a few periods of air-breathing and the steady-state responses to 8% CO_2 and 6% O_2 arterial blood (0.1 ml) was sampled to measure arterial PO_2, PCO_2 and pH and, from the fractional difference in inlet and outlet gas flowing past the trachea, O_2 consumption (VO_2) and CO_2 production (VCO_2) were calculated. All tests were performed before and after carotid body denervation (CBD) which was achieved by bilateral transection of the IXth cranial nerves close to their emergence from the basioccipital bone. Data are expressed as means ± SEM's and statistical significance was evaluated with paired Student's *t*-tests.

3. RESULTS

In air, the ventilation (V_E) was 30.2 ± 1.2 ml/min/100 g, with a tidal volume (V_T) of 0.606 ± 0.042 ml/100 g and frequency (f) of 49.9 ± 3.7 breaths/min. These variables were unaltered by either 15 s of 100% O_2 or CBD. Other variables during air-breathing were MABP 56 ± 3 Torr, HR 258 ± 3 beats/min, PaO_2 80 ± 2 Torr, $PaCO_2$ 34 ± 1 Torr, pHa 7.45 ± 0.01, VO_2 1.06 ± 0.06 ml/min/100 g and VCO_2 0.84 ± 0.05 ml/min/100 g. All were unaffected by CBD.

In response to 8% CO_2, V_E increased after a latency of 8.0 ± 0.2 s and reached by 4 min a steady state of 116 ± 10 ml/min/100 g, *i.e.*, a 385% increase in V_E due to greater increases in V_T (250%) than f (150%). The rate of development of the V_E response was such that 60% had occurred by 1 min and 90% by 2 min. $PaCO_2$ and pH_a at steady state (10 min) were 49 ± 1 Torr and 7.31± 0.1, respectively and because of the hyperventilation PaO_2 rose to 120 ± 3 Torr; MABP, HR and VO_2 were not altered. Carotid body denervation prolonged ($p < 0.05$) the V_E latency to 11.4 ± 1.3 s and reduced ($p < 0.05$) the steady-state V_E to 94.8 ± 13.4 ml/min/100 g, without altering the time course of the V_E increase. The lower V_E at steady-state after CBD was entirely due to a smaller f response. No other variables were affected by CBD.

The 15 s 40% CO_2 test, used to produce a rapid and severe CO_2 stimulus, caused a short V_E latency (1.9 ± 0.2 s) in the CB-intact state and by 15 s a 200% increase in V_E (comprised of V_E 85.3 ± 3.5 ml/min/100 g, V_T 1.319 ± 0.079 ml/100 g and f 73.1 ± 3.2 breaths/ min). Carotid body denervation not only prolonged ($p < 0.05$) the V_E latency (4.6

$\pm$ 0.3 s) but also reduced ($p < 0.05$) by 55% the rate of V_E increase over the next 10 s, entirely by abolishing the f response. In both CB-intact and CB-denervated states, 40% CO_2 with a latency of ~5 s caused by 15 s some hypotension (Δ10 Torr) and bradycardia (Δ20 beats/min).

In response to 6% O_2, the V_E increase occurred after a long latency (20.5 $\pm$ 3.9 s), reaching by 1 min a sustained value of only 40.9 $\pm$ 2.6 ml/min/100 g, which was primarily due to an increase in V_T. PaO_2 at steady state (5 min) was 12.8 $\pm$ 0.3 Torr and, because of both hyperventilation and metabolic depression (VO_2 0.79 $\pm$ 0.03 ml/min/100 g), $PaCO_2$ fell to 28.9 $\pm$ 1.0 Torr and pHa rose to 7.53 $\pm$ 0.01. There was some hypotension (Δ15 Torr), which commenced after a latency of ~10 s, but no significant bradycardia. The severe 10 s 100% N_2 test increased V_E after a shorter latency (7.3 $\pm$ 0.7 s), but the depressing effects of anoxia curtailed the maximum V_E (35.1 $\pm$ 2.1 ml/min/100 g), in which only the V_T not the f increase was significant. By 10 s of 100% N_2, no bradycardia and only Δ8 Torr of hypotension had developed. Carotid body denervation had no effect on the response of any variable to either 6% O_2 or 100% N_2.

In contrast, the V_E response to iv NaCN was not only rapid (latency 5.6 $\pm$ 0.4 s) but also substantial (74.8 $\pm$ 7.3 ml/min/100 g, the peak response occurring ~10 s after injection and lasting for ~5 s); it was due to equal increases in V_T and f. Furthermore, CBD increased the latency (7.4 $\pm$ 0.3 s) and reduced the maximum V_E response (55.5 $\pm$ 4.2 ml/min/100 g) by affecting only the V_T response ($p < 0.05$). In both CB-intact and CB-denervated states, NaCN caused slight hypotension (Δ15 Torr) but no bradycardia. Lower doses of NaCN (50–200 μg/kg) also stimulated V_E but did not cause hypotension.

4. DISCUSSION

The absence of rapid hypoventilation during the "Dejours" 15 s 100% O_2 test indicates that, unlike rats (Cragg & Khrisanapant, 1989) and other species, the carotid bodies of Guinea-pigs are not contributing a drive to V_E through their detection of normoxia. This is also confirmed by the absence of hypoventilation in air following CBD. Guinea-pig carotid bodies also appear insensitive to hypoxia, as sectioning their nerves had no effect on the hyperventilatory response, even to a hypoxia as severe as 100% N_2. Alternatively, the carotid bodies could be sensitive to hypoxia, but either the sensory input is ignored centrally in a hypoxic situation, or there is efferent inhibition of the carotid bodies during hypoxia, or hypoxia elicits a strong suprapontine inhibition of V_E (Bisgard & Neubauer, 1995).

Those possibilities aside, the delayed and blunted V_E response to hypoxia of CB-intact Guinea-pigs is of a latency and magnitude typical of the CB-denervated rat, except that in Guinea-pigs it is the V_T and in rats the f component that increases (Khrisanapant & Cragg, 1984; Cragg & Leonard, 1995). In CBD rats, the residual V_E response to hypoxia can be abolished by sectioning nerves supplying the aortic bodies, abdominal chemoreceptors and other carotid body-like paraganglia (Khrisanapant & Cragg, 1987, 1988); the site of detection for the V_T response to hypoxia in Guinea-pigs has still to be identified.

In contrast, the carotid bodies of the Guinea-pig are sensitive to CO_2 and, as shown by the 40% CO_2 test, are also capable of monitoring CO_2 rapidly. Overall their contribution to steady-state V_E is small (~20% of the 10 min response to 8% CO_2) and the component affected is f not V_T - characteristics also typical of rats (Cragg & Schwenke, unpublished).

Although insensitive to hypoxia, the carotid bodies of the Guinea-pig are powerfully stimulated by the metabolic poison NaCN, producing increases in V_T and f of equal magnitude and similar to those in the rat (Cárdenas & Zapata, 1983; Cragg & Leonard, 1995). In both species, CBD abolishes all of the V_T response to NaCN; however, whereas most of the f response in the rat is abolished, it remains unaltered in the Guinea-pig. Extracarotid peripheral chemoreceptors are presumed to be responsible for the residual response to NaCN (Cárdenas & Zapata, 1983).

The apparent insensitivity of the carotid bodies to hypoxia and the similarity of the overall V_E response to NaCN and 40% CO_2 (ignoring the different effects on f and V_T) suggests that NaCN may stimulate the carotid bodies through intracellular acidification (González et al, 1994) rather than by mimicking hypoxia and thus causing either inhibition of the mitochondrial electron transport chain or stimulation of the hypoxic-sensitive K^+-dependent cell membrane channel.

Support for our hypothesis that Guinea-pigs are preadapted to high altitude can be gained from evidence that altitude-acclimated rats (Lagneaux, 1994) and our sea-level Guinea-pigs both show a normal V_E response to NaCN but a blunted V_E response to hypoxia. Furthermore, Guinea-pigs have other characteristics typical of high altitude adaptation, for example, a low P_{50} (Turek et al, 1980) and a low MABP (Brown et al, 1989).

5. REFERENCES

Alarie Y & Stock MF (1988) Arterial blood gas measurements in Guinea-pigs and inspired CO_2 concentrations for ventilatory performance challenges. Fundam Appl Toxicol 11: 268–276

Bisgard GE & Neubauer JA (1995) Peripheral and central effects of hypoxia. In: Dempsey JA & Pack AI (eds) Regulation of Breathing. 2nd ed. (Lung Biology in Health and Disease, vol 79). New York: Dekker. pp 617–668

Blake CI & Banchero N (1985a) Ventilation and oxygen consumption in the Guinea-pig. Respir Physiol 61: 347–355

Blake CI & Banchero N (1985b) Effects of cold and hypoxia on ventilation and oxygen consumption in awake Guinea-pigs. Respir Physiol 61: 357–368

Brown JN, Thorne PR & Nuttall AL (1989) Blood pressure and other physiological responses in awake and anaesthetized Guinea-pigs. Lab Anim Sci 39: 142–148

Cárdenas H & Zapata P (1983) Ventilatory reflexes originated from carotid and extracarotid chemoreceptors in rats. Am J Physiol 244: R119-R125

Cragg PA & Khrisanapant W (1989) Rat carotid bodies: surgical denervation versus chemical 'denervation' by 100% O_2. Proc Univ Otago Med Sch 67: 11–12

Cragg PA & Menzies KJ (1992) Ventilatory responses of Guinea-pigs to hypercapnia and hypoxia. Proc Physiol Soc NZ 12: 17

Cragg PA & Leonard BL (1995) Unilateral carotid body denervation in rats - effect on ventilatory responses to transient hypoxia and cyanide. Proc Physiol Soc NZ 14: 17

González C, Almaraz L, Obeso A & Rigual R (1994) Carotid body chemoreceptors: From natural stimuli to sensory discharges. Physiol Rev 74: 829–898

Khrisanapant W & Cragg PA (1984) Transient stimulation of breathing frequency and ventilation by hypoxia after glossopharyngeal nerve section in the anaesthetized rat. Proc Univ Otago Med Sch 62: 84–86

Khrisanapant W & Cragg PA (1987) The sensory pathways and respiratory function of abdominal chemoreceptors in the anaesthetized rat. Proc Univ Otago Med Sch 65: 13–14

Khrisanapant W & Cragg PA (1988) Contribution of carotid body and vagal chemoreceptors to ventilatory sensitivity to normocapnic hypoxia in anaesthetised rats. Proc Univ Otago Med Sch 66: 55–56

Kummer W, Gibbins IL & Heym Ch (1989) Peptidergic innervation of arterial chemoreceptors. Arch Histol Cytol 52 (suppl): 361–364

Lagneaux D (1994) Ventilatory responses to brief hypoxic stimuli after simulated altitude exposure in rat. Respir Physiol 97: 157–173

Mir AK, Al-Neamy K, Pallot DJ & Nahorski SR (1982) Cathecholamines in the carotid body of several mammalian species: Effects of surgical and chemical sympathectomy. Brain Res 252: 335–342

Monge C & Leon-Velarde F (1991) Physiological adaptation to high altitude: Oxygen transport in mammals and birds. Physiol Rev 71: 1135–1172

Peebles KC & Cragg PA (1995) Ventilation in response to hypoxia in newborn and mature Guinea-pigs. Proc Physiol Soc NZ 14: 15

Turek Z, Ringnalda BEM, Moran O & Kreuzer F (1980) Oxygen transport in Guinea-pigs native to high altitude. Pflügers Arch 384: 109–115

EFFECTS OF CONTINUOUS INTRACAROTID INFUSION OF DOPAMINE DURING LONG-TERM HYPOXIA IN AWAKE GOATS

P. L. Janssen, M. R. Dwinell, J. Pizarro, and G. E. Bisgard

Department of Comparative Biosciences
School of Veterinary Medicine
University of Wisconsin, Madison, Wisconsin 53706

1. INTRODUCTION

Ventilatory acclimatization to hypoxia (VAH) is the time-dependent increase in ventilation that occurs in mammals (including humans) during prolonged exposure to hypoxic environments. Goats acclimatize rapidly, reaching a ventilatory plateau within 4–6 hours of breathing hypoxic gas (Engwall & Bisgard, 1990). Evidence strongly suggests that VAH is caused by a time-dependent increase in carotid body (CB) sensitivity to hypoxia in goats (Nielsen et al, 1988). However, the mechanism for increased CB hypoxic sensitivity remains unknown.

The role of neurotransmitters within the CB has been of great interest in the study of VAH. A current hypothesis is that an increase in CB excitatory neurotransmitter activity, or decreased inhibitory activity, causes increased hypoxic sensitivity during VAH. The role of dopamine (DA) in CB function has been studied extensively, it being the most abundant neurotransmitter contained in CB glomus cells. The majority of evidence suggests that DA is an inhibitory neuromodulator in the CB. Exogenous administration of DA inhibits ventilation and carotid body discharge (Engwall & Bisgard, 1990; González et al, 1994) while CB DA receptor blockade stimulates ventilation and CB neural activity (Zapata & Torrealba, 1984; Kressin et al, 1986). Furthermore, acute hypoxia causes release of DA from the CB (Fidone et al, 1982), but the effect of long-term exposure to hypoxia may be suppression of release (Olson et al, 1983). Therefore, a time-dependent reduction in dopaminergic influence on the CB during prolonged hypoxia may account for the time-dependent increase in ventilation observed during VAH. Conversely, a continuous supply of DA at the CB during long-term hypoxia could possibly attenuate or prevent VAH. We sought to determine whether a constant infusion of DA during prolonged hypoxia could prevent VAH in awake goats.

Frontiers in Arterial Chemoreception, edited by Zapata *et al.*
Plenum Press, New York, 1996

2. METHODS

The effect of DA infusion on VAH was studied in 4 awake, carotid artery translocated goats. The animals were fitted with a face mask attached to a low resistance breathing valve, and expired air was collected in a spirometer for measurement of expired minute ventilation ($\dot{V}_E$). Arterial blood gases were monitored from samples drawn from the translocated carotid artery loops. After collection of baseline $\dot{V}_E$ and blood gas data, infusions of either DA (5.0 μg/kg/min; 1.0 ml/min ic) or saline (control; 1.0 ml/min ic) were begun in normoxia. Approximately 30 minutes into the infusion period, when stable $\dot{V}_E$ and blood gases were attained, the goats were exposed to hypoxia (PaO_2 *ca.* 40 Torr). Hypoxia, during DA (or saline) infusion, was maintained for 4 hours. During hypoxia $PaCO_2$ was maintained isocapnic to the level attained during the infusion in normoxia by adding CO_2 to the inspired air. Blood samples were collected frequently during the hypoxia/infusion period for close monitoring of PaO_2, $PaCO_2$, and pH.

3. RESULTS

3.1. Effects of DA Infusion on Breathing during Normoxia

During normoxia $\dot{V}_E$ was reduced 50% from baseline, and $PaCO_2$ was increased by 3.9 Torr after 1 minute of DA infusion (Table 1). After 30 min of DA infusion $\dot{V}_E$ had returned to within 7% of baseline, while $PaCO_2$ remained elevated by 4.7 Torr. Normoxic blood gases and $\dot{V}_E$ were not affected by saline infusion.

3.2. Effects of DA Infusion on Breathing during Hypoxia

The effects of DA infusion on ventilation during prolonged hypoxia are illustrated in Figure 1. $\dot{V}_E$ increased in a time-dependent manner during the 4 h hypoxia/infusion period in both DA-infused (Fig 1A) and control animals (Fig 1B). The time-course and magnitude of the ventilatory response to hypoxia were similar in control and DA-infused goats. The hypercapnia elicited by DA infusion during normoxia was maintained throughout the hypoxia/infusion period (Fig 1A). Likewise, the level of $PaCO_2$ that control animals attained during saline infusion in normoxia was maintained during hypoxia (Fig 1B).

Table 1. Expiratory minute ventilation and blood gas data from goats during dopamine or saline infusion in normoxia

Time	V_E (L/min)	$PaCO_2$ (Torr)	PaO_2 (Torr)	pH
Dopamine				
Baseline	8.03 ± 1.1	38.9 ± 1.9	82.6 ± 3.3	7.37 ± 0.01
1 min inf.	4.07 ± 0.8	42.8 ± 1.6	67.8 ± 2.3	7.34 ± 0.01
30 min inf.	7.47 ± 1.6	43.6 ± 2.1	78.1 ± 5.6	7.32 ± 0.01
Saline				
Baseline	11.37 ± 1.0	37.5 ± 0.9	95.7 ± 2.4	7.38 ± 0.03
1 min inf.	10.13 ± 1.3	37.1 ± 1.6	94.3 ± 2.8	7.39 ± 0.02
30 min inf.	11.80 ± 1.3	37.8 ± 0.7	95.6 ± 0.5	7.39 ± 0.03

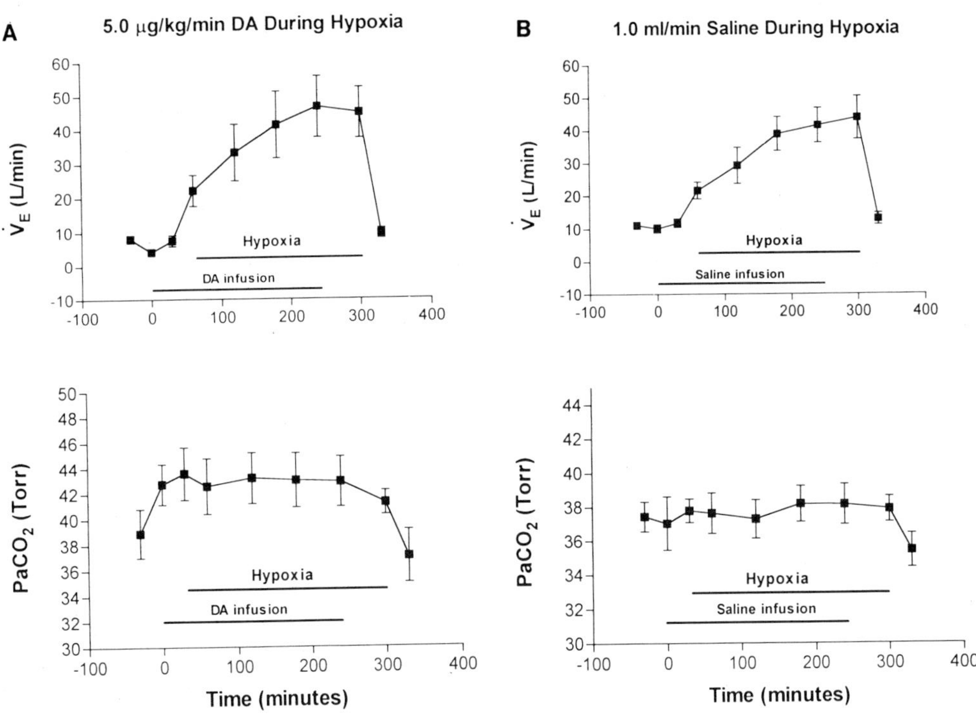

Figure 1. Time-course of $\dot{V}_E$ and $PaCO_2$ in goats during 4 h hypoxia while infused with either dopamine (A) or saline (B).

4. DISCUSSION

These results suggest that a continuous intracarotid infusion of DA during prolonged hypoxia does not prevent VAH in awake goats. Both DA-infused and control animals responded to 4 hours of isocapnic hypoxia with a time-dependent increase in ventilation that exceeded the acute response. The magnitude and time-course of ventilatory change were not different between control and DA-infused goats. However, due to hypercapnia caused by the DA infusion during normoxia, DA-infused goats were exposed to a higher level of $PaCO_2$ than control animals during the 4 hour hypoxia period. Unpublished data in our lab has shown that if $PaCO_2$ is allowed to fall to baseline (pre-infusion) values during 4 hours of hypoxia and DA infusion, the magnitude of ventilatory change is reduced, but acclimatization is not prevented.

A current hypothesis is that VAH is the result of a decrease in CB inhibitory mechanisms during prolonged hypoxia. Tatsumi et al (1995) showed that CB DA receptor blockade with domperidone increased ventilation and CB responses to hypoxia before, but not after, acclimatization to hypoxia in cats. It was suggested that the activity of inhibitory CB dopaminergic mechanisms were decreased by hypoxic exposure, and that the lessened inhibition may contribute to VAH (Tatsumi et al, 1995). Diminished DA inhibition could be caused by reduced DA receptor sensitivity or decreased availability of DA within the CB. However, current evidence does not support a change in CB DA receptor sensitivity during VAH in goats (Engwall & Bisgard, 1990). Providing the dose of DA was sufficient, the present data suggest that VAH occurs despite a continuous supply of DA to the CB which disputes the hypothesis that a decrease in the availability of DA causes VAH.

DA infusion caused acute hypoventilation during normoxia. While carotid sinus nerve recording studies show that CB activity remains suppressed throughout DA infusion, after 30 minutes of DA infusion $\dot{V}_E$ had returned to near baseline values but $PaCO_2$ remained elevated. Previous unpublished work in our lab showed that a 4 hour infusion of DA (5.0 μg/kg/min, ic) during normoxia caused a transient depression of ventilation followed by prolonged hypercapnia in the face of normal values for $\dot{V}_E$. Possible explanations for this discrepancy between $\dot{V}_E$ and $PaCO_2$ include changes in metabolic rate, dead space ventilation, or V_A/Q matching brought on by DA infusion. In our studies, we saw no changes in metabolic rate or dead space ventilation during DA infusion. However DA is a vasodilator in the lung (Polak et al, 1992) and therefore DA infusion could possibly lead to V_A/Q mismatch and subsequent hypercapnia.

In summary, our results show that a continuous intracarotid infusion of DA does not prevent VAH in awake goats, and hence do not support the hypothesis that a reduction in dopaminergic influence on the CB during prolonged hypoxia contributes to acclimatization.

5. ACKNOWLEDGMENTS

Work supported by NIH grants HL15473 and HL07654.

6. REFERENCES

Engwall MJA & Bisgard GE (1990) Ventilatory responses to chemoreceptor stimulation after hypoxic acclimatization in awake goats. J Appl Physiol 69: 1236–1243

Fidone S, González C & Yoshizaki K (1982) Effects of low oxygen on the release of dopamine from the rabbit carotid body *in vitro*. J Physiol, London 333: 93–110

González C, Almaraz L, Obeso A & Rigual R (1994) Carotid body chemoreceptors: From natural stimuli to sensory discharges. Physiol Rev 74: 829–898

Kressin NA, Nielsen AM, Laravuso R & Bisgard GE (1986) Domperidone-induced potentiation of ventilatory responses in awake goats. Respir Physiol 65: 169–180

Nielsen AM, Bisgard GE & Vidruk EH (1988) Carotid chemoreceptor activity during acute and sustained hypoxia in goats. J Appl Physiol 65: 1796–1802

Olson EB Jr, Vidruk EH, McCrimmon DR & Dempsey JA (1983) Monoamine neurotransmitter metabolism during acclimatization to hypoxia in rats. Respir Physiol 54: 79–96

Polak MJ, Kennedy LA & Drummond WH (1992) Manipulation of dopamine receptors alters hypoxic pulmonary vasoconstriction in isolated perfused rat lungs. Life Sci 51: 1317–1323

Tatsumi K, Pickett CK & Weil JV (1995) Possible role of dopamine in ventilatory acclimatization to high altitude. Respir Physiol 99: 63–73

Zapata P & Torrealba F (1984) Blockade of dopamine-induced chemosensory inhibition by domperidone. Neurosci Lett 51: 359–364

THE ROLE OF CAROTID BODY CO_2 DURING VENTILATORY ACCLIMATIZATION TO HYPOXIA IN THE GOAT

Melinda R. Dwinell, Patrick L. Janssen, Josue Pizarro, and Gerald E. Bisgard

Department of Comparative Biosciences
School of Veterinary Medicine
University of Wisconsin
Madison, Wisconsin 53706

1. INTRODUCTION

During a prolonged exposure to hypoxia, ventilation ($\dot{V}_E$) increases in a time-dependent manner. Ventilatory acclimatization to hypoxia (VAH) is associated with an increase in carotid body (CB) hypoxic sensitivity (Engwall & Bisgard, 1990; Ryan et al, 1993). The increased hypoxic sensitivity has been demonstrated under both systemic isocapnic or poikilocapnic conditions (Engwall & Bisgard, 1990). However, carotid body (CB) hypocapnia has a fairly strong inhibitory influence on normoxic ventilation in the awake goat (Daristotle et al, 1990) and dog (Smith et al, 1995). The objective of this study was to determine whether the increase in CB hypoxic sensitivity is dependent on the level of CB CO_2 pressure ($P_{cb}CO_2$) during the hypoxic exposure.

2. METHODS

Seven adult goats were trained to stand quietly in a stanchion while breathing through a face mask attached to a low resistance, one way breathing valve. Prior to the study, two surgeries, both done under general anesthesia (halothane, nitrous oxide, and oxygen), were performed on separate days to prepare the goats for CB perfusion by an extracorporeal circuit. This procedure has been described in detail previously (Busch et al, 1985). The initial surgery consisted of unilateral ligation of the internal maxillary and lingual arteries on the CB perfusion side and, contralaterally, excision of the CB and ligation of the occipital artery on the brain perfusion side. The second surgery involved inserting catheters into the common carotid artery (CB perfusion) and jugular vein (venous blood access) on the side with an intact CB. Goats were heparinized daily (40,000 units) and studied no sooner than six days after the second surgery.

Frontiers in Arterial Chemoreception, edited by Zapata *et al.*
Plenum Press, New York, 1996

On the day of the study, inspired ventilation was measured using a pneumotachograph. Expired gases were collected in a spirometer (120 l). Ventilation, end-tidal CO_2, systemic blood pressure and perfusion blood pressure were measured throughout the study. The perfusion circuit drew blood from the right atrium via the jugular vein. Blood was pumped through an oxygenator and blood filter and into the carotid artery for CB perfusion. Blood gases perfusing the CB were controlled by adjusting the relative concentrations of O_2, CO_2, and N_2 flowing through the oxygenator.

After control ventilation was collected during normoxic-normocapnic CB perfusion, the CB was perfused with hypoxic-normocapnic blood while maintaining systemic isocapnia by adding CO_2 to the inspiratory flow. The CB perfusion circuit was returned to normoxic-normocapnic conditions to allow the goats to return to baseline ventilation. The response to 4 h of CB hypoxia was then measured by adjusting the perfusion circuit to a $P_{cb}O_2$ of 40 Torr. In one group of goats (n= 7), CB normocapnia was maintained throughout the CB hypoxic period while maintaining systemic isocapnia. In the second group of goats (n= 5), $P_{cb}CO_2$ was progressively lowered to prevent any reflex hyperventilation. At the end of the 4 h CB hypoxic period, all animals were perfused with normoxic-normocapnic blood while breathing room air for 30 minutes. The acute CB hypoxic-normocapnic response was repeated following the prolonged hypoxic exposure.

3. RESULTS

During the CB hypoxic-normocapnic perfusion, $\dot{V}_E$ increased in the expected time-dependent manner throughout the 4 h hypoxic exposure (Fig 1A). When $P_{cb}CO_2$ was progressively lowered (CB hypocapnia), V_E remained at control levels throughout the

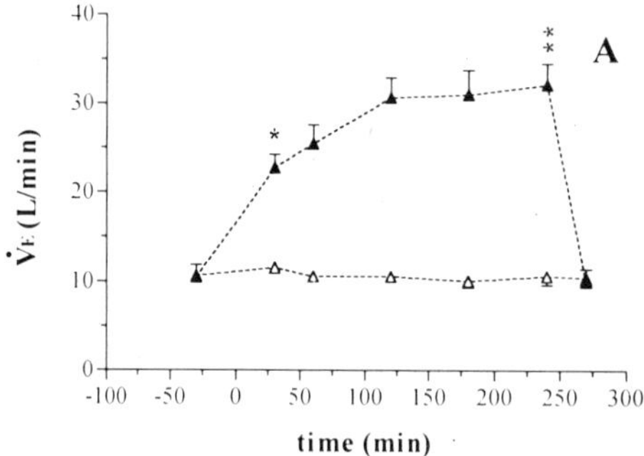

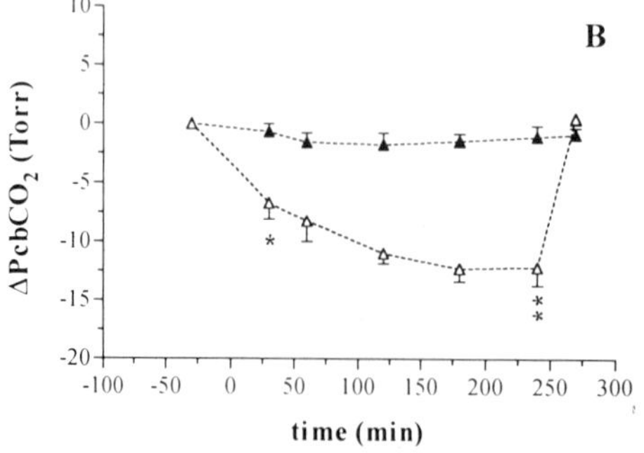

Figure 1. **A**: Ventilatory response to 4 h of CB hypoxia with either CB normocapnia-systemic isocapnia (filled triangles) or CB hypocapnia-systemic normocapnia (open triangles). **B**: Change in $P_{cb}CO_2$ during 4 h of CB hypoxia with CB normoxia-isocapnia (filled triangles) or CB hypocapnia-systemic normocapnia (open triangles). C, control value; R, return to CB normoxia-normocapnia. *Significantly different from control ($p < 0.05$). **Significantly different from 30 min ($p < 0.05$).

hypoxic exposure. To prevent the time-dependent increase in $\dot{V}_E$, $P_{cb}CO_2$ was lowered in a time-dependent manner (Fig 1B).

Both groups of animals had a brisk increase in $\dot{V}_E$ during the initial CB perfusion with hypoxic-normocapnic blood. Following the prolonged hypoxic exposure, after 30 minutes of normoxic-normocapnic conditions, the ventilatory responses of both groups to isocapnic CB hypoxia were significantly greater than the acute response prior to the prolonged hypoxic exposure. No significant differences between the group exposed to CB normocapnia or the group exposed to CB hypocapnia were found following prolonged hypoxic exposure.

4. DISCUSSION

The results of this study indicate that the increase in CB hypoxic sensitivity is not dependent on the level of $P_{cb}CO_2$ during the hypoxic exposure. Both groups of goats, exposed to either CB normocapnia or CB hypocapnia, had a significantly increased isocapnic hypoxic response following the 4 h CB hypoxic exposure. The increase in CB hypoxic sensitivity was not eliminated by progressively lowering $P_{cb}CO_2$ throughout the hypoxic exposure, preventing any time-dependent increase in $\dot{V}_E$.

The time-dependent increase in $\dot{V}_E$ during the CB hypoxia-normocapnia perfusion is consistent with previous findings in the awake goat demonstrating that CB hypoxia alone will elicit VAH (Busch et al, 1985). In addition, the magnitude of the ventilatory response during the 4 h exposure is analogous to the response when the whole animal, in-

Table 1. Mean ventilation and blood gas values during normoxia and hypoxia before (PRE) and after (POST) 4 h of CB hypoxia

	CB Normocapnia (n = 7)			
	PRE		POST	
	Normoxia	Hypoxia	Normoxia	Hypoxia
$\dot{V}_E$ (L/min)	10.4 ± 1.2	21.6 ± 2.2*	10.2 ± 1.3	25.1 ± 4.6*‡
freq (min^{-1})	17.7 ± 2.1	23.9 ± 2.1*	19.7 ± 3.9	30.6 ± 3.9*‡
V_T (ml)	646.0 ± 66	922.0 ± 112*	568.0 ± 65	1006.0 ± 114*
P_aCO_2 (Torr)	40.9 ± 0.9	40.6 ± 0.9	40.8 ± 1.3	41.1 ± 1.0
P_aO_2 (Torr)	88.6 ± 5.2	125.5 ± 4.9	91.5 ± 2.3	133.8 ± 4.2
$P_{cb}CO_2$ (Torr)	39.8 ± 1.1	39.5 ± 1.2	40.6 ± 1.3	40.9 ± 1.0
$P_{cb}O_2$ (Torr)	112.8 ± 3.9	42.2 ± 1.2*	109.4 ± 3.9	40.9 ± 0.4*
	CB Hypocapnia (n = 5)			
	PRE		POST	
	Normoxia	Hypoxia	Normoxia	Hypoxia
$\dot{V}_E$ (L/min)	9.8 ± 1.2	18.9 ± 3.1*	9.5 ± 1.1	27.9 ± 3.5*‡
freq (min^{-1})	20.7 ± 1.7	25.9 ± 1.0*	20.0 ± 1.7	29.7 ± 1.7*
V_T (ml)	479.0 ± 53	725.0 ± 104*	494.0 ± 42	944.0 ± 120*‡
P_aCO_2 (Torr)	42.4 ± 1.3	41.4 ± 1.1	40.5 ± 1.2	40.7 ± 1.1
P_aO_2 (Torr)	85.0 ± 4.1	116.6 ± 6.6	93.3 ± 3.9	130.4 ± 6.4
$P_{cb}CO_2$ (Torr)	40.9 ± 1.1	41.2 ± 1.0	41.4 ± 1.3	40.6 ± 1.2
$P_{cb}O_2$ (Torr)	107.1 ± 2.5	41.4 ± 0.5*	104.9 ± 2.0	41.1 ± 0.4*

* Significantly different than corresponding normoxia.
‡ Significantly different than PRE hypoxia value.

cluding both peripheral and central chemoreceptors, is exposed to hypoxia (Engwall & Bisgard, 1990; Ryan et al, 1993).

To prevent the characteristic time-dependent increase in $\dot{V}_E$ during CB hypoxia, it was necessary to gradually lower $P_{cb}CO_2$ in the CB hypocapnic group throughout the hypoxic exposure. This provides further evidence that the CB was becoming progressively more sensitive to hypoxia resulting in a greater drive to breathe.

We conclude that the level of $P_{cb}CO_2$ during prolonged exposure to hypoxia does not play a role in the gain in CB hypoxic sensitivity following VAH. An increase in $\dot{V}_E$ is not necessary to elicit an increase in the CB hypoxia-normocapnia ventilatory response.

5. ACKNOWLEDGMENTS

The authors thank Gordon Johnson for his assistance in these studies. The research was supported by NIH grants HL 15473 and HL 07654.

6. REFERENCES

Busch MA, Bisgard GE & Forster HV (1985) Ventilatory acclimatization to hypoxia is not dependent on arterial hypoxemia. J Appl Physiol 58: 1874–1880

Daristotle L, Berssenbrugge A, Engwall MJ & Bisgard GE (1990) The effects of carotid body hypocapnia on ventilation in goats. Respir Physiol 79: 123–136

Engwall MJA & Bisgard GE (1990) Ventilatory responses to chemoreceptor stimulation after hypoxic acclimatization in awake goats. J Appl Physiol 69: 1236–1243

Ryan ML, Hedrick MS, Pizarro J & Bisgard GE (1993) Carotid body noradrenergic sensitivity in ventilatory acclimatization to hypoxia. Respir Physiol 92: 77–90

Smith CA, Saupe KW, Henderson KS & Dempsey JA (1995) Ventilatory effects of specific carotid body hypocapnia in dogs during wakefulness and sleep. J Appl Physiol 79: 689–699

61

DYNAMIC SENSITIVITY OF CAROTID CHEMORECEPTORS TO CO_2 IN THE NEWBORN LAMB

Nicole Calder,[1] Prem Kumar,[2] and Mark Hanson[1]

[1] Department of Obstetrics and Gynaecology
University College London Medical School
London WC1E 6HX, United Kingdom
[2] Department of Physiology
University of Birmingham
Birmingham B15 2TT, United Kingdom

1. INTRODUCTION

In previous studies we examined the development of the response of carotid and aortic chemoreceptors to hypoxia in the lamb and kitten (Blanco et al, 1984; Hanson et al, 1989; Kumar & Hanson, 1989). Recently we have been examining the question of whether the response of the arterial chemoreceptors to CO_2 also develops post-natally. The issue is important because, whilst elevation in arterial PCO_2 (P_aCO_2) stimulates fetal chemoreceptors and fetal breathing movements, the effect of rapid changes in P_aCO_2 on chemoreceptors in the neonate is largely unknown. Because CO_2 production is linked to metabolism, it provides an important component of the drive to breathe in the neonate, especially at an age when the response to hypoxia is poor. This might be an important consideration in apnoea and respiratory failure in the neonate. Environmental temperature will, of course, affect metabolism and overheating has been proposed to play a role in the aetiology of certain types of respiratory failure, including sudden infant death syndrome. In previous studies (Watanabe et al, 1993) we found that environmental temperatures affected the gain of respiratory chemoreflex responses to changes in P_aO_2 and P_aCO_2. However, without direct information on chemoreceptor responses to CO_2, the mechanisms underlying such effects cannot be determined. For this reason we embarked on a study of the maturation of carotid chemoreceptor responses to CO_2 in the lamb. Preliminary data on the maturation of steady state and dynamic responses to CO_2 has already been published (Calder et al, 1995). In this report we concentrate on the adaptive nature of the chemoreceptor response to CO_2.

A step increase in P_aCO_2 increases chemoreceptor discharge rapidly but it then adapts down to a steady state level which depends on the PO_2 (Torrance et al, 1993). The

Frontiers in Arterial Chemoreception, edited by Zapata *et al.*
Plenum Press, New York, 1996

question of whether the rapid response to CO_2 constitutes true dynamic sensitivity, or whether it indicates that the carotid chemoreceptor is primarily a proportional receptor which adapts, has been discussed (Kumar et al, 1994). From these considerations, it could be predicted that if P_aCO_2 rises sharply and then continues to rise more slowly, the resulting pattern of chemoreceptor discharge will depend on two interacting factors - the rate of change of P_aCO_2 and the rate of adaptation. If the rate of increase of P_aCO_2 is relatively slower than that of the declining discharge due to adaptation, then discharge will reach a peak after the change in P_aCO_2 and then decline. If the rate of increase in P_aCO_2 is relatively faster than that of the adaptation, then discharge will rise rapidly following the initial increase in P_aCO_2 and then continue to increase more slowly. Lastly, if the two processes are equal and opposite in rate, then discharge will increase rapidly and be maintained, like a step function. Under this last set of conditions, the rate of adaptation can be measured from the rate of change of P_aCO_2. If the stimulus is administered via the inspired gas, then the rate of chemoreceptor adaptation can be measured from that of $P_{ET}CO_2$ or $F_{ET}CO_2$, because it is only necessary to define the rate of change in stimulus, not its absolute level in the arterial blood. This is the basis for our method.

2. METHOD

Nine lambs aged 4–17 days were anaesthetized (1.5–2.0% halothane, then alpha-chloralose 60–70 mg/kg iv) tracheotomised, paralysed and artificially ventilated. Depth of anaesthesia was checked from the stability of the arterial blood pressure and heart rate and the absence of any change in these variables on a noxious pinch of the foot. Repeated ramps in $F_{ET}CO_2$ were produced over 15 breaths by addition of 8–10% CO_2 to one of two inspirate lines. $F_{ET}CO_2$ was measured by a mass spectrometer. A ventilator switched between the two inspirates at the start of expiration every 15 breaths (respiratory frequency = *ca.* 2 Hz) during normoxia (NX: P_aO_2 80–100 mm Hg) and moderate hypoxia (MOD HX: P_aO_2 40–60 mm Hg). Few or multi- carotid chemoreceptor preparations (n= 12) were recorded from the left carotid sinus nerve (CSN) and discharge was summed in 200 msec bins repeatedly over the alternation period. Oscillations in CSN discharge were normalised to % maximum discharge (obtained during N_2 breathing with P_aCO_2 held constant), smoothed by 5 or 10 point moving average and viewed for evidence of a plateau in discharge at the peak or trough of the oscillation.

3. RESULTS

Figure 1 shows an example of a run in which 15 breath cycles in $F_{ET}CO_2$ were produced. A rapid rise in $F_{ET}CO_2$ produced by raising the inspired FCO_2 is followed by a slower rise in $F_{ET}CO_2$ of slope shown by A. $F_{ET}O_2$ is held nearly constant. Figure 2 shows an example of the resulting chemoreceptor oscillation from such an alternation in $F_{ET}CO_2$. In this trial, discharge increases rapidly after raising the CO_2, and then adapts down. Thus in this run, the rate of change in $F_{ET}CO_2$ after the initial increase was relatively slower than that of chemoreceptor adaptation. In Figure 3, the rate of increase in $F_{ET}CO_2$ was relatively faster, and so discharge increases continuously in a ramp function. Figure 4 shows an example of a step-shaped oscillation in chemoreceptor discharge, and the change in $F_{ET}CO_2$ which produced it. Taking all fibres together, we found that to hold chemoreceptor discharge constant as such a step function, the mean rate of increase in $F_{ET}CO_2$ was

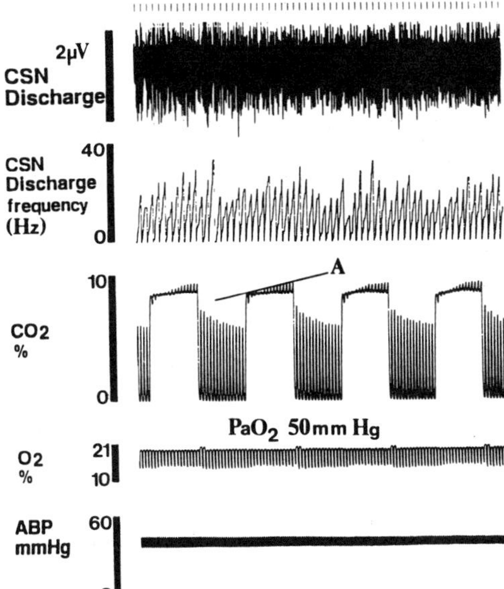

Figure 1. Example of an experimental run in a lamb aged 12 days in mild hypoxia. The rapid rise in $F_{ET}CO_2$ is followed by a slower rise, of slope A. $F_{ET}O_2$ remains relatively constant. Time (s) indicated at the top.

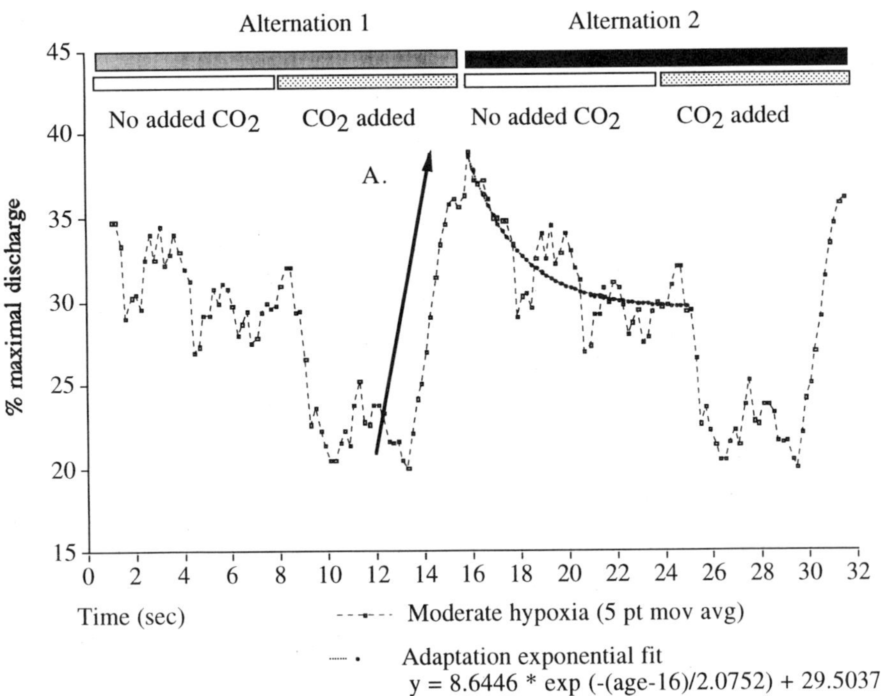

Figure 2. Carotid chemoreceptor discharge (% maximum discharge) plotted over two alternation periods during MOD HX in a lamb aged 12 days. Discharge frequency increases rapidly *ca.* 4–5 s after addition of CO_2 (A). As the CO_2 rises relatively slowly, adaptation to a lower level approaching steady-state occurs over *ca.* 6–8 s and is described by an exponential with a time constant of 2.1 s.

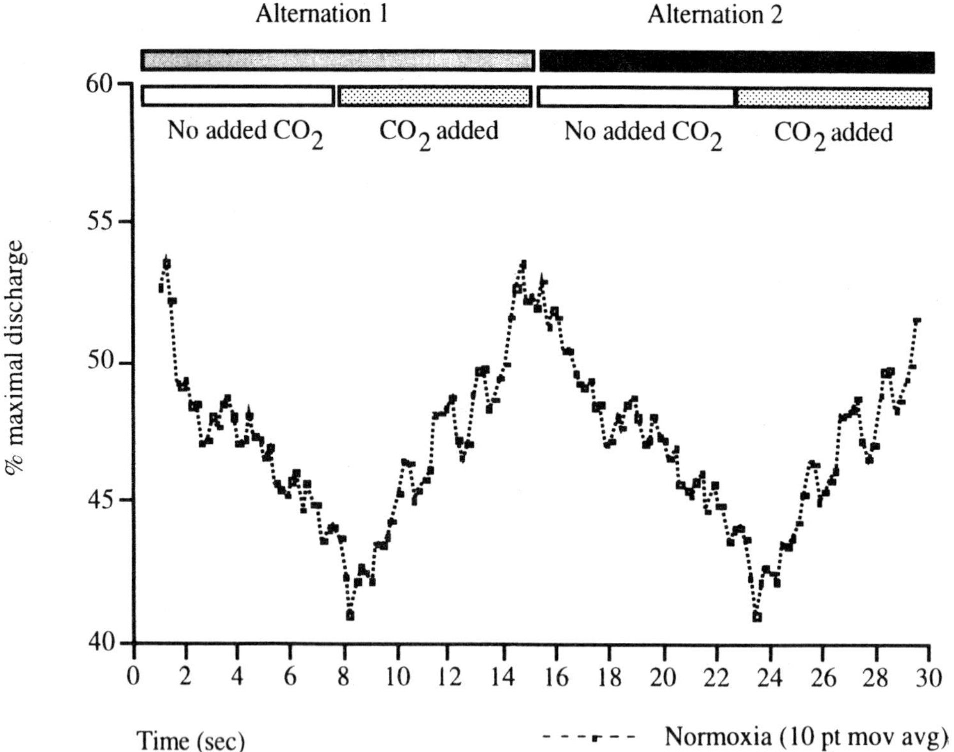

Figure 3. Carotid chemoreceptor discharge (% maximum discharge) plotted over two alternation periods for a saw-toothed oscillation during NX in a lamb aged 7 days. Discharge frequency increases slowly as CO_2 is added to the inspirate. As the CO_2 rises relatively fast, adaptation is not seen.

0.131 ± 0.013% $F_{ET}CO_2$/s (for a plateau at the peak of the oscillation) and -0.149 ± 0.026% $F_{ET}CO_2$/s (for a plateau at the trough of the oscillation).

Figure 5 shows the absolute rate of change of $F_{ET}CO_2$ which produced such a plateau, expressed as a function of post-natal age. There was no correlation with age (by linear regression $R^2 = 0.05$, $p > 0.4$).

4. DISCUSSION

Our results agree with those of previous workers in finding that the carotid chemoreceptors adapt to a rapid sustained rise in CO_2 (McCloskey, 1968). Moreover the rate of this adaptation does not change with age. This reinforces the idea that the responses to changes in CO_2 are present at birth and do not mature, unlike those to hypoxia. Thus the dynamic response to changes in P_aCO_2 is independent of the degree of hypoxia sensitivity and the level of P_aCO_2, both in terms of the initial response when CO_2 changes and the rate of adaptation which occurs, as suggested by Torrance et al (1993). Only the steady state, adapted level of discharge to a new steady P_aCO_2 level depends on the P_aO_2 level.

The results have implications for understanding the processes by which ventilation is matched to metabolism in the neonate. In addition, this simple method can be used to

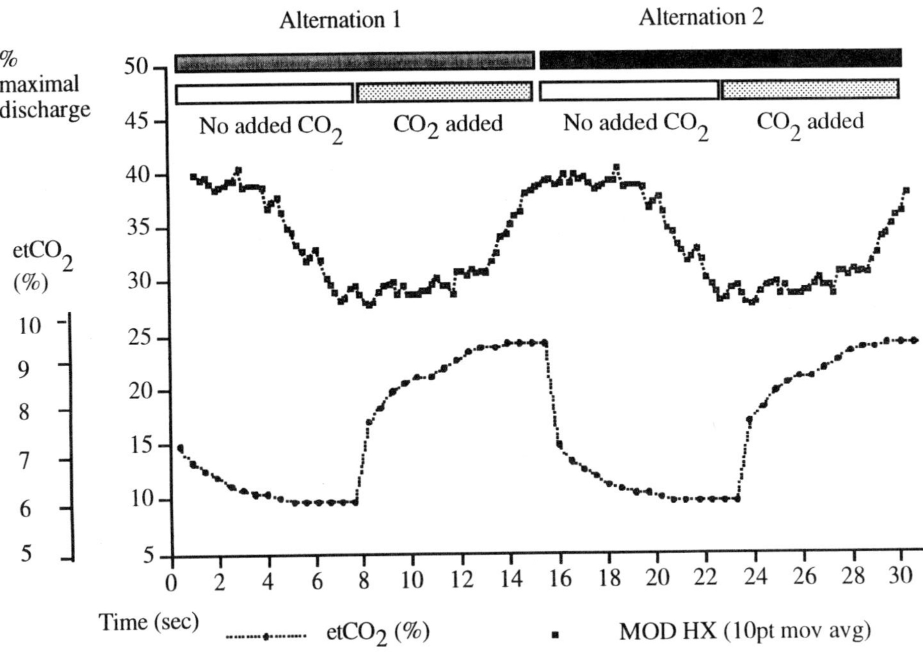

Figure 4. Carotid chemoreceptor discharge (% maximum discharge) plotted over two alternation periods for a step-shaped oscillation during MOD HX in a lamb aged 6 days. Discharge frequency increases rapidly *ca.* 4–5 s after addition of CO_2, and then reaches a plateau for *ca.* 3–4 s. At this time any decline in discharge due to adaptation must be offset by an increase due to the rising CO_2. When CO_2 is removed, discharge frequency falls more slowly, but here it does show some sign of adaptation, as it increases slowly for *ca.* 6 s before increasing briskly again when CO_2 is added.

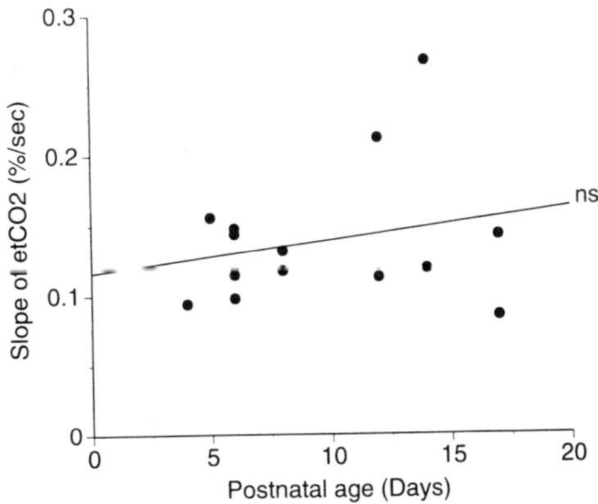

Figure 5. Plot of the absolute rate at which it was necessary to increase or decrease $F_{ET}CO_2$, in order to maintain chemoreceptor discharge constant for several seconds at the peak or trough of the oscillation, against post-natal age in lambs. There is no correlation between rate and age.

investigate mechanisms by which the carotid body detects changes in CO_2, since it obviates the need to produce maintained step changes in P_aCO_2, for example by perfusion of the carotid body.

5. ACKNOWLEDGMENTS

We are grateful to SPARKS and the Wellcome Trust for financial support.

6. REFERENCES

Blanco CE, Dawes GS, Hanson MA & McCooke HB (1984) The response to hypoxia of arterial chemoreceptors in fetal sheep and newborn lambs. J Physiol, London 351: 15–37

Calder NA, Kumar P & Hanson MA (1995) Maturation of carotid chemoreceptor responses to CO_2 in the anaesthetized newborn lamb. J Physiol, London 489: 162P

Hanson MA, Kumar P & Williams BA (1989) The effect of chronic hypoxia on the development of respiratory chemoreflexes in the newborn kitten. J Physiol, London 411: 563–574

Kumar P & Hanson MA (1989) Re-setting of the hypoxia sensitivity of the aortic chemoreceptors in the new-born lamb. J Dev Physiol 11: 199–206

Kumar P, Nye PCG & Torrance RW (1994) Proportional sensitivity of arterial chemoreceptors to CO_2. In: O'Regan RG, Nolan P, McQueen DS & Paterson DJ (eds). Arterial Chemoreceptors. New York: Plenum. pp 237–239

McCloskey DI (1968) Carbon dioxide and the carotid body. In: Torrance RW (ed) Arterial Chemoreceptors. London: Blackwell. pp 279–295

Torrance RW, Bartels EM & McLaren A (1993) Update on the bicarbonate hypothesis. Adv Exp Med Biol 337: 241–250

Watanabe T, Kumar P & Hanson MA (1993) Effect of warm environmental temperature on the gain of the respiratory chemoreflex in the kitten. J Physiol, London 459: 336P

A PHOSPHOLIPASE C INHIBITOR IMPEDES THE HYPOXIC VENTILATORY RESPONSE IN THE CAT

M. Pokorski,[1] M. Walski,[1] and Z. Matysiak[2]

[1] Medical Research Center and
[2] Institute of Biochemistry and Biophysics
Polish Academy of Sciences, Warsaw, Poland

1. INTRODUCTION

Arterial hypoxemia increases the chemosensory discharge of the carotid body (CB), which in turn stimulates the central respiratory output. The mechanisms of transduction of the hypoxic stimulus in the CB are not fully known.

Phospholipase C (PLC) is an enzyme that cleaves the phosphoinositols (PI). The cleavage of phosphatidylinositol-4,5-bisphosphate (PIP_2) leads to the formation of the second messengers 1,4,5-inositol triphosphate (IP_3), which mobilizes intracellular Ca^{2+}, and 1,2-diacylglycerol (DG), which activates protein kinase C (Nahorski, 1988). We have previously reported that PLC acting against PIP_2 may be involved with the hypoxic signal transduction, as its activity is enhanced in the hypoxic CB (Pokorski & Strosznajder, 1992). We have further shown that the PLC activation was coupled to a G-protein and might be a receptor-mediated process in the CB (Pokorski & Strosznajder, 1994). Both a stimulus-induced release of neurotransmitters, notably dopamine, and a rise of intracellular Ca^{2+} are at the core of contemporary theories of the mechanism of chemotransduction (Peers & Buckler, 1995), albeit the exact determinants and interactions of these processes are unclear. It seems therefore possible that the hypoxic activation of PLC may be an intermediary linking the two processes. If that is the case, then inhibition of PLC ought to affect the ventilatory response to hypoxia. In the present study we addressed this issue by examining the effects on the hypoxic ventilatory response (HVR) and on the CB ultrastructure of phenylmethylsulfonyl fluoride (PMSF), an inhibitor of PLC. We found that PMSF suppressed the ventilatory response to hypoxia.

2. METHODS

Four adult cats were used in the study which was performed in three stages.

Frontiers in Arterial Chemoreception, edited by Zapata *et al.*
Plenum Press, New York, 1996

Stage I. The cats were anesthetized with medetomidin HCl (Domitor; Orion-Famos, Finland), 0.4 mg/kg i.m., intubated, and the ventilatory response to 7% O_2 in N_2 was recorded, using a Fleisch head #00 and pneumotachograph (Mercury, England). This response was taken as control. The cats were then given 100 mg/kg PMSF mixed in 4% arabic gum suspension (two cats) or the vehicle suspension alone (one cat), i.p. in a volume of 5 ml/kg, or nothing (one cat) and were extubated and rapidly awakened with the anesthetic's antidote atipamezol HCl (Anisedan, Orion-Famos, Finland), 0.4 mg/kg, i.m. The ventilatory response was presented as changes of minute ventilation ($\dot{V}_E$), the product of respiratory rate and tidal volume. PMSF was purchased from the Sigma Chemical Co. The cats were housed in room air in separate cages for 7 days, obtaining food and water ad libitum. No significant behavioral or somatic signs of disease were noticeable, except for sporadic episodes of emesis in one PMSF-treated animal towards the end of the observation period.

Stage II. On day 8, the cats were reanesthetized and the HVR was reinvestigated under exactly the same conditions. Each cat served therefore as its own control. The carotid bodies were then exposed bilaterally, fixed *in situ* with a mixture of 2% paraformaldehyde and 2.5% glutaraldehyde in a 0.1 M kakodylan buffer of pH 7.4, excised rapidly, and postfixed in the same mixture.

Stage III. The organs were further processed for the electron microscopic study. The postfixation was completed with osmium tetroxide and potassium ferricyanide (McDonald, 1984). After dehydration in ethanol and propylene oxide, the specimens were embedded in Spurr resin. The study of the ultrathin sections was carried out with a JEM 1200 Ex electron microscope.

3. RESULTS

Figure 1 shows the HVR before and 7 days after the injection of PMSF (Panel A & B) and after the vehicle alone (Panel C) in three separate cats. The control, pre-injection response was stimulatory in all three cats and consisted of a 28–44% peak increase in $\dot{V}_E$ at 2 min; the response abating thereafter. The post-injection response was of a similar pattern but its magnitude differed, depending on the agent administered. In the PMSF-treated cats, the peak $\dot{V}_E$ increase was from 0.887 to 0.960 l/min (Panel A) and from 0.861 to 0.943 l/min (Panel B), the mere 8.2% and 9.5% increases as opposed to the respective increases of 28.4% and 43.8% in the pre-injection state in the same animals. In the vehicle-treated cat (Panel C), the $\dot{V}_E$ response was not appreciably affected after a 7 day of lapse, which was also the case in the control, uninjected cat (not shown). The HVR response was thus blunted in the PMSF-treated cats.

In all, 4 carotid bodies dissected from the PMSF-treated cats were studied under the electron microscope and compared with 4 control ones (1 vehicle-injected and 1 uninjected cat). Figure 2 shows the structural features of a carotid body of the vehicle-treated cat. There are cross-sections of 3 glomus cells (I) containing numerous dense-cored vesicles, a typical pattern of endoplasmic reticulum (ER), clearly visible Golgi elements (↓), and mitochondria with clearly defined cristae. A nucleus is visible in two of these cells. A sustentacular cell (II) is seen in the middle bottom. The picture shows the normal CB structure.

In contrast, micrographs (Figs 3 and 4) from the carotid bodies of PMSF-treated cats show a substantial degree of parenchymal damage. Figure 3 shows a section of glomus cells (I) that contain giant phagolysosomes (PL) and swollen mitochondria in their cyto-

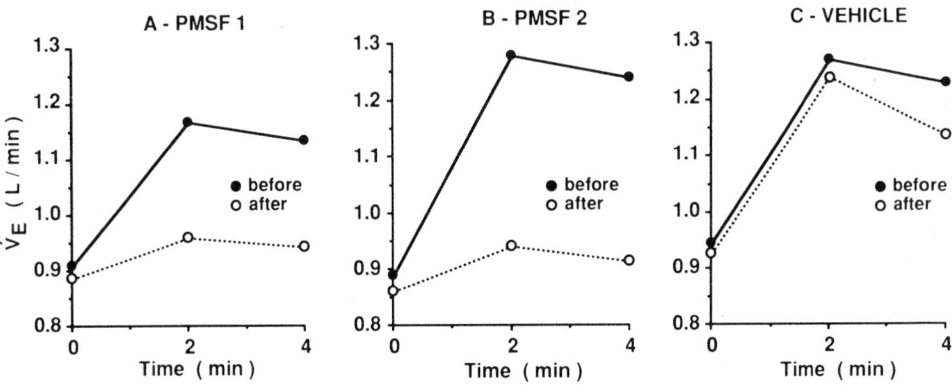

Figure 1. The ventilatory response to 7% O_2 (A) before and (B) 7 days after the injection of PMSF (100 mg/kg, ip) and (C) after the vehicle alone. Each panel represents a separate cat. PMSF suppressed the response.

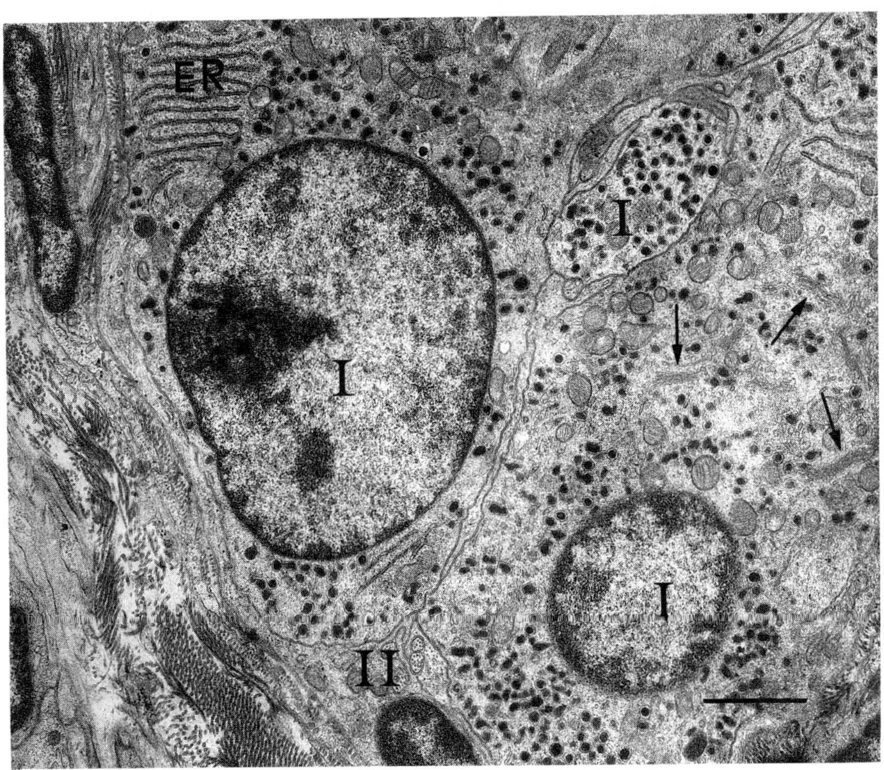

Figure 2. Electron micrograph of a carotid body of a vehicle-treated cat showing the normal parenchymal structure. Cross-sections of 3 glomus cells (I) are seen, two of which contain large nuclei. A characteristic endoplasmic reticulum (ER), Golgi elements (↓), and dense-cored vesicles of various sizes are seen. A sustentacular cell (II) can be seen in the middle bottom. Bar, 2 μm.

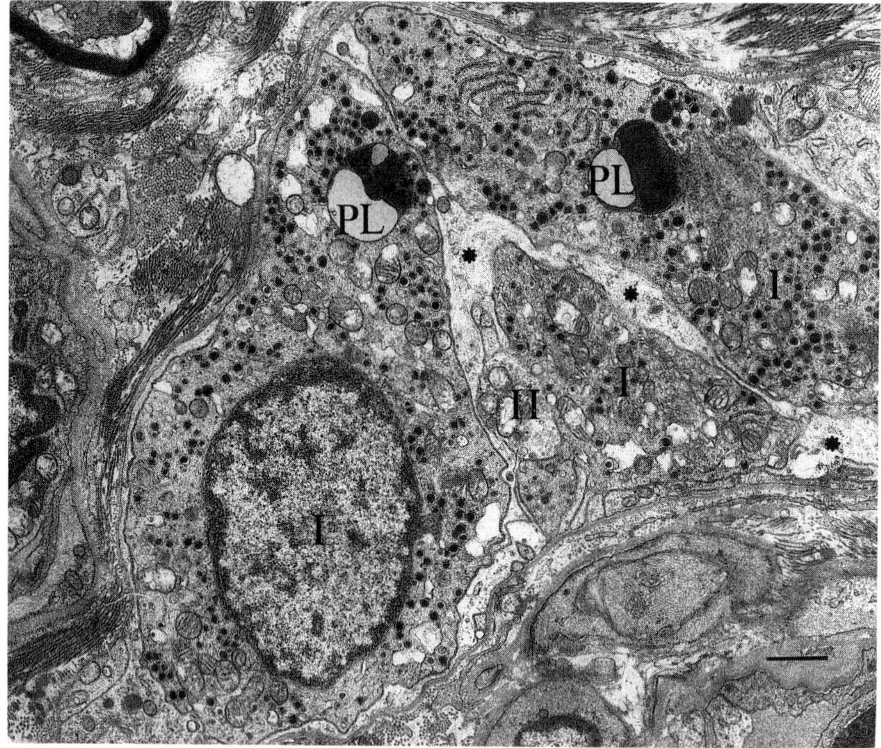

Figure 3. Electron micrograph of a carotid body of a PMSF-treated cat. There are cross-sections of 3 glomus cells (I) with giant phagolysosomes (PL) and swollen mitochondria in their cytoplasm. The space between the glomus cells is widened (*). The dense-cored vesicles are present. The sustentacular cell (II), in the middle of the picture, shows swollen mitochondria and clearing of the cytoplasm. Bar, 2 μm.

plasm. The space between the glomus cells is markedly widened (*) and filled with a fine fibrillar material. The sustentacular cell (II) also shows swollen mitochondria and clearing of the cytoplasm. Figure 4 shows another section of glomus cells (I) whose cytoplasm contains large vacuolar spaces (*). There is a reduced number of intracellular organelles but dense-cored vesicles abound. The cytoplasm of sustentacular cells (II) is unchanged.

4. DISCUSSION

This study demonstrates that PMSF suppressed the ventilatory response to hypoxia in the cat. PMSF is an inhibitor of serine esterase. It blocks the stimulus-induced release of arachidonic acid in platelets (Walenga et al, 1980) and in rat neocortex (Unemura et al, 1979) by inhibiting PI-specific PLC. The carotid body PIP_2-specific PLC is activated in hypoxia (Pokorski & Strosznajder, 1992). Activation of PLC seems to take place at an early stage of the response to hypoxia, since it is a G-protein-linked process (Pokorski & Strosznajder, 1994), probably initiated by a neurotransmitter-receptor interaction. If PMSF blocked PLC in the carotid body, as it does in the brain, then production of IP_3 and DG, the signaling molecules that control cellular responses, from PIP_2 would be inhibited.

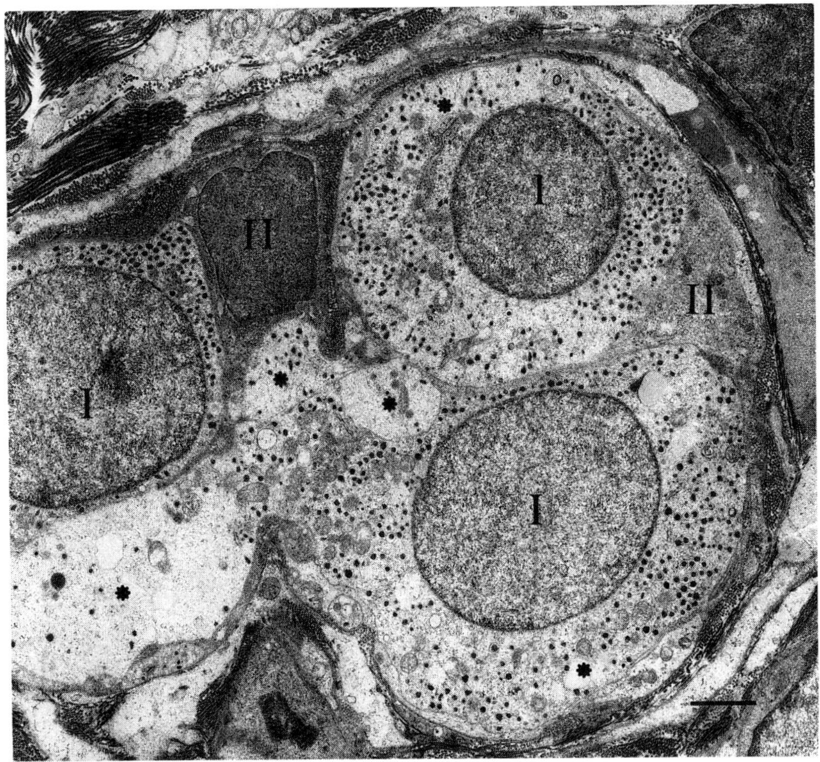

Figure 4. Electron micrograph of another PMSF-treated carotid body showing advanced parenchymal damage. There are cross-sections of 3 glomus cells (I) containing large vacuolar spaces (*) in their cytoplasm. There is a reduced number of intracellular organelles but the dense-cored vesicles are there. Sustentacular cells (II) show unchanged cytoplasm. Bar, 2 µm.

The suppression of the ventilatory response might thus have to do with the blockage of cytosolic Ca^{2+} increase in the glomus cells, either IP_3-mediated or due to the loss of modulation of calcium channels by PLC, which is required for chemosensory activation by hypoxia (Peers & Buckler, 1995).

The carotid bodies of the cats that showed the suppressed hypoxic ventilatory response exhibited substantial degenerative changes in their parenchyma. The structural damage caused by PMSF is not readily explainable. This damage apparently requires a prolonged action of PMSF, since it was not noticeable in the carotid bodies dissected 24 h after the PMSF treatment (not shown). All parenchymal elements of the carotid body structure were vulnerable to PMSF action. The changes most commonly seen concerned the glomus cell. Interestingly, the dense-cored vesicles and synapses apposed to glomus cells were usually spared (Fig 5), which implies that other elements are also vital for the preservation of the carotid chemosensory response.

In most fields selected randomly for microscopic evaluation, there was a whole spectrum of damage to the glomus cells; from little damaged cells to dark-type degeneration and ghost cells, intermingled with intact cells. The number of intact glomus cells that is sufficient to uphold the chemosensory response to hypoxia is unknown. Nor are the effects of protracted inhibition of PI breakdown by PLC or the delayed effects on PI metabolism of a brief period

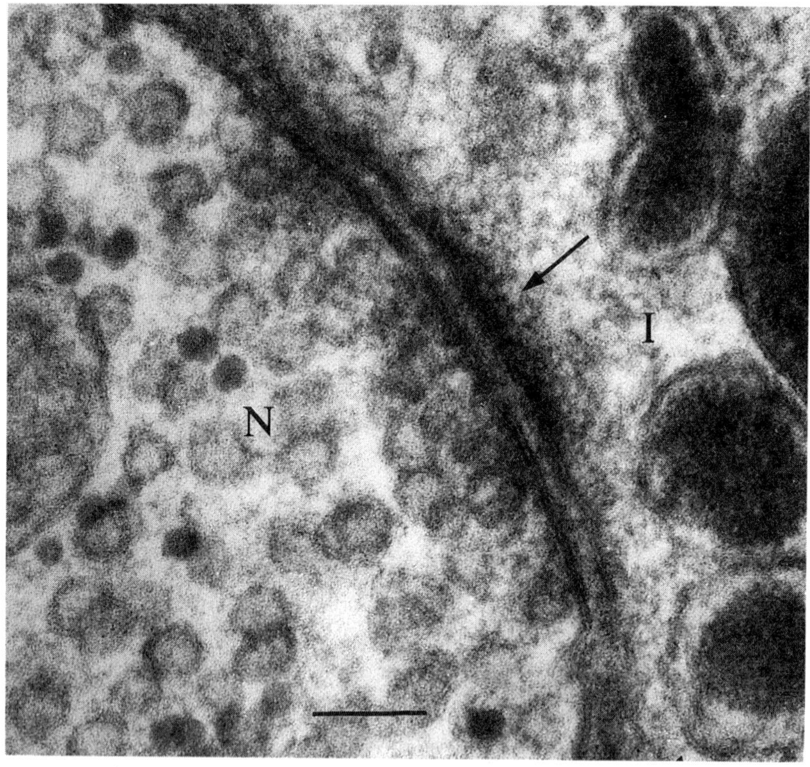

Figure 5. Electron micrograph of a PMSF-treated carotid body showing the normal synaptic cleft between a glomus cell (I) and a nerve fiber (N). The arrow is placed in the presynaptic part. Bar, 100 nm.

of hypoxia in the carotid body. In the gerbil hippocampus, arachidonic acid increase probably due to the breakdown of PI by PLC continues for over a day after reperfusion of the ischemic insult (Abe et al, 1989). Such a long PLC activation may serve the intracellular repair processes. It may therefore be surmised that the structural damage to the carotid body parenchyma developing over a period of days involves the inhibition of the enzyme and a subsequent intramolecular derangement in the cascade of events that follows the receptor-mediated PLC activation. PMSF may also have different intrinsic activities that cause damage to cellular structures. Regardless of the exact determinants of PMSF action, the suppression of the hypoxic ventilatory response observed in this study may be attributed to dysfunction of the carotid bodies, even though PMSF crosses the blood-brain barrier (Turini et al, 1969) and might affect the central integration of carotid body input and respiratory output.

In conclusion, the results of this study lend support to the suggestion that the phosphoinositide cascade is germane to hypoxia transduction in the carotid body.

5. ACKNOWLEDGMENTS

This study was supported by the statutory budget of the Polish Academy of Sciences Medical Research Center. Dr R Strosznajder is thanked for help at the preliminary stage of the study and Ms Kinga Sroczynska for skillful technical assistance.

6. REFERENCES

Abe K, Yoshidomi M & Kogure K (1989) Arachidonic acid metabolism in ischemic neuronal damage. Ann N Y Acad Sci 559: 259–268

McDonald K (1984) Osmium ferricyanide fixation improves microfilament preservation and membrane visualization in a variety of animal cell types. J Ultrastruct Res 86: 107–118

Nahorski SR (1988) Inositol polyphosphates and neuronal calcium homeostasis. Trends Neurosci 11: 444–448

Peers C & Buckler KJ (1995) Transduction of chemostimuli by the type I carotid body cell. J Membr Biol 144: 1–9

Pokorski M & Strosznajder R (1992) Phosphoinositides and signal transduction in the cat carotid body. In: Honda Y, Miyamoto Y, Konno K & Widdicombe JG (ed) Control of Breathing and Its Modeling Perspective. New York: Plenum. pp 367–370

Pokorski M & Strosznajder R (1994) G proteins in chemotransduction of the carotid body. J Neurochem 63 (suppl 1): S70C

Turini P, Kurooka S, Steer M, Corbascio AN & Singer TP (1969) The action of phenylmethylsulfonyl fluoride on human acetylcholine esterase, chymotrypsin and trypsin. J Pharmacol Exp Ther 167: 98–104

Unemura A, Mabe H, Nagai H & Sugino F (1992) Action of phospholipase A_2 and C on free fatty acid release during complete ischemia in rat neocortex. J Neurosurg 76: 648–651

Walenga R, Vanderhoek JY & Feinstein MB (1980) Serine esterase inhibitors block stimulus-induced mobilization of arachidonic acid and phosphatidylinositol-specific phospholipase C activity in platelets. J Biol Chem 255: 6024–6027

63

MODELLING THE PERIPHERAL CHEMOSENSORY DRIVE OF VENTILATION ON BASIS OF HOMOGENOUS SENSORY UNITS

Jaime Eugenín

Facultad de Ciencias Médicas
Universidad de Santiago de Chile
Santiago, Chile

1. INTRODUCTION

Depth and timing of breath are supposed to be the result of the interaction of two functional compartments forming the respiratory pattern generator ("Inspiratory off-switch Hypothesis"). The first compartment generates the central inspiratory activity (CIA). The second one, the inspiratory off-switch (IO-S), has control of the inspiratory duration; when IO-S activity overpasses certain threshold the activity of the CIA is inhibited (Bradley et al, 1975; Cohen & Feldman, 1977; von Euler, 1977, 1986).

The peripheral arterial chemoreceptors constitute one of the most important systems modulating the respiratory pattern generator. Peripheral chemosensory units increase their rate of firing in response to several stimuli like hypoxia, hypercarbia, and acidosis. Once activated, chemosensory units trigger, among others, ventilatory reflexes (Eyzaguirre et al, 1983; Trzebski, 1983). Typically, activation of chemosensory units increases tidal volume and decreases inspiratory duration (Clark & von Euler, 1972).

The contribution of chemosensory units innervating carotid bodies to the ventilatory reflexes differs from those innervating aortic bodies in both magnitude and delay of apparition of chemoreflexes. Disparities likely arise from intrinsic properties of each kind of chemoreceptor organ, and at some extension, from differences in their central connections. In spite of quantitative differences, it has been largely considered that the pattern of ventilatory responses elicited by carotid and aortic body stimulation is qualitatively identical. That is, once activated, they would act upon similar mechanisms. In other terms, carotid and aortic inputs would arrive into the same functional compartments of the respiratory pattern generator.

In the present work, simulations were focused to explore whether the contribution of carotid and aortic chemosensory units to the ventilatory chemoreflexes can be described on basis of a common input to the respiratory pattern generator. Two main assumptions were done: i) Chemosensory units innervating a same kind of chemoreceptor organ (*i.e.*, carotid or

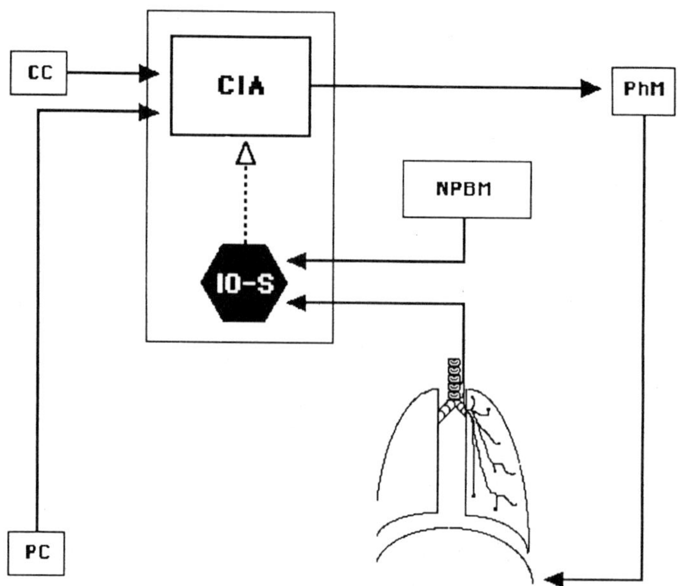

Figure 1. Scheme of the functional organization of the inspiratory pattern generator based on the inspiratory off-switch hypothesis. CIA, central inspiratory activator; CC, central chemoreceptors; IO-S, inspiratory off-switch; NPBM, nucleus pontine parabrachialis medialis; PC, peripheral chemoreceptors; PhM, phrenic motoneurons. Solid lines and filled triangles indicate excitation; broken lines and open triangle indicate inhibition. Note that only CIA receives chemosensory input.

aortic bodies) constitute an homogenous group of sensory cells; and ii) Chemosensory units excite directly and specifically the structures that originate the central inspiratory activity.

2. MODEL

2.1. Description of the Respiratory Pattern Generator

The general structure of the model is illustrated in Figure 1.

Description of the relationship between depth and timing of respiratory cycles was implemented on the theoretical framework of the inspiratory off-switch hypothesis using equations from a recent model in which integration is the essential function of the inspiratory off-switch (see details in Eugenín, 1995). That means that the inhibition of the CIA will occur when the activity within the inspiratory off-switch, "S", exceeds a certain threshold, "Th", which is reached through the integration of the incoming activity arriving to the inspiratory off-switch. This is,

$$S = K_{NPB} \cdot Ti + K_{dv} \cdot V_T + K_v \cdot \int_0^{Ti} V(t)\,dt \quad \geq Th \tag{1}$$

Where K_{NPB}, K_{dv} and K_v are constants; Ti, inspiratory duration; V_T, tidal volume; V(t), lung volume at the time "t". V(t) is obtained from the solution to the following differential equation

$$V(t) = (a/R) \cdot [\exp(-t/\tau)] \cdot \int t^b \cdot [\exp(t/\tau)]\, dt \tag{2}$$

where "a", index of the rate of rise of the inspiratory activity; "t", time in seconds; R and E, active resistance and elastance of the respiratory system, respectively; $\tau = R \cdot (1/E)$, time constant; b, dimensionless index of the shape of the curve of tracheal occlusion (details in Eugenín, 1995).

2.2. Input of Chemoafferents

It is assumed that peripheral chemosensory units excite directly only the central inspiratory activator and no input from chemosensory units to the inspiratory off-switch was considered. Such organization can be described making "a", index of the rate of rise of the inspiratory activity (eq. 2), a lineal function of chemosensory input originated from carotid and aortic bodies. The magnitude of ventilatory chemoreflex was defined as a function of the number of primary chemoafferents able to activate central structures, their firing rate, their central inhibition, and the "strength" of their central synapses acting directly upon CIA. A diagram of components and interactions considered in the model as relevant features of the peripheral chemoreceptor system are depicted in Figure 2.

Chemosensory input to the CIA, E(x), is defined by

$$E(x) = G(S)\sum_{i=1}^{n} f_i(x) \cdot m_i(x) \quad i = 1,2\ldots,n \tag{3}$$

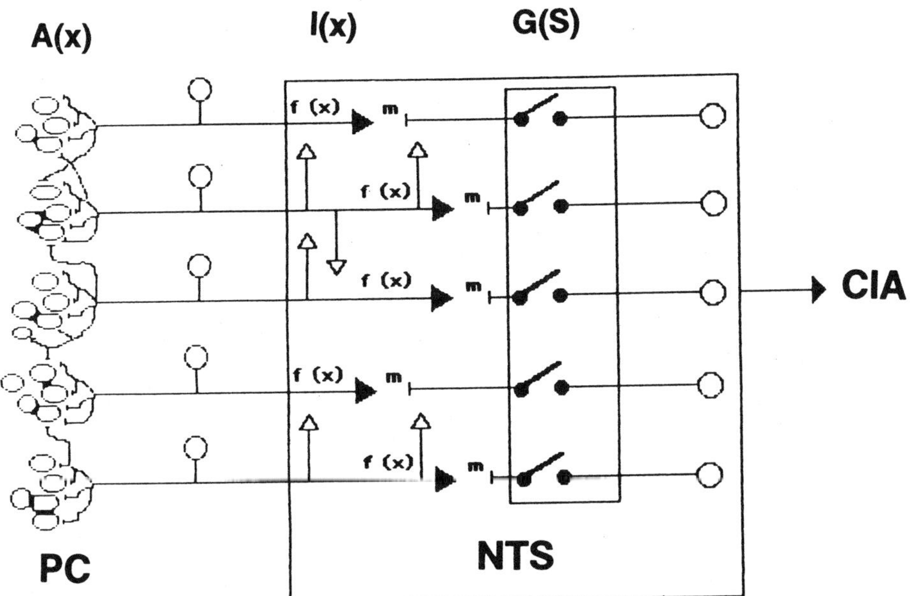

Figure 2. Scheme of structures, their interactions, and functions considered in the description of carotid chemosensory input to the central inspiratory activator. A peripheral chemosensory unit is constituted by a primary afferent and the chemoreceptor cells which it innervates; A(x), activation function for peripheral chemosensory units; f(x), frequency of discharge of chemosensory unit; G(S), gating function; I(x), inactivation function depending on pre- and postsynaptic interactions; m, synaptic strength; NTS, nuclear complex of the solitary tract.

where G(S) is a gating function taking values G(S)=1 if S ≤ Th or G(S)=0 if S > Th. The gating function G(S) was introduced to indicate that chemosensory stimulation increases inspiratory activity only when applied during inspiratory phase (Eldridge & Millhorn, 1986); $f_i(x)$, frequency of discharge of chemosensory unit "i" in function of dose of chemical stimulus "x"; it was described as a sigmoidal function. Maximal and minimal frequencies were obtained from available data (Eyzaguirre et al, 1983; Fitzgerald & Lahiri, 1986); $m_i(x)$, "strength" of chemosensory unit "i" to activate CIA; it was assumed constant for all the chemosensory units acting effectively on CIA.

2.3. Recruitment of Chemosensory Units

As illustrated in Figure 2, the number of primary chemoafferents to be activated will depend on the dose of chemical stimuli "x", the number of chemoreceptor cells which innervate them and their intrinsic properties of activation, activation function A(x). In turn, the increase in the rate of rise of central inspiratory activity will depend on the number of primary chemoafferents which are able to activate the CIA. The extension to what activity from chemosensory units is propagated to central structures can be modified by pre- or postsynaptic interactions (Felder & Heesch, 1987). This factor will be considered as the inactivation function I(x). Since it is assumed that chemosensory units constitute an homogenous group of sensory cells (Goodman, 1974), the functions A(x) and I(x) should take similar values in all the units. It will be considered that A(x) is constant, that is, A(x) = A, and I(x) is proportional to the number "n" of recruited chemosensory units, that is, I(x) = I n. Let "N_T" be the total number of chemosensory units, then the recruitment process can be described through a "population growth model" of the form

$$dn / dx = K \cdot [N_T - n] \cdot [A - I \cdot n] \tag{4}$$

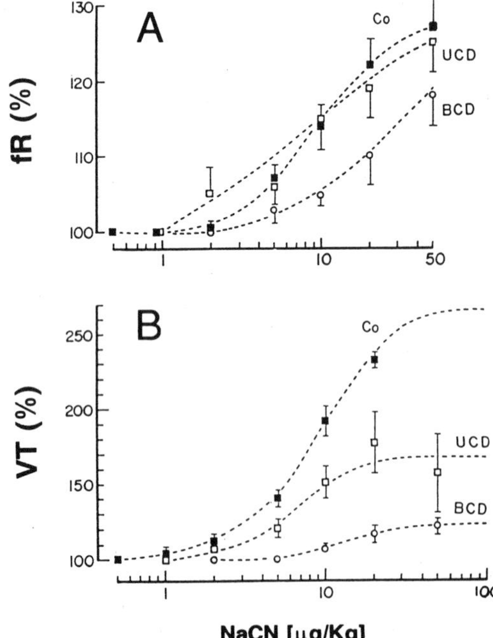

Figure 3. Dose-response curves for changes in respiratory frequency (**A**) and tidal volume (**B**) evoked by iv injections of NaCN in six anaesthetized cats with intact buffer nerves (Co, control), unilateral carotid deafferentation (UCD) and bilateral carotid deafferentation (BCD). Changes expressed as percentages of corresponding basal values. Means and SEM's, symbols and vertical lines. Curves adjusted to sigmoidal function. (Redrawn from Eugenín et al, 1989).

where K, constant. This is a differential equation of the Ricatti's form which can be solved analytically.

3. SIMULATIONS

Dose-response curves for changes in tidal volume and respiratory frequency in anaesthetized cats are illustrated in Figure 3.

Three conditions were simulated (Fig 4): intact buffer nerves (Co), unilateral carotid deafferentation (UCD), and bilateral carotid deafferentation (BCD). Contribution of carotid and aortic afferents were assumed to be independent. Thus, the function of che-

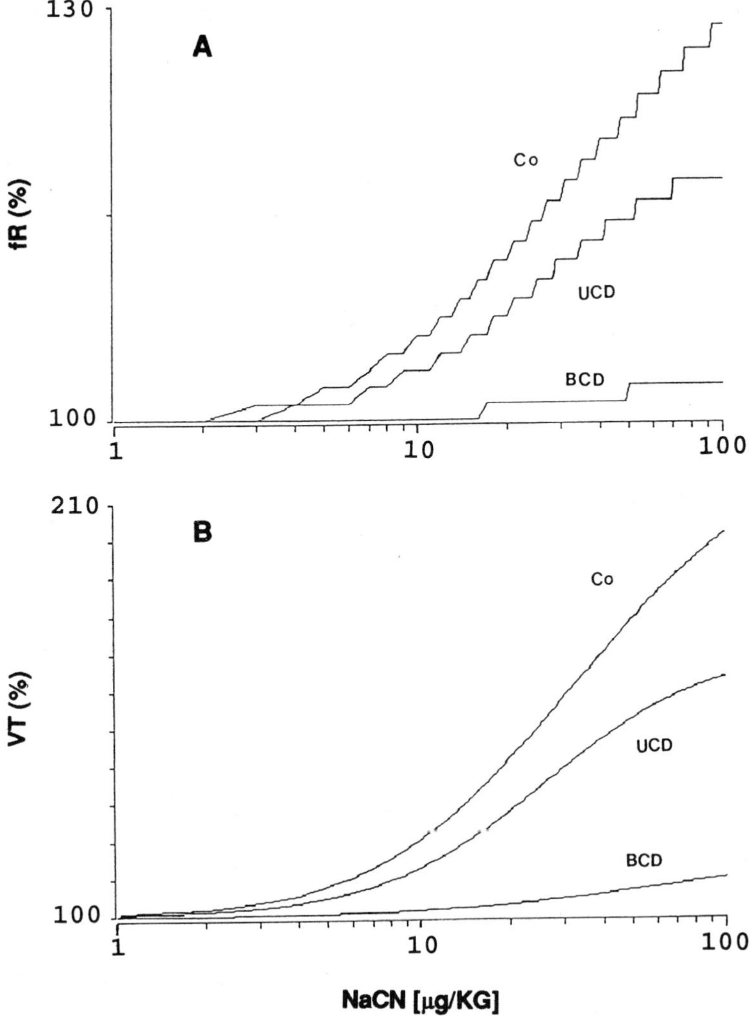

Figure 4. Simulation of dose-response curves for reflex changes in instantaneous respiratory frequency (**A**) and tidal volume (**B**). Conditions as in Figure 3. Co, control; unilateral (UCD) and bilateral (BCD) carotid deafferentation.

mosensory input to CIA for carotid afferents was linearly added to that for aortic afferents. Unilateral carotid deafferentation was simulated decreasing N_T to half and, since "I" factor depends on the number of active chemoafferents, its value was reduced in Eq. 4. Comparison with experimental curves (Fig 3) indicates that dose-response curves for tidal volume under the three conditions are well approached on basis of the main assumptions of the model. In contrast, simulated changes in respiratory frequency were partially reproduced (compare Figs 3A and 4A).

4. DISCUSSION

The present model provides adequate simulation of the contribution of carotid and aortic chemosensory units to the reflex changes in amplitude of breathing evoked by a wide range of iv injections of sodium cyanide in anaesthetized cats. The results support the notion that the magnitude of changes in tidal volume in response to cytotoxic hypoxia can be explained on basis of the assumptions of functional homogeneity of chemosensory units innervating a same chemoreceptor organ and their direct excitatory action upon the central inspiratory activator. In contrast, reflex changes in respiratory frequency after unilateral or bilateral carotid deafferentation were not adequately reproduced. This major deviation from experimental data suggests that the simple assumption of one common input to the respiratory pattern generator for both carotid and aortic chemoafferents should be reviewed. It should be remarked that an important weakness of the present model is the absence of information about properties of input of peripheral chemosensory to central structures. In that respect, this model should be regarded as an effort to explain some functional properties of ventilatory chemoreflexes quantitatively.

5. REFERENCES

Bradley GW, von Euler C, Marttila I & Roos B (1975) A model of the central and reflex inhibition of inspiration in the cat. Biol Cybernet 19: 105–116

Clark FJ & von Euler C (1972) On the regulation of depth and rate of breathing. J Physiol, London 222: 267–295

Cohen MI & Feldman JL (1977) Models of respiratory phase-switching. Fed Proc 36: 2367–2374

Eldridge FL & Millhorn DE (1986) Oscillation, gating, and memory in the respiratory control system. In: American Physiological Society: Handbook of Physiology, sect 3, vol 2. Baltimore, MD: Williams & Wilkins. pp 93–114

Eugenín J (1995) Generation of the respiratory rhythm: modelling the inspiratory off switch as a neural integrator. J Theor Biol 172: 107–120

Eugenín J, Larraín C & Zapata P (1989) Correlative contribution of carotid and aortic afferences to the ventilatory chemosensory drive in steady-state normoxia and to the ventilatory chemoreflexes induced by transient hypoxia. Arch Biol Med Exp 22: 395–408

Eyzaguirre C, Fitzgerald RS, Lahiri S & Zapata P (1983) Arterial Chemoreceptors. In: American Physiological Society: Handbook of Physiology, sect 2, vol 3. Baltimore, MD: Williams & Wilkins. pp 557–621

Felder RB & Heesch CM (1987) Interactions in nucleus tractus solitarius between right and left carotid sinus nerves. Am J Physiol 253: H1127-H1135

Fitzgerald RS & Lahiri S (1986) Reflex responses to chemoreceptor stimulation. In: American Physiological Society: Handbook of Physiology, sect 3, vol 2. Baltimore, MD: Williams & Wilkins. pp 313–362

Goodman NW (1974) Some observations on the homogeneity of responses of single chemoreceptor fibers. Respir Physiol 20: 271–281

Trzebski A (1983) Central pathways of the arterial chemoreceptor reflex. In: Acker H & O'Regan RG (eds) Physiology of the Peripheral Arterial Chemoreceptors. Oxford: Elsevier. pp 431–464

von Euler C (1977) The functional organization of the respiratory phase-switching mechanisms. Fed Proc 36: 2375–2380

von Euler C (1986) Brain stem mechanisms for generation and control of breathing pattern. In: American Physiological Society: Handbook of Physiology, sect 3, vol 2. Baltimore, MD: Williams & Wilkins Co. pp 1–68

64

FUNCTIONAL ACTIVATION OF CEREBRAL GLUCOSE UPTAKE AFTER CAROTID BODY STIMULATION

Ramón Alvarez-Buylla,[1] Alberto Huberman,[2] Sergio Montero,[1] and Elena Roces de Alvarez-Buylla[3]

[1] Centro Universitario de Investigaciones Biomédicas
Universidad de Colima
Colima, Col, México
[2] Departamento de Bioquímica
Instituto Nacional de la Nutrición "Salvador Zubirán", México, DF, México
[3] Departamento de Fisiología, Biofísica y Neurociencias
CINVESTAV, México, DF, México

1. INTRODUCTION

Our laboratory is interested in the mechanism of glucose homeostasis (Alvarez-Buylla & Roces de Alvarez-Buylla, 1975) and in particular in how appropriate levels of glucose are ensured for brain metabolism. The central nervous system (CNS) relies on a large and sustained supply of glucose for its functional activity (Erecinska & Silver, 1989; Ueki et al, 1988). However, the mechanisms that regulate the transfer of glucose from blood to brain are not well understood. Insulin increases membrane transfer of glucose in many tissues, but it does not regulate glucose uptake by the brain (LeMay et al, 1988). Besides its neuroendocrine function, the hypothalamus has an important role in integrating the activity of the autonomic nervous system (Chen et al, 1994), but its possible participation in regulating brain glucose uptake is unknown. In a previous study we have shown that changes in blood glucose concentration in the carotid body modify brain glucose retention (Alvarez-Buylla & Roces de Alvarez-Buylla, 1994). The role of the cerebrospinal fluid (CSF) in neuroendocrine functions, and as a conduit of communication between hypothalamus, pituitary and brain has been established (Jackson, 1984). In this paper we show that after carotid body receptor (CBR) stimulation a putative bioactive substance appears in the CSF that increases glucose retention in the brain. We further study the pituitary and adrenal glands participation in this reflex effect caused by CBR stimulation.

Frontiers in Arterial Chemoreception, edited by Zapata *et al.*
Plenum Press, New York, 1996

2. METHODS

2.1. Animals and Surgical Procedures

Experiments were performed on 37 mongrel dogs (8–12 kg weight), and 58 Wistar rats (250–300 g weight). Anesthesia was induced and maintained by intraperitoneal administration of sodium pentobarbital (30 mg/kg in dogs, and 3 mg/100 g in rats). Respiration and body temperature were artificially controlled. The left carotid sinus was temporarily isolated from the cephalic circulation during injections of sodium cyanide (NaCN) by a method previously described (Alvarez-Buylla & Roces de Alvarez-Buylla, 1988). With this technique only the carotid sinus is exposed to NaCN during the injection. Carotid body receptor stimulation was performed by slowly injecting NaCN (50 µg/kg in 0.25 ml saline). In order to ensure that homeostatic responses were triggered by NaCN reaching the left isolated carotid sinus, both aortic nerves and the right carotid nerve were sectioned. In control experiments the left carotid nerve was cut to denervate this carotid body region. Electrical stimulation of the sectioned carotid nerve was performed by placing its central stump on platinum bipolar electrodes connected to a stimulus isolation unit and a stimulator (square pulses applied for 5 min, 2 msec, 2–4 V, 20 c/sec). The time of NaCN injection or CSF injections was considered as t= 0 (indicated as an arrow in the figures). Blood samples were obtained from catheters inserted into the femoral artery and jugular sinus. The jugular sinus catheter was also used when intravenous (iv) injections were done. At each sample time, 0.2 ml of blood from each catheter was collected at t = -4 min, t = 0 min (basal values), and after the stimulation at t = 2, t = 4, t = 8 and t = 16 min. CSF was collected from silastic cannulas chronically inserted into the cisterna magna. The cisterna magna was also chosen as the site for central administration (ic) of CSF taken from donor dogs. At each collection time 2 ml of CSF were collected from donor dogs, at t= -5 min (control CSF) and after the CBR stimulation at t = 2–4 min, t = 4–8 min, t = 8–16 min and t = 16–32 min. CSF samples at the same times from different dogs were pooled for biological assay (2 ml of CSF drawn at each interval were tested in dogs and 0.5 ml in rats). CSF samples contaminated with blood were discarded. Hypophysectomies were performed in 15 rats by a previously described technique (Alvarez-Buylla et al, 1991). Adrenalectomies were done in 5 rats by dorsal retroperitoneal approach.

2.2. Analytical Methods

Glucose concentration in plasma and the CSF was determined by the glucose oxidase method (Beckman Autoanalyzer, Fullerton CA, USA). Glucose uptake by the brain was recorded by measuring blood flow and arterio-venous (a-v) glucose difference across the brain (Hawkinset al, 1974). Blood flow was monitored with an ultrasonic pulsed doppler flowmeter (Bioengineering, Univ. Iowa, USA) placed around the right common carotid without altering blood circulation.

2.3. Purification of CSF Extracts

The first step consisted in concentrating (66.5 times) 133 ml of CSF from various stimulated dogs in a dialysis bag covered with Aquacide II (Calbiochem, San Diego, CA, USA) in the cold room (4° C). Samples were taken before (50µl) and after concentration (25 µl) for activity determination (bioassay). The second purification step consisted of a HPLC gel filtration performed with a Beckman-Altex (Berkeley, CA, USA) system. The detector was a LKB Uvicord-S (Bromma, Sweden) provided with a 8 µl flow-through cell. A Protein-Pak I-125 column (7.8 x 300 mm) (Waters, Milford, MA, USA) was washed with 120 ml of H_20, pH 7.0, at 1 ml/min, equilibrated with 120 ml of a 0.1 M K_2HPO_4, adjusted to pH 7.0 with H_3PO_4, at a flow rate of 1 ml/min. Two hundred µl were injected into the column and the elution under isocratic conditions effected with the same buffer at 1 ml/min. The absorbance of the fractions thus separated was measured at 277 nm. The effluent collection was begun after 5 min, at 1 min/tube. Aliquots from each tube were submitted to bioassay. The contents of active tubes were pooled, concentrated in Aquacide II as above, and dialyzed *vs* the above mentioned buffer during 1.5 h, with three changes (one every 0.5 h). Final volume: 1.2 ml. These concentrated active fractions were submitted to a second gel filtration on the same Protein-Pak I-125 column, after filtering through a 0.2 µm microcentrifugal device provided with a regenerated cellulose filter (Model MF-1, Bioanalytical Systems Inc, West Lafayette, IN, USA) under the same isocratic conditions as above, but only 150 µl were injected at a time. Active 1 min fractions were again identified by means of the bioassay. The contents of the active tubes of the second gel filtration were pooled, concentrated with Aquacide II and dialyzed *vs* a 0.015 M Na_2HPO_4 + 0.15 M NaCl buffer, adjusted to pH 6.5 with H_3PO_4. Final volume: 500 µl. The active fractions were submitted to the last HPLC gel filtration on a Spherogel-TSK 2000 SW column (7.5 x 600 mm) (Altex-Beckman, Fullerton, CA, USA), washed with 120 ml of H_20 and equilibrated with 120 ml of the above mentioned sodium buffer at a flow rate of 1 ml/min. Detection absorbance was 277 nm and injection volume was 250 µl. Elution was isocratic with the above mentioned sodium buffer and absorbance peaks were collected manually. Active peaks (Fig 1) were identified by bioassay.

2.4. Experimental Protocol

Animals were subjected to one of the following procedures: (a) chemoreceptor stimulation of the carotid body in normal, hypophysectomized and adrenalectomized rats;

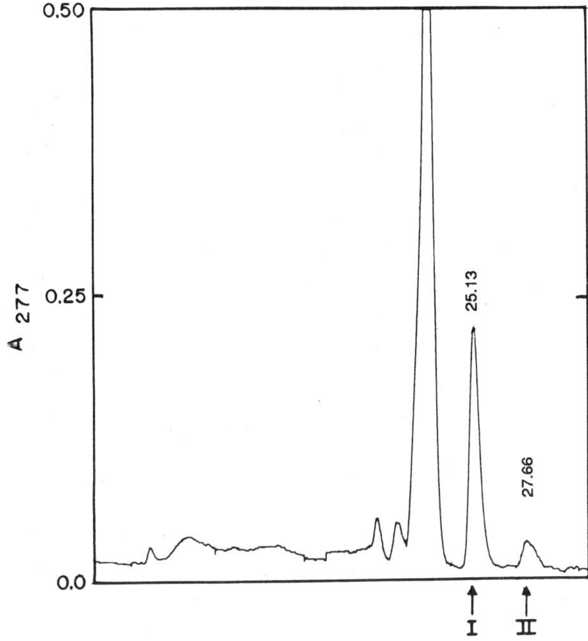

Figure 1. Last purification step by gel filtration on a Spherogel-TSK 2000 SW column. The column was equilibrated with 120 ml 0.015 M Na_2HPO_4 + 0.15 M NaCl buffer, pH 6.5 at a flow rate of 1 ml/min. Two hundred fifty µl of the concentrated active fractions from the second Protein-Pak I-125 column gel filtration were injected, eluted isocratically, and collected manually per peak of absorbance at 277 nm. Activity was detected only at the peaks marked as I and II (25.13 min and 27.66 min, respectively). A standard marker of tryptophan (MW 204) eluted at the same position as active peak II.

(b) chemoreceptor stimulation of the carotid body in normal dogs and in denervated-control dogs; (c) electrical stimulation of the carotid nerve in normal dogs and rats; (d) CSF (taken from normal donor dogs after CBR stimulation) ic-injections in normal dogs or rats; (e) active purified CSF collected from dogs (peaks I and II) iv-injections in normal rats.

3. RESULTS

3.1. CBR Stimulation in Normal, Hypophysectomized, and Adrenalectomized Rats

When the carotid body chemoreceptors were stimulated with NaCN injected into the temporarily isolated carotid sinus in 10 normal rats, brain glucose retention increased (Fig 2A). This response was maximal 4 min after injection, when glucose retention reached 0.41 ± 0.05 μmol/g/min compared to a basal level 0.13 ± 0.02 μmol/g/min ($p < 0.01$). These results confirmed our previous observations (Alvarez-Buylla & Roces de Alvarez-Buylla, 1990). We tested next whether glucose retention by the brain after CBR stimulation was affected by hypophysectomy or adrenalectomy. CBR stimulation in 10 rats one week after complete hypophysectomy yielded similar results to those obtained in control rats (Fig 1B), brain glucose retention increased above basal levels at 2, 4 and 8 min after injection ($p < 0.05$). In the same way, when CBR stimulation was done in 5 adrenalectomized rats, brain glucose retention increased from 0.12 ± 0.05 μmol/g/min to a maximum level of 0.44 ± 0.10 μmol/g/min 4 min after injection ($p < 0.001$), and remained above basal levels until 8 min after ($p < 0.05$).

3.2. Cerebrospinal Fluid

CBR stimulation also induced a noticeable elevation of glucose concentration in CSF both in rats and in dogs. When CBR stimulation was done in rats, CSF glucose increased from 3.65 ± 0.40 μmol/ml to 4.80 ± 0.35 μmol/ml, and this effect lasted for at least 8 min. Similar results were observed in dogs, brain glucose uptake increased from 3.08 ± 0.18 μmol/ml to 4.85 ± 0.16 μmol/ml (Table I). In contrast, CBR stimulation in dogs after sectioning the carotid nerve (denervated dogs), did not change significantly the glucose concentration in CSF. Electrical stimulation of the central stump (square pulses of 2 msec, 2–4 V, 20 c/sec, during 5 min) of a previously sectioned carotid nerve in rats and dogs, produced results similar to those obtained with NaCN injections in normal animals. Four min after the end of the stimulus, CSF glucose concentration had risen from 3.41 ± 0.20 μmol/ml to 4.50 ± 0.27 μmol/ml in rats and from 3.44 ± 0.16 μmol/ml to 4.18 ± 0.16 μmol/ml in dogs, and the values remained high for 8 min (Table 1).

In order to test whether the CSF might contain a neurosecretory substance capable of eliciting cerebral glucose uptake after CBR stimulation, the following experiments were performed. In 10 donor dogs 10 ml samples of CSF were drawn in the course of the test of CBR stimulation (see Methods). When 2 ml samples of CSF collected 2–8 min after CBR stimulation, were injected ic in normal dogs (n=10), glucose retention by the brain increased significantly. This response was maximal 4 min after injection, glucose retention rising from 0.45 ± 0.09 μmol/g/min to 1.50 ± 0.35 μmol/g/min. Control experiments with boiled CSF (100°C) from the same times had no significant effect (Table 2).

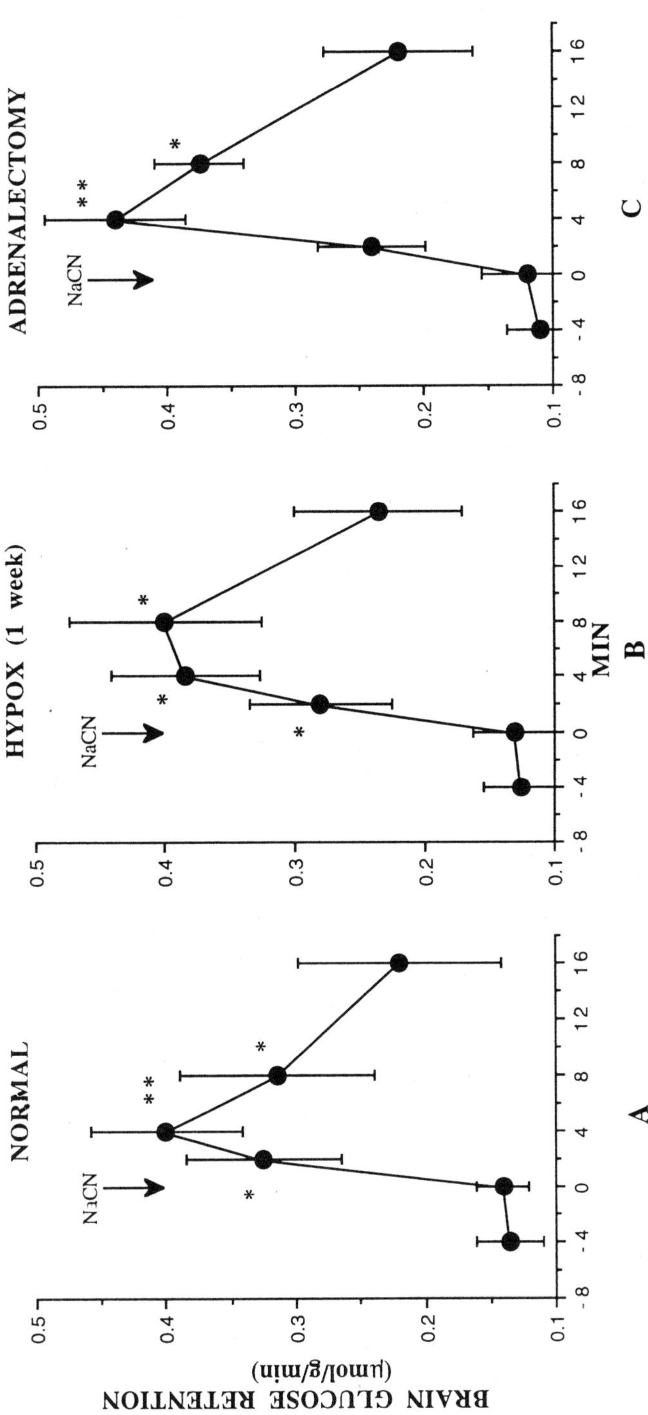

Figure 2. Changes in brain glucose retention after carotid body receptor stimulation with cyanide (NaCN 50 μg/kg injected into the vascularly isolated carotid sinus) in rats. (A) normal rats (n=10); (B) hypophysectomized rats (n= 10); (C) adrenalectomized rats (n= 5). Mean ± SEM, *$p < 0.05$, **$p < 0.01$.

Table 1. The effect of carotid body receptor stimulation (NaCN 50 μg/kg) or electrical stimulation (ST; 2–4 V, 2 ms, 20 Hz) of cephalic stump of cut carotid nerve on CSF glucose concentration (μmol/ml)

	NaCN			ST	
Time (min)	Rats (8)	Dogs (12)	Den Dogs (5)	Rats (8)	Dogs (12)
- 4	3.85 ± 0.37	3.61 ± 0.18	3.88 ± 0.21	3.53 ± 0.21	3.48 ± 0.15
0	3.65 ± 0.40	3.08 ± 0.18	3.95 ± 0.24	3.41 ± 0.20	3.44 ± 0.16
+ 2	4.18 ± 0.36	3.50 ± 0.17*	3.85 ± 0.31	3.78 ± 0.15	3.85 ± 0.13
+ 4	4.80 ± 0.35*	4.85 ± 0.16**	4.25 ± 0.32	4.50 ± 0.13*	4.18 ± 0.16*
+ 8	4.67 ± 0.39*	3.35 ± 0.24	4.12 ± 0.25	4.84 ± 0.27*	3.91 ± 0.23*
+ 16	4.15 ± 0.50	3.16 ± 0.32	4.06 ± 0.25	3.75 ± 0.46	3.60 ± 0.26

Den dogs, denervated dogs (left carotid nerve cut). Numbers of animals per experiment in parentheses.
*$p < 0.05$; **$p < 0.01$.

We tested next whether the CSF collected from donor dogs after CBR stimulation, increased brain glucose retention when injected ic in normal rats. Receptor rats (n=10) that received 0.5 ml CSF ic injections drawn in dogs 2–8 min after CBR stimulation, showed a clear increase in brain glucose uptake. Four min after the injection the glucose uptake rose from 0.11 ± 0.02 μmol/g/min up to 0.23 ± 0.02 μmol/g/min, and remained high up to 8 min postinjection ($p < 0.05$) (Figs 3B and 3C). The CSF samples collected after 8 min were ineffective in increasing brain glucose retention in rats (Figs 3D and 3E). In the same way, the control CSF collected before CBR stimulation was ineffective in increasing glucose retention by the brain in 5 normal rats (Fig 3A). When we registered the maximal responses obtained in brain glucose uptake after each CSF injection, we found that efficiency of the CSF samples in increasing glucose retention reached a maximum at t= 4–8 min after CBR stimulation. This effect was transient and no longer observed with CSF samples collected from dogs t= 8–16 min after CBR stimulation (Fig 3E). When we plotted time vs maximal effects observed with each CSF samples, a temporal course curve of brain glucose retention was obtained (Fig 3F).

The purification of CSF samples, collected 2–8 min after CBR stimulation, resulted in three main absorbance peaks. Only peaks I (25.15 min) and II (27.66 min) were clearly

Table 2. The effect of CSF [taken from donor dogs 2–8 min after carotid body receptor stimulation (NaCN 50 μg/kg injection into the cisterna magna)] on brain glucose uptake (μmol/g/min) of normal dogs

	Dogs (n = 10)	
Time (min)	CSF before boiling	CSF after boiling
- 4	0.44 ± 0.12	0.50 ± 0.14
0	0.45 ± 0.09	0.49 ± 0.12
+ 2	1.09 ± 0.38*	0.68 ± 0.25
+ 4	1.50 ± 0.35**	0.71 ± 0.32
+ 8	0.85 ± 0.38	0.58 ± 0.21
+ 16	0.55 ± 0.46	0.46 ± 0.31
+ 32	0.38 ± 0.32	0.58 ± 0.36

* $p < 0.05$; ** $p < 0.01$.

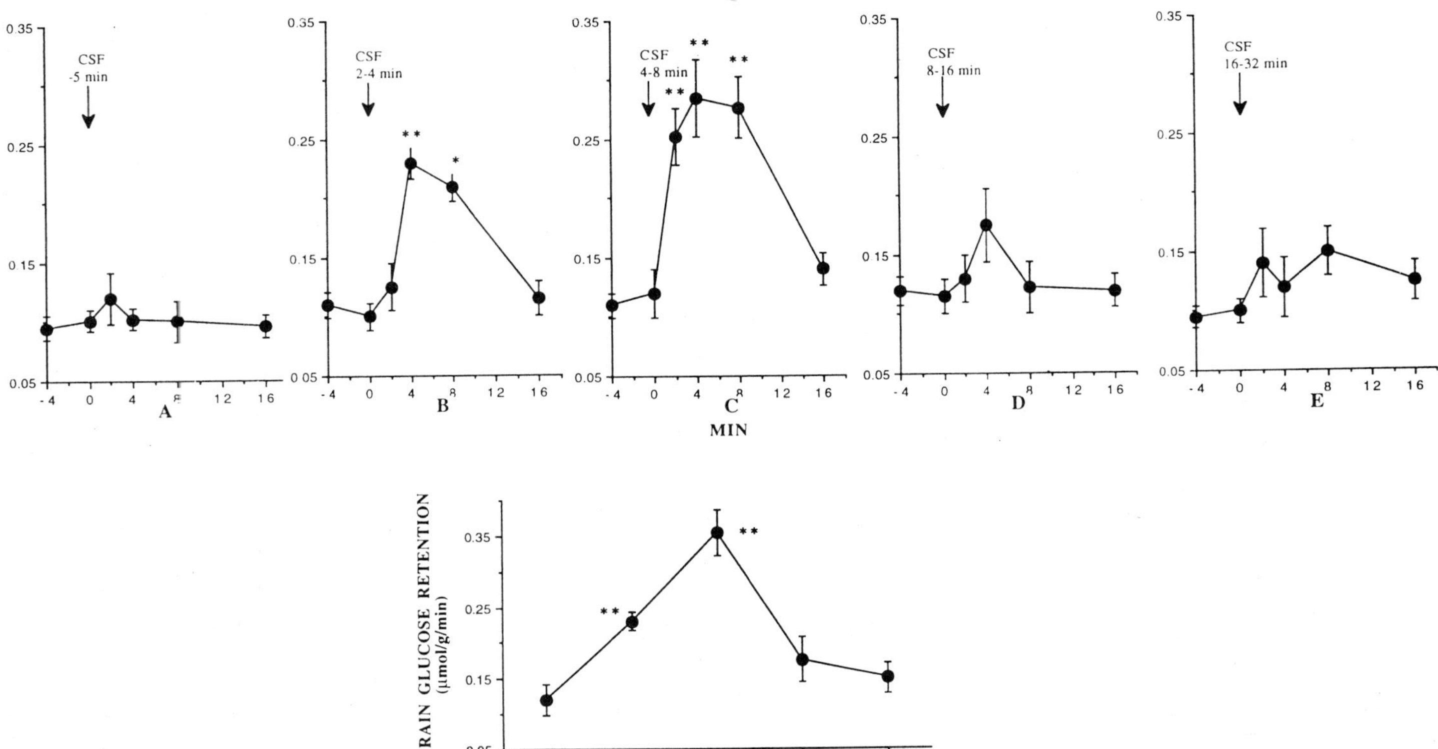

Figure 3. Changes in brain glucose retention after CSF injections (0.5 ml of CSF taken from donor dogs after carotid body receptor stimulation was injected into the cisterna magna of rats). (A) normal rats received control CSF taken at t= -5 min (n= 5); (B) normal rats received CSF taken between 2–4 min after stimulation (n= 5); (C) normal rats received CSF taken between 4–8 min after stimulation (n= 5); (D) normal rats received CSF taken between 8–16 min after stimulation (n= 5), (E) normal rats received CSF taken between 16–32 min after stimulation (n= 5); (F) brain glucose retention after CSF injection (taken from donor dogs at: t= -5 min, t= 2–4 min, t= 4–8 min, t= 8–16 min and t= 16–32 min after carotid body receptor stimulation), maximal effects with each CSF injections were plotted. Mean ± SEM, * $p < 0.05$; ** $p < 0.01$.

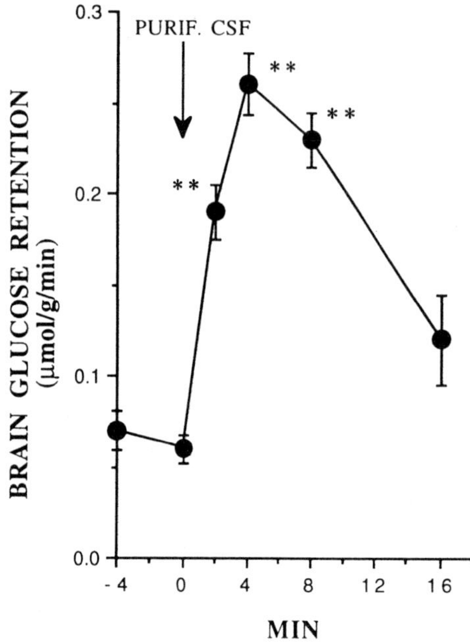

Figure 4. Changes in brain glucose retention after purified-active CSF iv injections (see Fig 1). Fractions from peaks I and II were pooled and 0.5 ml was injected iv into normal rats. Mean ± SEM, $^{*}p < 0.05$, $^{**}p < 0.01$.

active in the bioassay. When active fractions (peaks I and II) were injected iv into recipient rats a clear increase in brain glucose retention was observed (Fig 4). Four min after the injection brain glucose retention increased from 0.07 ± 0.01 µmol/g/min to 0.26 ± 0.03 µmol/g/min. At 8 min the values began to decrease, but they were still significantly above basal levels. A tryptophan marker (MW 204) eluted in the same position as peak II of the Spherogel TSK- 2000 SW filtration. In view of this, a provisional MW of approximately 500 can be ascribed to peak I and of 200 to peak II.

4. DISCUSSION

Results from the first series of experiments showed that the increase in glucose uptake by the brain produced by the anoxic stimulus in the temporarily isolated carotid sinus was not affected either by hypophysectomy or adrenalectomy. We have previously shown that these glands intervene in the effector mechanism of the hyperglycemic effect (Alvarez-Buylla et al, submitted). CBR stimulation also increased glucose concentration in the CSF both in rats and dogs (Table 1). Denervation of the carotid sinus body region abolished these reflex responses and led us to rule out the possibility that NaCN entering the general circulation had direct effects on nervous tissue. Also, the positive results obtained with electrical stimulation of the carotid nerve (Table 1) indicated an afferent role of the carotid reflexogenic zones that reaches the brain and stimulates its glucose retention. Previous studies support the existence of multiple pathways by which peripheral chemoreceptor inputs may influence central respiratory neurons (Finley & Katz, 1992).

When a sample of CSF was drawn from donor dogs 2–8 min after the anoxic stimulus, and injected ic into normal recipient dogs or rats, an increase in brain glucose retention was observed (Table 2). The purified-active fractions of CSF (collected from the last purification step) taken from stimulated dogs, induced a significant more robust effect in brain glucose retention when injected iv in recipient rats (Fig 4). If the glucose uptake by the brain is not caused by insulin secreted by the pancreas (LeMay et al, 1988), it may be supposed to be a response to the action of some other neurosecreted substance. The presence in the CNS of a large number of peptides has been known for several years (Krieger & Martin, 1981). Many of them have been recognized as participating in glucoregulation (Baile et al, 1986). These facts suggest that the putative role of some of these factors is to enhance CNS glucose uptake. The hypothalamus is the critical CNS locus for metabolic integration and it has been shown to play a major role in the integration of baroreceptor and chemoreceptor reflexes. Single unit recording in the region of the supraoptic and paraventricular nucleus indicates that individual neurons alter their rate of discharge during selective activation of carotid baro- or chemoreceptors (Calaresu & Ciriello, 1980). Here we are postulating that the CBR stimulation elicits the secretion of some substance that favors brain glucose retention. Work underway in our laboratory focuses on the biochemical characterization of the putative substance regulating this activity in CSF.

5. ACKNOWLEDGMENTS

This project was supported by the Consejo Nacional de Ciencia y Tecnología PO19CCOL-904045.

6. REFERENCES

Alvarez-Buylla R & Roces de Alvarez-Buylla E (1975) Hypoglycemic conditioned reflex in rats: preliminary study of its mechanism. J Comp Physiol Psychol 88: 155–160.

Alvarez-Buylla R & Alvarez-Buylla RE (1988) Carotid sinus receptors participate in glucose homeostasis. Respir Physiol 72: 347–360

Alvarez-Buylla R & de Alvarez-Buylla E (1990) Carotid sinus receptors participate in glucose homeostasis. In: Eyzaguirre C, Fidone SJ, Fitzgerald RS, Lahiri S, McDonald DM (eds) Arterial Chemoreception. New York: Springer-Verlag. pp 330–336

Alvarez-Buylla R & Roces de Alvarez-Buylla E (1994) Changes in blood glucose concentration in the carotid body-sinus modify brain glucose retention. Brain Res 654: 167–170

Alvarez-Buylla R, Quintanar-Stephano A, Quintanar-Stephano JL & Alvarez-Buylla E (1991) Removal of the unfragmented pituitary gland (hypophysectomy) in the rat. Bol Inst Med Biol (México) 39: 33–38

Alvarez-Buylla R, Roces de Alvarez-Buylla E, Mendoza H, Montero SA & Alvarez-Buylla A (1996) Pituitary and adrenals are required for the hyperglycemic reflex initiated by stimulation of the carotid body receptors with cyanide. Am J Physiol (Submitted)

Baile CA, McLaughlin CL & Della-Fera MA (1986) Role of cholecystokinin and opioid peptides in control of food intake. Physiol Rev 66: 172–234

Calaresu FR & Ciriello J (1980) Projections to the hypothalamus from buffer nerves and nucleus tractus solitarius in the cat. Am J Physiol 239: R130-R136

Chen I-LI, Weber JT & Yates RD (1994) Synaptic connections of central carotid sinus afferents in the nucleus of the tractus solitarius of the rat. II. Connections with substance P-immunoreactive neurons. J Neurocytol 23: 313–322

Erecinska M & Silver IA (1989) ATP and brain function. J Cereb Blood Flow Metab 9: 2–19

Finley JC & Katz DM (1992) The central organization of carotid body afferent projections to the brainstem of the rat. Brain Res 572: 108–116

Hawkins RA, Miller AL, Cremer JE & Veech RL (1974) Measurement of the rate of glucose utilization by rat brain in vivo. J Neurochem 23: 917–923

Jackson I (1984) Neuropeptides in the cerebrospinal fluid. In: Muller EE, MacLeod RM (eds) Neuroendocrine Perspectives. New York: Elsevier. pp 121–159

Krieger DT & Martin JB (1981) Brain peptides. N Engl J Med 304: 876–885

LeMay DR, Gehua L, Zelenock GB & D'Alecy LG (1988) Insulin administration protects neurologic function in cerebral ischemia in rats. Stroke 19: 1411–1419

Ueki M, Linn F & Hossman KA (1988) Functional activation of cerebral blood flow and metabolism before and after global ischemia of rat brain. J Cereb Blood Flow Metab 8: 486–494

65

PROLONGED HEMODYNAMIC EFFECTS OF INTERMITTENT, BRIEF CHEMORECEPTOR STIMULATION IN HUMANS

Andrzej Trzebski and Maciej Smietanowski

Department of Physiology
Medical Academy
00–325 Warsaw, Poland

1. INTRODUCTION

Augmented arterial chemoreceptor reflex tonic drive was observed in human subjects with essential mild hypertension and it was suggested as a sympatho-excitatory mechanism contributing to elevated blood pressure (Trzebski et al, 1982; Trzebski, 1992). Human subjects are exposed to repetitive episodic nocturnal hypoxic chemoreceptor stimulation in obturative sleep apnea syndrome (OSAS). In agreement with the original hypothesis on the role of the chemoreceptor reflex in hypertension, OSAS is usually accompanied by systemic arterial hypertension (Jeong et al, 1989; Hla et al, 1994) which is reversed by tracheostomy (Guilleminault et al, 1981). Repetitive, brief hypoxia produces in rats a sustained blood pressure elevation (Fletcher et al, 1992a) prevented by carotid chemoreceptor or sympathetic denervation (Fletcher et al, 1992b,c). In contrast to baroreceptors, chemoreceptors do not exhibit adaptation with long-lasting stimulation. On the contrary, their responsiveness appears to be enhanced with prolonged hypoxia (Smith et al, 1986; Barnard et al, 1987; Vizek et al, 1987; Nielsen et al, 1988; but Tatsumi, 1991). In awake OSAS patients resting sympathetic vasoconstrictor activity is augmented (Carlson et al, 1993). Morgan et al (1995) found long-lasting vasoconstrictor sympathetic activation in healthy human subjects after termination of a 20 min period of combined hypoxia and hypercapnia.

Borderline or labile hypertension in young subjects of genetic family background depends on augmented cardiac output (CO), a feature of the alerting response (Birkenhagen, 1991). This is regarded as an early stage, usually preceding mild and established hypertension characterized by elevated total peripheral resistance (TPR) with normal CO (Folkow, 1982; Julius, 1988). If repetitive apneas, mimicking OSAS and applied to awake subjects do facilitate the sympatho-excitatory chemoreceptor reflex and induce sustained hypertension, one could speculate that exposure to this procedure would shift the dynamic control of mean arterial blood pressure from a CO to a TPR dominated pattern. The pre-

Frontiers in Arterial Chemoreception, edited by Zapata *et al.*
Plenum Press, New York, 1996

sent study addressed this hypothesis by continuous beat-to-beat computation of the relative contribution of CO versus TPR to the instantaneous blood pressure changes.

2. METHODS

Thirty three subjects of both sexes, medical students aged 19–24 year, normotensive and free from cardiovascular or any other diseases, provided informed consent and were used for this study. Continuous recordings were collected in a sitting position over a 1 hour period divided into three experimental sections: 20 min control, 20 min of 10 1 min voluntary apneas each separated by 1 min intervals of free breathing, and a 20 min free breathing recovery period. Subjects maintained voluntary apnea in quiet inspiration to avoid hemodynamic consequences of negative intrathoracic pressure (Morgan et al, 1993). To inactivate peripheral arterial chemoreceptors, hyperoxia was produced by breathing continuously a 70% O_2 30% N_2 gas mixture over the whole period before, during and after apneic episodes. Finger systolic (SP) diastolic (DP) and mean (MAP) arterial blood pressure and heart interbeat interval (IBI) were recorded. CO and TPR were computed indirectly and continuously on line by a Portapres-2 TNO BMI system based on a nonlinear three-element model of aortic blood flow in humans (Wesseling et al, 1993). The relative contribution of CO (Pco) and TPR (P_{TPR}) to dynamic changes of MAP was computed on line from the formula MAP = CO x TPR and expressed as an index COT (Fig 1).

Negative values of COT indicate predominance of TPR over CO mediated control of the mean arterial blood pressure changes. All recordings, including arterial blood hemoglobin oxygen saturation (SP O_2) and respiratory rate, monitored by nasal thermistor probe, were digitalized and sent to mass memory SPIKE-2 v.4 (CED) for off-line analysis by MATLAB v. 4.0 and FAST mf/c^2 system (TNO BMI). Prior to spectral analysis, SP, DP, IBI and respiratory rate were low-pass filtered, demeaned, detrended and resampled with 4 Hz effective sampling frequency. Power spectra (PDS) were computed as component spectra zoomed around continuously traced respiratory rhythm and mid-frequency band 0.1 Hz.

P -mean arterial pressure
CO -cardiac output
TPR -total peripheral resistance

(1) $P = CO*TPR$;
(2) $dP = TPR*dCO+CO*dTPR$;
(3) $dP/P = dCO/CO+dTPR/TPR$;
(4) $dPP = dP_{CO}+dP_{TPR}$; where $dPP = dP/P$, $dP_{CO} = dCO/CO$, $dP_{TPR} = dTPR/TPR$;

$$COT = \frac{|dP_{CO}|-|dP_{TPR}|}{|dP_{CO}|+|dP_{TPR}|}; \quad (5)$$

Figure 1. Algorithm for continuous on-line computation of cardiac output versus total peripheral resistance contribution to dynamic changes of the mean arterial blood pressure.

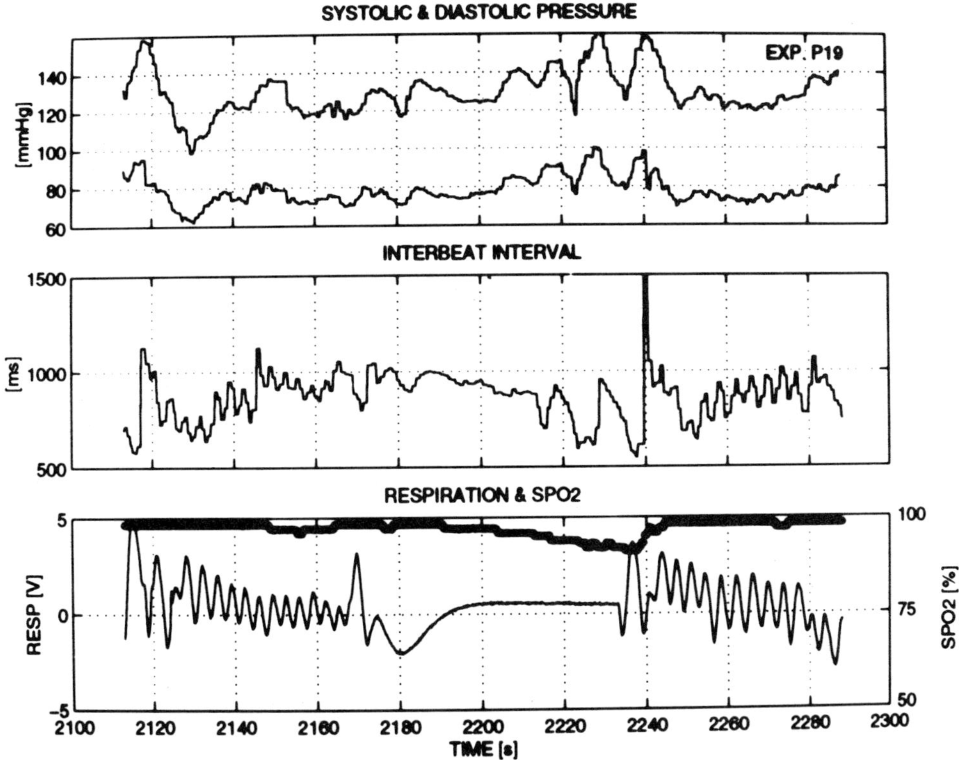

Figure 2. Voluntary apnea marked by arrest of respiratory movements (lower record). From the top: systolic and diastolic blood pressure, cardiac interbeat interval, hemoglobin oxygen saturation in arterial blood (SP O_2).

3. RESULTS

During each apneic period SP, DP and MAP rose and reached a peak at, or immediately after, resumption of breathing, IBI was prolonged and TPR increased (Fig 2).

The increase in the arterial blood pressure continued for over 10 min after termination of asphyxic protocol (Fig 3).

High oxygen breathing prevented or attenuated significantly the pressor and hemodynamic effects and aftereffects of repetitive asphyxias. By itself high oxygen inhalation produced an increase in TPR due to a peripheral vasoconstrictor effect of oxygen and a slight bradycardia (Cassuto et al, 1979; Tafil-Klawe et al, 1985).

The dynamic contribution of CO to MAP fluctuations was shifted to TPR during apnea and in the 20 min recovery period. The COT value for the apneic period was calculated as a mean computed over the whole 20 min period including ten consecutive apneas and ten intervals of free breathing (Fig 4). During an individual apnea there was a significant increase in TPR and a decrease in CO (Trzebski & Smietanowski, 1996) and the COT index was significantly more negative than the mean COT value computed over ten combined averaged apneas and ten intervals in a 20 min period.

Figure 5 shows the scatter-plot of COT *vs.* control COT for all subjects. Each point represents a 20 min average of COT value in control (o), apnea (*A) and recovery (xR). Although a clear correlation between the points obtained in control and those in apnea and

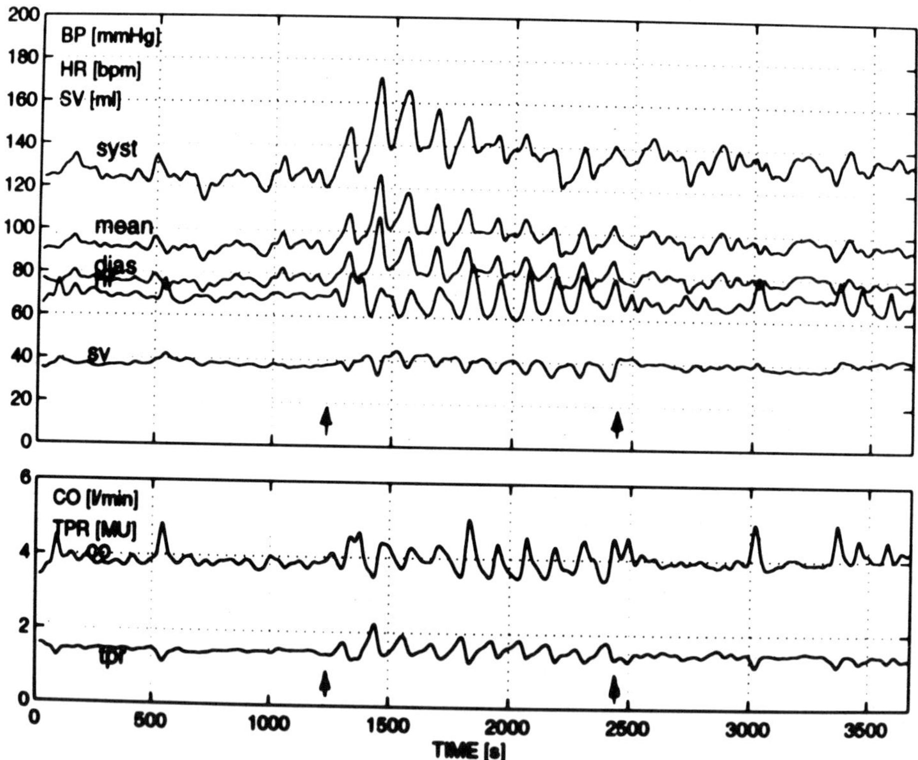

Figure 3. 1 hour recording: 20 min free breathing at rest, 20 min of ten repetitive voluntary apneas and 20 min free breathing recovery. Arrows mark the onset and termination of repetitive apnea period. From the top: continuous record of systolic, mean and diastolic blood pressure, heart rate, stroke volume, cardiac output and total peripheral resistance.

recovery can not be established because of points dispersion, most of the subjects (2/3) responded by shifting COT to more negative values (*i.e.* to TPR-dependent pressure changes). This effect becomes more evident when analysing the position of theoretical straight lines (C, A, R), which are the best linear fits to corresponding points (in least squares sense). The equations, together with correlation coefficients (goodness of fit) are shown in the upper left corner of the figure. The slope for the control, which by default equals 1, differs very much (0.5, 0.6) from that in apnea and the recovery period suggesting some tendency in direction and magnitude of subjects response to apnea. The more positive was the initial COT, the more prominent the response and/or long lasting the aftereffect. Bisection points between R, A lines and C line divides all subjects into two subsets. The first group (26 persons) responded to apneas and in the recovery period by augmenting vascular (TPR) control of blood pressure. The second group (7 persons) with very large negative initial COT values (predominance of TPR control) did not change the pattern in similar manner during the apneic and the recovery period.

In resting conditions the pattern of CO versus TPR control of MAP was equally distributed among subjects: in 17 subjects the COT index was positive and in 16 negative. Therefore we accepted an arbitrary COT value >-0.2 separating those exhibiting at rest a distinct predominance of TPR control of MAP fluctuations (11 subjects COT<-0.2) from

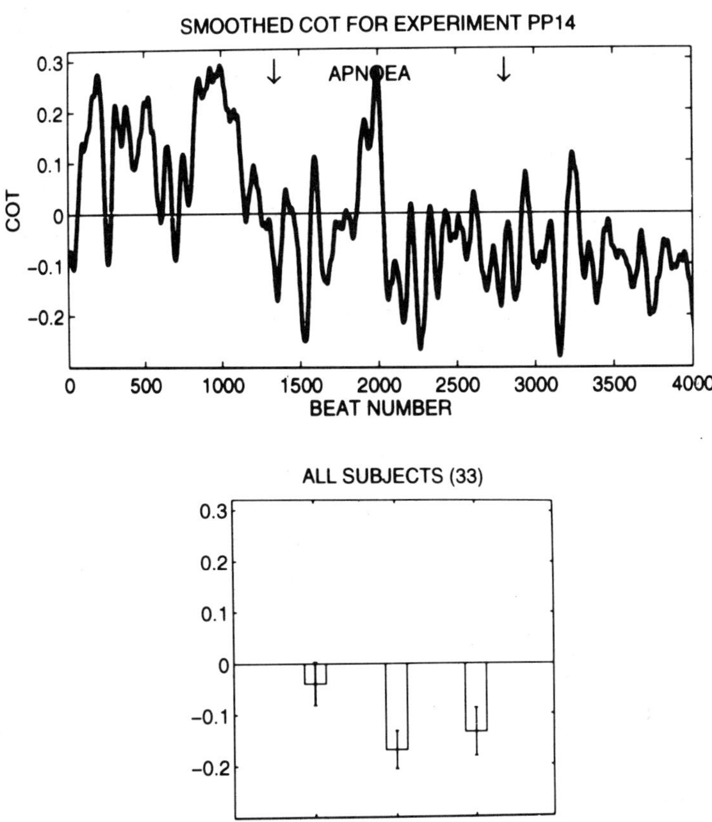

Figure 4. On the top: COT values before, during and after a single apnea. On the bottom: mean COT control values at rest (C), during a whole apneic period (A) and over a 20 min recovery period after apneas (R).

those with a significant CO contribution to MAP fluctuations (22 subjects COT>-0.2). 22 subjects with CO predominance of MAP dynamic control at rest, except for one subject, showed a significant shift to TPR-type of MAP control during a 20 min period after repetitive apneas (Fig 6, left). Seven out of 11 remaining subjects who exhibited a dominating TPR-type of MAP control in resting conditions accentuated or preserved a similar pattern in the post-apneic recovery period (Fig 6, right).

PDS of IBI, SP and DP oscillations exhibited three main patterns: A) concentration of power mainly in the respiratory frequency band (13 subjects); B) the power dominating in mid-frequency band of 0.1 Hz (3 subjects); and C) a dominating power within the respiratory frequency band in PDS of IBI and SP yet in PDS of DP fluctuations a significant power around 0.1 Hz (17 subjects) (Fig 7). The pattern of PDS remained relatively similar in individual subjects examined over several weeks. After termination of the apneic protocol the PDS pattern of either type did not change significantly over the 20 min period of recovery and remained similar to that of the resting control conditions characterizing each individual subject (Fig 7).

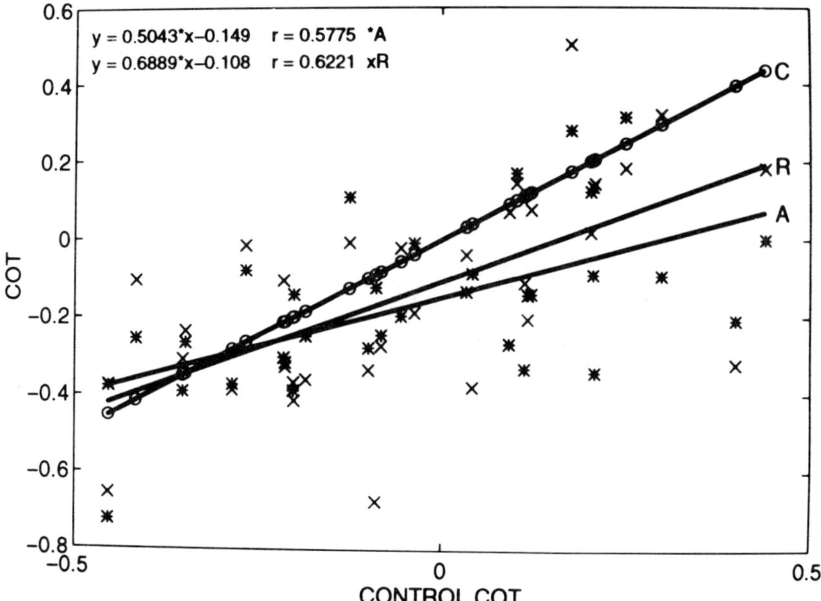

Figure 5. Correlation of COT computed during control (C) apneic (A) and recovery (R) period with initial COT computed at rest. Explanation in text.

4. DISCUSSION

The major and novel finding of this study is a significant increase in TPR control of the mean arterial blood pressure during the 20 min period after termination of repetitive asphyxias in those subjects who exhibited a dominating CO pattern of blood pressure control at rest. We believe that a shift from CO to TPR control of blood pressure fluctuations suggests a tendency to sustained hypertension after repetitive apneas. A slight increase in the arterial blood pressure during the post-apneic period was observed. Morgan et al.

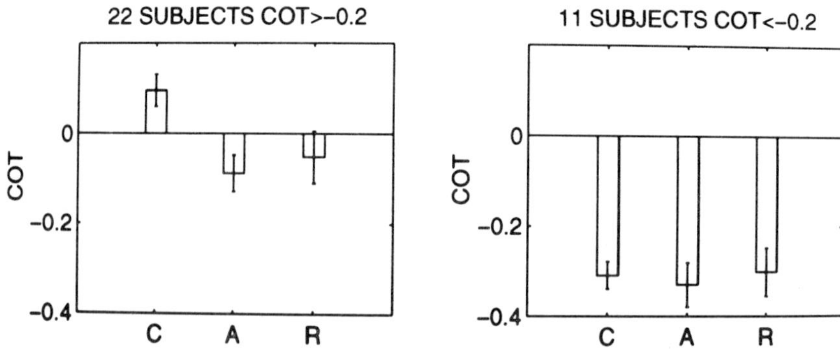

Figure 6. Mean COT value in the control at rest (C), during 20 min apneic period (A) and during 20 min recovery (R) in 22 subjects with a CO pattern of MAP control at rest (left) and in 11 subjects with TPR pattern of MAP control at rest (right).

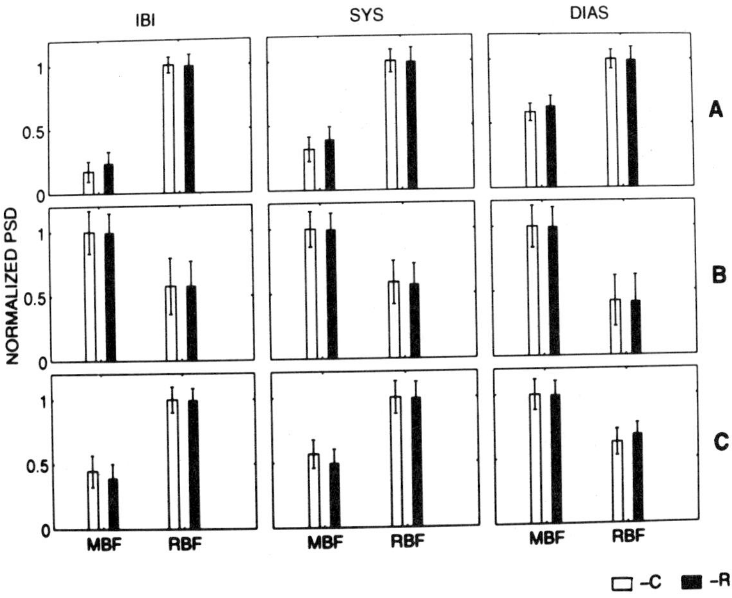

Figure 7. Mean power of PDS computed in all 33 subjects in 0.1 Hz mid-frequency band (MBF) and in respiratory frequency band (RBF) at rest (C, white bars) and in the post-apneic recovery period (R, black bars) for cardiac interbeat fluctuations (IBI), systolic (sys) and diastolic (dias) blood pressure. A, B and C represent three different patterns of power density spectra.

(1995) did not find any significant increase in the arterial blood pressure during the 20 min which followed free breathing in combined hypoxia and hypercapnia. However, vigorous free breathing, and consequently stimulation of cardio-respiratory mechanoreceptors, induces a reflex attenuation of pressor and sympatho-excitatory effects of hypoxic and hypercapnic chemoreceptor stimulation in humans (Trzebski et al, 1995). Voluntary apneas mimick more effectively OSAS. In order to check if sustained hypertension could be produced in healthy subjects by repetitive apneas, an experimental protocol would have to be applied regularly for weeks, a project not acceptable for ethical reasons.

"Memory" or long-term sensitization of carotid chemoreceptors and of the chemoreceptor reflex by prolonged and repetitive stimulation appears to apply not only to the respiratory (Millhorn et al, 1980; Cao et al, 1992) but evidently also to the pressor reflex response. In OSAS patients with arterial hypertension a tonic respiratory drive from arterial chemoreceptors is augmented as compared to OSAS patients without hypertension but, interestingly, the ventilatory response to brief acute hypoxia is attenuated (Tafil-Klawe et al, 1995). This dissociation of tonic drive and responsiveness to acute hypoxia may resemble a controversial and still debated "hypoxic desensitization" or blunting of the ventilatory response to acute hypoxia after the exposure to very prolonged hypoxia of native and nonnative residents of high altitude (Severinghaus, 1971; Lahiri et al, 1978). Hypoxia is considered as a factor which delays chemoreceptor maturation (resetting up) in neonates (Hanson & Kumar, 1993). The mechanism of resetting seems to depend on postnatal emergence of multiplicative CO_2-O_2 interaction at the carotid body and is delayed by hypoxia (Landauer et al, 1995). OSAS patients differ significantly from those exposed to prolonged hypoxia as hypoxia is combined with hypercapnia in OSAS. Multiplicative combination of repetitive brief hypoxic and hypercapnic stimuli creates a situation different from high altitude chronic hypoxemia. Prolonged systemic hypoxia attenuates systemic arterial hypertension and the incidence of essential hypertension is significantly lower among the native highlanders (Hultgren, 1970; Mirakhimov, 1992). Chronic hypoxemia induces a large spectrum of adaptative changes in the vascular system which apparently compensate for reduced tissue oxygen supply and may override vasoconstrictor sympatho-excitatory chemoreceptor reflex (for discussion Trzebski, 1992).

Power density spectra were proposed as a marker of sympatho-vagal interaction in man and the power within mid-frequency band 0.1 Hz was suggested as an index of sympathetic activity (Pagani et al, 1986). However the patterns of PDS computed over the 20 min post-apneic period do not differ significantly from those computed during normoxia at rest. They are relatively constant and characterize individual subjects (Fig 6). As in most of the subjects a prolonged sympathetic overactivity persists for 20 min or more after return from hypoxia/hypercapnia to room breathing (Morgan et al, 1995), the usefulness of PDS as a reliable index of sympathetic activity remains in question.

5. ACKNOWLEDGMENTS

This work was supported by the KBN grant 4 PO5A 059 09.

6. REFERENCES

Barnard P, Andronikou S, Pokorski M, Smatresk N, Mokashi A & Lahiri S (1987) Time-dependent effect of hypoxia on carotid body chemosensory function. J Appl Physiol 63: 685–691

Birkenhager WH (1991) A critical interpretation of juvenile borderline hypertension. J Hypertension 9 (suppl 6): S2-S9

Cao KY, Zwilich CW, Berthon-Jones M & Sullivan CE (1992) Increased normoxic ventilation induced by repetitive hypoxia in conscious dogs. J Appl Physiol 73: 2083–2088

Carlson JT, Hedner J, Elam M, Ejnel H, Sellgren J & Wallin BG (1993) Augmented resting sympathetic activity in awake patients with obstructive sleep apnea. Chest 103: 1763–1768

Cassuto Y & Fahri LE (1979) Circulatory responses to arterial hyperoxia. J Appl Physiol 46: 973–987

Fletcher EC, Lesske J, Qian W, Miller CC & Unger T (1992a) Respective episodic hypoxia causes diurnal elevation of blood pressure in rats. Hypertension 19: 555–561

Fletcher EC, Lesske J, Behm R, Miller CC, Strauss H & Unger T (1992b) Carotid chemoreceptors, systemic blood pressure and chronic episodic hypoxia mimicking sleep apnea. J Appl Physiol 72: 1978–1984

Fletcher EC, Lesske J, Culman CC, Miller CC & Unger T (1992c) Sympathetic denervation blocks blood pressure elevation in episodic hypoxia. Hypertension 20: 612–619

Folkow B (1982) Physiological aspects of primary hypertension. Physiol Rev 62: 347–504

Guilleminault C, Simon B, Motta J, Cumiskey J, Rosekind M, Schroeder JS & Dement WC (1981) Obstructive sleep apnea syndrome and tracheostomy. Long-term follow-up experience. Arch Int Med 141: 985–997

Hanson M & Kumar P (1994) Chemoreceptor function in the fetus and neonate. In: O'Regan RG, Nolan P, McQueen DS & Paterson DJ (eds) Arterial Chemoreceptors: Cell to System. NY: Plenum. Adv Exp Med Biol 360: 99–108

Hla KM, Young TB, Bidwell T, Palta M & Skatrud JB (1994) Sleep apnea and hypertension. Ann Int Med 120: 382–388

Hultgren HN (1970) Reduction of systemic arterial blood pressure at high altitudes. Adv Cardiol 5: 49–53

Jeong DU & Dimsdale JE (1989) Sleep apnea and essential hypertension: a critical review of the epidemiological evidence for co-morbidity. Clin Exp Hypertens A11: 1301–1323

Julius S (1988) Transition from high cardiac output to elevated vascular resistance in hypertension. Am Heart J 116: 600–606

Lahiri S, Brody JS, Motoyama EK & Velasquez TM (1978) Regulation of breathing in newborns at high altitude. J Appl Physiol 44: 673–678

Landauer RC, Pepper DR & Kumar P (1995) Effect of chronic hypoxemia from birth upon chemosensitivity in the adult rat carotid body in vitro. J Physiol, London 485: 543–550

Millhorn DE, Eldridge FL & Waldrop TG (1980) Prolonged stimulation of respiration by a new central neural mechanism. Respir Physiol 41: 87–103

Mirrakhimov M (1992) The treatment of hypertension by adaptation to high-altitude hypoxia. Kardiol 32: 5–10

Morgan BJ, Denahan T & Ebert TJ (1993) Neurocirculatory consequences of negative intrathoracic pressure *vs* asphyxia during voluntary apnea. J Appl Physiol 74: 2969–2975

Nielsen AM, Bisgard GE & Vidruk EH (1988) Carotid chemoreceptor activity during acute and sustained hypoxia in goats. J Appl Physiol 65: 1796–1802

Pagani M, Lombardi F, Guzetti S, Rimoldi O, Furlan R, Pizinelli P, Sandrone G, Malfato G, Dell'Orto S, Piccaluga E, Turiel M, Baselli G, Cerutti S & Malliani A (1986) Power spectral analysis of heart rate and arterial pressure variabilities as a matter of sympatho-vagal interaction in man conscious dog. Circ Res 59: 178–193

Severinghaus JW (1971) Hypoxic respiratory drive and its loss during chronic hypoxia. Clin Physiol, Oxf 2: 57–79

Smith CA, Bisgard GE, Nielsen AM, Daristotle L, Kressin N, Forster HV & Dempsey JA (1986) Carotid bodies are required for ventilatory acclimatization to moderate and severe hypoxemia. J Appl Physiol 60: 1003–1010

Tafil-Klawe M, Trzebski A, Klawe J & Palko T (1985) Augmented chemoreceptor tonic drive in early human hypertension and in normotensive subjects with family background of hypertension. Acta Physiol Polon 36: 51–58

Tafil-Klawe M, Klawe J, Moog R, Schneider H, Grote L, Janicki J, Raschke F, Penzel T, Peter JH & Hildebrandt G (1995) Arterielle Baro- und Chemorezeptorenreflexe bei Schlafapnoepatienten. In: Peter JH, Penzel T, Cassel W & Wiechert von P (eds) Schlaf-Atmung-Kreislauf. Germany: Springer Verlag. pp 142–163

Tatsumi K, Pickett CK & Weil JV (1991) Attenuated carotid body hypoxic sensitivity after prolonged hypoxic exposure. J Appl Physiol 70: 748–755

Trzebski A (1992) Arterial chemoreceptor reflex and hypertension. Hypertension 19: 562–566

Trzebski A, Tafil M, Zoltowski M & Przybylski J (1982) Increased sensitivity of the arterial chemoreceptor drive in young men with mild hypertension. Cardiovasc Res 16: 163–172

Trzebski A, Smith ML, Beightol LA, Fritch-Yelle JM, Rea RF & Eckberg DL (1995) Modulation of human sympathetic periodicity by mild, brief hypoxia and hypercapnia. J Physiol Pharmacol 46: 17–35

Trzebski A & Smietanowski M (1996) Cardiovascular periodicities in healthy humans in the absence of breathing and under reduced chemical drive of respiration. J Aut Nerv Syst (in press)

Vizek M, Pickett CK & Weil JV (1987) Increased`carotid body hypoxic sensitivity during acclimatization in hypobaric hypoxia. J Appl Physiol 63: 2403–2410

Wesseling KH, Jansen RC, Settels JJ & Schreuder JJ (1993) Computation of aortic flow from pressure in humans using a nonlinear, three-element model. J Appl Physiol 74: 2566–2573

66

INTERACTION BETWEEN THE BRADYCARDIC RESPONSES TO UPPER AIRWAY NEGATIVE PRESSURE AND CAROTID CHEMORECEPTOR STIMULATION IN THE ANAESTHETISED RABBIT

Philip Nolan, Miriam G. Langdon, and Ronan G. O'Regan

Department of Human Anatomy and Physiology
University College, Dublin, Ireland

1. INTRODUCTION

Collapse of the pharyngeal airway, leading to obstructive apnoea, is a relatively common event during sleep in adult and infant life. Obstructive apnoea is associated with progressive and often profound bradycardia. The fall in heart rate is thought to be a reflex response to asphyxic stimulation of the peripheral arterial chemoreceptors (Bonsignore et al, 1994). However, the failure of some studies to demonstrate a clear association between apnoeic bradycardia and oxyhaemoglobin desaturation has led to the suggestion that there may be other mechanisms involved (Guilleminault et al, 1984; Andreas et al, 1992).

The larynx is exposed to large negative transmural pressures during obstructed respiratory efforts. Our laboratory (Langdon et al, 1995) and others (Sant'Ambrogio et al, 1985) have shown that subatmospheric pressure in the lumen of the upper airway causes bradycardia. This response is absent after topical anaesthesia of the mucosa of the upper airway or following bilateral section of the superior laryngeal nerves. We propose that this reflex mechanism may contribute to the bradycardia of upper airway obstruction.

We were interested in the effect of upper airway negative pressure on the heart rate response to activation of the peripheral arterial chemoreceptors, given that these two stimuli occur together during obstructive apnoea. Electrical stimulation of the superior laryngeal nerve is known to alter the cardiorespiratory response to activation of the carotid chemoreceptors (Kordy et al, 1975). The increase in respiratory activity that normally follows carotid body stimulation is abrogated, while the chemoreflex bradycardia is markedly exaggerated (Elsner et al, 1977; Daly et al, 1978, 1983). We hypothesised that upper airway negative pressure would also exaggerate the bradycardic response to stimulation of the carotid body.

2. METHODS

Experiments were performed on six adult New Zealand White rabbits of either sex, 2.5 to 3.6 kg in weight. Anaesthesia was induced by injection of propofol (Diprivan, Zeneca 10 mg/kg) into a marginal ear vein and maintained with halothane (1–3% inhaled concentration, F_IO_2 0.6). Animals were placed in the supine position and rectal temperature recorded and maintained at 38–40°C with a heating blanket and infra-red lamp. A low cervical tracheostomy was performed, and tracheal pressure (Validyne DP45, Validyne, Northridge, CA) and end-tidal CO_2 (Engstrom Eliza, Gambro, Sweden) continuously monitored. The right femoral vein and artery were cannulated, and the arterial cannula attached to a pressure transducer (P23Db, Statham, Hato Rey, Puerto Rico) to record systemic arterial pressure. Arterial blood gas determinations were made at regular intervals (Corning 278). A lead II electrocardiogram was recorded. The upper airway was isolated by tying a second cannula into the upper trachea, directed cranially, with its tip just below the cricoid cartilage, and by sealing two short cannulae into the external nares. The mouth and nose were sealed around these cannulae with cyanoacrylate adhesive and rapid-setting epoxy cement. The isolated upper airway was connected, via a solenoid valve, to a reservoir which was evacuated to a controlled subatmospheric pressure by a vacuum pump. Upper airway pressure was continuously recorded (Validyne DP45). A small nylon vascular cannula (2FG nylon, 0.63 mm o.d., 0.5 mm i.d., Portex, UK) was inserted via the right lingual artery so that its tip lay in the common carotid artery 5 to 10 mm below the carotid bifurcation. This cannula was attached, via a three-way tap, to a Hamilton syringe of 100 μL capacity, filled with a 0.01% w/v solution of sodium cyanide (NaCN, Sigma, UK) in heparinised saline (Heparin, Leo, 250 IU/ml). A potentiometer attached to the syringe plunger allowed the volume and timing of injections to be accurately recorded. The right phrenic nerve was isolated low in the neck, cut, and its desheathed central end placed across a bipolar silver recording electrode. The signal was amplified, band pass filtered (30–1000 Hz), rectified and 'integrated' (Neurolog NL100, NL104A, NL125 and NL500, Digitimer, Welwyn Garden City, UK). Systemic arterial pressure (SAP), tracheal pressure (P_{tr}), upper airway pressure, raw and 'integrated' phrenic nerve activity, Hamilton syringe volume, and ECG signals were digitized at 500 samples per second, and RR interval derived on-line (Biopac MP100 and Acknowledge software, Linton Instrumentation, UK). When all surgical procedures were complete, a stable plane of anaesthesia (0.6% to 0.8% inhaled halothane) was established; paralysis was then induced with vecuronium (Norcuron, Organon, 200 μg/kg plus 5 μg/kg/min i.v.) and the animals artificially ventilated (F_IO_2 0.6). Adequacy of anaesthesia in the paralysed state was assured by the absence of changes in heart rate, phrenic nerve activity or systemic arterial pressure in response to paw pinch. All animals were given atenolol (Sigma, UK, 1 mg/kg plus 0.25 mg/kg/hr).

All experimental interventions were performed while artificial ventilation was temporarily withheld for a period of 10 seconds to eliminate the effects of phasic pulmonary stretch receptor activity. We recorded the response to (i) laryngeal negative pressure by applying -40 cm H_2O pressure to the isolated upper airway for the entire 10 seconds of a ventilator disconnection, (ii) carotid body stimulation by rapid intra-carotid injection of 25 to 100 μL 0.01% w/v NaCN in the third second of a similar ventilator disconnection, with no pressure applied to the upper airway, and (iii) carotid body stimulation while exposing the upper airway to negative pressure. The responses to these interventions were compared to a control intervention where artificial ventilation was withheld for 10 seconds but no carotid body or upper airway stimulus was applied. These four interventions were performed in random order, separated by 5 minutes.

The maximum RR interval following intra-carotid cyanide was identified; inspiratory time (T_I) and total respiratory cycle duration (T_{TOT}) were recorded for the respiratory cycle during which this maximum RR interval occurred. We also computed off-line the true mathematical integral of the rectified digitized raw signal of this phrenic burst (∫PHR), and divided this by inspiratory time as an index of respiratory drive (∫PHR /T_I). We then identified the respiratory cycle occurring at a time-matched point during the other interventions, and recorded the maximum RR interval within this cycle, along with T_I, T_{TOT} and ∫PHR /T_I. Mean SAP was recorded over the last three cardiac cycles of each 10 second intervention.

Differences between the means of these variables across the four interventions were assessed for statistical significance using analysis of variance and Student-Newman-Keuls post-hoc test, with $P<0.05$ taken to indicate a statistically significant difference. The results are presented as differences from values recorded during the control intervention where artificial ventilation was withheld for 10 seconds, except for ∫PHR /T_I which is expressed as a percentage of the value recorded during the control intervention.

3. RESULTS

Baseline values (mean, range) for relevant physiological variables during the experimental period were as follows: pH_a 7.386 (7.338–7.43), P_aCO_2 33.7 (29.1–40.9) mm Hg, P_aO_2 308 (275–335) mm Hg, mean SAP 66 (44–79) mm Hg, peak inspiratory P_{tr} 9.6 (7.2–13.6) cm H_2O, RR interval 271 (230–296) msec.

Original records, from one experimental animal, of the responses to all four experimental interventions, are shown (Fig 1). Ventilator disconnection alone caused little change in RR interval and an increase in phrenic nerve activity. The application of negative pressure to the upper airway caused a small bradycardia and reductions in respiratory frequency and the rate of rise of phrenic nerve activity. Stimulation of the carotid body also caused bradycardia, but this was accompanied by an increase in phrenic nerve activity. Stimulation of the carotid body while the upper airway is exposed to negative pressure results in a large bradycardia, which is greater than could be accounted for by simple summation of the separate responses to airway negative pressure and intra-carotid cyanide. There was a marked reduction in respiratory frequency, similar to that observed in response to upper airway negative pressure alone, while peak phrenic nerve activity was increased.

Carotid body stimulation caused a mean prolongation of RR interval of 143 ± 54 msec (mean ± S.E.M.), while upper airway negative pressure caused an increase of 77 ± 33 msec; neither of these changes was statistically significant (see Fig 2). Combined upper airway and carotid body stimulation caused a statistically significant increase in cardiac interval of 404 ± 88 msec ($P = 0.0005$, n=6). This response was significantly greater than the arithmetic sum of the separate responses to intra-carotid cyanide and upper airway negative pressure, which was 220 ± 81 msec ($P = 0.02$, paired *t*-test, n=6). These changes in heart rate were accompanied by small changes in mean SAP which were not statistically significant

Quantitative analysis of phrenic discharge was performed in only five experiments due to a technical error. Carotid chemoreceptor excitation had no statistically significant effect on respiratory timing, but evoked an increase in respiratory drive so that ∫PHR /T_I rose to 153 ± 26% of control (see Fig 2). Upper airway negative pressure significantly prolonged both T_I and T_{TOT}, and caused a small, non-significant depression of ∫PHR /T_I.

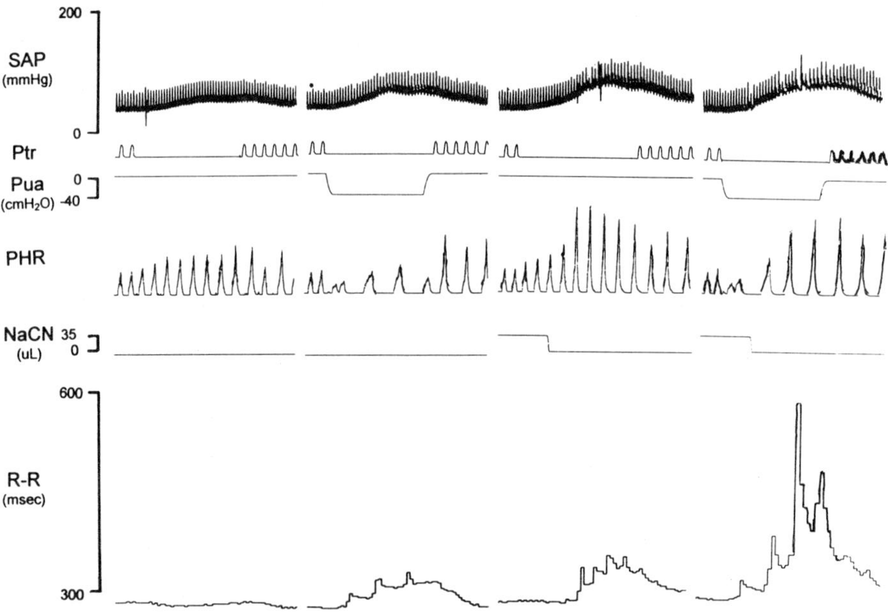

Figure 1. Responses to upper airway negative pressure and carotid chemoreceptor excitation in the anaesthetised paralysed rabbit. Four original non-continuous records are shown from one experiment. The leftmost panel shows the response to temporary cessation of artificial ventilation for 10 seconds, second from left is the response to -40 cm H_2O upper airway pressure applied during a similar ventilator disconnection, third from left is the response to intra-carotid injection of 35μL of 0.01% w/v sodium cyanide in the third second of ventilator disconnection, and the rightmost panel shows the effect of conjoint application of these latter two stimuli. Traces are, from top to bottom, systemic arterial pressure (SAP) tracheal pressure (P_{tr}) upper airway pressure (P_{ua}), 'integrated' phrenic nerve activity (PHR), volume of sodium cyanide solution in the injecting syringe (NaCN) and RR interval (R-R).

When the carotid body was stimulated together with the upper airway, the effect of upper airway negative pressure on respiratory timing was not affected by the chemoreceptor excitation: T_I and T_{TOT} were again significantly increased, and the extent to which these were prolonged was not significantly different from the response to upper airway negative pressure alone. Furthermore, with simultaneous activation of chemoreceptor and laryngeal inputs, the chemoreflex stimulation of respiratory drive was not altered by upper airway negative pressure; $\int PHR / T_I$ thus increased to 167 ± 24% control, which was not significantly different from the response to intra-carotid cyanide alone.

4. DISCUSSION

The major finding of this work is that negative pressure applied to the isolated upper airway of the anaesthetised paralysed rabbit potentiates the reflex bradycardia that occurs in response to stimulation of the carotid body by intra-carotid injection of sodium cyanide. The decreases in heart rate in response to upper airway negative pressure alone and to carotid body stimulation alone were not statistically significant; this reflects the fact that in the experiments reported here the level of anesthesia was deepened and the dose of sodium cyanide adjusted so that these primary bradycardias were similar and small.

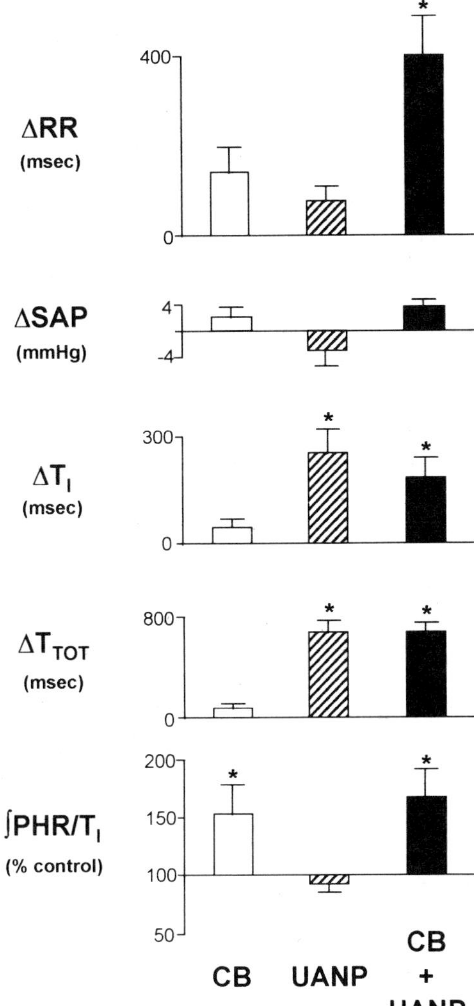

Figure 2. Group mean responses to carotid chemoreceptor stimulation, upper airway negative pressure, and the combination of these two stimuli. Unfilled bars show the response to intra-carotid injection of sodium cyanide (CB), hatched bars the response to -40 cm H_2O upper airway negative pressure (UANP) and filled bars the response to concurrent stimulation of carotid body and upper airway (CB+UANP). All responses are expressed as differences from control (Δ), except for the mean slope of the integral of phrenic nerve activity (∫PHR /T_I), which is expressed as a percentage of control. n=6 for RR interval (RR) and mean systemic arterial pressure (SAP). n=5 for inspiratory time (T_I), total respiratory cycle time (T_{TOT}) and ∫PHR /T_I. * indicates a significant difference from control, $P < 0.05$, ANOVA and Student-Newman-Keuls test.

Electrical stimulation of the superior laryngeal nerve has been shown to exaggerate carotid chemoreflex bradycardia in the dog (Kordy et al, 1975), cat (Daly et al, 1983) seal (Elsner et al, 1977) and monkey (Daly et al, 1978). In human infants, laryngeal stimulation with water causes a fall in heart rate which is much more marked when hypoxaemia is induced by lowering inspired O_2 to 15% (Wennergren et al, 1989). The exact mechanism by which laryngeal stimuli might synergistically interact with carotid chemoreceptor inputs in the brain stem is not certain. There appears to be little convergence of mechanosensitive laryngeal afferents and chemosensitive carotid sinus afferents in the nucleus tractus solitarius (Dawid-Milner et al, 1995). However, mechanical, chemical and electrical stimulation of laryngeal afferent fibres all inhibit inspiration and stimulate post-inspiratory neurones (Remmers et al, 1986). These effects will serve to increase the excitability of cardioinhibitory vagal preganglionic neurones (Gilbey et al, 1984); such a promotion of post-inspiratory activity by upper airway negative pressure appears to be the most likely explanation for the potentiation of the carotid chemoreflex bradycardia observed in these experiments. This raises the possibility that the augmented effect of carotid body excitation on heart rate with upper airway negative pressure may be entirely secondary to the changes in respiratory timing that occur in response to the latter stimulus. We do not know whether or not upper airway negative pressure can potentiate the carotid body-heart rate reflex in the absence of changes in respiratory timing.

Peripheral arterial chemoreceptor stimulation and negative airway pressure occur together during obstructive apnoea in humans, and a synergistic interaction similar to that reported here may explain the marked bradycardia that can occur under these circumstances (Bonsignore et al, 1994). Bradycardia with continuing respiratory effort is reported to be the predominant event in the hours preceding sudden infant death (Meny et al, 1994); obstructive apnoea, hypoxaemia or both have been proposed as likely mechanisms. Our results support the suggestion (Daly et al, 1979) that an interaction between these two stimuli could induce profound slowing of the heart and perhaps cause cardiac arrest.

The combined effects of upper airway negative pressure and carotid body stimulation on respiratory drive and timing are also of interest. We found that carotid chemoreceptor excitation did not alter the degree to which upper airway negative pressure prolonged T_I and T_{TOT}. This correlates well with the observation that the effects of upper airway negative pressure on respiratory timing persist in the presence of high central chemoreceptor drive (van Lunteren, 1987; Woodall & Mathew, 1988). The ability of carotid body excitation to increase respiratory drive, as assessed by $\int PHR / T_I$ was unaffected by airway negative pressure. In this respect the effect of upper airway negative pressure differs from that of electrical stimulation of the superior laryngeal nerve, which greatly suppresses or completely abolishes the ventilatory response to stimulation of the carotid body (Elsner et al, 1977; Daly et al, 1978, 1983).

5. ACKNOWLEDGMENTS

PN is supported by the North American Medical Alumni of University College, Dublin, as a Newman Scholar. MGL is supported by the Health Research Board, Ireland.

The presentation of this paper by PN received the Heymans-deCastro-Neil Young Scientist Award.

6. REFERENCES

Andreas S, Hajak G, v Breska B, Ruther E & Kreuzer H (1992) Changes in heart rate during obstructive sleep apnoea. Eur Respir J 5: 853–857

Bonsignore MR, Marrone O, Insalaco G & Bonsignore G (1994) The cardiovascular effects of obstructive sleep apnoeas: analysis of pathogenic mechanisms. Eur Respir J 7: 786–805

Daly M de Burgh, Korner PI, Angell-James JE & Oliver JR (1978) Cardiovascular-respiratory reflex interactions between carotid bodies and upper-airways receptors in the monkey. Am J Physiol 234: H293-H299

Daly M de Burgh, Angell-James JE & Elsner R (1979) Role of carotid-body chemoreceptors and their reflex interactions in bradycardia and cardiac arrest. Lancet i: 764–767

Daly M de Burgh, Litherland AS & Wood LM (1983) The modification of the respiratory, cardiac and vascular responses to stimulation of the carotid body chemoreceptors by a laryngeal input in the cat. IRCS Med Sci 11: 861–862

Dawid-Milner MS, Silva-Carvalho L, Goldsmith GE & Spyer KM (1995) Hypothalamic modulation of laryngeal reflexes in the anaesthetised cat: role of the nucleus tractus solitarii. J Physiol, London 487: 739–749

Elsner R, Angell-James JE & Daly M de Burgh (1977) Carotid body chemoreceptor reflexes and their interactions in the seal. Am J Physiol 232: H517-H525

Gilbey MP, Jordan D, Richter DW & Spyer KM (1984) Synaptic mechanisms involved in the inspiratory modulation of vagal cardio-inhibitory neurones in the cat. J Physiol, London 356: 65–78

Guilleminault C, Connolly S, Winkle R, Melvin K & Tilkian A (1984) Cyclical variation of the heart rate in sleep apnoea syndrome. Lancet i: 126–131

Kordy MT, Neil E & Palmer JF (1975) The influence of laryngeal afferent stimulation on cardiac vagal responses to carotid chemoreceptor excitation. J Physiol, London 247: 24P-25P

Langdon M, Nolan P, McKeogh, D & O'Regan RG (1995) Heart rate responses to upper airway negative pressure in the anaesthetized paralysed rabbit. J Physiol, London 487: 171P-172P

van Lunteren E (1987) Interactive effects of CO_2 and upper airway negative pressure on breathing pattern. J Appl Physiol 63: 229–237

Meny RG, Carroll JL, Carbone MT & Kelly D (1994) Cardiorespiratory recordings from infants dying suddenly and unexpectedly at home. Paediatrics 93: 44–49

Remmers JE, Richter DW, Ballantyne D, Bainton CR & Klein JP (1986) Reflex prolongation of stage I of expiration. Pflügers Arch 407: 190–198

Sant'Ambrogio FB, Mathew OP, Clark WD & Sant'Ambrogio G (1985) Laryngeal influences on breathing pattern and posterior cricoarytenoid muscle activity. J Appl Physiol 58: 1298–1304

Wennergren G, Hertzberg T, Milerad J, Bjure J & Lagercrantz H (1989) Hypoxia reinforces reflex bradycardia in infants. Acta Paediatr Scand 78: 11–17

Woodall DL & Mathew OP (1988) Interaction between upper airway negative pressure pulses and CO_2 on breathing pattern. J Appl Physiol 65: 205–209

67

CHEMORECEPTORS IN AUTONOMIC RESPONSES TO HYPOXIA IN CONSCIOUS RATS

Y. Hayashida, H. Hirakawa, T. Nakamura, and M. Maeda

Department of Systems Physiology
University of Occupational and Environmental Health
Yahatanishi, Kitakyushu 807, Japan

1. INTRODUCTION

It has been suggested that the cardiovascular responses to hypoxia are produced as integrated interactions between the effects of the autonomic nervous system and the direct effect of hypoxia on the central nervous system (CNS) and the cardiovascular system (Daly, 1986; Marshall, 1994). However, hypoxic exposure has been delivered for relatively short periods of time before attaining a steady state in many works. Therefore, such responses may have resulted before integrated interactions began operating. There is also no information on the behavior of the autonomic nervous activities during hypoxia in conscious animals, which may be relevant to the study of an integrated function. In this study, the autonomic nervous activities are examined during the cardiovascular responses of the chemoreceptor-intact and of denervated conscious rats to systemic hypoxia, in order to determine the contribution of the arterial chemoreceptors to these responses.

2. MATERIALS AND METHODS

Wistar male rats, weighing between 400 and 500 g, were divided into two groups: intact and sinoaortic denervated (SAD). Under pentobarbital anesthesia and using aseptic techniques, a skull plate was attached to all rats, and electrodes and catheters were implanted. The femoral artery and vein were cannulated for blood pressure (BP) measurement and for administering drugs. ECG was recorded through electrodes implanted under the skin at midchest. Stainless steel bipolar electrodes were used to record the renal sympathetic nerve activity (RSNA). The nerve and electrodes were stabilized with a two-component silicone rubber gel. After the gel hardened, the incision was closed. In order to denervate the peripheral chemo- and baroreceptors, the sinus nerves and the aortic nerves were bilaterally sectioned (SAD) in accordance with the procedure of Krieger (1964). The rat was then instrumented two weeks after the denervation as in the intact one. All leads

Frontiers in Arterial Chemoreception, edited by Zapata *et al.*
Plenum Press, New York, 1996

and catheters were routed subcutaneously to exit at the nape, and the leads were attached to a miniature pin socket that was then cemented to the skull plate. The socket and a slip ring were connected with flexible wires so that the rat could move, eat and drink freely.

The hypoxic exposure experiment made up of 3 sessions, hypocapnic, isocapnic and hypercapnic hypoxia, was carried out more than 2 days after the surgery in an air-tight box (40 L), where the rat was allowed free movement. Each session consisted of 3 experimental periods each of 30 min: control, hypoxic exposure and recovery periods. The temperature of the chamber was maintained at 25°C. Arterial blood samples taken during each session were analyzed for pH and gas tension by a gas analyzer (ABL-30, Radiometer, Copenhagen).

3. RESULTS

3.1. Arterial Blood Gas Tension and pH

P_aO_2 and P_aCO_2 of each rat were adjusted to a certain range for each hypoxic condition by changing the composition of the gas mixture in the exposure chamber. Table 1 shows the mean values of P_aO_2, P_aCO_2 and pH of the control and the three hypoxic groups (n= 6) in the intact rats. Similar ranges of P_aO_2, P_aCO_2 and pH levels were obtained in the SAD conscious rats, but the hypocapnic state could not be obtained, because of the absence of central and peripheral drives in the SAD rats to expel CO_2 through tachypnea.

3.2. Responses to Hypoxia in SAD Rats

Typical recordings of BP, HR and integrated renal sympathetic nerve activity during the control, isocapnic hypoxia and recovery periods for each 30 min are shown in Figure 1, together with the changes in gas tension of the exposure chamber in an SAD conscious rat. Isocapnic hypoxia induced a decrease in BP, HR and RSNA. BP of 97.2 ± 0.7 mm Hg (mean ± SE) in the control decreased to 79.9 ± 1.2 mm Hg during the isocapnic hypoxia. HR of 383 ± 1 beats/min in the control decreased to 353 ± 2 beats/min during the isocapnic hypoxia. RSNA decreased to 93.1 ± 0.6% of the control during the isocapnic hypoxia. In the recovery period, BP, HR and RSNA increased by 12.9%, 4.7% and 4.6%, respectively, when compared to the control period. There was a slight increase of 6% in the respiration rate in the steady state of the isocapnic hypoxia.

3.3. Responses to Hypoxia in Intact Rats

Figure 2 shows recordings of BP, HR and integrated renal sympathetic nerve activity during the control period, three kinds of hypoxia (hypocapnic, isocapnic and hypercapnic)

Table 1. Mean values of P_aO_2, P_aCO_2 and pH in each session of intact rats

	P_aO_2 (mm Hg)	P_aCO_2 (mm Hg)	pH
Control	94.2	34.3	7.43
Hypocapnic Hypoxia	38.7	21.5	7.56
Isocapnic Hypoxia	50.5	35.4	7.43
Hypercapnic Hypoxia	56.4	45.0	7.33

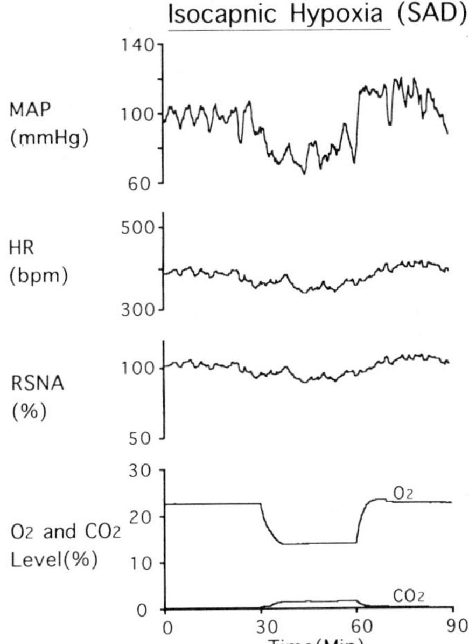

Figure 1. Effects of isocapnic hypoxia on mean arterial pressure (MAP), heart rate (HR) and renal sympathetic nerve activity (RSNA) in a sino-aortic denervated (SAD) rat. Gas tensions (%) of exposure chamber are also shown.

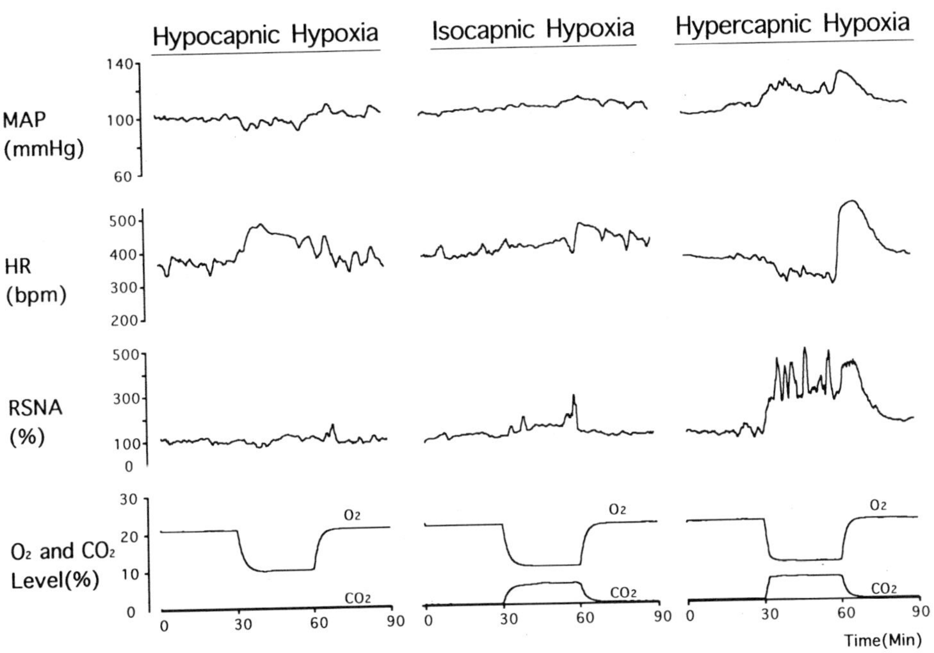

Figure 2. Effects of hypocapnic (left column), isocapnic (middle column) and hypercapnic (right column) hypoxia on mean arterial pressure (MAP), heart rate (HR) and renal sympathetic nerve activity (RSNA) in an intact conscious rat. Gas tensions (%) of exposure chamber are also shown.

and recovery periods for each 30 min. Isocapnic hypoxia induced a slight increase in BP from 100.6 ± 0.1 mm Hg to 104.4 ± 0.3 mm Hg, and HR from 380 ± 1 beats/min to 406 ± 2 beats/min, and a significant increase of 169.8% in RSNA. Hypocapnic hypoxia induced significant increases in HR from 365 ± 1 beats/min to 435 ± 2 beats/min and RSNA to 110.6%, but a significant decrease in BP from 99.5 ± 0.2 mm Hg to 94.5 ± 0.4 mm Hg. Hypercapnic hypoxia elicited significant increases in BP from 98.5 ± 0.2 mm Hg to 110.2 ± 0.4 mm Hg and RSNA to 300.8%, but a significant decrease in HR from 355 ± 1 beats/min to 292 ± 2 beats/min. The respiration rate increased to 52.0%, 43.4% and 72.1%, respectively, during steady states of isocapnic, hypocapnic and hypercapnic hypoxia. In the recovery period of isocapnic hypoxia, BP and HR increased significantly by 4.5% and 12.6%, respectively, when compared to the control period. In the recovery period of hypercapnic hypoxia, BP, HR and RSNA increased significantly by 8.9%, 20% and 90%, respectively, when compared to the control period. However, there were no significant increases in BP, HR and RSNA in the recovery period of hypocapnic hypoxia when compared to the control period. Atropine sulfate reversed the change in HR during hypercapnic hypoxia.

4. DISCUSSION

The major findings of this study were:

a) a direct action of hypoxia upon the cardiovascular and autonomic nervous systems elicited decreases in BP, HR and RSNA, as observed in the SAD rats.
b) all three kinds of the hypoxic challenge induced an activation of RSNA in the peripheral chemo- and baroreceptor intact rats. It was shown in the experiment with isocapnic hypoxia that the direct effect of hypoxia was counterbalanced in the intact rats by the activation of the sympathetic nervous system via peripheral chemoreceptors.
c) atropine pretreatment reversed HR changes during hypercapnic hypoxia, indicating that hypercapnia increased cardiac parasympathetic activity to induce bradycardia.

In this study, respiratory frequencies were observed to increase during the steady state of hypoxia according to the P_aCO_2 levels, and bradycardic and tachycardic responses were also observed to be dependent on P_aCO_2 levels but not on respiratory frequency.

It is interesting that BP and HR during the recovery periods after isocapnic and hypercapnic hypoxia were sustained significantly, remaining increased for more than 10 min, in comparison to those of the control period. It is reasonable to assume that the cardiovascular system and CNS would have attained a steady state of hypoxia in 30 min.

No attempts were made in this study to analyze any humoral factors and vasoactive hormones, which would modify the cardiovascular responses through chemoreceptor activation during hypoxia.

5. REFERENCES

Daly M de B (1986) Interactions between respiration and circulation. In: Handbook of Physiology, Sect 3: The Respiratory System, Vol II: Control of Breathing. Bethesda, Maryland: Am Physiol Soc. pp 529–594
Krieger EM (1964) Neurogenic hypertension in the rat. Circ Res 15: 511–521
Marshall JM (1994) Peripheral chemoreceptors and cardiovascular regulation. Physiol Rev 74: 543–594

THE EFFECT OF SYMPATHETIC NERVE STIMULATION ON VENTILATION AND UPPER AIRWAY RESISTANCE IN THE ANAESTHETIZED RAT

K. D. O'Halloran, A. K. Curran, and A. Bradford

Department of Physiology
Royal College of Surgeons in Ireland, Dublin, Ireland

1. INTRODUCTION

We have previously demonstrated that moderate cooling of the isolated upper airway (UA) causes a substantial fall in UA resistance in anaesthetized rats (O'Halloran et al, 1994). This effect is partly of reflex origin but a large fall in resistance still persists following elimination of reflex effects. We have proposed that this residual effect is due to a direct effect of cooling on the UA mucosal vasculature, causing a reduction in mucosal blood flow, a thinning of the mucosa and therefore, an increase in UA cross-sectional area and a fall in resistance. If such a mechanism were responsible for the fall in resistance, then we might expect that activation of sympathetic vasoconstrictor fibres in the cervical sympathetic trunk would also reduce UA resistance in the same preparation. The present experiments examine the effects of electrical stimulation of the cervical sympathetic trunk on the airflow resistance of the isolated UA in anaesthetized rats breathing spontaneously through a low-cervical tracheostomy. Spontaneously breathing animals were used because we also wished to examine the effects of sympathetic stimulation on ventilation. The influence of the cervical sympathetic nerves on ventilation are complex and controversial and very little is known about their effects in the rat.

2. METHODS

Experiments were performed in 34 male, Wistar rats (300–450 g) anaesthetized with chloralose (100 mg/kg) and urethane (1 g/kg) ip. Body temperature was maintained at 37°C using a rectal probe and thermostatically-controlled heating blanket. Animals were placed supine and allowed to breath room air spontaneously through a cannula inserted into a low-cervical tracheostomy. Airflow was measured with a pneumotachograph attached to this cannula and the signal integrated to give tidal volume. Warmed (37°C), humidified air was blown at a rate of 10–20 ml/sec/kg through a cannula inserted into a high-cervical tracheostomy to exit through the mouth and nose or mouth only (the nose having been sealed). Upper airway temperature, airflow and subglottic pressure were recorded. The oesophagus was tied off. Both cervical sympathetic trunks were cut low in the neck and the peripheral ends stimulated using bipolar electrodes (10 V, 1 msec, 20 Hz) for 20–40 sec. Cannulae were placed in an external jugular vein for administration of supplemental anaesthetic, propranolol (1 mg/kg) and phentolamine (1 mg/kg) and into a femoral or common carotid artery to record arterial blood pressure. Upper airway resistance was calculated from measurements of UA airflow and subglottic pressure. Values, expressed as mean ± SD, for UA resistance and ventilatory variables were compared for the last 10 breaths before stimulation and for 10 breaths when effects were maximal using Student's *t* test with p less than 0.05 considered significant.

3. RESULTS

3.1. Effect of Sympathetic Stimulation on UA Resistance

In 34 animals, stimulation of the cervical sympathetic trunks had variable effects on arterial blood pressure, *i.e.*, either no change (n = 10), an increase (n = 7) or a decrease (n = 17). However, in 29 out of the 34 animals, there was a reproducible fall in UA resistance with the nose open (see Fig 1). In the remaining 5 animals, there were no changes in UA resistance.

The fall in resistance was usually immediate and return to pre-stimulus values in the post-stimulus period was either immediate or required 1–2 min for complete recovery. When the nose was sealed, there was an increase in UA resistance and the fall in UA resistance caused by sympathetic stimulation was significantly reduced compared to nose open values. This response was not significantly affected by propranolol but was abolished by phentolamine. Both of these drugs reduced blood pressure but did not affect baseline UA resistance values. The fall in resistance caused by sympathetic stimulation was not related to changes in blood pressure or ventilation (see later) because it was observed in tests

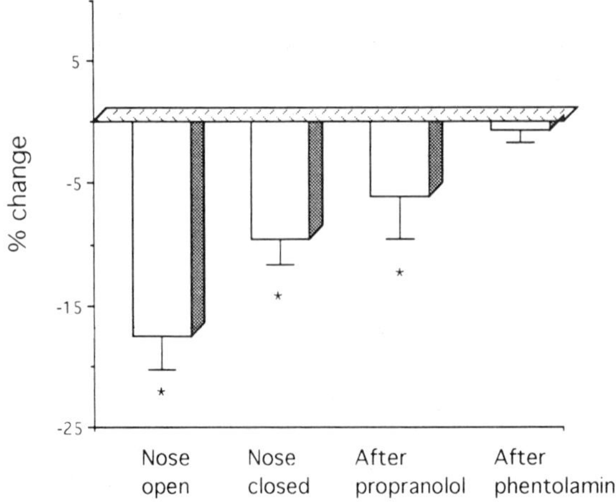

Figure 1. Effect of sympathetic nerve stimulation on UA resistance. Values are mean ± SD % change from before stimulation in animals with the nose open (n = 29), nose closed (n =29), after propranolol (n = 16) and after phentolamine (n = 16). *indicates significant difference from before stimulation.

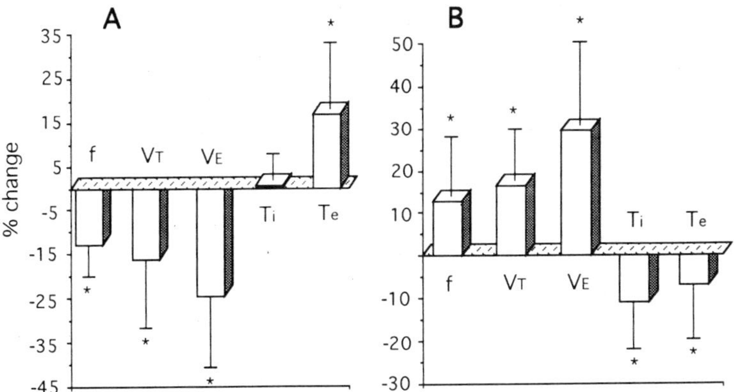

Figure 2. Effect of sympathetic nerve stimulation on ventilation. **A** and **B** show changes in respiratory frequency (f), tidal volume (V_T), minute ventilation (V_E), inspiratory time (T_i) and expiratory time (T_e) expressed as mean ± SD % change from before stimulation during the inhibitory and excitatory phases, respectively, of the ventilatory response. * indicates significant difference from before stimulation.

where these variables were unaffected. The fall was also observed in 5 animals which had their sinus nerves cut at the beginning of the experiment.

3.2. Effect of Sympathetic Stimulation on Ventilation

Sympathetic stimulation had no effect on ventilation in 7 out of 34 animals. In the remaining 27, there was an immediate inhibition of breathing which either persisted for the duration of stimulation or was followed during the stimulus period by an excitation. The excitation (14 out of 27) usually persisted for 1–2 min after the end of the stimulus period and sometimes appeared only when the stimulus was removed. These effects are quantified in Fig 2.

All ventilatory effects were absent following section of both sinus nerves (10 animals). The effects of propranolol on ventilatory responses were examined in 21 animals of which all 21 showed the inhibitory response prior to propranolol and 9 of these also showed the subsequent excitation. Propranolol had no effect on the inhibitory component but enhanced the excitatory component in 5 of the 9 animals in which this effect was obtained. Furthermore, in 7 of the 12 animals which did not initially have the excitatory component, excitation was now observed following propranolol. All 21 animals treated with propranolol were then given phentolamine which had no effect on the inhibitory response and very little effect on the excitatory response. The excitatory effect obtained in the 16 animals following propranolol was unaffected in 11 but was absent in the remaining 5 animals.

4. DISCUSSION

The present results demonstrate that electrical stimulation of the cervical sympathetic trunks causes a fall in UA resistance in anaesthetized rats. This effect was independent of the changes in blood pressure and ventilation which occurred. It is known that carotid chemoreceptor activity influences UA muscle activity (Brouillette & Thach,

1980). Therefore it is possible that changes in carotid chemoreceptor activity brought about by the sympathetic stimulation could have reflexly affected UA muscle activity and therefore resistance. However, this is an unlikely mechanism since the effect was also present in animals with sectioned sinus nerves. We believe that the decrease in resistance is due to activation of vasoconstrictor fibres to the airway mucosa causing a reduction in mucosal thickness, an increase in airway cross-sectional area and a fall in resistance. The finding that the effect was resistant to beta-adrenoceptor blockade but was abolished by alpha-adrenoceptor blockade is consistent with this view. Our results are also consistent with a previous report that cervical sympathetic nerve stimulation increases nasal vascular resistance and decreases nasal airway resistance in anaesthetized dogs (Lung & Wang, 1989). The fall in resistance caused by sympathetic stimulation in the present work was less when the nose was bypassed, indicating that nasal resistance is reduced when the nose is open but that resistance is also reduced elsewhere in the UA.

Sympathetic stimulation also caused changes in ventilation usually consisting of a biphasic response with initial inhibition followed by excitation. This is reminiscent of the well-described initial inhibition followed by excitation of carotid chemoreceptor activity caused by exogenous noradrenaline (Llados & Zapata, 1978). Although, there are several reports to the contrary, it is generally believed that the inhibition is alpha-adrenoceptor-mediated whereas the excitation is beta-adrenoceptor-mediated (Prabhakar & Kou, 1994). The inefficacy of alpha- and beta-adrenoceptor antagonists to prevent the ventilatory changes in the present experiments does not support such a mechanism in the rat carotid body. However, this assumes that the ventilatory effects are due to activation of noradrenergic nerves ending in the carotid body. Although the changes in ventilation were abolished by cutting the sinus nerves, we cannot exclude the possibility that these effects are due to activation of sympathetic fibres coursing centrally in the sinus nerve (Eyzaguirre & Uchizono, 1961). The effects are unlikely to be due to changes in sinus baroreceptor activity since there was no relationship between the ventilatory and blood pressure changes. Another possible cause of the ventilatory changes is the possible presence of vagal afferents in the cervical sympathetic trunk as proposed by Lung & Wang (1989) in order to explain the small increases in respiratory frequency which they occasionally observed during sympathetic stimulation in anaesthetized dogs. However, for this to be true for the present experiments, it would also be necessary to postulate that such afferents pass centrally through the sinus nerves.

5. ACKNOWLEDGMENTS

Supported by the Royal College of Surgeons in Ireland, Health Research Board (Ireland) and Wellcome Trust.

6. REFERENCES

Brouillette RT & Thach BT (1980) Control of genioglossus muscle inspiratory activity. J Appl Physiol 49: 801–808

Eyzaguirre C & Uchizono K (1961) Observation on the fibre content of nerves reaching the carotid body of the cat. J Physiol, London 159: 268–281

Llados F & Zapata P (1978) Effects of adrenoceptor stimulating and blocking agents on carotid body chemosensory inhibition. J Physiol, London 274: 501–509

Lung MA & Wang JCC (1989) Autonomic nervous control of nasal vasculature and airflow resistance in the anaesthetized dog. J Physiol, London 419: 121–139

O'Halloran KD, Curran AK & Bradford A (1994) Ventilatory and upper-airway resistance responses to upper-airway cooling and CO_2 in anaesthetized rats. Eur J Physiol 429: 262–266

Prabhakar NR & Kou YR (1994) Inhibitory sympathetic action on the carotid body responses to sustained hypoxia. Respir Physiol 95: 67–79

VENTILATORY AND UPPER AIRWAY MUSCLE RESPONSES TO UPPER AIRWAY CO_2 IN ANAESTHETIZED NEONATAL GUINEA-PIGS

A. K. Curran, K. D. O'Halloran, and A. Bradford

Department of Physiology
Royal College of Surgeons in Ireland, Dublin, Ireland

1. INTRODUCTION

In adult animals, CO_2 confined to the isolated upper airway (UA) lumen reflexly inhibits breathing and excites genioglossus muscle activity (Nolan et al, 1990) by affecting the activity of CO_2-sensitive receptors in the superior laryngeal nerves (Bradford et al, 1993). These effects may be important in the regulation of breathing and UA patency since the genioglossus is a major UA dilator muscle. There is some evidence that superior laryngeal nerve (SLN) reflexes are more potent in neonates than in adults (Al-Shway & Mortola, 1982; Boggs & Bartlett Jr, 1982). Therefore, the present investigation examines the effects of UA CO_2 on ventilation and geniohyoid (GH) muscle activity in neonatal Guinea-pigs. We chose to study the GH muscle because of its ease of access and because, like the genioglossus, it exerts an important influence on UA patency. Contraction of the GH causes anterior displacement of the hyoid bone and stiffening of the hypopharynx (Brouillette & Thach, 1979), a site which is vulnerable to collapse (Shepard Jr et al, 1991).

2. METHODS

Experiments were performed on anaesthetized (urethane, 2 g/kg ip) 10–21 day-old, one-month-old and three-month-old Guinea-pigs placed supine and breathing spontaneously through a cannula inserted into a low-cervical tracheostomy and attached to a pneumotachograph to record tracheal airflow. Body temperature was maintained at 37°C using a rectal probe and a thermostatically-controlled heating blanket and radiant heat. A steady flow of 10 ml/sec/kg of warmed (37°C), humidified (100% relative humidity) air containing 0,5% and 10% CO_2 was applied to the UA through a cannula inserted into a high-cervical tracheostomy to just below the cricoid cartilage (see Fig 1). The flow exited through the mouth and nose or mouth only (having sealed the nose). UA airflow, subglottic pressure and temperature were recorded. Electrodes were inserted into the GH muscle and dia-

Frontiers in Arterial Chemoreception, edited by Zapata *et al.*
Plenum Press, New York, 1996

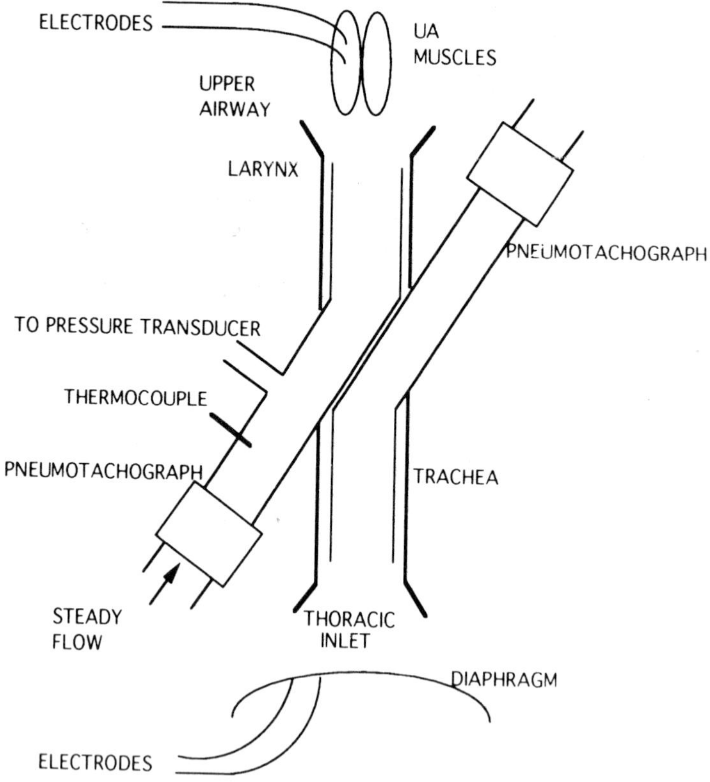

Figure 1. Schematic representation of the experimental set-up.

phragm (DIA) to record raw and integrated GH and DIA EMG activity. Mean respiratory frequency, inspiratory time, expiratory time, peak inspiratory flow and peak integrated GH and DIA activity were calculated for 10 breaths before, during and after application of CO_2 and expressed as % change ± SE with respect to control. Values were compared statistically using Student's *t* test with $p < 0.05$ taken as significant.

3. RESULTS

3.1. Effect of UA CO_2 on Ventilation

In 8 animals, the application of 5% and 10% CO_2 to the isolated UA with the nose closed caused an increase in respiratory frequency (+8.6 ± 2.1% and 12.9 ± 2.5%, respectively, values are mean ± SE % change from control) due to a decrease in expiratory time (-6.9 ± 2.1% and -11.9 ± 2.1%, respectively) but had no effect on peak inspiratory flow. An example of the tachypnoea is shown in Fig 2.

The effects were also present in 7 separate animals with sectioned SLN in which 5% and 10% CO_2 increased respiratory frequency (+11.7 ± 3.8% and +18.2 ± 3.5%, respectively) and reduced expiratory time (-10.2 ± 3.8% and -14.9% ± 3.0%, respectively). In a separate group of 8 animals with the nose sealed and the SLN, glossopharyngeal and va-

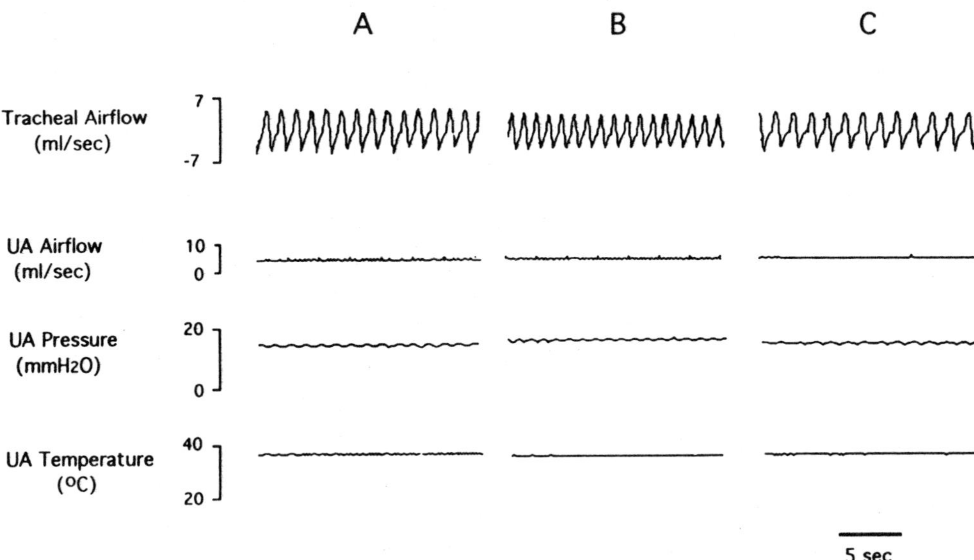

Figure 2. Effect of 10% CO_2 applied to the isolated UA on ventilation. **A**, **B** and **C** show records of spontaneous tracheal airflow and UA airflow, pressure and temperature before, during and after, respectively, the application of 10% CO_2. CO_2 caused an increase in respiratory frequency with no change in UA airflow, pressure or temperature.

gus nerves cut, 10% CO_2 still caused a significant increase in respiratory frequency (+24.3 ± 10.2%) due to a decrease in expiratory time (-22.5 ± 9.2%). However, these effects were abolished by topical anaesthesia of the UA with a 2% xylocaine solution applied by means of a cannula inserted through the mouth. The tachypnoea was also present in 5 one-month old animals but was absent in 5 three-month old animals.

3.2. Effect of UA CO_2 on DIA and GH EMG Activity

In a separate group of 17 animals with the nose open, GH activity was absent in all animals but became apparent in 12 out of the 17 animals following mid-cervical vagotomy. Overall, application of 10% CO_2 caused a significant decrease in GH and DIA ac-

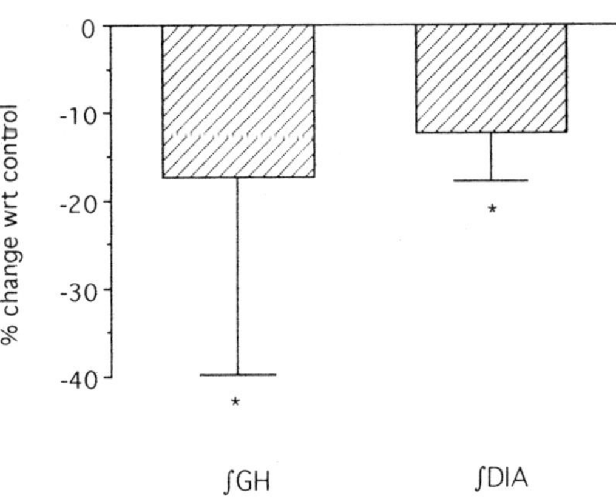

Figure 3. The effects of passing 10% CO_2 over the isolated UA on peak integrated geniohyoid (∫ GH) and diaphragm (∫ DIA) EMG activity in the neonatal Guinea-pig following bilateral section of the vagus nerves. Values are mean ± SE % changes with respect to (wrt) air control (n = 17). * indicates significant difference from control.

tivity (see Fig 2) although significant increases in GH activity were observed in a small number of trials. These effects were present following section of the SLN and glossopharyngeal nerves but were abolished by topical anaesthesia of the entire UA.

4. DISCUSSION

These results show that rather than inhibiting ventilation and exciting UA muscle activity as is the case in adult cats (Nolan et al, 1990), UA CO_2 causes a tachypnoea and usually inhibits GH muscle activity in neonatal Guinea-pigs. Furthermore, these effects are not due to SLN-mediated reflexes unlike those in adult cats. However, UA CO_2 has been shown to have no effect on breathing in neonatal cats and dogs (Al-Shway & Mortola, 1982) and inspired CO_2 inhibits breathing in preterm infants, a response which has been suggested to be due to an UA reflex (Alvaro et al, 1992). In the present experiments, the responses were present following section of the SLN and glossopharyngeal nerves but were abolished following topical anaesthesia of the entire UA suggesting a reflex from CO_2-sensitive receptors outside of the larynx. However, the effects of UA CO_2 on UA receptors have not been studied in the neonate. These results may have implications for the control of breathing and UA patency in the neonate, especially since they appear to be attenuated by maturation.

5. ACKNOWLEDGMENTS

Supported by the Royal College of Surgeons in Ireland, Health Research Board (Ireland) and Wellcome Trust.

6. REFERENCES

Al-Shway SF & Mortola JP (1982) Respiratory effects of airflow through the upper airways in newborn kittens and puppies. J Appl Physiol 53: 805–814

Alvaro RE, Weintraub Z, Kwiatkowski K, Cates DB & Rigatto H (1992) A respiratory sensory reflex in response to CO_2 inhibits breathing in preterm infants. J Appl Physiol 73: 1558–1563

Boggs DF & Bartlett Jr D (1982) Chemical specificity of a laryngeal apneic reflex in puppies. J Appl Physiol 53: 455–462

Bradford A, Nolan P, O'Regan RG & McKeogh D (1993) Carbon dioxide-sensitive superior laryngeal nerve afferents in the anaesthetized cat. Exp Physiol 78: 787–798

Brouillette RT & Thach BT (1979) A neuromuscular mechanism maintaining extrathoracic airway patency. J Appl Physiol 46: 772–779

Nolan P, Bradford A, O'Regan RG & McKeogh D (1990) The effects of changes in laryngeal airway CO_2 concentration on genioglossus muscle activity in the anaesthetized cat. Exp Physiol 75: 271–274

Shepard JW Jr, Gefter WB, Guilleminault C, Hoffman EA, Hoffstein V, Hudgel DW, Surrat PM & White DP (1991) Evaluation of the upper airway in patients with obstructive sleep apnea. Sleep 14: 361–371

NEUROGENIC INFLAMMATION

A Model for Studying Efferent Actions of Sensory Nerves

Donald M. McDonald,[1,2] Jeffrey J. Bowden,[1,2] Peter Baluk,[1,2] and Nigel W. Bunnett[3,4]

[1] Cardiovascular Research Institute and
[2] Department of Anatomy
[3] Department of Physiology
[4] Department of Surgery
University of California
San Francisco, California 94143

1. INTRODUCTION

Cytoplasmic vesicles, resembling synaptic vesicles of efferent nerve fibers,* are a distinctive feature of sensory nerve fibers that innervate glomus cells of the carotid body (Biscoe et al, 1970; Kobayashi & Uehara, 1970; McDonald & Mitchell, 1975). Ultrastructural studies have shown that some vesicles cluster at synaptic junctions where sensory nerves are presynaptic to glomus cells (McDonald & Mitchell, 1975; Verna, 1979; Pallot, 1987). This finding has led to speculation that substances from sensory nerves influence glomus cells (McDonald & Mitchell, 1975). Indeed, the phenomenon of "efferent inhibition" (Neil & O'Regan, 1969, 1971), in which electrical stimulation of the carotid sinus nerve inhibits chemoreceptor firing, has been interpreted as an efferent action of sensory nerves on glomus cells (McDonald & Mitchell, 1981). Although there are other interpretations of the mechanism underlying efferent inhibition (Biscoe, 1971; Sampson et al, 1976; O'Regan, 1977, 1981; Acker & O'Regan, 1981), the morphological evidence that sensory nerves are presynaptic to glomus cells is compelling.

---

* For the purpose of this review, the term **efferent nerve fibers** refers to axons that carry impulses away from the central nervous system to effector cells, as with efferent nerve fibers that activate skeletal muscle, smooth muscle, or gland cells. The term **sensory (afferent) nerve fibers** refers to axons that carry impulses into the central nervous system, whether or not they mediate conscious sensations. The **efferent actions of sensory nerve fibers** refer to local effects of sensory nerves on target cells in peripheral tissues. In the case of efferent inhibition of chemoreceptors, glomus cells are the putative target cells, whereas in neurogenic inflammation, endothelial cells are the target cells.

More recently, we have used the phenomenon of neurogenic inflammation as a model for studying the efferent actions of sensory nerves (McDonald, 1994a, 1996). This review highlights what has been learned about efferent functions of sensory nerves from studies of neurogenic inflammation. The review focuses on neurogenic inflammation of the respiratory tract, which has been studied in particular detail.

2. DEFINITION OF NEUROGENIC INFLAMMATION

The term neurogenic inflammation describes the increase in vascular permeability produced by substances released from sensory nerves. The concept of neurogenic inflammation evolved from observations made by Jancsó in experiments with capsaicin, which is the substance that makes red peppers taste hot (Jancsó, 1960; Jancsó et al, 1967, 1968). Jancsó used the term neurogenic inflammation to describe the plasma leakage and edema that develops when capsaicin is applied to the skin or mucous membranes of rats or guinea pigs. Antidromic electrical stimulation of sensory nerves and irritating substances such as mustard oil, formaldehyde, and hypertonic saline have the same effect. Jancsó deduced that sensory nerves play an essential role because neurogenic inflammation does not occur after the nerves are desensitized with capsaicin or destroyed by surgical transection (Jancsó, 1960; Jancsó et al, 1967, 1968). Jancsó speculated that intense sensory nerve stimulation evokes the release of a neural mediator that can increase vascular permeability (Jancsó et al, 1967).

3. TRIGGERS OF NEUROGENIC INFLAMMATION

Neurogenic inflammation can be triggered in the airway mucosa of rats and guinea pigs by inhalation of capsaicin, cigarette smoke, ether, formaldehyde, hypertonic saline, or sodium metabisulphite (Lundberg & Saria, 1983; Umeno et al, 1990; Sakamoto et al, 1992). Neurogenic inflammation can also be evoked by hyperventilation of dry air (Garland et al, 1991). Electrical stimulation of the vagus nerve has the same effect (Lundberg & Saria, 1983; McDonald, 1988a). In addition, the plasma leakage produced by histamine and bradykinin is partly dependent on sensory nerves (Lundberg & Saria, 1983). Prior desensitization with capsaicin prevents the neurogenic inflammatory response in the respiratory mucosa (Lundberg & Saria, 1983), just as it does in the skin and eye (Jancsó, 1961; Jancsó et al, 1967).

4. ROLE OF ENDOTHELIAL GAPS IN POSTCAPILLARY VENULES

In respiratory tract of rats and guinea pigs, neurogenic inflammation occurs in the nose, larynx, trachea, and first through fourth order bronchi but not in the lung alveoli (Lundberg & Saria, 1983; McDonald, 1988a; Petersson et al, 1993). The plasma leakage results from an increase in the permeability of postcapillary venules (about 7 to 40 μm in diameter) and collecting venules (about 40 to 80 μm in diameter) (McDonald, 1988a); arterioles and capillaries do not become leaky (Fig 1A). In this respect, neurogenic inflammation resembles the immediate inflammatory response evoked by histamine, bradykinin, and serotonin (Majno et al, 1961; Joris et al, 1982).

In neurogenic inflammation, as in other immediate inflammatory responses, the leakage occurs through focal gaps that form between endothelial cells (Majno & Palade, 1961; McDonald, 1994b). In blood vessels of the rat trachea, endothelial gaps have an average diameter of 0.3 to 0.5 μm (Hirata et al, 1995; Baluk et al, 1996). Within a minute of the onset of neurogenic inflammation, some 15 gaps form around each endothelial cell in postcapillary venules. Fewer gaps form in collecting venules. Despite their small size, endothelial gaps can be localized by light microscopy after staining with silver nitrate (Fig 1B) (McDonald, 1994b). The gaps are transient, and the leakage ends in a few minutes (McDonald, 1994b; Baluk et al, 1996).

5. ROLE OF SUBSTANCE P FROM SENSORY NERVE FIBERS

Neurogenic inflammation is mediated by substance P and perhaps other peptides released from unmyelinated sensory axons (Lembeck & Holzer, 1979; Lundberg et al, 1985). Nerve fibers with substance P-immunoreactivity are abundant in tissues in which neurogenic inflammation occurs (Lundberg et al, 1984; Baluk et al, 1992; Kummer et al, 1992). In the respiratory mucosa, such nerve fibers form a dense plexus at the base of the epithelium (Fig 1C) (Baluk et al, 1992). The nerve fibers are destroyed by capsaicin pretreatment (Lundberg et al, 1984; Baluk et al, 1992).

Experiments using selective denervation, vagal ligation, retrograde tracers, and electrical stimulation have shown that most sensory nerve fibers that mediate neurogenic inflammation in the respiratory tract travel in the vagus nerve and have their cell body in vagal sensory ganglia (Lundberg & Saria, 1983; Terenghi et al, 1983; McDonald et al, 1988; Kummer et al, 1992). Sensory nerve fibers from dorsal root ganglia make a smaller contribution (Dalsgaard & Lundberg, 1984; Springall et al, 1987).

6. ROLE OF NK1 RECEPTORS ON ENDOTHELIAL CELLS

Substance P mediates neurogenic inflammation through its action on NK1 receptors, also known as neurokinin-1 or substance P receptors. The role of NK1 receptors has been documented by using selective agonists and antagonists (Abelli et al, 1991; Delay-Goyet & Lundberg, 1991; Lei et al, 1992; Sakamoto et al, 1993). NK2 receptors may contribute in some species (Tousignant et al, 1993).

The issue of whether substance P increases vascular permeability through a direct action on blood vessels was first addressed by localizing binding sites with iodinated Bolton-Hunter-coupled substance P (Carstairs & Barnes, 1986; Hoover & Hancock, 1987). Some small vessels are labeled by this approach (Sertl et al, 1988), but it is unclear whether they are sites of plasma leakage. Another approach is to localize substance P binding sites by using immunohistochemistry with an anti-idiotypic antibody raised against an anti-substance P antibody (Kummer et al, 1990, 1991). No blood vessels are labeled by this approach.

We addressed this issue by using immunohistochemistry with an antibody against a 15-amino acid portion of the carboxy terminus of the rat NK1 receptor (Vigna et al, 1994). This approach revealed abundant NK1 receptor-immunoreactivity on venules that leak in neurogenic inflammation but little or no immunoreactivity on capillaries or arterioles (Bowden et al, 1994a, 1996). Our studies showed that binding of substance P to NK1 receptors on endothelial cells rapidly triggers the internalization of the receptors into en-

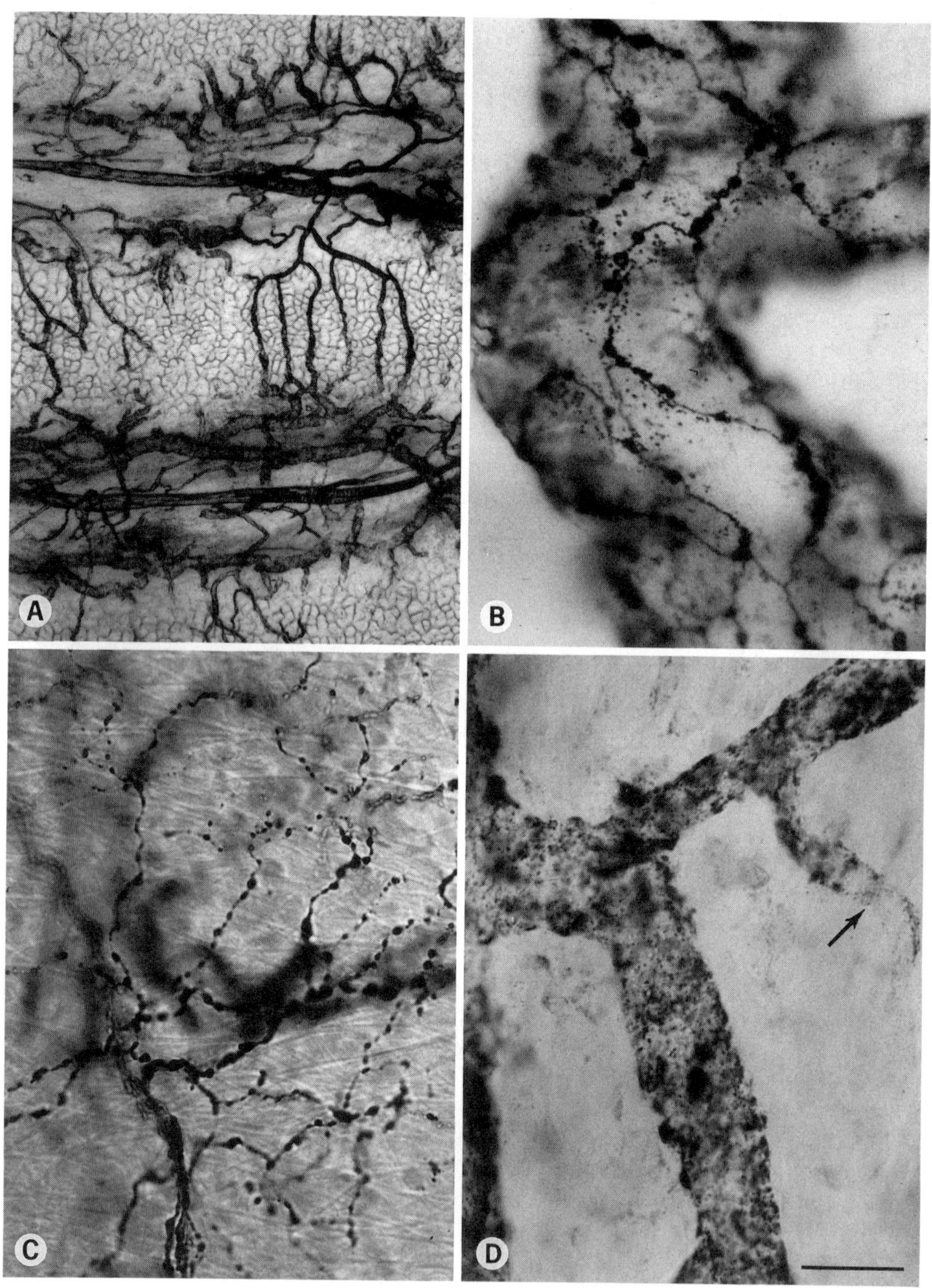
A
B
C
D

dosomes, and that most of the NK1 receptor immunolabeling is due to the presence of labeled endosomes (Fig 1D). Postcapillary venules and collecting venules have the largest number of labeled endosomes (some 70 to 80 endosomes per endothelial cell at 5 minutes after the stimulus) and the largest amount of leakage (Bowden et al., 1996). Arterioles have no labeled endosomes and no leakage. Both the plasma leakage and the receptor internalization are blocked by the selective NK1 receptor antagonist SR 140333 (Bowden et al., 1996). Exogenous substance P and platelet activating factor cause plasma leakage, but only substance P induces NK1 receptor internalization (Bowden et al., 1996).

Binding of substance P to its receptor results in desensitization to subsequent exposure to the peptide (Bowden et al., 1994a). The rapid removal of NK1 receptors from the cell surface after ligand binding contributes to the desensitization and thereby limits the amount of plasma leakage. It could also participate in the resensitization of endothelial cells to substance P and in the restoration of the neurogenic inflammatory response after a period of desensitization (Bowden et al., 1994a).

The receptor localization studies show that the cellular targets of substance P from sensory nerves can be identified by the presence of immunoreactive endosomes. Although it may seem predictable that the NK1 receptor localization studies show that substance P causes plasma leakage through a direct action on endothelial cells, this finding was actually unexpected because substance P-containing nerves are not closely associated with venules (McDonald et al., 1988; Baluk et al., 1992).

7. EXACERBATION BY AIRWAY INFECTIONS

Several years ago, we discovered that airway infections can exacerbate neurogenic inflammation (McDonald, 1988b). In particular, we found that *Mycoplasma pulmonis* infection, a common respiratory disease in rats, can increase the plasma leakage evoked by substance P, capsaicin, or vagal stimulation as much as 30-fold (McDonald, 1988b; McDonald et al, 1991). Some infected rats are so sensitive to capsaicin that they can be killed by a dose that is readily tolerated by pathogen-free rats (McDonald et al., 1991). Untreated *M. pulmonis* infection is lifelong (Bowden et al., 1994b).

Several processes participate in the abnormal sensitivity of the infected airway mucosa to stimuli that evoke neurogenic inflammation. There are increases in the number of blood vessels that become leaky in neurogenic inflammation and in the leakiness of indi-

Figure 1. Whole mounts of rat tracheas illustrating several features of neurogenic inflammation in the respiratory mucosa. **A** shows abnormally leaky postcapillary venules and collecting venules that extravasated as a result of neurogenic inflammation triggered by electrical stimulation of the vagus nerve. Arterioles and capillaries did not become leaky in neurogenic inflammation. **B** shows a postcapillary venule. Focal regions, which are located along endothelial borders, mark endothelial gaps produced by an intravenous injection of substance P. **C** shows part of a plexus of substance P-immunoreactive nerves located at the base of the tracheal epithelium. Postcapillary venules are out of focus because they are located in a plane beneath the nerve plexus. **D** shows NK1 receptor immunoreactivity of endothelial cells of postcapillary venules 5 minutes after an injection of substance P. NK1 receptor immunoreactive endosomes are abundant in the endothelium of the venules but are sparse in the endothelium of a capillary (arrow). Scale bar, 250 μm in A, 20 μm in B, 75 μm in C, and 20 μm in D. For a color representation of this figure, see the color insert facing page 458.

vidual vessels (McDonald et al, 1991). The increased number of leaky vessels is a consequence of angiogenesis associated with the chronic inflammation. The abnormal sensitivity of the vessels results in part from increased expression of NK1 receptors on the endothelial cells of the newly formed blood vessels (Baluk et al, 1995).

Like some human airway diseases, *M. pulmonis* infection in rats can be exacerbated by viral infections or exposure to irritants (Schoeb et al, 1982; Schoeb & Lindsey, 1987). The exacerbated *M. pulmonis* infection further increases the amount of plasma leakage occurring in neurogenic inflammation (McDonald et al, 1991).

8. OTHER EFFERENT ACTIONS OF SENSORY NERVE FIBERS

Neurogenic inflammation, as defined by Jancsó's original criteria, has been identified in the dura, conjunctiva, eye lid, middle ear, oral mucosa, dental pulp, salivary gland ducts, esophagus, biliary system, anal mucosa, ureter, urinary bladder, skin, joints, nose, larynx, trachea, and bronchi of rats and guinea pigs (reviewed by McDonald, 1994a, 1996). However, each organ exhibits its own unique collection of effects of mediators released from sensory nerves. In the respiratory tract, sensory nerve stimulation not only can trigger plasma leakage but also can cause neutrophil adhesion, vasodilatation, submucosal gland secretion, ion transport, bronchial smooth muscle contraction, increased cholinergic transmission, and cough (Barnes, 1991a; Nadel, 1992). Similarly, sensory nerves in the eye can mediate plasma leakage, miosis, vasodilatation in the anterior uvea, breakdown of the blood-aqueous barrier, and increased intraocular pressure (Stjernschantz et al, 1982; Krootila et al, 1992).

9. OCCURRENCE IN HUMAN DISEASE

The possible involvement of neurogenic inflammation in human airway disease has been examined by studying the actions of sensory neuropeptides (Barnes, 1992), the mechanism of sensory nerve-mediated changes (Barnes, 1991b; Solway & Leff, 1991), and the involvement of sensory nerves in mucosal edema (Persson, 1991; Yager et al, 1991). Because most approaches used to characterize neurogenic inflammation in the airways of rats and guinea pigs cannot be applied to humans, other strategies have been used (reviewed by McDonald, 1994a, 1996). The effect of tachykinins and capsaicin on the airway mucosa has been tested in humans, and the release of tachykinins into airway fluids has been measured. Furthermore, the action of endogenous tachykinins has been blocked with selective antagonists, and the breakdown of tachykinins has been blocked with neutral endopeptidase inhibitors. Also, the number of tachykinin-immunoreactive nerves in mucosal biopsies from normal subjects has been compared with the number in subjects with airway disease. The bottom line is that sensory nerves clearly participate in local responses of the human respiratory tract, but the extent of their role in the pathophysiology of airway diseases such as asthma and chronic bronchitis is still unknown.

10. SUMMARY AND CONCLUSIONS

Several lines of evidence suggest that sensory nerves of the carotid body have an efferent function in addition to their afferent function of conducting chemoreceptive im-

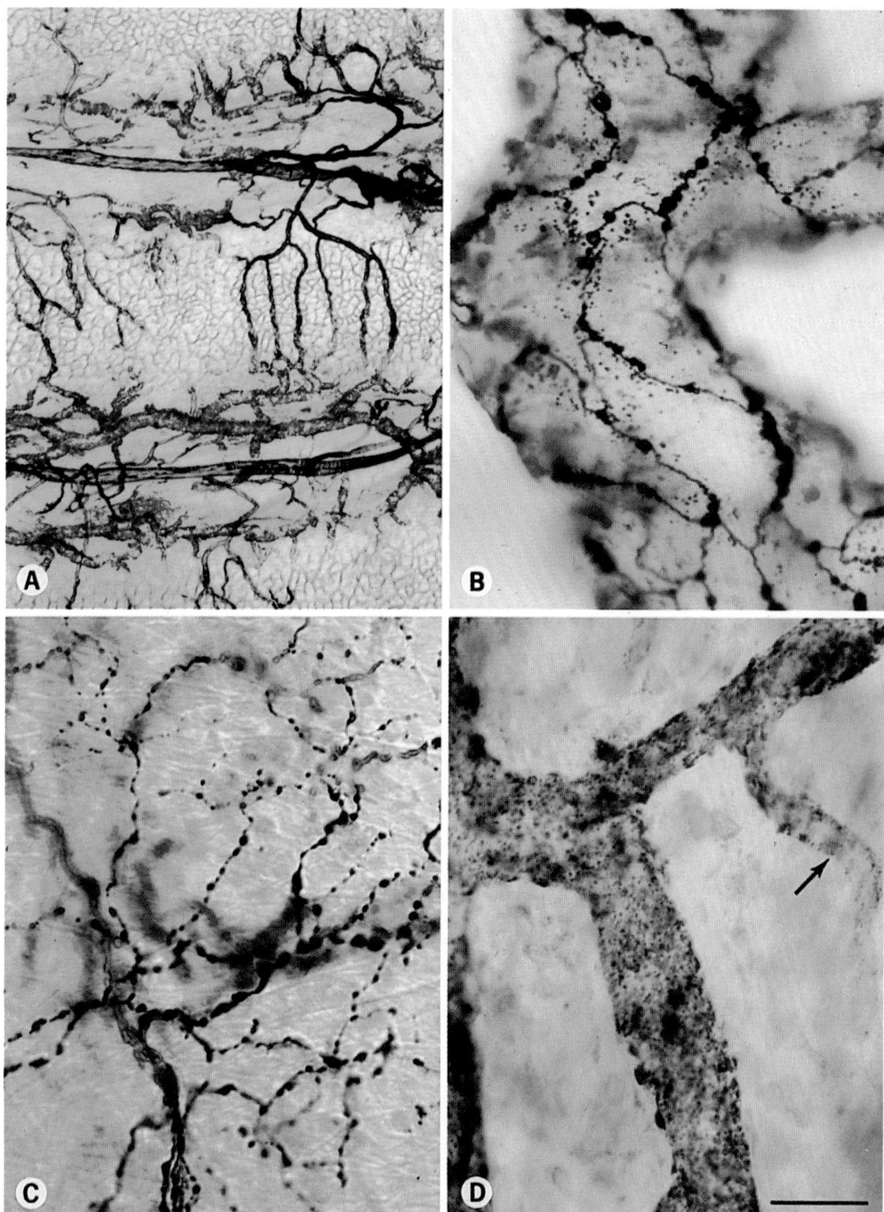

Figure 1. Whole mounts of rat tracheas illustrating several features of neurogenic inflammation in the respiratory mucosa. **A** shows abnormally leaky postcapillary venules and collecting venules, which are labeled by Monastral blue that extravasated as a result of neurogenic inflammation triggered by electrical stimulation of the vagus nerve. Arterioles and capillaries, not labeled by Monastral blue but stained black by perfusion of silver nitrate, did not become leaky in neurogenic inflammation. **B** shows a postcapillary venule stained with silver nitrate to mark endothelial cell borders and intercellular gaps. Focal black regions, which are located along endothelial borders, mark endothelial gaps produced by an intravenous injection of substance P. The presence of Monastral blue in the vessel wall indicates that the endothelium was leaky. **C** shows part of a plexus of substance P-immunoreactive nerves (brown) located at the base of the tracheal epithelium. Monastral blue-labeled postcapillary venules are out of focus because they are located in a plane beneath the nerve plexus. **D** shows NK1 receptor immunoreactivity of endothelial cells of postcapillary venules 5 minutes after an injection of substance P. NK1 receptor immunoreactive endosomes (brown spots) are abundant in the endothelium of the venules but are sparse in the endothelium of a capillary (arrow). Vessel leakiness is shown by the presence of extravasated Monastral blue. Scale bar, 250 μm in A, 20 μm in B, 75 μm in C, and 20 μm in D.

pulses to the brain. However, it has been difficult to document the release of substances from sensory nerve terminals on glomus cells and to determine whether such an efferent function plays a role in chemoreception. By comparison, the phenomenon of neurogenic inflammation has been relatively easy to study in rats and guinea pigs and has proven to be an informative model system for analyzing efferent actions of sensory nerves.

The main characteristic of neurogenic inflammation is plasma leakage. Chemical irritants that activate unmyelinated sensory nerves cause plasma leakage in the skin, respiratory tract, and other organs by triggering the release of substances from sensory nerve fibers. Substance P, which is synthesized and released by some sensory neurons, appears to be the main active mediator, although other tachykinins, calcitonin gene-related peptide, and perhaps other peptides may also participate.

Neurogenic inflammation results from the action of substance P on NK1 receptors, as demonstrated by selective NK1 receptor agonists and antagonists. The NK1 receptors involved in plasma leakage are located on the endothelial cells of postcapillary venules and collecting venules. Within seconds of the activation of NK1 receptors by substance P, gaps form in the endothelium of target vessels. The endothelial gaps are transient, and the leak normally ends in a few minutes. However, the magnitude of the response can increase in pathological conditions such as *Mycoplasma pulmonis* infection in rats, which results in a chronic inflammatory disease of the respiratory tract. The infected airway mucosa becomes abnormally vascular as a result of angiogenesis, and the endothelial cells of the newly formed vessels express increased numbers of NK1 receptors and thus are abnormally sensitive to substance P.

Studies of neurogenic inflammation not only have helped to understand the efferent actions of sensory nerves but also have given insight into the mechanism and consequences of inflammatory changes in endothelial cells and in the plasma leakage that follows.

11. ACKNOWLEDGMENTS

The research described in this review was supported in part by Grants HL-24136 (DMcD, PB), DK-39957 (NWB), and DK-43207 (NWB) from the US National Institutes of Health.

12. REFERENCES

Abelli L, Maggi CA, Rovero P, Del Bianco E, Regoli D, Drapeau G & Giachetti A (1991) Effect of synthetic tachykinin analogues on airway microvascular leakage in rats and guinea-pigs: evidence for the involvement of NK-1 receptors. J Auton Pharmacol 11: 267–275

Acker H & O'Regan RG (1981) The effects of stimulation of autonomic nerves on carotid body blood flow in the cat. J Physiol, London 315: 99–110

Baluk P, Nadel JA & McDonald DM (1992) Substance P-immunoreactive sensory axons in the rat respiratory tract: a quantitative study of their distribution and role in neurogenic inflammation. J Comp Neurol 319: 586–598

Baluk P, Bowden JJ, Lefevre PL & McDonald DM (1995) Increased expression of substance P (NK1) receptors on airway blood vessels of rats with *Mycoplasma pulmonis* infection. Am J Respir Crit Care Med 151: A719

Baluk P, Hirata A, Fujiwara T, Neal CR, Michel CC & McDonald DM (1996) Endothelial gaps in inflamed venules of rat airways: Time course of changes in permeability and morphology. Submitted for publication

Barnes PJ (1991a) Neurogenic inflammation in airways. Intl Arch Allergy Appl Immunol 94: 303–309

Barnes PJ (1991b) Sensory nerves, neuropeptides, and asthma. Ann NY Acad Sci 629: 359–370

Barnes PJ (1992) Neural mechanisms in asthma. Br Med Bull 48: 149–168

Biscoe TJ (1971) Carotid body: structure and function. Physiol Rev 51: 427–495

Biscoe TJ, Lall A & Sampson SR (1970) Electron microscopic and electrophysiological studies on the carotid body following intracranial section of the glossopharyngeal nerve. J Physiol, London 208: 133–152

Bowden JJ, Garland A, Baluk P, Lefevre P, Grady E, Vigna SR, Bunnett NW & McDonald DM (1994a) Direct observation of substance P-induced internalization of neurokinin 1 (NK1) receptors at sites of inflammation. Proc Natl Acad Sci USA 91: 8964–8968

Bowden JJ, Schoeb TR, Lindsey JR & McDonald DM (1994b) Dexamethasone and oxytetracycline reverse the potentiation of neurogenic inflammation in airways of rats with *Mycoplasma pulmonis* infection. Am J Respir Crit Care Med 150: 1391–1401

Bowden JJ, Baluk P, Lefevre PM, Vigna SR & McDonald DM (1996) Substance P (NK1) receptor immunoreactivity on endothelial cells of the rat tracheal mucosa. Am J Physiol 270: L404-L414

Carstairs J & Barnes P (1986) Autoradiographic mapping of substance P receptors in lung. Eur J Pharmacol 127: 295–296

Dalsgaard CJ & Lundberg JM (1984) Evidence for a spinal afferent innervation of the guinea pig lower respiratory tract as studied by the horseradish peroxidase technique. Neurosci Lett 23: 117–122

Delay-Goyet P & Lundberg JM (1991) Cigarette smoke-induced airway oedema is blocked by the NK1 antagonist, CP-96,345. Eur J Pharmacol 2: 157–158

Garland A, Ray DW, Doerschuk CM, Alger L, Eappon S, Hernandez C, Jackson M & Solway J (1991) Role of tachykinins in hyperpnea-induced bronchovascular hyperpermeability in guinea pigs. J Appl Physiol 70: 27–35

Hirata A, Baluk P, Fujiwara T & McDonald DM (1995) Location of focal silver staining at endothelial gaps in inflamed venules examined by scanning electron microscopy. Am J Physiol (Lung Cell Mol Physiol 13) 269: L403-L418

Hoover D & Hancock J (1987) Autoradiographic localization of substance P binding sites in guinea-pig airways. J Auton Nerv Syst 19: 171–174

Jancsó N (1960) Role of the nerve terminals in the mechanism of inflammatory reactions. Bull Millard Fillmore Hosp, Buffalo, NY 7: 53–77

Jancsó N (1961) Inflammation and the inflammatory mechanisms. J Pharm Pharmacol 13: 577–594

Jancsó N, Jancsó-Gábor A & Szolcsányi J (1967) Direct evidence for neurogenic inflammation and its prevention by denervation and by pretreatment with capsaicin. Br J Pharmacol Chemother 31: 138–151

Jancsó N, Jancsó-Gábor A & Szolcsányi J (1968) The role of sensory nerve endings in neurogenic inflammation induced in human skin and in the eye and paw of the rat. Br J Pharmacol Chemother 33: 32–41

Joris I, DeGirolami U, Wortham K & Majno G (1982) Vascular labelling with Monastral blue B. Stain Technol 57: 177–183

Kobayashi S & Uehara M (1970) Occurrence of afferent synaptic complexes in the carotid body of the mouse. Arch Histol Jap 32: 193–201

Krootila K, Oksala O, Zschauer A, Palkama A & Uusitalo H (1992) Inhibitory effect of methysergide on calcitonin gene-related peptide-induced vasodilatation and ocular irritative changes in the rabbit. Br J Pharmacol 106: 404–408

Kummer W, Fischer A, Preissler U, Couraud J-Y & Heym C (1990) Immunohistochemistry of the guinea-pig trachea using an anti-idiotypic antibody recognizing substance P receptors. Histochemistry 93: 541–546

Kummer W, Fischer A, Couraud J-Y & Heym C (1991) Immunohistochemistry of peptides (substance P and VIP) and peptide receptors in the trachea. J Auton Nerv Syst 33: 121–123

Kummer W, Fischer A, Kurkowski R & Heym C (1992) The sensory and sympathetic innervation of guinea-pig lung and trachea as studied by retrograde neuronal tracing and double-labelling immunohistochemistry. Neuroscience 49: 715–737

Lei YH, Barnes PJ & Rogers DF (1992) Inhibition of neurogenic plasma exudation in guinea-pig airways by CP-96,345, a new non-peptide NK1 receptor antagonist. Br J Pharmacol 105: 261–262

Lembeck F & Holzer P (1979) Substance P as neurogenic mediator of antidromic vasodilation and neurogenic plasma extravasation. Naunyn-Schmiedeberg's Arch Pharmacol 310: 175–183

Lundberg JM & Saria A (1983) Capsaicin-induced desensitization of airway mucosa to cigarette smoke, mechanical and chemical irritants. Nature 302: 251–253

Lundberg JM, Saria A, Theodorsson-Norheim E, Brodin E, Hua X-Y, Martling C-R, Gamse R & Hökfelt TG (1985) Multiple tachykinins in capsaicin-sensitive afferents: occurrence, release and biological effects with special reference to irritation of the airways. In: Håkanson R & Sundler F (eds) Tachykinin Antagonists. New York: Elsevier North-Holland. pp 159–169

Lundberg JM, Hökfelt T, Martling CR, Saria A & Cuello C (1984) Substance P-immunoreactive sensory nerves in the lower respiratory tract of various mammals including man. Cell Tiss Res 235: 251–261

Majno G & Palade GE (1961) Studies on inflammation. I. The effect of histamine and serotonin on vascular permeability: an electron microscopic study. J Biophys Biochem Cytol 11: 571–604

Majno G, Palade GE & Schoefl GI (1961) Studies on inflammation. II. The site of action of histamine and serotonin along the vascular tree: a topographic study. J Biophys Biochem Cytol 11: 607–625

McDonald DM (1988a) Neurogenic inflammation in the rat trachea. I. Changes in venules, leucocytes and epithelial cells. J Neurocytol 17: 583–603

McDonald DM (1988b) Respiratory tract infections increase susceptibility to neurogenic inflammation in the rat trachea. Am Rev Respir Dis 137: 1432–1440

McDonald DM (1994a) The concept of neurogenic inflammation in the respiratory tract. In: Kaliner MA, Barnes PJ, Kunkel GHH & Baraniuk JN (eds) Neuropeptides in Respiratory Medicine. New York: Marcel Dekker. pp 321–349

McDonald DM (1994b) Endothelial gaps and permeability of venules in rat tracheas exposed to inflammatory stimuli. Am J Physiol 266: L61-L83

McDonald DM (1996) Neurogenic inflammation in the airways. In: Barnes P (ed) Autonomic Control of the Respiratory System. London: Harwood Academic Publishers. In press

McDonald DM & Mitchell RA (1975) The innervation of glomus cells, ganglion cells and blood vessels in the rat carotid body. A quantitative ultrastructural analysis. J Neurocytol 4: 177–230

McDonald DM & Mitchell RA (1981) The neural pathway involved in "efferent inhibition" of chemoreceptors in the cat carotid body. J Comp Neurol 201: 457–476

McDonald DM, Mitchell RA, Gabella G & Haskell A (1988) Neurogenic inflammation in the rat trachea. II. Identity and distribution of nerves mediating the increase in vascular permeability. J Neurocytol 17: 605–628

McDonald DM, Schoeb TR & Lindsey JR (1991) *Mycoplasma pulmonis* infections cause long-lasting potentiation of neurogenic inflammation in the respiratory tract of the rat. J Clin Invest 87: 787–799

Nadel JA (1992) Regulation of neurogenic inflammation by neutral endopeptidase. Am Rev Respir Dis 145: S48-S52

Neil E & O'Regan RG (1969) Effects of sinus and aortic nerve efferents on arterial chemoreceptor function. J Physiol, London 200: 69P-71P

Neil E & O'Regan RG (1971) The effects of electrical stimulation of the distal end of the cut sinus and aortic nerves on peripheral arterial chemoreceptor activity in the cat. J Physiol, London 215: 15–32

O'Regan RG (1977) Control of carotid body chemoreceptors by autonomic nerves. Irish J Med Sci 146: 199–205

O'Regan RG (1981) Responses of carotid body chemosensory activity and blood flow to stimulation of sympathetic nerves in the cat. J Physiol, London 315: 81–98

Pallot DJ (1987) The mammalian carotid body. Adv Anat Embryol Cell Biol 102: 1–91

Persson CGA (1991) Plasma exudation in the airways: mechanisms and function. Eur Respir J 4: 1268–1274

Petersson G, Bacci E, McDonald DM & Nadel JA (1993) Neurogenic plasma extravasation in the rat nasal mucosa is potentiated by peptidase inhibitors. J Pharmacol Exp Ther 264: 509–514

Sakamoto T, Elwood W, Barnes PJ & Chung KF (1992) Pharmacological modulation of inhaled sodium metabisulphite-induced airway microvascular leakage and bronchoconstriction in the guinea-pig. Br J Pharmacol 107: 481–487

Sakamoto T, Barnes PJ & Chung KF (1993) Effect of CP-96,345, a non-peptide NK1 receptor antagonist, against substance P-induced, bradykinin-induced and allergen-induced airway microvascular leakage and bronchoconstriction in the guinea pig. Eur J Pharmacol 231: 31–38

Sampson SR, Aminoff MJ, Jaffe RA & Vidruk EH (1976) A pharmacological analysis of neurally induced inhibition of carotid body chemoreceptor activity in cats. J Pharmacol Exp Ther 197: 119–125

Schoeb TR & Lindsey JR (1987) Exacerbation of murine respiratory mycoplasmosis by sialodacryoadenitis virus infection in gnotobiotic F344 rats. Vet Pathol 24: 392–9

Schoeb TR, Davidson MK & Lindsey JR (1982) Intracage ammonia promotes growth of *Mycoplasma pulmonis* in the respiratory tract of rats. Infect Immun 38: 212–7

Sertl K, Wiedermann CJ, Kowalski ML, Hurtado S, Plutchok J, Linnoila I, Pert CB & Kaliner MA (1988) Substance P: the relationship between receptor distribution in rat lung and the capacity of substance P to stimulate vascular permeability. Am Rev Respir Dis 138: 151–159

Solway J & Leff AR (1991) Sensory neuropeptides and airway function. J Appl Physiol 71: 2077–2087

Springall DR, Cadieux A, Oliveira H, Su H, Royston D & Polak JM (1987) Retrograde tracing shows that CGRP-immunoreactive nerves of rat trachea and lung originate from vagal and dorsal root ganglia. J Auton Nerv Syst 20: 155–166

Stjernschantz J, Sears M & Mishima H (1982) Role of substance P in the antidromic vasodilation, neurogenic plasma extravasation and disruption of the blood-aqueous barrier in the rabbit eye. Naunyn-Schmiedeberg's Arch Pharmacol 321: 329–335

Terenghi G, McGregor GP, Bhuttacharji S, Wharton J, Bloom SR & Polak JM (1983) Vagal origin of substance P-containing nerves in the guinea pig lung. Neurosci Lett 36: 229–239

Tousignant C, Chan C-C, Guevremont D, Brideau C, Hale JJ, MacCoss M & Rodger IW (1993) NK2 receptors mediate plasma extravasation in guinea-pig lower airways. Br J Pharmacol 108: 383–386

Umeno E, McDonald DM & Nadel JA (1990) Hypertonic saline increases vascular permeability in the rat trachea by producing neurogenic inflammation. J Clin Invest 85: 1905–1908

Verna A (1979) Ultrastructure of the carotid body in the mammals. Intl Rev Cytol 60: 271–330

Vigna SR, Bowden JJ, McDonald DM, Fisher J, Okamoto A, McVey DC, Payan DG & Bunnett NW (1994) Characterization of antibodies to the rat substance P (NK-1) receptor and to a chimeric substance P receptor expressed in mammalian cells. J Neurosci 14: 834–845

Yager D, Shore S & Drazen JM (1991) Airway luminal liquid. Sources and role as an amplifier of bronchoconstriction. Am Rev Respir Dis 143: S52-S54

EFFECTS OF HYPERCAPNIA ON STEADY STATE, PHENYLEPHRINE-INDUCED TENSION IN ISOLATED RINGS OF RAT PULMONARY ARTERY

M. Sweeney, R. G. O'Regan, and P. McLoughlin

Department of Human Anatomy and Physiology
University College, Dublin 2, Ireland

1. INTRODUCTION

One of the primary functions of the lung is the exchange of oxygen and carbon dioxide with the environment. In order for this task to be carried out, matching of regional blood flow to ventilation is essential. To achieve this matching, the pulmonary vasculature has developed functional properties, which are significantly different from those of the systemic circulation. The best known of these is hypoxic pulmonary vasoconstriction; the response of systemic vessels to a reduction in PO_2 is dilatation (Fishman, 1985). Standard teaching suggests that a second specialization seen in the pulmonary circulation is a vasoconstrictor response to hypercapnic acidosis (Barnes & Liu, 1995). However, review of the original literature reveals much disagreement on this issue. Acidosis has been variably reported as potentiating (Rudolph & Yuan, 1966), inhibiting (Marshall et al, 1984), or having no effect on HPV (Housley et al, 1970). Alkalosis has been found to leave HPV unaffected (Silove et al, 1968) to reduce (Marshall et al, 1984) or to enhance it (Gordon et al, 1993). Brimioulle et al (1979) have suggested that elevation of PCO_2 exerts a pH independent vasodilator effect on the pulmonary circulation. This finding is similar to the vasodilator effect of CO_2 reported in systemic arteries (Carr et al, 1993) but contrasts with the enhanced contraction seen in other smooth muscle preparations in these circumstances (Liston et al, 1991).

It is difficult to reconcile these conflicting findings. They may be due to differing experimental protocols and techniques. Much of the previous work in this area has been carried out in whole animal preparations. The well known difficulties in measuring pulmonary vascular resistance *in vivo* (McGregor & Sniderman, 1985) together with the confounding effects of reflex mechanisms and release of non-specific mediators (Orr et al, 1987) during infusions of acid and alkali have probably led to these apparently contradictory results.

Frontiers in Arterial Chemoreception, edited by Zapata *et al.*
Plenum Press, New York, 1996

More recently, it has been reported that, under suitable conditions, the unique vasoconstrictor response of the pulmonary circulation may be reproduced in isolated rings of pulmonary artery (Bennie et al, 1991). This suggests that the same preparation will allow an examination of the direct effects on the pulmonary vasculature of changes in pH and PCO_2, isolated from the potentially confounding variables outlined above.

The purpose of this study was to examine the effects of hypercapnia and acidosis on isometric tension development in isolated rings of rat pulmonary artery.

2. METHODS

Male Sprague-Dawley rats (400–600 g) were sacrificed by stunning and cervical dislocation. The extrapulmonary branches of the main pulmonary artery were dissected free and cut into rings, 2–3 mm in length. Each vessel segment was mounted in a tissue bath by gently threading the arterial ring onto a horizontally oriented, fixed position, surgical steel wire (300 μm in diameter). Once anchored, a second wire, of the same dimensions, connected to a force transducer (F30, Hugo-Sachs Electronik, March, Germany) was introduced into the lumen, above the first wire. The rings were left to equilibrate for 1 hour. The tissue baths were filled with 50 ml of control physiological saline solution (PSS) (122.6 mM NaCl, 5.4 mM KCl, 20 mM $NaHCO_3$, 0.9 mM Na_2HPO_4, 0.8 mM $MgSO_4$, 2.4 mM $CaCl_2$ and 5.5 mM D-glucose) thermostatically maintained at 37°C, and equilibrated with 95% air-5% CO_2. Isometric tension was recorded as a function of time using an analogue to digital system (Biopac MP100 WS, Linton Instrumentation, Norfolk, England) connected to a desk top computer (Apple Macintosh Performa 475). Syringe samples of the bathing fluid were taken intermittently for analysis of PO_2, PCO_2 and pH using an automated blood-gas analyzer (Corning Model 278).

After equilibration, the rings were set at an optimal pre-tension (0.5–1.8 g) and left for about 30 min. The pre-tension selected for each ring was determined from its wet weight using a formula derived in preliminary experiments. Each ring was maximally contracted by three successive exposures to 80 mM KCl (iso-osmotically substituted for NaCl). The tension developed 7 min after the onset of the third 80 mM KCl induced contraction was taken as the maximal depolarization induced response. The rings were then relaxed back to pre-tension by rinsing with control PSS. A first cumulative concentration-response curve for phenylephrine (10^{-10} to 10^{-4} M) was obtained. The presence of an intact endothelium was tested by exposing the maximally contracted rings to acetylcholine (bath concentration 10^{-5} M). The rings were then allowed to relax by rinsing with control PSS.

The concentration of phenylephrine required to give half maximal contraction (Ec50 phe) was calculated for each individual ring, based on the initial concentration-response curve. This concentration of phenylephrine was used to elicit submaximal contraction in that ring and was present in all solutions subsequently used in the experimental protocol. Arterial rings were submaximally tensioned using Ec50 phe in control PSS at normal pH and PCO_2. After approximately 10 min, when tension was steady, the switch to the experimental conditions for that ring was made. After a further 90 min, the experimental solution was exchanged for control PSS with Ec50 phe.

Three test conditions were examined (See Table I): (a) hypercapnic acidotic conditions, produced by switching to a control PSS equilibrated with 9% CO_2 in air; (b) hypercapnic conditions at normal pH, produced by switching to a modified PSS ($NaHCO_3$ iso-osmotically substituted for NaCl) equilibrated with 9% CO_2 in air; (c) normocapnic acidotic conditions, produced by switching to a modified PSS ($NaHCO_3$ isosmotically replaced by NaCl) equilibrated with 5% CO_2 in air. The solution was modified so that the reduction in pH was approximately equal to that which occurred during hypercapnic acidosis.

A paired design was used in all experiments so that for each test condition examined an arterial ring dissected from the same pulmonary artery branch in the same animal underwent a control protocol. The control conditions consisted of introducing fresh Ec50 phe equilibrated with 5% CO_2 in air.

Following the experimental protocol, the rings were rinsed with control PSS and allowed to relax to pre-tension. A second cumulative concentration-response curve to phenylephrine was recorded and the response to ACh (10^{-5} M) was again examined. Finally, the response to 80 mM KCl was determined. If the maximal response of a ring to phenylephrine following the experimental protocol was less than 90% of the first maximal response, the results from that ring were discarded. Similarly, if the relaxation induced by ACh was less than 20% of the maximal phenylephrine-induced tension, the rings were discarded.

All active tensions developed (total tension developed minus pre-tension) were expressed as a percentage of the maximal response to phenylephrine, of that ring determined from its first concentration-response curve. The average tension developed in the 5 min before the preswitch to the experimental conditions in each ring was calculated and all tensions developed during the experimental period were expressed as difference (+ or -) from this pre-preswitch level.

All values shown are means ± SEM. To test for statistical differences between mean values paired *t* tests were used where appropriate. For multiple comparison of means across all experimental groups, analysis of variance was carried out and where a significant F-value was found Student-Newman-Keuls post-hoc test was used to assess the significance of the differences between means. A value of $P < 0.05$ was accepted as statistically significant.

3. RESULTS

Figure 1 illustrates the protocol in a single control ring. Figure 2 shows reproductions of the original records of a single ring during each of the three experimental interventions. Switching to hypercapnic acidotic conditions (Panel A) led to decline in tension which reached a minimum in approximately 7- 8 min. The mean minimum tension (n = 9) was -19 ± 2.6%. Following this, tension increased slightly and achieved a steady value from 15–20 min onwards. Typical response to a change to hypercapnia at normal pH (n = 8) was a slight reduction in tension (-4.3 ± 1.3%) with a subsequent recovery (Fig 2, Panel B) to a value very similar to that seen in control rings. No early relaxation was seen during control switches. Normocapnic acidosis (n = 8) caused an abrupt relaxation to a minimum value (-28.8 ± 3.7%) at approximately 5 min (Fig 2, Panel C). Subsequently tension increased slightly towards the pre-preswitch value.

Since, in all rings, tension had reached a steady value within 15–20 min of the solution change, the average tension between 20 and 80 min in each ring was taken as an index of the steady state response to the experimental intervention. The means of these values are illustrated in Figure 3.

Table 1 shows the mean PCO_2, pH and PO_2 during each of the experimental conditions.

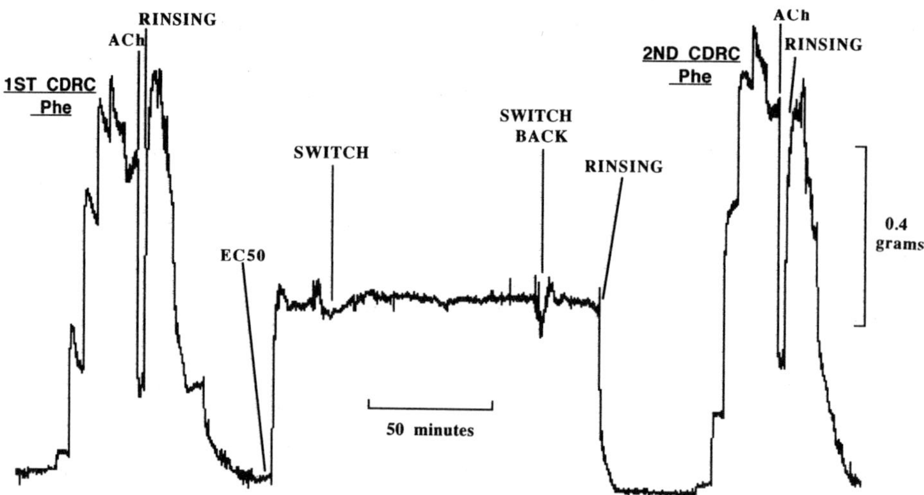

Figure 1. Typical original recording of tension development by a control ring. CCRC Phe = cumulative concentration-response curve for phenylephrine. -10 to -4 = logarithm of bath concentration of phenylephrine (M). ACh = 10^{-5} M acetylcholine in bath. Ec50= control PSS with Ec50 phe (concentration of phenylephrine giving half maximal contraction). Switch = introduction of fresh control PSS with Ec50 phe. Switch back = return to control PSS with Ec50 phe.

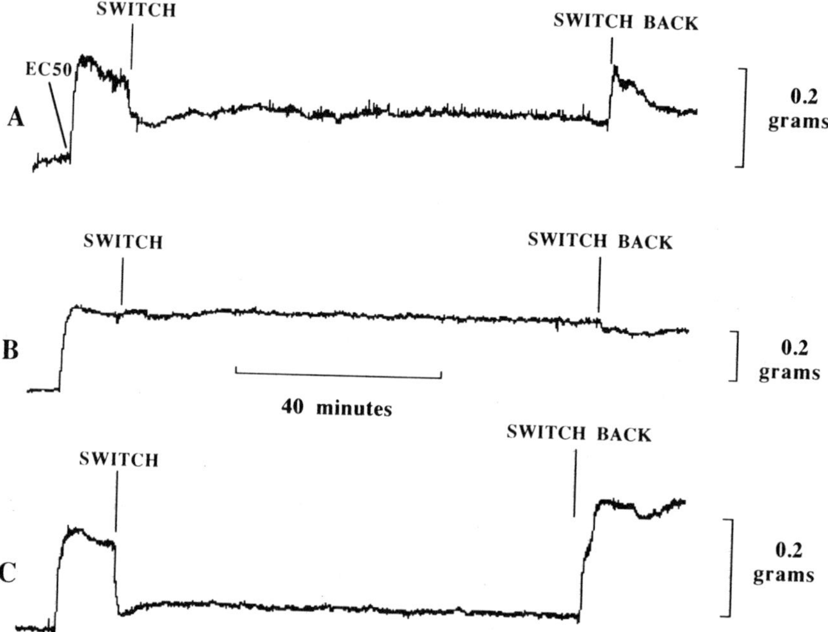

Figure 2. Original recordings of tension development during the three test conditions. Rings were contracted with Ec50 phe in control PSS. Panel A = switch to hypercapnic acidosis. Panel B = switch to hypercapnia at normal pH. Panel C = switch to normocapnic acidosis.

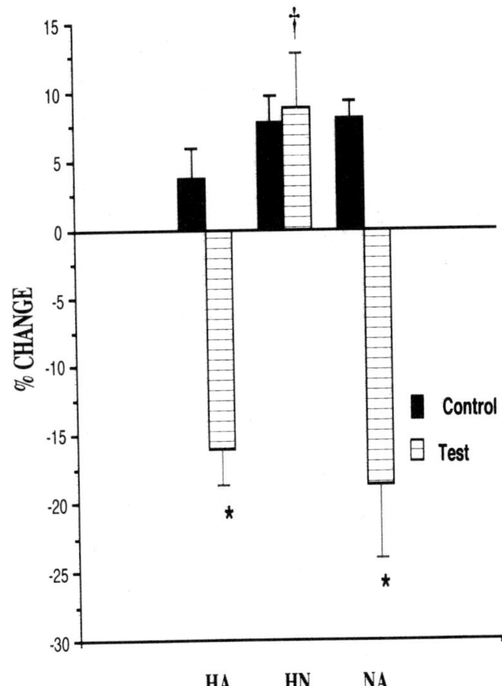

Figure 3. Changes in steady state tension in test conditions compared to paired controls. HA = hypercapnic acidosis. HN = hypercapnia at normal pH. NA = normocapnic acidosis. * = significantly different from control group ($p < 0.001$; paired *t* test). † = significantly different from other test conditions ($p < 0.01$; Student-Newman-Keuls post-hoc test).

4. DISCUSSION

In the present study, we found that hypercapnic acidosis caused a sustained relaxation of isolated pulmonary arterial rings. Hypercapnia at normal pH had no significant effect on tension development while normocapnic acidosis caused a significant sustained relaxation that was similar to the steady state response obtained with hypercapnic acidosis.

These data suggest that intracellular acidosis, caused by elevated extracellular PCO_2, does not alter tension development in isolated rings of pulmonary artery. In contrast, ex-

Table 1. Mean PCO_2, pH and PO_2 values in the baths during the experimental conditions

Protocol	Group	PCO_2 (mm Hg)	pH	PO_2 (mm Hg)
Hypercapnic Acidosis (n = 9 pairs)	Control	34.3 (± 0.3)	7.390 (± 0.005)	145.7 (+ 0.6)
	Test	55.0 (± 0.6)	7.199 (± 0.012)	141.8 (± 0.7)
Hypercapnia normal pH (n = 8 pairs)	Control	34.3 (± 0.3)	7.406 (± 0.006)	141.7 (± 0.6)
	Test	54.1 (± 0.7)	7.395 (± 0.007)	137.3 (± 1.0)
Normocapnic Acidosis (n = 8 pairs)	Control	35.1 (± 0.4)	7.413 (± 0.120)	139.6 (± 1.0)
	Test	33.9 (± 0.4)	7.154 (± 0.010)	142.2 (± 0.9)

tracellular acidosis, whether at normal or elevated PCO_2, causes relaxation. In isolated rings of systemic arteries, it is reported that both the above conditions cause relaxation. The regulation of pH_i in systemic vascular smooth muscle cells is markedly different from that of most other cells examined to date. The majority of cell types demonstrate a fall in pH_i following extracellular acidification and the ratio of change in pH_i to change in pH_e is approximately 0.3 (Ellis & Thomas, 1976). In systemic vascular smooth muscle cells the ratio of pH_i/pH_e change is 0.7 (Austin & Wray, 1993b). These large changes in pH_i are the result of the high permeability of the smooth muscle cell membrane to hydrogen ions (Austin & Wray, 1993a). This high value of pH_i/pH_e is similar to that reported in carotid body Type I cells, the chemotransductive elements of the carotid arterial chemoreceptors (Buckler et al, 1991). It has been suggested that the high permeability of the systemic vascular smooth muscle membrane also serves a chemotransductive function, providing an intracellular signalling mechanism which leads to vasodilatation and increased blood flow in poorly perfused tissues (Austin & Wray, 1993b). This hypothesis suggests a central role for intracellular pH in regulating vascular smooth muscle tone. The findings of the present study suggest that pulmonary vascular smooth muscle cells regulate intracellular pH in a fundamentally different manner or that tension development in these cells is insensitive to intracellular pH changes.

More recently, it has been demonstrated that relaxation in response to hypercapnia in systemic arteries is, at least in part, due to increased endothelial production of nitric oxide (Carr et al, 1993; Fukuda et al, 1990). In isolated mesenteric vessels, both endothelial removal and inhibition of nitric oxide synthase markedly reduce the relaxation produced by increased CO_2 at constant extracellular pH. Fukuda et al (1990) have reported that hypercapnia reduces the tension development in aortic rings in response to vasoconstrictor agents by increasing endothelial production of nitric oxide. Our finding that hypercapnia, at constant extracellular pH, does not cause relaxation of pulmonary arteries suggests that the pulmonary endothelium responds to this stimulus in a manner essentially different from that of endothelium in systemic vessels. This suggestion is supported by other, recently published, data from this laboratory (Beddy & McLoughlin, In Press).

The data reported here were obtained using conduit pulmonary arteries. These vessels show responses to hypoxia and vasoconstrictor agents which are qualitatively similar to those of smaller intrapulmonary vessels (Leacht et al, 1992). This suggests that the responses reported may also be observed in the resistance vessels within the lungs. Further work is needed to directly examine this issue.

The chemotransductive mechanisms which underlie the responses to changes in extracellular pH and PCO_2 in the pulmonary endothelial and/or pulmonary vascular smooth muscle cells are largely unexplored. They may be similar to those which have been reported in the peripheral arterial chemoreceptors (Buckler et al, 1991).

In conclusion, our findings suggest that isolated rings of pulmonary artery respond to changes in intracellular and extracellular pH in a manner which is markedly different to the response of arterial rings from the systemic circulation. The mechanisms of these differences warrant further investigation.

5. ACKNOWLEDGMENTS

We wish to acknowledge the financial support of Forbairt (Ireland) and The Irish Lung Foundation.

6. REFERENCES

Austin C & Wray S (1993a) Changes of intracellular pH in rat mesenteric vascular smooth muscle with high K^+ depolarization. J Physiol, London 469: 1–10

Austin C & Wray S (1993b) Extracellular pH signals affect rat vascular tone by rapid transduction into intracellular pH changes. J Physiol, London 466: 1–8

Barnes PJ & Liu SF (1995) Regulation of pulmonary vascular tone. Pharmacol Rev 47: 87–131

Beddy D & McLoughlin P (1996) Effects of hypercapnia on phenylephrine induced tension and endothelium dependent relaxation in isolated rings of rat pulmonary artery. J Physiol, London (Abstract) (In Press)

Bennie RE, Packer CS, Powell DR, Jin N & Rhoades RA (1991) Biphasic contractile response of pulmonary artery to hypoxia. Am J Physiol 261: L156-L163

Buckler KJ, Vaughn-Jones RD, Peers C, Lagadic-Gossman C & Nye PCG (1991) Effects of extracellular pH, PCO_2 and HCO^-_3 on intracellular pH in isolated type-1 cells of the neonatal rat carotid body. J Physiol, London 444: 703–721

Carr P, Graves JE & Poston L (1993) Carbon dioxide induced vasorelaxation in rat mesenteric small arteries precontracted with noradrenaline is endothelium dependent and mediated by nitric oxide. Pflügers Arch 423: 343–345

Ellis D & Thomas RC (1976) Direct measurement of the intracellular pH of mammalian cardiac muscle. J Physiol, London 262: 755–771

Fishman AP (1985) Pulmonary circulation. In: Handbook of Physiology, sect 3: Respiration, vol I: Circulation and Nonrespiratory Functions (Fishman AP & Fisher AB, eds). Bethesda, Maryland: American Physiological Society. pp 93–153

Fukuda S, Matsumoto M, Nishimura N, Fujiwara N, Shimoji K, Takeshita H & Lee TJF (1990) Endothelial modulation of norepinephrine-induced constriction of rat aorta at normal and high CO_2 tensions. Am J Physiol 258: H1049-H1054

Gordon JB, Fernando RM, Keller PA, Tod ML & Madden JA (1993) Differing effects of acute and prolonged alkalosis on hypoxic pulmonary vasoconstriction. Am Rev Respir Dis 148: 1651–1656

Housley E, Clarke SW, Hedworth-Whitty RB & Bishop JM (1970) Effect of acute and chronic acidemia and associated hypoxia on the pulmonary circulation of patients with chronic bronchitis. Cardiovasc Res 4: 482–489

Leach RM, Twort CHC, Cameron IR & Ward JPT (1992) A comparison of the pharmacological and mechanical properties *in vitro* of large and small pulmonary arteries of the rat. Clin Sci 82: 55–62

Liston TG, Palfrey ELH, Raimbach SJ & Fry CH (1991) The effects of pH changes on human and ferret detrusor muscle function. J Physiol, London 432: 1–21

Marshall C, Lindgren L & Marshall BE (1984) Metabolic and respiratory hydrogen ion effects on hypoxic pulmonary vasoconstriction. J Appl Physiol 5: 545–550

McGregor M & Sniderman A (1985) On pulmonary vascular resistance: the need for more precise definition. Am J Cardiol 55: 217–221

Orr JA, Shams HM, Fredde R & Scheid P (1987) Cardiorespiratory changes during HCl infusion unrelated to decreases in circulating blood pH. J Appl Physiol 62: 2362–2370

Rudolph AM & Yuan S (1966) Response of the pulmonary vasculature to hypoxia and H^+ ion changes. J Clin Invest 4: 399–411

Silove ED, Inoue T & Grover RF (1968) Comparison of hypoxia, pH, and sympathomimetic drugs on bovine pulmonary vasculature. J Appl Physiol 24: 355–365

PARTICIPANTS LIST

Verónica Abudara, Departamento de Fisiología, Facultad de Medicina, Universidad de la República, Montevideo, URUGUAY

Helmut Acker, Max-Planck Institut für molekulare Physiologie, 44026 Dortmund, GERMANY

Julio Alcayaga, Laboratorio de Neurobiología, Departamento de Biología, Facultad de Ciencias, Universidad de Chile, Santiago, CHILE

Ramón Alvarez-Buylla, Centro Universitario de Investigaciones Biomédicas, Universidad de Colima, Colima, Col 28040, MEXICO

Aida Bairam, Laboratoire de Néonatologie, Centre de Recherche, Centre Hospitalier Universitaire de Québec, Québec, P.Q., CANADA G1L-3L5

Carlos Belmonte, Departamento de Fisiología, Instituto de Neurociencias, Facultad de Medicina, Universidad de Alicante, 03080 Alicante, SPAIN

Gerald E Bisgard, Department of Comparative Biosciences, School of Veterinary Medicine, University of Wisconsin, Madison, Madison, WI 53706–1102, USA

Aidan Bradford, Department of Physiology, Royal College of Surgeons in Ireland, Dublin 2, IRELAND

Keith J Buckler, University Laboratory of Physiology, Oxford University, Oxford, OX1 3PT, ENGLAND, UK

Nicole Calder, Department of Obstetrics & Gynaecology, University College London Medical School, London, WC1E 6HX, ENGLAND, UK

Hugo Cárdenas, Departamento de Química, Facultad de Ciencias, Universidad de Santiago de Chile, Santiago, CHILE

Elisabeth Carpenter, Institute for Cardiovascular Research, Research School of Medicine, University of Leeds, Leeds LS2 9JT, ENGLAND, UK

John L Carroll, Children's Center, Pediatric Pulmonary Division, Johns Hopkins Hospital, Baltimore, MD 21205–2182, USA

Neil S Cherniack, New Jersey Medical School, University of Medicine and Dentistry of New Jersey, Newark, New Jersey, USA

Luis Constandil, Ph.D. Program in Physiological Sciences, Catholic University of Chile, Santiago 1, CHILE

Anneli Conway, Department of Physiology, Medical School, University of Birmingham, Birmingham B15 2TT, ENGLAND, UK

Patricia Ann Cragg, Department of Physiology, University of Otago Medical School, Dunedin, NEW ZEALAND

Leonardo Dasso, University Laboratory of Physiology, Oxford University, Oxford OX1 3PT, ENGLAND, UK

Marco Delpiano, Max-Planck-Institut für molekulare Physiologie, 44139 Dortmund, GERMANY

Bruce Dinger, Department of Physiology, University of Utah School of Medicine, Salt Lake City, UT 84108, USA

David F Donnelly, Division of Respiratory Medicine, Department of Pediatrics, Yale University School of Medicine, New Haven, CT 06510, USA

Melinda Dwinell, Department of Comparative Biosciences, School of Veterinary Medicine, University of Wisconsin - Madison, Wisconsin, Madison 53706, USA

Jaime Eugenín, Facultad de Ciencias Médicas, Universidad de Santiago de Chile, Santiago 2, CHILE

Carlos Eyzaguirre, Department of Physiology, University of Utah School of Medicine, Salt Lake City, UT 84108, USA

Salvatore J Fidone, Department of Physiology, College of Medicine, University of Utah, Salt Lake City, UT 84108, USA

Xavier Figueroa, Ph.D. Program in Physiological Sciences, Catholic University of Chile, Santiago 1, CHILE

Robert S Fitzgerald, Department of Environmental Health Sciences, School of Hygiene & Public Health, Johns Hopkins University, Baltimore, MD 21205, USA

Pedro Gallardo, Ph.D. Program in Physiological Sciences, Catholic University of Chile, Santiago 1, CHILE

Roberto Gallego, Departamento de Fisiología, Facultad de Medicina, Universidad de Alicante, E03080 Alicante, SPAIN

Estelle B Gauda, Division of Neonatology, Department of Pediatrics, Johns Hopkins Institution, Baltimore, MD 21287–3200, USA

Constancio González, Departamento de Bioquímica y Biología Molecular y Fisiología, Facultad de Medicina, Universidad de Valladolid, 47005 Valladolid, SPAIN

Arcadi Gual, Laboratori de Neurofisiología, Facultat de Medicina, Universitat de Barcelona, 08028-Barcelona, SPAIN

Bernard Hannhart, INSERM - Unité 14, Physiopathologie Respiratoire, 54511 Vandoeuvre-lès-Nancy, Cedex, FRANCE

Mark A Hanson, Department of Obstetrics & Gynæcology, University College London Medical School, London WC1E 6HX, ENGLAND, UK

Chris J Hatton, Institute for Cardiovascular Research, University of Leeds, Leeds LS2 9JT, ENGLAND, UK

Yoshiaki Hayashida, Department of Systems Physiology, University of Occupational & Environmental Health, Kitakyushu 807, JAPAN

Yoshiyuki Honda, Professor Emeritus of Physiology, Chiba University, Chiba 264, JAPAN

Yumiko Ishizawa, Department of Environmental Health Sciences, The Johns Hopkins Medical Institutions, Baltimore, MD 21205, USA

Rodrigo Iturriaga, Laboratory of Neurobiology, Catholic University of Chile, Santiago 1, CHILE

Patrick L Janssen, Department of Comparative Biosciences, School of Veterinary Medicine, University of Wisconsin, Madison, Madison, WI 53706–1102, USA

Homayoun Kazemi, Chief, Pulmonary and Critical Care Unit, Massachusetts General Hospital, Boston, MA 02114, USA

Hisatake Kondo, Department of Anatomy, School of Medicine, Tohoku University, Sendai 980, JAPAN

Ganesh Kumar, Department of Biochemistry, Case Western Reserve University, Cleveland, OH 44106–2333, USA

Prem Kumar, Department of Physiology, Medical School, University of Birmingham, Birmingham B15 2TT, ENGLAND, UK

Tatsumi Kusakabe, Department of Anatomy, School of Medicine, Yokohama City University, Yokohama 236, JAPAN

Sukhamay Lahiri, Department of Physiology, School of Medicine, University of Pennsylvania, Philadelphia, PA 19104, USA

Rachel C Landauer, Department of Physiology, Medical School, Birmingham University, Birmingham B15 2TT, ENGLAND, UK

Miriam Langdon, Department of Physiology, University College, Dublin 2, IRELAND

Carolina Larraín, Laboratory of Neurobiology, Catholic University of Chile, Santiago 1, CHILE

Donald McDonald, Cardiovascular Research Institute, Medical Center, University of California, San Francisco, San Francisco, CA 94143–0130, USA

Paul McLoughlin, Department of Physiology, University College, Dublin 2, IRELAND

Daniel S McQueen, Department of Pharmacology, Medical School, University of Edinburgh, Edinburgh, EH8 9JZ, SCOTLAND, UK

Mart Mojet, Department of Physiology, University College London, London WC1E 6BT, ENGLAND, UK

Emilia C Monteiro, Department of Pharmacology, Faculty of Medical Sciences, New University of Lisbon, 1198 Lisbon, PORTUGAL

Philip Nolan, Department of Human Anatomy and Physiology, University College, Dublin 2, IRELAND

Colin Nurse, Department of Biology, McMaster University, Hamilton, Ontario, CANADA L8S 4Kl

Ana Obeso, Departamento de Bioquímica y Biología Molecular y Fisiología, Facultad de Medicina, 47005-Valladolid, SPAIN

Ronan G O'Regan, Department of Physiology, University College, Dublin 2, IRELAND

Jose M Panisello, Department of Pediatrics, Section of Critical Care Medicine, Yale University School of Medicine, New Haven, CT 06520, USA

Chris Peers, Institute for Cardiovascular Research, Leeds University, Leeds LS2 9JT, ENGLAND, UK

David R Pepper, Department of Physiology, Medical School, University of Birmingham, Birmingham B15 2TT, ENGLAND, UK

Mieczyslaw Pokorski, Department of Neurophysiology, Polish Academy of Sciences, Medical Research Center, 00.784 Warsaw, POLAND

Nanduri R Prabhakar, Department of Physiology & Biophysics, School of Medicine, Case Western Reserve University, Cleveland, OH 44106, USA

Beatriz Ramírez, Facultad de Ciencias Médicas, Universidad de Santiago de Chile, Santiago 2, CHILE

Elena Roces de Alvarez-Buylla, Departamento de Fisiología, Biofísica y Neurociencias, CINVESTAV, Mexico, DF, MEXICO

Machiko Shirahata, Departments of Physiology & Environmental Health Sciences, Johns Hopkins University, Baltimore, MD 21205, USA

Luc J Teppema, Department of Physiology, Leiden University, Leiden, THE NETHERLANDS

Roger J Thompson, Department of Biology, McMaster University, Hamilton, Ontario, CANADA L8S 4Kl

Robert W Torrance, St John's College, Oxford University, Oxford OX2 7BD, ENGLAND, UK

Fernando Torrealba, Departamento de Ciencias Fisiológicas, Facultad de Ciencias Biológicas, P. Universidad Católica de Chile, Santiago 1, CHILE

Andrezej Trzebski, Department of Physiology, Institute of Physiological Sciences, Medical Faculty, Medical Academy Warsaw, 00–325 Warsaw, POLAND

Nirit Weiss, Department of Pediatrics, Section Respiratory Medicine, Yale University School of Medicine, New Haven, CT 06520, USA

Katsuki Yoshizaki, Department of Physiology, Akita University School of Medicine, Akita City 010, JAPAN

Patricio Zapata, Laboratory of Neurobiology, Catholic University of Chile, Santiago 1, CHILE

INDEX